COLOR ATLAS
AND SYNOPSIS
OF CLINICAL
DERMATOLOGY

Adam McDiarmid.

Thomas B. Fitzpatrick, M.D., Ph.D., D.Sc. (Hon.)

Wigglesworth Professor of Dermatology, Emeritus
Chairman, Emeritus
Department of Dermatology, Harvard Medical School
Chief Emeritus, Dermatology Service
Massachusetts General Hospital
Boston, Massachusetts

Richard Allen Johnson, M.D.C.M.

Clinical Instructor in Dermatology
Harvard Medical School
Clinical Associate in Dermatology
Massachusetts General Hospital
Associate in Dermatology
Beth Israel Hospital
Associate Physician (Dermatology)
Brigham and Women's Hospital
Dermatologist
New England Deaconess Hospital
Boston, Massachusetts

Klaus Wolff, M.D.

Professor and Chairman
Department of Dermatology
University of Vienna Medical School
Head, Division of General Dermatology
Vienna General Hospital
Vienna, Austria

Machiel K. Polano, M.D.

Professor Emeritus and Chairman
Department of Dermatology, University Hospital
Leiden, The Netherlands

Dick Suurmond, M.D.

Professor Emeritus and Chairman
Department of Dermatology, University Hospital
Leiden, The Netherlands

Third Edition

COLOR ATLAS AND SYNOPSIS OF CLINICAL DERMATOLOGY

COMMON AND SERIOUS DISEASES

Thomas B. Fitzpatrick, M.D.
Richard Allen Johnson, M.D.
Klaus Wolff, M.D.

Machiel K. Polano, M.D.
Dick Suurmond, M.D.

McGraw-Hill
HEALTH PROFESSIONS DIVISION

New York St. Louis San Francisco Auckland Bogotá
Caracas Lisbon London Madrid Mexico City Milan Montreal
New Delhi San Juan Singapore Sydney Tokyo Toronto

McGraw-Hill

*A Division of The **McGraw·Hill** Companies*

Color Atlas and Synopsis of Clinical Dermatology

234567890 DOC DOC 98

ISBN 0-07-021388-7

This book was set in Times Roman by York Graphic Services, Inc. The editors were Martin J. Wonsiewicz, Mariapaz Ramos Englis, and Peter A. McCurdy; editing assistant was Daniel Green.

The production supervisor was Robert Laffler; the text and cover designer was Marsha Cohen of Parallelogram.

The index was prepared by Irving Conde Tullar.

The color photographs were processed by T. B. Fitzpatrick, Jr., of Streamline Studios, Carlisle, Massachusetts.

R. R. Donnelley and Sons, Inc., was printer and binder.

This book is printed on acid-free paper.

Library of Congress Cataloging-in-Publication Data

Color atlas and synopsis of clinical dermatology / Thomas B.
  Fitzpatrick . . . [et al.]. —3rd ed.
      p.   cm.
  Includes bibliographical references and index.
  ISBN 0-07-021388-7
    1. Dermatology—Atlases.   I. Fitzpatrick, Thomas B. (Thomas
Bernard), (date)
    [DNLM: 1. Skin Diseases—atlases.   WR 17 C718 1997]
RL81.C65   1997
616.5—dc20
DNLM/DLC
for Library of Congress   96-41318

To Pat Novak

Mrs. Patricia Knowles Novak was a master craftswoman of words.

For one person to have skillfully guided to publication the three editions of this *Atlas* and four editions of the comprehensive, contributed textbook of dermatology, *Dermatology in General Medicine,* is a record of accomplishment. Pat did this quietly and with aplomb—with her unusual talents, her Yankee rectitude, and, because she was a lady in the highest sense of the word, she never lost her "cool," was tolerant, generous, understanding, and virtually indefatigable.

Pat passed away on November 1, 1996. *Requiescat in pace.*

NOTICE

CONTENTS

Part I

DISORDERS PRESENTING IN THE SKIN AND MUCOUS MEMBRANE

Section 9

MELANOMA PRECURSORS AND PRIMARY CUTANEOUS MELANOMA 180

Section 10

PRECANCEROUS LESIONS AND CUTANEOUS CARCINOMAS 208

Section 11

PHOTOSENSITIVITY AND PHOTOINDUCED DISORDERS 228

Part II

DERMATOLOGY AND INTERNAL MEDICINE

Part III

DISEASES DUE TO MICROBIAL AGENTS

Section 33

MUCOCUTANEOUS MANIFESTATIONS OF HUMAN IMMUNODEFICIENCY VIRUS DISEASE 918

Appendices

Indexes

Subject Index 1009

PREFACE

Changes in health care delivery around the world are creating new challenges for the primary care physician because referral to specialists is being severely restricted. Diagnosis is often perplexing in patients with diseases of the skin. To keep pace with the much expanded role of dermatology in general medical practice, we have assembled this new practical clinical tool: a richly illustrated color atlas with juxtaposed précis of the skin disease or the systemic disease with a skin manifestation.

THE PRESENT NEED FOR DERMATOLOGIC DIAGNOSIS

Familiarity with dermatology is now necessary because of the increasing number of patients presenting with skin lesions as incidental findings or as major complaints who are being seen by a wide circle of "health care providers": primary care physicians, pediatricians, internists (allergists, rheumatologists, infectious disease consultants) and nurse practitioners. These care providers are now being forced to become "paraspecialists" in dermatology. Just as a chest physician must look at and attempt to interpret chest films or the orthopedist the bone films, so the general physician must now be able to "read" skin lesions and make a decision about referral to a dermatologist or to manage the patient by her or himself.

THE GOAL OF THIS COLOR ATLAS-SYNOPSIS

Recognition of skin diseases is not easy exercise and is difficult to teach. The correct diagnosis assures the best therapy. Our goal is to provide a "management manual" of skin diseases, as a tool for all health care providers, to acquaint members of the health professions with the principal lesions of the skin in order to facilitate dermatologic diagnosis. As dermatologic diagnosis is a visual task, a logical approach is to carefully study a color photograph of typical lesions, and simultaneously, while viewing the lesions, to consult across the page a succinct summary (précis) of the major features of the disease. For the primary care physician or the medical student the précis may be new knowledge, for the dermatologist these précis can, however, serve as a recall of the essential facts. With this aim in mind, we have placed large color photographs of skin lesions opposite a synopsis of the essential facts of diagnosis and treatment of the common skin disorders and the skin signs of many of the serious systemic diseases.

This third edition contains over 400 more photographs and over 100 more précis than the first edition in 1983 of *Color Atlas and Synopsis of Clinical Dermatology*. The first and second editions were used by thousands of health care providers—both new and repeat buyers of each edition. This edition has been extensively revised with largely new photographs, and virtually every précis has been updated.

The *Atlas* can only supplement the complete presentations of dermatology provided in *Dermatology in General Medicine,* published by McGraw-Hill, and available in the United States and internationally.

This book has been a cooperative effort of three dermatology departments: Boston (United States), Vienna (Austria), and Leiden (The Netherlands). The color plates are from the collections of the Department of Dermatology, University of Vienna, the Department of Dermatology, Harvard Medical School/Massachusetts General Hospital, Boston, and the University Hospital, Leiden.

ACKNOWLEDGMENTS

We are grateful to CIBA-Geigy for their permission to use certain photographs in this book. A few color plates for this edition were prepared in the lithographic institute Sturm of Basel, Switzerland, on appointment by CIBA-Geigy.

Also we would like to thank our colleagues: Arthur J. Sober, MD; Arthur R. Rhodes, MD; Kenneth H. Kraemer, MD; Joop Grevelink, MD; Suzanne Virnelli-Grevelink, MD; Amy Wong, MD; Ann Taylor, MD; Charles R. Taylor, MD; and John Hawk, MD; who helped prepare the précis and/or provided critical assessment of the précis; Kathryn E. Bowers, MD; Richard Langley, MD; Peter Lee, MD; K.C. Tan, MBBS; Arthur Tong, MD; and Hensin Tsao, MD, PhD; for their assistance in the preparation of some of the précis; Gail Burroughs, who prepared the line drawings and halftones except for the three halftones depicting primary melanoma, which were done by Gail Cooper, MD.

Oclassen Pharmaceuticals of California made an educational grant for the preparation of the color plates and we are grateful for this generous gesture to help in the education of the health care professionals.

The Health Professions Division of McGraw-Hill made the publication of this book possible. Especially important was Mariapaz Ramos Englis who gave her heart and head to this book. Also, we thank Martin Wonsiewicz, Editorial Director, for his support; his predecessor, the redoubtable J. Dereck Jeffers, who worked with us on the first two editions of the *Atlas;* and Robert Laffler, Production Director.

The Editors

INTRODUCTION

APPROACH TO DERMATOLOGIC DIAGNOSIS[1]

"The art of being wise is the art of knowing what to overlook"

William James

Too often, it seems that many health professionals make no serious attempt to identify skin lesions promptly. Although accurate recognition is usually possible, asymptomatic skin lesions are considered trivial and are overlooked. Undiagnosed asymptomatic lesions are treated for months with topical and oral corticosteroids and/or antibiotics; this postponement of appropriate treatment prolongs discomfort, aids and abets disfigurement, and leads, not uncommonly, to an irreversible generalization of the disorder or, most critically, to a delay in diagnosis that can result in multisystem illness or death.

One must be aware that robust *well* people can have asymptomatic skin lesions that are signs of serious multisystem disease, and these lesions cannot be overlooked without endangering the patient's health. Certain skin changes that may be encountered during a routine physical examination are just as important to detect as are enlarged lymph nodes, for example, early malignant melanoma in a curable stage of evolution, or the small yellow papules of hyperlipoproteinemic xanthomas, a potentially fatal but, treatable disease.

Similarly, for acute and chronically ill patients, ambulatory or in hospital, identification of skin lesions[2] and frequently a skin biopsy[2] are necessary. Of all the organs, the skin is the easiest from which one can obtain material for the study of the pathologic changes that are the basis of the clinical lesion. In this manner, puzzling multisystem disorders—such as sarcoidosis, deep fungal infections, cutaneous infarcts in septicemia, or the characteristic tender nodules on the leg that occur in acute pancreatitis—can be diagnosed.

"What's the use of a book," thought Alice, "without pictures or conversations?"

Lewis Carroll

This *Atlas* plus text is proposed as a "field guide" to the recognition of skin disorders. The skin is a treasury of important lesions that can usually be clinically recognized. At present, gross morphology in the form of skin lesions remains the hard core of dermatologic diagnosis. Skin lesions are visible to the unaided eye, just as pulmonary and brain lesions are gross pathology but visible only with imaging. Both types of lesions require a differential diagnosis and both can often lead the clinician to the correct diagnosis—and thus the proper management of the patient.

---

[1]See page xxii for Outline of an Approach to Dermatologic Diagnosis.
[2]See Appendices A and B for illustrations of Types of Skin Lesions and Special Clinical and Laboratory Aids to Dermatologic Diagnosis.

OUTLINE OF AN APPROACH TO DERMATOLOGIC DIAGNOSIS

HOW TO APPROACH A PATIENT WITH SKIN LESIONS

There are two distinct clinical situations regarding the nature of skin changes:

A. The skin changes are *incidental* findings in *well* people noted during the routine general physical examination

    1. <u>"Bumps and blemishes"</u>: See figures on pages 1006 and 1007 for the location of many of those lesions that are present in well people but are not the reason for the visit to the physician; every general physician should be able to recognize each of these diseases and disorders.

    2. <u>Important skin lesions</u> *not* noted by the patient but that cannot be overlooked by the physician:

    Dysplastic nevi
    Lesion >1.5 cm (not a melanoma or dysplastic nevus but likely a congenital
        melanocytic nevus)
    Early melanoma
    Xanthomatoses
    Basal cell carcinoma
    Squamous cell carcinoma
    Café-au-lait macules in von Recklinghausen's disease

B. The skin changes are the *chief complaint* of the patient

    1. Minor problems:
    Localized itchy rash, "rash," warts, common moles, seborrheic keratosis, rash in groin, and so on

    2. "4-S" = Serious Skin Signs in Sick Patients:[1]

    Generalized Red Rash: with Fever
        MEASLES
        RUBELLA
        ROCKY MOUNTAIN SPOTTED FEVER (PALMS AND SOLES FIRST)
        VIRAL EXANTHEM

---

[1]Requires complete search for multisystem disease: history, general physical examination, biopsy, basic laboratory studies, possibly immunofluorescence, imaging.

Generalized Red Rash: with Bullae and Prominent Mouth Lesions
ERYTHEMA MULTIFORME (MAJOR)
TOXIC EPIDERMAL NECROLYSIS
PEMPHIGUS VULGARIS
BULLOUS PEMPHIGOID
DRUG ERUPTIONS

Generalized Red Rash: with Pustules
PUSTULAR PSORIASIS (VON ZUMBUSCH)
DRUG ERUPTIONS

Generalized Vesicular Lesions
DISSEMINATED HERPES SIMPLEX
GENERALIZED HERPES ZOSTER
VARICELLA
DRUG ERUPTIONS

Multiple Bullous Lesions with Mouth Lesions
PEMPHIGUS
DRUG ERUPTIONS

Generalized Pustules
DRUG ERUPTIONS
PUSTULAR PSORIASIS

Generalized Dermatitis over Whole Body
EXFOLIATIVE ERYTHRODERMA

Facial Inflammatory Edema with Fever
ERYSIPELAS
LUPUS ERYTHEMATOSUS

Generalized Purpura
THROMBOCYTOPENIA
PURPURA FULMINANS
DRUG ERUPTIONS

Palpable Purpura
VASCULITIS
BACTERIAL ENDOCARDITIS

Multiple Skin Infarcts
MENINGOCOCCEMIA
GONOCOCCEMIA
DISSEMINATED INTRAVASCULAR COAGULOPATHY

Generalized Skin Necrosis
DISSEMINATED INTRAVASCULAR COAGULOPATHY

Generalized Urticaria and Angioedema
DRUG ERUPTIONS

I. Epidemiology and Etiology
Age, race, sex, occupation

II. History
A. Duration of onset of skin lesions: days, weeks, months, years
B. Relationship of skin lesions to season, travel history, heat, cold, previous treatment, drug ingestion, occupation, hobbies, effects of menses, pregnancy
C. Skin symptoms: pruritus, pain, paresthesia
D. Constitutional symptoms
1. "Acute illness" syndrome: headaches, chills, feverishness, weakness
2. "Chronic illness" syndrome: fatigue, weakness, anorexia, weight loss, malaise
E. Systems review

III. Physical Examination
A. Appearance of patient: uncomfortable, "toxic," well
B. Vital signs: pulse, respiration, temperature
C. Skin—four major skin signs: (1) type, (2) shape, (3) arrangement, (4) distribution of lesions
1. **Type** of lesions (see Appendix A)

Basic lesions	Telangiectasia
Macule	Infarct
Papule-plaque	Purpura
Wheal	
Nodule	*Sequential lesions*
Cyst	Scale
Vesicle-bulla	Hyperkeratosis
Pustule	Exudation: dry (crust), wet (weeping)
Ulcer (also sequential)	Erosion
Hyperkeratosis (also sequential)	Ulcer
Sclerosis	Scar
Atrophy (also sequential)	Lichenification

Color of lesions or of the skin if diffuse involvement: *"skin color"*: white: leukoderma, hypomelanosis; red: erythema; pink; violaceous; brown: hypermelanosis or hemosiderin; black; blue; gray; orange; yellow. Red or purple purpuric lesions do not blanch with pressure (diascopy).
Palpation
Consistency (soft, firm, hard, fluctuant, boardlike)
Deviation in temperature (hot, cold)
Mobility
Presence of tenderness
Estimate the depth of lesion (i.e., dermal or subcutaneous)

2. **Shape** of individual lesions
Round, oval, polygonal, polycyclic, annular (ring-shaped), iris, serpiginous (snakelike), umbilicated
3. **Margination,** well-defined (can be traced with the tip of a pencil), ill-defined
4. **Arrangement** of multiple lesions

Grouped: herpetiform, zosteriform, arciform, annular, reticulated (net-shaped), linear, serpiginous (snakelike)

Disseminated: scattered discrete lesions or diffuse involvement (i.e., without identifiable borders)

5. **Distribution** of lesions

Extent: isolated (single lesions), localized, regional, generalized, universal

Pattern: symmetrical, exposed areas, sites of pressure, intertriginous area, follicular localization, random

Characteristic patterns: secondary syphilis, atopic dermatitis, acne, erythema multiforme, candidiasis, lupus erythematosus, pemphigus, pemphigoid, porphyria cutaneous tarda, xanthoma, necrotizing angiitis (vasculitis). Rocky Mountain spotted fever, Lyme disease, rubella, rubeola, AIDS, scarlet fever, toxic shock syndrome, typhoid, Kawasaki's disease, herpes zoster, varicella, scalded-skin syndrome, toxic epidermal necrolysis, Kaposi's sarcoma (epidemic)

D. Hair and nails

E. Mucous membranes

F. General medical examination

IV. Differential Diagnosis
V. Laboratory and Special Examinations

A. Dermatopathology
1. Light microscopy: site, process, cell types
2. Immunofluorescence
3. Special techniques: stains, transmission electron microscopy, and so on

B. Microbiologic examination of skin material: scales, crusts, exudate, or tissue
1. Direct microscopic examination of skin (see Appendix B)
   For yeast and fungus: 10% postassium hydroxide preparation
   For bacteria: Gram's stain
   For virus: Tzanck smear
   For spirochetes: dark-field examination
   For parasites: scabies mite from a burrow
2. Culture
   Bacterial
   Viral
   Parasitic
   Mycologic
   For granulomas, culture of minced tissue

C. Laboratory examination of blood
   Bacteriologic: culture
   Serologic: ANA, STS, serology
   Hematologic: hematocrit or hemoglobin, cells, differential smear
   Chemistry: fasting blood sugar, blood urea nitrogen, creatinine, liver function, and thyroid function tests (if indicated)

D. Imaging (x-ray, CT scan, MRI, ultrasound)

E. Urinalysis

F. Stool examination (for occult blood, for example, in vasculitis syndromes; for ova and parasites, for porphyrins)

G. Wood's lamp examination
Urine: pink-orange fluorescence in porphyria cutanea tarda (add 1.0 ml of 5.0% hydrochloric acid)
Hair (in vivo): green fluorescence in tinea capitis (hair shaft)
Skin (in vivo):
Erythrasma: coral-red fluorescence
Hypomelanosis: decrease in intensity
Brown hypermelanosis: increase in intensity
Blue hypermelanosis: no change in intensity
H. Patch testing
I. Acetowhitening—whitening of sublinical penile warts after application of 5% acetic acid

VI. Diagnosis

Based on a synthesis and analysis of history, physical examination, laboratory findings.

VII. Pathophysiology
VIII. Course and Prognosis
IX. Treatment

COLOR ATLAS AND SYNOPSIS OF CLINICAL DERMATOLOGY

Section 1

DISORDERS OF SEBACEOUS AND APOCRINE GLANDS

ACNE VULGARIS (COMMON ACNE) AND CYSTIC ACNE

Acne is an inflammation of the pilosebaceous units of certain body areas (face and trunk) that occurs most frequently in adolescence and manifests itself as comedones *(comedonal acne)*, papulopustules *(papulopustular acne),* or nodules plus cysts *(nodulocystic acne* and *acne conglobata)*. Pitted, depressed, or hypertrophic scars may follow all types but especially nodulocystic acne and acne conglobata. *Severe acne* includes one or more of the following: persistent or recurrent inflammatory nodules, extensive papulopustular lesions, active scarring, and/or presence of sinus tracts.

Epidemiology and Etiology

Age 10 to 17 years in females; 14 to 19 in males; may appear first at 25 years or older.

Sex More severe in males than in females

Race Lower incidence in Asians and blacks; rare in China

Occupation Exposure to acnegenic mineral oils, dioxin, others

Drugs Lithium, hydantoin, topical and systemic corticosteroids, and oral contraceptives may cause exacerbation.

Genetic Aspects Multifactorial; severe acne is associated with XYY syndrome.

Other Factors *Endocrine factors* (see Pathophysiology, below). *Emotional stress* definitely can cause exacerbations. *Occlusion* and *pressure on the skin* by leaning face on hands or on a telephone are very important and often unrecognized exacerbating factors. Acne is not caused by chocolate or fatty foods or, in fact, by any kind of food.

History

Duration of Lesions Weeks to months to years

Season Often worse in fall and winter

Symptoms Pain in lesions (especially nodulocystic type)

Physical Examination

Skin Lesions

TYPES

Comedones—open (blackheads) or closed (whiteheads) (Figure 1-1)
Papules and papulopustules—with (red) (Figure 1-2) or without inflammation
Nodules, noduloulcerative lesions, or cysts—1 to 4 cm in diameter (Figures 1-3 and 1-4). The soft nodules are not cysts but large secondary comedones from repeated ruptures and reencapsulations with inflammation and abscess formation.

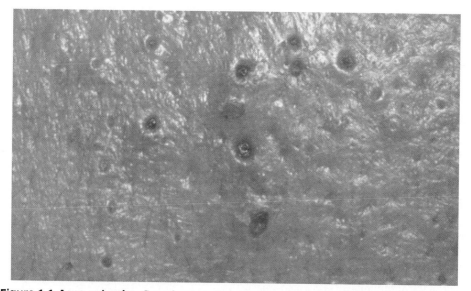

Figure 1-1 Acne vulgaris *Comedones are keratin plugs that form within follicular ostia, frequently associated with surrounding erythema and pustule formation. Comedones associated with small ostia are referred to as closed comedones or "white heads"; those associated with large ostia, open comedones or "black heads."*

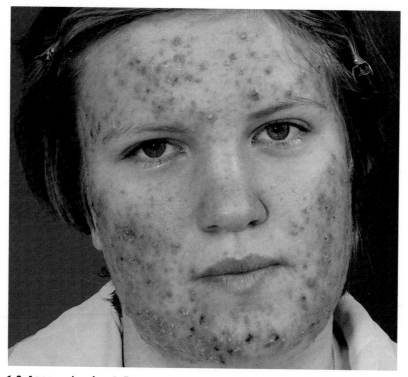

Figure 1-2 Acne vulgaris *Inflammatory papules, pustules, crusting on the forehead, cheeks, and chin.*

Sinuses—draining epithelial-lined tracts, usually with nodular acne

Scars—atrophic depressed (often pitted) or hypertrophic (at times, keloid) scars

Seborrhea of the face and scalp is often present and sometimes severe.

SHAPE Round; nodules may coalesce to form linear mounds or sinus tracts.

ARRANGEMENT Isolated single lesion (e.g., nodule) or scattered discrete lesions (papules, cysts, nodules)

SITES OF PREDILECTION Face, neck, upper arms, trunk, buttocks

Special Forms

Acne in the Adult Woman Persistent acne in a hirsute female with or without irregular menses needs an evaluation for hypersecretion of adrenal and ovarian androgens: total testosterone, free testosterone, and/or dehydroepiandrosterone sulfate (e.g., polycystic ovary syndrome). Also, recalcitrant acne can be related to partial 11- or 12-hydroxylase block.

Acne Conglobata Severe cystic acne (Figure 1-4) with more involvement of the trunk than the face. Coalescing nodules, cysts, and abscesses. Spontaneous remission is long delayed. Rarely, acne conglobata is the type seen in XYY genotype (tall males, slightly mentally retarded, with aggressive behavior) or in the polycystic ovary syndrome.

Acne Fulminans Young males (ages 13 to 17). *Acute onset* severe cystic acne with concomitant suppuration and always *ulceration;* also, there is malaise, fatigue, fever, generalized arthralgias, leukocytosis, and increased ESR.

Differential Diagnosis

Face: Staphylococcus aureus folliculitis, pseudofolliculitis barbae, rosacea, perioral dermatitis. *Trunk: Pityrosporum* folliculitis, "hot-tub" folliculitis, *S. aureus* folliculitis. *Single painful* *"cyst":* staphylococcal abscess, furuncle, ruptured inclusion cyst.

Laboratory Examination

Hormone Workup for Detecting Polycystic Ovary Syndrome Includes:

Free testosterone—ovarian source in females

FSH and LH; if ratio of LH/FSH is >3:1, highly suggestive

DHEA-S—adrenal source of androgens

Note: In the overwhelming majority of acne patients hormones are normal.

Pathophysiology

The lesions of acne (comedones) are the result of complex interaction between hormones (androgens) and bacteria *(Propionibacterium acnes)* in the pilosebaceous units of individuals with appropriate genetic backgrounds. Androgens (which are qualitatively and quantitatively normal) stimulate sebaceous glands to produce larger amounts of sebum; bacteria contain lipase that converts lipid into fatty acids. Both sebum and fatty acids cause a sterile inflammatory response in the pilosebaceous unit; this results in hyperkeratinization of the lining of the follicle with resultant plugging. The enlarged follicular lumen contains inspissated keratin and lipid debris (the whitehead). When the follicle has a portal of entry at the skin, the semisolid mass protrudes, forming a plug (the blackhead). The black color is due to oxidation of tyrosine, contained in the follicular orifice, to melanin. The distended follicle walls may break, and the contents (sebum, lipid, fatty acids, keratin, etc.) may enter the dermis, provoking a foreign-body response (papule, pustule, nodule). Rupture plus intense inflammation leads to scars.

Course

Acne may persist to age 35 or older.

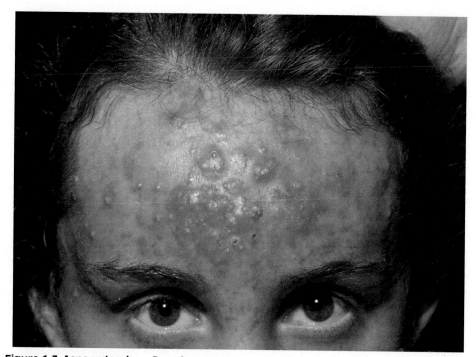

Figure 1-3 Acne vulgaris *Comedones rupturing into the dermis give rise to an intense inflammatory response with pustule and abscess formation (so-called "cystic" or nodulocystic acne).*

Management

The psychological impact of acne (perceived cosmetic disfigurement) should be assessed individually in each patient and therapy modified accordingly.

Mild Acne

Topical antibiotics (clindamycin and erythromycin)

Benzoyl peroxide gels (2 %, 5 %, or 10 %)

Topical retinoids (tretinoin) are effective in comedonal and papulopustular acne but require detailed instructions regarding gradual increases in concentration:

0.025 % cream **or** 0.01 % gel
↓
0.05 % cream **or** 0.025 % gel
↓
0.1 % cream
↓
0.05 % liquid
↓
lowest effective maintenance

Improvement occurs over a period of months (2 to 5) and may take even longer for noninflamed comedones. Topical retinoids are applied in the evening. Topical antibiotics and benzoyl peroxide gels are applied during the day.

Moderate Acne Oral tetracyclines added to the preceding regimen. Minocycline, 50 to 100 mg b.i.d., and this can be tapered to 50 mg/day as acne lessens. Antibiotics are additive and should not be the sole treatment. In females, moderate acne can be controlled with *high* doses of oral estrogens combined with progesterone or antiandrogens. However, cerebrovascular disorders are a serious risk.

Severe Acne Isotretinoin is a retinoid that inhibits sebaceous gland function and keratinization and has proved to be a very effective treatment for severe acne.

INDICATIONS For severe, recalcitrant, nodular acne. The nodules should be ≥5.0 mm, and there should be many, not a few. Also, the patient must have been resistant to other acne therapies, including systemic antibiotics.

CONTRAINDICATIONS Isotretinoin is a teratogenic drug. Therefore, pregnancy should be avoided at all costs. In females who may become pregnant, contraception is necessary. Both tetracycline and isotretinoin may cause pseudotumor cerebri (benign intracranial swelling); therefore the two medications should never be used together.

WARNINGS Blood lipids should be determined before starting therapy. About 25 % of patients can develop *increased plasma triglycerides*. Also, 15 % of patients develop a *decrease in high-density lipoproteins* and about 7 % show an *increase in cholesterol levels*. This may increase the cardiovascular risk. Also, when levels of serum triglycerides above 800 mg/dl are noted, the patient may develop acute pancreatitis. Therefore, every attempt should be made to control the triglyceride levels through such measures as weight reduction, dietary fat reduction, restriction of alcohol, and actual reduction of the dose of isotretinoin. Patients should not take vitamin supplements containing vitamin A. *Hepatotoxicity* has been very rarely reported in the form of clinical hepatitis. In one study, 15 % of patients developed mild to moderate elevation of hepatic enzymes that normalized with reduction of the dose of the drug. Although the clinical experience has not confirmed this in one large series, hepatic enzymes should be determined before beginning therapy. *Eye:* The patient should be advised that *night blindness* has been reported, and patients should be warned about driving at night. Also, patients may have *decreased tolerance to contact lenses* during and after therapy. *Skin:* An eczema-like rash can appear, and this responds dramatically to Class I corticosteroids. For additional rare possible complications, consult the package insert.

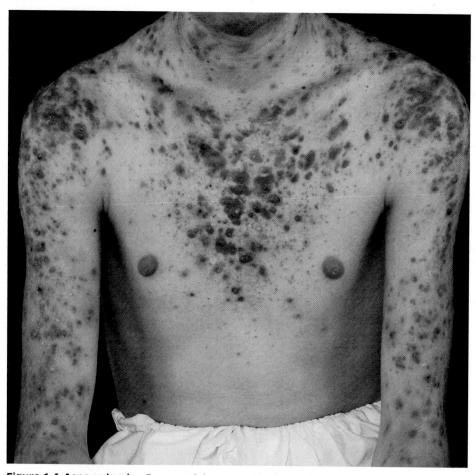

Figure 1-4 Acne vulgaris *Severe nodular acne with abscess formation and many recent red scars following resolution of inflammatory lesions on the upper chest, neck, arms.*

DOSAGE Isotretinoin, 0.5 to 2.0 mg/kg given in two divided doses *with food*, for 15 to 20 weeks. Most patients improve with 1.0 mg/kg. For severe disease, especially on the trunk, a dose of 2.0 mg/kg may be required.

If the nodule count has been reduced by more than 70 % prior to completing 15 to 20 weeks, the drug may be discontinued. After an interval of 2 months, a second course may be given if necessary.

HIDRADENITIS SUPPURATIVA

Hidradenitis suppurativa is a chronic, suppurative, cicatricial disease of apocrine gland–bearing skin in the axillae, the anogenital region, and rarely, the scalp (this is called *cicatrizing perifolliculitis*). Sometimes the disease is associated with severe nodulocystic acne and pilonidal sinuses (termed *follicular occlusion syndrome*).

Synonyms: Apocrinitis, hidradenitis axillaris, abscess of the apocrine sweat glands.

Epidemiology and Etiology

Race All races. Severe involvement is seen more often in blacks.

Age From puberty to climacteric

Sex Males more often have anogenital and females axillary involvement.

Heredity While no data are available, mother-daughter transmission has been observed repeatedly. Also, families may give a history of nodulocystic acne and hidradenitis suppurativa occurring separately or together in blood relatives.

Etiology Unknown. Predisposing factors: obesity, genetic predisposition to acne, apocrine duct obstruction, secondary bacterial infection

History

Symptoms: Intermittent pain and marked point tenderness related to abscess formation in axilla(e) and/or anogenital area

Physical Examination

Skin Findings

TYPES OF LESIONS Initial lesion: inflammatory nodule/abscess (Figure 1-5) that may resolve or point to surface and drain purulent/sero-purulent material; relationship to hair follicle usually not apparent. Eventually, sinus tracts form. Fibrosis, "bridge" scars, hypertrophic and keloidal scars, contractures (Figure 1-6). Subsequently, open comedones, at times double comedones, form (Figure 1-5) and these are highly characteristic of the disease. Comedones that are double, with two adjacent black comedones, may be present, even when active nodules are absent, and these can serve as a marker for a patient with hidradenitis suppurativa. Rarely, lymphedema of associated limb may develop.

COLOR Erythematous nodules

PALPATION Lesions moderately to exquisitely tender. Pus drains from opening of abscess and sinus tracts.

DISTRIBUTION OF LESIONS Axillae (Figures 1-5 and 1-6), breasts, anogenital area, groin. Often bilateral in axillae and/or anogenital area; may extend over entire back, buttocks, and scalp.

ASSOCIATED FINDINGS Cystic acne, pilonidal sinus

General Examination Often obesity

Differential Diagnosis

Early: furuncle, carbuncle, lymphadenitis, ruptured inclusion cyst, cat-scratch disease. *Late:* lymphogranuloma venereum, donovanosis, scrofuloderma, actinomycosis, sinus tracts and fistulas associated with ulcerative colitis and regional enteritis.

Laboratory and Special Examinations

Bacteriology A variety of pathogens may secondarily colonize or "infect" lesions. These include *Staphylococcus aureus*, streptococci, *Escherichia coli*, *Proteus mirabilis*, and *Pseudomonas aeruginosa*.

Dermatopathology *Early:* keratin occlusion of apocrine duct and hair follicle, ductal/tubu-

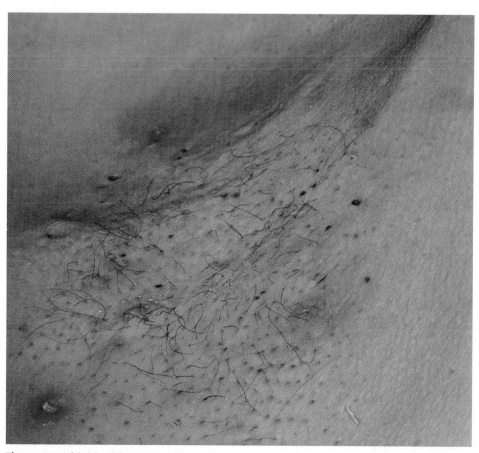

Figure 1-5 Hidradenitis suppurative *Many comedones, some of which are paired, are a characteristic finding, associated with several deep exquisitely painful abscesses and old scars in the axilla.*

lar dilatation, inflammatory changes limited to a single apocrine gland. *Late:* destruction of apocrine/eccrine/pilosebaceous apparatus, fibrosis, pseudoepitheliomatous hyperplasia in sinuses

Diagnosis

Clinical diagnosis

Pathophysiology

The pathogenesis is unknown. The following sequence may be the mechanism of the development of the lesions: keratinous plugging of the apocrine duct → dilatation of the apocrine duct and hair follicle → severe inflammatory changes limited to a single apocrine gland → bacterial growth in dilated duct → ruptured duct/gland resulting in extension of inflammation/infection → extension of suppuration/tissue destruction → ulceration and fibrosis, sinus tract formation

Course and Prognosis

The severity of the disease varies considerably. Many patients have only mild involvement with recurrent self-healing tender red nodules and do not seek therapy. The disease usually undergoes a spontaneous remission with age (>35 years). In some individuals, the course can be relentlessly progressive, with marked morbidity related to chronic pain, draining sinuses, and scarring. Complications (rare): fistulas to urethra, bladder, and/or rectum; anemia, amyloidosis.

Management

It should be emphasized that hidradenitis suppurativa is not simply an infection and that systemic antibiotics are only part of the treatment program. Combinations of (1) intralesional corticosteroids, (2) surgery, (3) oral antibiotics, and (4) isotretinoin are used.

Medical Management

ACUTE PAINFUL LESIONS *Nodule* Intralesional triamcinolone (3 to 5 mg/ml): diluted with lidocaine

> *Abscess* Intralesional triamcinolone (3 to 5 mg/ml): diluted with lidocaine into the wall followed by incision and drainage of abscess fluid

CHRONIC LOW-GRADE DISEASE Oral antibiotics: erythromycin (250 to 500 mg q.i.d.), or tetracycline (250 to 500 mg q.i.d.), or minocycline (100 mg b.i.d.) until lesions resolve; may take weeks. Intralesional triamcinolone (3 to 5 mg/ml) into early inflammatory lesions is helpful in hastening resolution of individual lesions.

PREDNISONE May be given concurrently if pain and inflammation are severe, 70 mg, tapered over 14 days.

ORAL ISOTRETINOIN Efficacy in severe disease is not established, but it appears to be useful in early disease and when combined with surgical excision of individual lesions.

Surgical Management

- Incise and drain acute abscesses.
- Excise chronic recurrent, fibrotic nodules or sinus tracts. If one or two nodules can be pinpointed with recurrent disease, these can be excised with a good result.
- With extensive, chronic disease, complete excision of axilla or involved anogenital area may be required. Excision should extend down to fascia and requires split skin grafting.

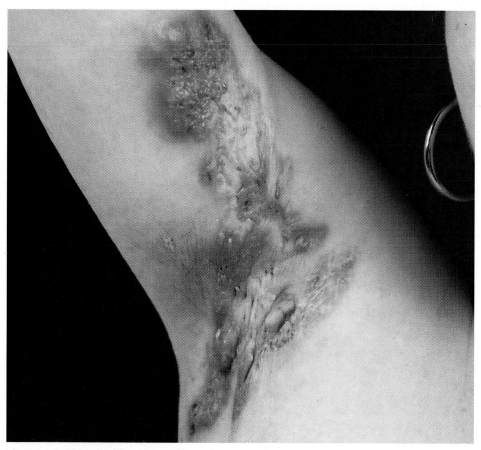

Figure 1-6 Hidradenitis suppurativa *Severe involvement of the axilla with multiple old hypertrophic and keloidal scars.*

ROSACEA

Rosacea (Latin: "like roses") is a chronic acneform disorder of the facial pilosebaceous units, coupled with an increased reactivity of capillaries to heat, leading to flushing and ultimately to telangiectasia. The disease was previously called *acne rosacea,* but it is unrelated yet quite often coexists with acne, which may have preceded the onset of rosacea. It is the cause of significant cosmetic disfigurement.

Epidemiology and Etiology

Age   30 to 50 years, peak incidence between 40 and 50 years

Sex   Females predominantly; rhinophyma occurs mostly in males

Race   Celtic peoples (skin phototypes I and II) but also in southern Italians; less frequent or rare in pigmented (brown and black) peoples

Other Factors   Patients with rosacea usually have a long history of episodic reddening of the face (flushing) with increases in skin temperature in response to heat stimuli in the mouth (hot liquids), spicy foods; alcohol (cold or hot) may be a precipitating factor in rosacea, possibly because it causes flushing. Exposure to sun and heat (such as chefs working near a hot stove) may cause exacerbations. Acne may have preceded the onset of rosacea by years; nevertheless, rosacea may and usually does arise *de novo* without any preceding history of acne or seborrhea.

History

Stages of Evolution (Plewig and Kligman Classification)

Episodic erythema, "flushing and blushing"—the rosacea diathesis

Stage I: Persistent erythema with telangiectases

Stage II: Persistent erythema, telangiectases, papules, tiny pustules

Stage III: Persistent deep erythema, dense telangiectases, papules, pustules, nodules; may rarely have persistent "solid" edema of the central part of the face, as occurs with acne

Duration of Lesions   Days, weeks, months

Skin Symptoms   Patients are concerned about their cosmetic facial appearance; they are often perceived as being alcoholic. Flushing, feeling of "heat" in the face.

Physical Examination

Skin Lesions

TYPE   ***Early*** Papules (2 to 3 mm), pustules [the pustule is often *small* (<1mm) and on the apex of the papule (Figure 1-7)]. Nodules. *No comedones*

  Late Telangiectases. Chronic rosacea can be associated with marked sebaceous hyperplasia and lymphedema, causing disfigurement of the nose, forehead, eyelids, ears, and chin.

COLOR   Red facies, papules and dusky-red nodules (Figure 1-7)

SHAPE   Papules and nodules are round, dome-shaped

ARRANGEMENT   Scattered, discrete lesions

DISTRIBUTION   Characteristic is a symmetrical localization on the face (cheeks, chin, forehead, glabella, nose). Rarely, neck, chest (V-shaped area), back, and scalp.

Special Lesions   *Rhinophyma* (enlarged nose, Figures 1-8 and 1-9), *metophyma* (enlarged cushion-like swelling of the forehead), *blepharophyma* (swelling of the eyelids related to marked sebaceous gland hyperplasia), *otophyma* (cauliflower-like swelling of the earlobes), *gnathophyma* (swelling of the chin).

Eye Lesions   "Red" eyes as a result of chronic blepharitis, conjunctivitis, and episcleritis.

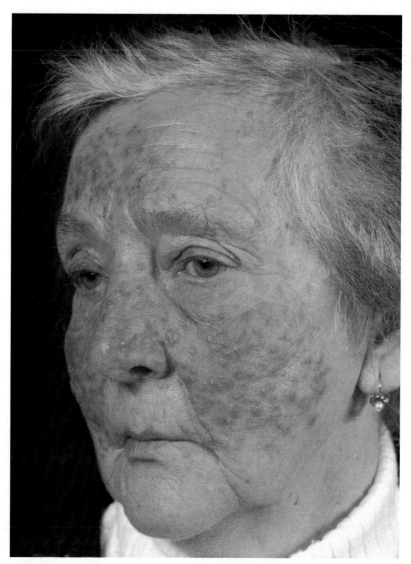

Figure 1-7 Rosacea *Typical moderately severe involvement with confluent erythematous papules and pustules on the forehead, cheeks, and nose. Note the absence of comedones that are typically seen with acne vulgaris.*

Rosacea keratitis is a serious problem because corneal ulcers may develop. *An ophthalmologist should follow the patient if there is a suspicion of eye involvement.*

Differential Diagnosis

Acne, perioral dermatitis, *Staphylococcus aureus* folliculitis, gram-negative folliculitis, *Demodex folliculorum* infestation, and SLE

Laboratory and Special Examinations

Bacterial Culture   Rule out *S. aureus* infection

Dermatopathology

STAGES OF ROSACEA

Stage I   Papules and telangiectases

Papules   Nonspecific perifollicular inflammatory infiltrate with occasional foci of "tuberculoid" granulomatous areas; epithelioid cells, lymphocytes, and few giant cells but no caseation

Telangiectasia   Dilated capillaries surrounded by a nonspecific inflammatory infiltrate

Stage II   Papules and pustules

Pustules   Foci of neutrophils high and within the follicle

Stage III   Papules, pustules, and nodules

Nodules   Diffuse hypertrophy of the connective tissue, marked sebaceous gland hyperplasia, epithelioid granuloma without caseation, and many foreign-body giant cells

RHINOPHYMA   *Glandular Type*   Enlarged nose is related to very marked lobular sebaceous hyperplasia.

Fibrous Type   There is a marked increase in the connective tissue with only a variable amount of sebaceous hyperplasia.

Fibroangiomatous Type   Copper-red nose is related to much enlarged edematous connective tissue with large ectatic veins.

Course

Prolonged. Recurrences are common. After a few years, the disease tends to disappear spontaneously. Men and rarely women may develop rhinophyma, which is treated successfully by surgery or laser surgery.

Management

Prevention   Marked reduction or elimination of alcoholic and hot beverages may be helpful in some patients; it is not the caffeine but the temperature ("hotness") of the tea and coffee that is the culprit. Emotional stress may be a factor in some individuals.

Topical

Metronidazole gel or cream, 0.75 %, twice daily is very effective.
Topical antibiotics (e.g., erythromycin gel) may be effective.

Systemic   If metronidazole fails, or for severe disease, add oral antibiotics:

Tetracycline, 1.0 to 1.5 g/day in divided doses until clear; then gradually reduce to once-daily doses of 250 to 500 mg.
Minocycline and doxycycline, 50 to 100 mg twice daily, are alternative antibiotics, especially minocycline because doxycycline is a phototoxic drug and this limits exposure to sunlight in summer.

MAINTENANCE   After control of papulopustules, a dose of 250 to 500 g tetracycline or 50 mg minocycline or doxycycline per day is given.

Oral Isotretinoin   Oral isotretinoin is an alternative in individuals with severe disease (especially stage II) not responding to antibiotics and topical treatments. A low-dose regimen of 0.1 to 0.2 mg/kg of body weight per day is effective in most patients but occasionally 1 mg/kg may be required.

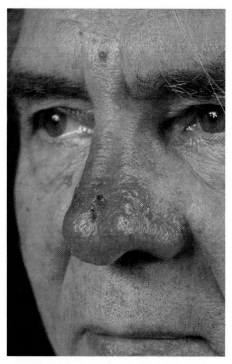

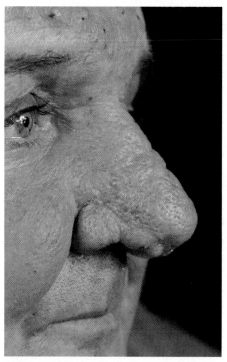

Figure 1-8 Rosacea *Mild involvement with few erythematous papules and crusts and striking erythema, edema, and telangiectasias on the nose (early rhinophyma).*

Figure 1-9 Rosacea *Long-standing disease with edema and hyperplasia of the tissues of the nose (rhinophyma), cheeks, and forehead.*

PERIORAL DERMATITIS

Perioral dermatitis is a pesky facial dermatosis occurring mainly in young women, characterized by discrete erythematous micropapules that often become confluent, forming inflammatory plaques, on the perioral and periorbital skin.

Synonym: Rosacea-like dermatitis.

Epidemiology and Etiology

Age   20 to 30 years; can occur in children

Sex   Females predominantly

Etiology   Unknown

Other Factors   May be markedly aggravated by potent topical (fluorinated) corticosteroids.

History

Duration of Lesions   Weeks to months

Skin Symptoms   Perceived cosmetic disfigurement; occasional itching or burning, feeling of tightness

Physical Examination

Skin Lesions

TYPE   Papulopustules on an erythematous background (Figure 1-10). Initial lesions are erythematous 1- to 2-mm micropapules on a patchy erythematous background. Papules increase in number with central confluence and satellite lesions, including papules, vesicles, and/or pustules. Confluent plaques may appear eczematous with erythema and scales (Figure 1-11). There are no comedones.

COLOR   Pink to red, "patchy redness"

ARRANGEMENT   Papules are irregularly grouped, symmetrical (Figures 1-10 and 1-11).

DISTRIBUTION   Initial lesions usually perioral. Rim of sparing around the vermilion border of lips. At times, micropapules (1 to 2 mm) and pustules in the periorbital area also occur. Uncommonly, only periorbital involvement is present. Occasionally, glabella and forehead are involved.

Differential Diagnosis

Allergic contact dermatitis, atopic dermatitis, seborrheic dermatitis, rosacea, acne vulgaris, steroid acne

Laboratory Examination

Culture   Rule out *Staphylococcus aureus* infection.

Diagnosis

Clinical diagnosis

Course

Appearance of lesions is usually subacute over weeks to months. Perioral dermatitis is, at times, misdiagnosed as an eczematous or a seborrheic dermatitis and treated with a potent topical corticosteroid preparation, aggravating perioral dermatitis or inducing steroid acne. Untreated, perioral dermatitis fluctuates in activity over months to years but is not nearly as chronic as rosacea. With adequate treatment for several months, mild recurrences do occur but usually are controlled with topical metronidazole gel or a low-dose tetracycline or minocycline.

Management

Topical

Metronidazole, 0.75 % gel or cream, or *ery-*

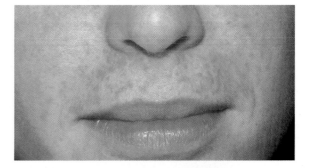

Figure 1-10 Perioral dermatitis
Mild early involvement with tiny erythematous nonpruritic papules on the upper lip, which is commonly misdiagnosed as eczematous dermatitis.

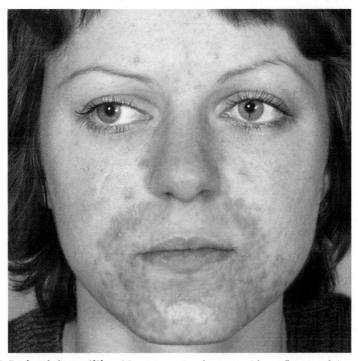

Figure 1-11 Perioral dermatitis   *More severe involvement with confluence of tiny papules and pustules in a wide perioral distribution. Note: Typical tiny papules/pustules can arise in the periorbital region, with or without perioral involvement.*

thromycin, 2.0 % gel, applied to involved areas b.i.d. may be effective in some cases.

Systemic

Minocycline, 100 mg b.i.d. until clear, then 100 mg daily for 1 month, then 50 mg daily for 1 additional month **or**

Doxycycline 100 mg b.i.d. until clear, then 100 mg daily for 1 month, then 50 mg daily for 1 additional month **or**
Tetracycline, 500 mg b.i.d. until clear, then 500 mg daily for 1 month, then 250 mg daily for 1 additional month.

Section 2

DISORDERS OF HAIR FOLLICLES AND RELATED DISORDERS

DISORDERS OF HAIR GROWTH

Loss of hair is termed *effluvium* or *defluvium,* and the condition resulting from this is called *alopecia* (baldness). Patients have a different perception of balding than the dermatologist, often aware and very concerned about subtle thinning of the hair. Disorders characterized by loss of hair are conveniently classified into *noncicatricial alopecia,* where, at least clinically, there is no sign of tissue inflammation, scarring, or atrophy of skin, and *cicatricial alopecia,* where evidence of tissue destruction such as inflammation, atrophy, and scarring is apparent.

Hair growth on the scalp occurs in cycles of intermittent activity; periods of growth are followed by periods of quiescence. The period of active growth is referred to as *anagen,* which is followed normally by a brief transition phase, called *catagen,* during which growth stops and follicles enter the resting, or *telogen,* phase. Telogen phase is prolonged in the eyebrows, eyelashes, and axillary and pubic hair compared with the relatively short telogen phase in the scalp and beard areas.

NONSCARRING ALOPECIA

ALOPECIA AREATA

Alopecia areata is a localized loss of hair in round or oval areas without any visible inflammation of the skin in hair-bearing areas; the most common presenting site is the scalp. *Alopecia totalis* is loss of all scalp hair and eyebrows. *Alopecia universalis,* the end stage of alopecia areata, is complete loss of all body hair.

Epidemiology and Etiology

Prevalence Relatively common. About 1 % of the U.S. population has at least one episode of alopecia areata by age 50.

Age Young adults (<25 years); children are affected more frequently.

Sex Equal in both sexes, although the male : female ratio is reported to be 2 : 1 in Italy and Spain.

Race All races

Etiology Unknown. Association with other autoimmune diseases suggests an anti-hair bulb autoimmune process.

Other Factors Not a sign of any multisystem disease but may be associated with other autoimmune disorders such as vitiligo, familial autoimmune polyendocrinopathy syndrome (hypoparathyroidism, Addison's disease, and mucocutaneous candidiasis), and thyroid disease (Hashimoto's disease).

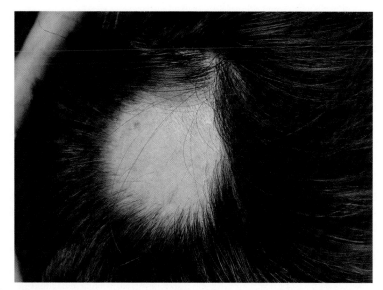

Figure 2-1 Alopecia areata *A sharply outlined portion of the scalp with complete alopecia without scaling, erythema, atrophy, or scarring. Empty follicles can still be seen on the involved scalp. The short, broken-off hair shafts (so-called exclamation point hair) appear as very short stubs emerging from the bald scalp.*

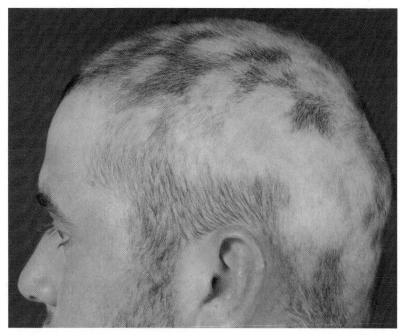

Figure 2-2 Alopecia areata *Multiple, confluent, involved sites on the scalp with evidence of regrowth in some areas. Newly regrowing hairs are fine and gray-white in color.*

History

Duration of Area of Hair Loss   Gradual over weeks to months. Patches of alopecia areata can be stable and often show spontaneous regrowth over a period of several months; new patches may appear while others resolve.

Skin Symptoms   No pain or itching. However, patients are often very concerned about a single area of hair loss and prognosis of continued, progressive balding.

Associated Findings   Hashimoto's thyroiditis, vitiligo, myasthenia gravis

Physical Examination

Skin Lesions   Usually none. Possibly erythema in the area of hair loss. The absence of clinical signs of inflammation is remarkable in that histopathologically there is always an inflammatory infiltrate around hair follicles in active lesions.

Hair   Alopecia, normal-appearing skin with follicular openings present (Figure 2-1). No scarring, no atrophy; occasionally, with diagnostic broken-off stubby hairs called *exclamation point hairs,* sharp margins. With regrowth of hair, new hairs are thin and often white or gray. Alopecia always sharply defined.

ARRANGEMENT   Scattered, discrete areas of alopecia (Figures 2-1 and 2-2) or confluent with total loss of scalp hair (alopecia areata totalis), or generalized resulting in generalized loss of body hair (including vellus hair) termed *alopecia areata universalis* (Figure 2-3). Sometimes hair loss in alopecia areata totalis may follow a diffuse (noncircumscribed) pattern.

SITES OF PREDILECTION   Scalp, eyebrows, eyelashes, pubic hair, beard

Nails   Dystrophic changes. The dorsal nail plate may have hundreds of tiny depressions simulating "hammered brass."

Differential Diagnosis

Nonscarring Alopecia   Secondary syphilis ("moth-eaten" appearance in beard or scalp), white-patch tinea capitis, trichotillomania, traction alopecia, early chronic cutaneous lupus erythematosus, androgenetic alopecia

Laboratory and Special Examinations

Serology   Antinuclear antibodies (to rule out lupus erythematosus); RPR (to rule out secondary syphilis)

KOH Preparation   To rule out tinea capitis

Dermatopathology   Follicles are reduced in size, arrested in anagen IV, and lie high in the dermis; perifollicular lymphocytic infiltrate with dilated vessels followed by degenerative changes in the blood vessels that lead to the hair papillae. Trichogram (see page 24): Hair roots have typical club shape; proximal portion of shaft shows dystrophic taper (exclamation point hairs). Dystrophic anagen hairs. Increase of telogen hair from normal (<20 %) to 40 % or more.

Course

If occurring after puberty, 80 % of patients regrow hair. Alopecia universalis is rare. Following the first episode of hair loss, about 33 % completely regrow the hair within a year. Recurrences of alopecia, however, are frequent. Repeated attacks, nail changes, and total alopecia before puberty are poor prognostic signs. Poor prognostic sign is also confluence of lesions in occipital region (ophiasis).

Management

No curative treatment is currently available. Efficacy of treatment in individual patients is difficult to assess in light of spontaneous regrowth. All in all, treatment for alopecia areata is unsatisfactory. In many cases, the most important factor in management of the patient is psycho-

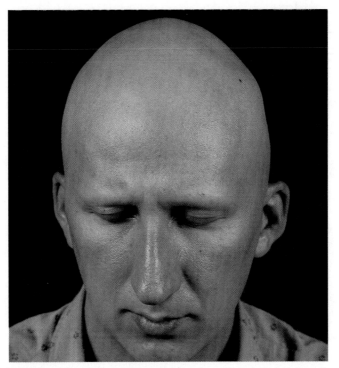

Figure 2-3 Alopecia universalis *This patient has lost all scalp hair (alopecia universalis), eyebrows, eyelashes, beard, and all body hair, and has dystrophic ("hammered brass") nails.*

logical support from the dermatologist, family, and support groups (The National Alopecia Areata Foundation, Tel. 1-415-456-4644).

Corticosteroids

TOPICAL   Superpotent agents may be effective.

INTRALESIONAL INJECTION   Few and small spots of alopecia areata can be treated with intralesional triamcinolone acetonide 3.5 mg/ml, which can be very effective temporarily.

SYSTEMIC CORTICOSTEROIDS   Usually induce regrowth, but alopecia frequently recurs upon discontinuation; risks of long-term therapy therefore preclude their use.

Systemic Cyclosporine Induces regrowth, but alopecia recurs when drug is discontinued.

Induction of Allergic Contact Dermatitis Dinitrochlorobenzene, squaric acid dibutylester, or diphencyprone can be used successfully, but local discomfort due to allergic contact dermatitis and swelling of regional lymph nodes poses a problem.

Oral PUVA (Photochemotherapy) Variably effective, as high as 30 %, and worth a trial in patients who are very distressed about the problem. The entire body must be exposed, in that the therapy is believed to be a form of systemic immune suppression.

ANDROGENETIC ALOPECIA

Androgenetic alopecia (AGA) is the common progressive balding that occurs through the combined effect of a genetic predisposition and the action of androgen on the hair follicles of the scalp. Pattern of hair loss in males varies from bitemporal recession, to frontal and/or vertex thinning, to loss of all hair except that along the occipital and temporal margins. In males, diffuse thinning occurs, worse centrally.

Synonyms: Male-pattern baldness, common baldness (males), hereditary thinning (females).

Epidemiology and Etiology

Age of Onset   *Males:* May begin any time after puberty, as early as the second decade; often fully expressed in forties. *Females:* Later—in about 40 % occurs in the sixth decade.

Sex   Males much more commonly than females

Race   Occurs in all races

Heredity   Polygenic or autosomal dominant in males; autosomal recessive in females

Etiology   Combined effects of androgen on genetically predisposed hair follicles

History

Skin Symptoms   Most patients present with complaints of gradually thinning hair or baldness. In males (Figure 2-4), there is a receding anterior hair line, especially in the parietal regions, which results in an M-shaped recession. Following this, a bald spot may appear on the posterior crown. If AGA progresses rapidly, some patients also complain of increased falling out of hair. In females, parietal and temporal recession is not usually a major feature and effluvium follows a pattern depicted in Figure 2-4; severe thinning is not common. The cosmetic appearance of AGA is very disturbing to many patients owing to the high value that our society places on a "healthy head of hair."

Systems Review   In young women, manifestations of androgen excess should be sought as significant: acne, hirsutism, irregular menses,

or virilization. However, most women with AGA are endocrinologically normal.

Physical Examination

Skin Lesions   No skin lesions are seen in AGA except seborrhea that may be present in severe cases. In young women, other signs of virilization should be sought, such as acne and excess facial or body hair or a male-pattern escutcheon.

Hair (Figures 2-5 and 2-6)   Hair in areas of AGA becomes finer in texture, i.e., shorter in length and of reduced diameter. In time, hair becomes vellus and eventually atrophies completely. With complete alopecia, scalp is smooth and shiny; orifices of follicles are barely perceptible with the unaided eye.

Associated Findings   Often associated with seborrheic dermatitis of the scalp (oily scalp)

DISTRIBUTION

Males usually exhibit patterned loss in the frontotemporal and vertex areas. The end result may be only a rim of residual hair on the lateral and posterior scalp (Figures 2-4 and 2-5). In these regions hair never falls in AGA. Paradoxically, males with extensive AGA may have excess growth of secondary sexual hair, i.e., axillae, pubic area, chest, and beard. Hamilton (*Am J Anat* 1941; 71:451) classified male-pattern hair loss into stages: type I, loss of hair along the frontal margin; type II, increasing frontal hair loss as well as onset of loss on the occipital scalp (crown); and types III, IV, and V, increasing hair loss in both regions with eventual confluent and

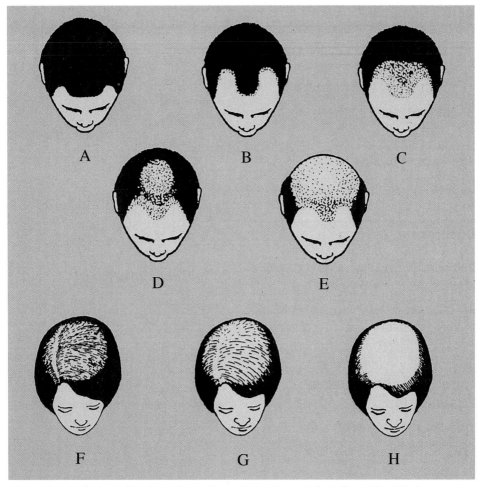

Figure 2-4 Androgenetic alopecia: patterns in males and females *The different patterns as they appear in males (A–E) (classification according to Hamilton) and females (F–H) (classification according to Ludwig).*

complete balding of the top of the scalp with sparing of the sides (Figure 2-4).

Females, including those who are endocrinologically normal, also lose scalp hair according to the male pattern, but hair loss is far less pronounced. Often hair loss is more diffuse in women following a pattern first described by Ludwig (*Br J Dermatol* 1977; 97:249). (Figure 2-4)

Systemic Findings In young women with AGA, signs of virilization such as clitoral hypertrophy, acne, and facial hirsutism should be sought to rule out endocrine dysfunction.

Differential Diagnosis

Diffuse Nonscarring Scalp Alopecia Diffuse pattern of hair loss with alopecia areata, telogen defluvium, secondary syphilis, systemic lupus erythematosus, iron deficiency, hypothyroidism, hyperthyroidism, trichotillomania, seborrheic dermatitis.

Laboratory and Special Examinations

Trichogram A trichogram determines the number of anagen and telogen hairs and is made by epilating (plucking) 50 hairs or more from the scalp with a needleholder and counting the number of anagen hairs (A) (growing hairs with a long encircling hair sheath) and the number of club or telogen hairs (T) (resting hairs with an inner root sheath and roots usually largest at the base). Normally, 80 % to 90 % of hairs are in anagen phase. In AGA, the earliest changes are an increase in the percentage of telogen hairs.

Dermatopathology Abundance of telogen-stage follicles is noted, associated with hair follicles of decreasing size and eventually nearly complete atrophy.

Hormone Studies In women with hair loss and evidence of increased androgens (menstrual irregularities, infertility, hirsutism, severe cystic acne, virilization), total testosterone, free testosterone, dehydroepiandrosterone sulfate (DHEAS), and prolactin should be determined.

Other Studies Treatable causes of thinning hair should be excluded with TSH, T_4, serum iron, serum ferritin, and/or total iron-binding capacity (TIBC), CBC.

Diagnosis

Clinical diagnosis is made on the history, pattern of alopecia, and family incidence of AGA.

Pathophysiology

The mechanism of action of androgen on follicular cellular processes that results in AGA is unclear, but in most cases it is a local phenomenon (increased expression of androgen receptors, changes in androgen metabolism) of the scalp hair follicles. *Consequently, most patients (male and female) are endocrinologically normal.* Terminal follicles are transformed into vellus-like follicles, which in turn undergo atrophy. During successive follicular cycles, the hairs produced are of shorter length and of decreasing diameter. Conversely, androgens induce vellus-to-terminal follicle production of secondary sexual hair. Males castrated before or during puberty do not develop AGA despite a strong family history; administration of androgen can produce baldness that does not progress if the drug is withdrawn. Dihydrotestosterone, an intracellular hormone, causes growth of androgen-dependent hair (e.g., pubic, beard) and loss of non-androgen-dependent scalp hair.

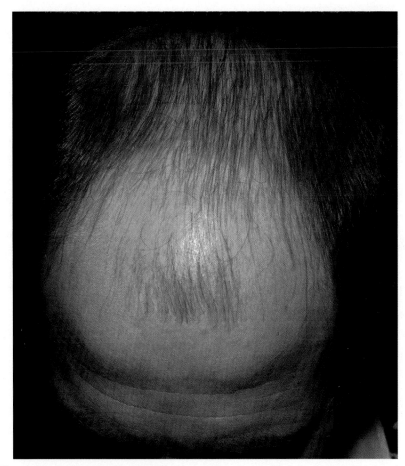

Figure 2-5 Androgenetic alopecia in a male *Loss of hair in the frontotemporal and vertex areas in a male corresponding to Hamilton types D and E.*

In males, testosterone produced by the testes is the major androgen. In females, androstenedione and dehydroepiandrosterone sulfate are the major peripheral androgens, and these two hormones are very slowly converted to dihydrotestosterone in the target cell (hair keratinocyte) by 5-alpha-testosterone reductase. The serum testosterone levels in men are much higher than in women, and there are higher tissue levels and greater conversion to dihydrotestosterone.

Course

The progression of alopecia is usually very gradual, over years to decades.

Management

There is no highly effective therapy to prevent the progression of AGA.

Topical Minoxidil   Topically applied minoxidil 2 % solution is helpful in reducing the rate of hair loss or in partially restoring lost hair in some patients; in large clinical trials, moderate growth has been noted at 4 and 12 months in 40 % of males. The efficacy of minoxidil in females is not yet known from large clinical trials. Combinations of higher concentrations of minoxidil with topical retinoic acid are promising improvements.

Antiandrogens   Spironolactone, cyproterone acetate, flutamide, and cimetidine, which bind to androgen receptors and block the action of dihydrotestosterone, have been reported to be effective in treating women with AGA who have elevated adrenal androgens; these are not used in men.

Wigs   A wide variety of hair pieces are used.

Hair Transplantation   Moving multiple punch grafts of follicles taken from androgen-insensitive hair sites (peripheral occipital and parietal hairy areas) to bald androgen-sensitive scalp areas is effective in some patients with AGA. These micrografts are a successful technique in many patients and help restore more normal appearance.

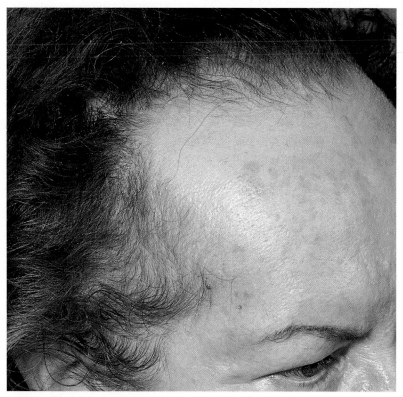

Figure 2-6 Androgenetic alopecia in a female   *This woman had pronounced diffuse thinning of hair on the crown but, in addition, also had thinning of the hair in the frontotemporal region of the scalp after treatment with androgens.*

TELOGEN EFFLUVIUM

Telogen defluvium is the transient increased shedding of normal club hairs (telogen) from resting scalp follicles secondary to accelerated shift of anagen (growth phase) into catagen and telogen (resting phase), which results clinically in increased daily hair loss and, if severe, thinning of hair. *Synonym:* Telogen defluvium.

Epidemiology and Etiology

Age   Any age

Sex   More common in women due to parturition, cessation of an oral contraceptive, and "crash" dieting

Incidence   Second most common cause of alopecia after androgenetic alopecia

Etiology   Factors that affect follicle growth resulting in telogen effluvium include pregnancy followed either by abortion or parturition, discontinuing or changing type of oral contraceptive, major surgical procedure, major traumatic injury, "crash" dieting with significant weight loss in a short period of time, and significant medical illness (especially with high fever).

History

Skin Symptoms   Patient presents with complaint of increased hair loss on the scalp that may be accompanied by varying degrees of hair thinning. Most patients are very anxious, fearing they will become bald. The physician is often presented with a plastic bag containing the shed hair. The precipitating event precedes the telogen defluvium by 6 to 16 weeks.

Physical Examination

Skin Lesions   No abnormalities of the scalp are detected.

Hair (Figure 2-7)   Diffuse shedding of the scalp hair is seen. In running the fingers through the patient's hair, several to many hairs may be shed with each passage. These hairs are all telogen or club hairs.

DISTRIBUTION   Hair loss occurs diffusely throughout the scalp and includes the sides and back of the head (Figure 2-7). If hair loss is significant enough to result in thinning of hair, alopecia is noted diffusely throughout the scalp. Short regrowing new hairs are present close to the scalp; these hairs are finer than older hairs and have tapered ends.

SITE OF PREDILECTION   Scalp

Nails   The precipitating stimulus for telogen defluvium also may affect the growth of nails, resulting in Beau's lines, which appear as transverse lines or grooves on the fingernail and toenail plates.

Differential Diagnosis

Increased Shedding of Scalp Hair ± Alopecia   That of nonscarring, noninflammatory alopecia: androgenetic alopecia, diffuse-pattern alopecia areata, hyperthyroidism, hypothyroidism, systemic lupus erythematosus, secondary syphilis, drug-induced alopecia (see Table 2-A).

Laboratory and Special Examinations

Trichogram   Compared with the normal trichogram, in which 80 % to 90 % of hair is in the anagen phase, telogen defluvium is characterized by a reduced percentage of anagen hairs, varying with the intensity of hair shedding. See page 24 for an explanation of the trichogram.

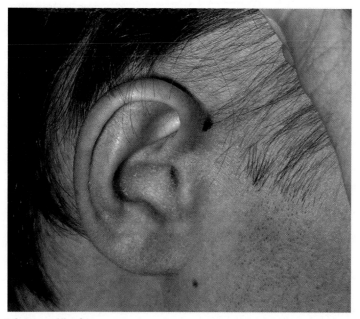

Figure 2-7 Telogen effluvium *A clump of hair in the hand, associated with striking thinning of scalp hair; the patient was HIV-infected and experienced* Pneumocystis carinii *pneumonia 10 weeks previously.*

CBC   Rule out iron deficiency anemia.

Chemistry   Serum iron, iron-binding capacity

TSH   Rule out thyroid disease.

Serology   Antinuclear antibodies (ANAs), RPR (to rule out syphilis)

Histopathology   No abnormality other than an increase in the proportion of follicles in telogen

Diagnosis

Made on history, clinical findings, and trichogram, excluding other causes

Pathophysiology

In the normal scalp, 80 % to 90 % of hairs are in anagen phase, 5 % in catagen phase, and 10 % to 15 % in telogen phase; 50 to 100 hairs are shed as they are replaced daily. With telogen defluvium, many more hairs than normal are shed daily. The precipitating stimulus for telogen effluvium results in a premature shift of anagen follicles into the telogen phase.

Course and Prognosis

Complete regrowth of hair is the rule. In postpartum telogen defluvium, if hair loss is severe and recurs after successive pregnancies, regrowth may never be complete. Telogen defluvium may continue for up to a year after the precipitating cause.

Management

No intervention is needed or required. The patient should be reassured that the process is part of a normal cycle of hair growth and shedding and that full regrowth of the hair is to be expected in most cases. High dose vitamin B and calcium have been reported to be beneficial, but this may be a placebo effect.

ANAGEN EFFLUVIUM

In anagen effluvium, the pattern of hair loss follows that of telogen effluvium—it is diffuse and involves the entire scalp—but is usually more rapid in onset and far more pronounced. It results from a rapid growth arrest or damage to anagen hairs that skip catagen and telogen and are shed. In most cases, anagen effluvium is caused by drugs, intoxication, or chemotherapy.

TABLE 2-A   DRUG-INDUCED ALOPECIA*

DRUGS	FEATURES OF ALOPECIA
ACE Inhibitors	
Enalapril	Probable telogen effluvium
Anticoagulants	
Heparin	Few reports
Warfarin	Reported incidence ranges from 19% to 70% but is probably much lower; diffuse shedding with increased number of hairs in telogen phase
Antimitotic Agents	
Colchicine	Diffuse hair loss; increased number of telogen hairs
Antineoplastic Agents	
Bleomycin	Anagen effluvium
Cyclophosphamide	Anagen effluvium
Cytarabine	Anagen effluvium
Dacarbazine	Anagen effluvium
Dactinomycin	Anagen effluvium
Daunorubicin	Anagen effluvium
Doxorubicin	Anagen effluvium
Etoposide	Anagen effluvium
Fluorouracil	Anagen effluvium
Hydroxyurea	Anagen effluvium
Ifosfamide	Anagen effluvium
Mechlorethamine	Anagen effluvium
Melphalen	Anagen effluvium
Methotrexate	Anagen effluvium
Mitomycin	Anagen effluvium
Mitoxantrone	Anagen effluvium
Nitrosourea	Anagen effluvium
Procarbazine	Anagen effluvium
Thiotepa	Anagen effluvium
Vinblastine	Anagen effluvium
Vincristine	Anagen effluvium
Antiparkinsonian Agents	
Levodopa	Probable telogen defluvium
Antiseizure Agents	
Trimethadione	Probable telogen defluvium
Beta Blockers	
Metoprolol	Probable telogen defluvium
Propanolol	Probable telogen defluvium
Birth Control Agents	
Oral contraceptives	Diffuse hair loss (telogen defluvium) 2 to 3 months after cessation of oral contraceptive

continued

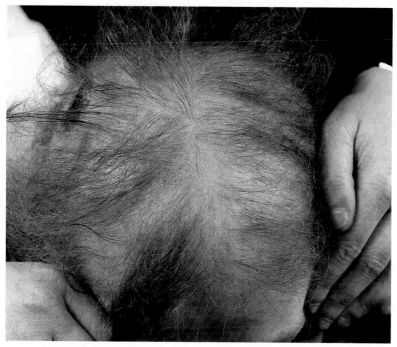

Figure 2-8 Anagen efluvium   *Massive, diffuse hair loss of the scalp following initiation of cancer chemotherapy.*

Drugs Used in Treatment of Bipolar Disorders
Lithium — Probable telogen defluvium

Ergot Derivatives (used in treatment of prolactinemia)
Bromocriptine — Probable telogen defluvium

H₂ Blockers
Cimetidine — Onset 1 week to 11 months; probable telogen effluvium

Heavy Metals (Poisoning)
Thallium — Diffuse shedding of abnormal anagen hair 10 days after ingestion; complete hair loss in 1 month; characteristic is pronounced hair loss on sides of head, also of lateral eyebrows

Mercury and lead — Diffuse hair loss with acute and chronic exposure

Cholesterol-Lowering Drugs
Clofibrate — Occasionally associated with hair loss

Pesticides
Boric acid — Total scalp alopecia reported after acute intoxication; with chronic exposure hair becomes dry and falls out

Retinoids
Etretinate — Increased hair shedding and plucked telogen count; decreased duration of anagen phase

Isotretinoin — Diffuse loss; probably same mechanism as above

*Prepared by Suzanne Virnelli-Grevelink, M.D.

SCARRING ALOPECIA

Scarring (cicatricial) alopecias result from damage or destruction of the hair follicles by inflammatory (infectious and noninfectious) or other pathologic processes, and healing occurs with scarring. A large number of dermatologic conditions, mostly inflammatory, that also occur on glabrous skin lead to cicatricial alopecia, and these are listed in Table 2-B, which has been restricted to conditions described elsewhere in this volume.

Practically all these bald (hairless) lesions are characterized by scarring and atrophy and complete loss of hair follicles. Skin lesions within or at the periphery of the alopecia may be characteristic for that given disease [e.g., chronic cutaneous lupus erythematosus (Figure 2-9) or tinea capitis (see Section 25)]. Idiopathic conditions (where the etiology or pathogenesis is unknown) confined to nonglabrous skin also can result in scarring and cicatricial alopecia, and most of these are exceedingly rare. Four conditions are a little more common and are therefore described briefly here.

Pseudopelade of Brocq (Figure 2-10)   This is a slowly progressive cicatricial alopecia that may represent the end stage of other inflammatory follicular diseases, such as lichen planus or lupus erythematosus. It does, however, occur as a primary noninflammatory scarring process without known cause. The scalp is usually smooth with atrophic or mildly scarred patches devoid of hair that may coalesce. Hair follicles are absent, but nonsuppurative inflammation may be seen around persisting follicles in the periphery of the lesions. Several hairs are often seen emerging from a single orifice within the scarred area.

Folliculitis Decalvans (Figure 2-11)   This is a circumscribed cicatricial alopecia on the scalp or beard area resulting from coalescing inflammation of hair follicles with pustulation that leads to crusting and atrophic or scarred areas devoid of hair.

Dissecting Perifolliculitis of the Scalp (Perifolliculitis Capitis Abscedens et Suffodiens) Manifested by deep and superficial abscess formation and extensive scarring. The disease is primarily not of bacterial etiology. Scarring leads to permanent alopecia.

Acne Keloidalis   Occurs most commonly in black men. Usually occurs on the nape of the neck, starting with a chronic papular or pustular eruption localized to the nape of the neck and occipital area and eventuating in hypertrophic keloidal scar formation (Figures 2-12 and 2-16).

Pseudofolliculitis Barbae   Because of the tight curls in beard of black men, hair often grows back into the skin, causing an inflammatory response, a pseudofolliculitis. *S. aureus* secondary infection is common (Figure 2-13).

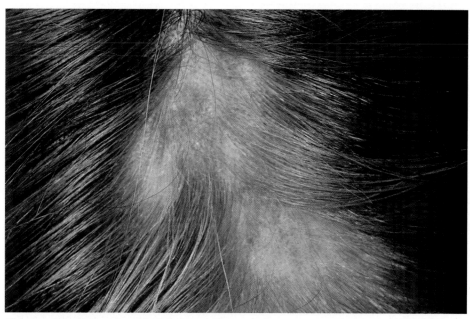

Figure 2-9 Scarring alopecia: chronic cutaneous lupus erythematosus *Residual erythema, follicular plugging, atrophy, and scarring alopecia of the scalp.*

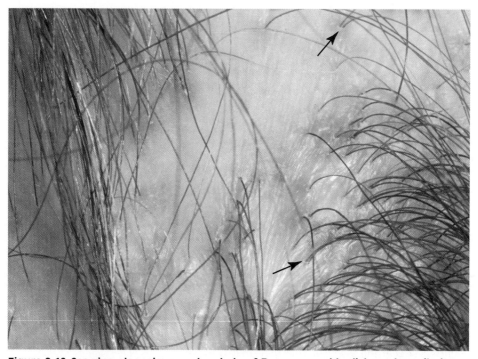

Figure 2-10 Scarring alopecia: pseudopelade of Brocq caused by lichen planopilaris
The scalp is smooth, shiny, devoid of hair and hair follicles in many areas; some of the remaining follicles are inflamed with perifollicular erythema and scale. Several hairs are seen emerging from a single site within the area of alopecia (arrows).

TABLE 2-B CLASSIFICATION OF CICATRICIAL ALOPECIAS

Developmental defects and hereditary disorders
  Recessive X-linked ichthyosis
  Epidermal nevi
  Epidermolysis bullosa (GAREB) (recessive dystrophic type)
Infections
  Staphylococcus aureus
  Tinea capitis: following kerion or favus
  Varicella zoster virus (VZV): following severe herpes zoster
Neoplasms
  Basal cell carcinoma
  Squamous cell carcinoma
  Metastatic tumors
  Lymphomas
  Adnexal tumors
Physical/chemical agents
  Mechanical trauma (including factitial: trichotillomania)
  Burns
  Radiation
  Caustic agents
  Other chemicals/drugs

Dermatoses of uncertain origin and clinical syndromes
  Lupus erythematosus: chronic cutaneous
  Lichen planus
  Sarcoidosis
  Scleroderma/morphea
  Lichen sclerosus et atrophicus
  Necrobiosis lipoidica diabeticorum
  Dermatomyositis
  Cicatricial pemphigoid
  Follicular mucinosis
  Acne keloidalis/sycosis nuchae
  Pseudofolliculitis barbae
  Pseudopelade of Brocq
  Folliculitis decalvans
  Dissecting perifolliculitis of the scalp (perifolliculitis capitis abscedens et suffodiens)
  Amyloidosis

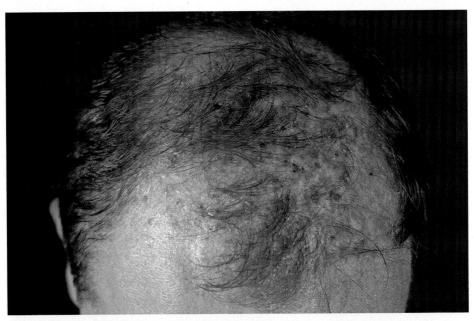

Figure 2-11 Scarring alopecia: folliculitis decalvans *Erythema, inflammatory papules, crusts, and scarring in a male who also has androgenetic alopecia.*

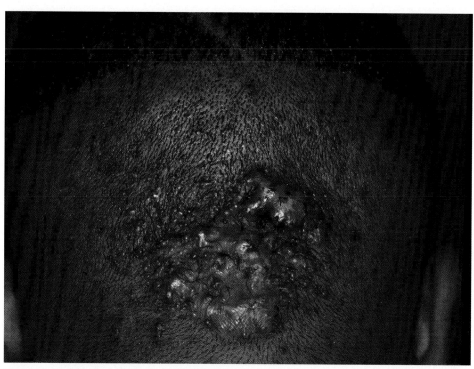

Figure 2-12 Scarring alopecia: follicular keloids *Papular and nodular scars becoming confluent on the occipital scalp of a black male; a few hairs emerging from within the scars.*

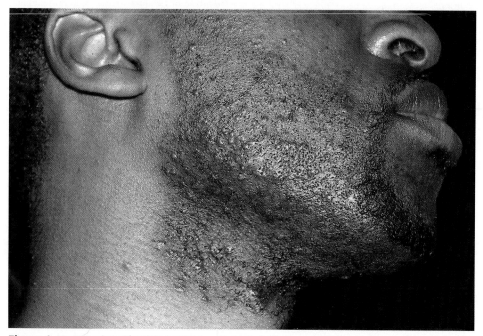

Figure 2-13 Pseudofolliculitis barbae *Multiple follicular papular scars in the beard area of a black male; the presence of follicular pustules usually is indicative of secondary* S. aureus *folliculitis.*

INFECTIOUS FOLLICULITIS

Infectious folliculitis is an infection of the upper portion of the hair follicle, characterized by a follicular papule, pustule, erosion, or crust at the follicular infundibulum; the involvement can extend deeper to the entire length of the follicle (sycosis).

Epidemiology and Etiology

Regions of the Pilosebaceous and Apocrine Apparatus

- *Infundibulum* Superior region extending down to the junction of the sebaceous duct with the follicle
- *Isthmus* Midregion between the sebaceous duct and the arrector pili muscle protuberance
- *Inferior region* Lower region below the arrector pili muscle protuberance

Classification of Infectious Folliculitis by Etiology

BACTERIAL

- *Staphylococcus aureus*
  Superficial (Bockhart's impetigo)
  Deep (sycosis); may progress to furuncle (boil) or carbuncle formation
- *Pseudomonas aeruginosa* ("hot tub") folliculitis
- Gram-negative folliculitis

FUNGAL
- Dermatophytic folliculitis: tinea capitis, tinea barbae, Majocchi's granuloma (see page 38)
- *Pityrosporum* folliculitis
- *Candida* folliculitis

VIRAL   Herpes simplex virus

SYPHILITIC   Secondary syphilis (acneform)

INFESTATION   Demodicidosis

Race *S. aureus* folliculitis on the legs of males: Indians, West Africans. Pseudofolliculitis and keloidal folliculitis in black men can be complicated by *S. aureus* infection.

Predisposing Factors Shaving hairy regions such as the beard area, axillae, or legs facilitates follicular infection; also extraction of hair such as plucking or waxing. Occlusion of hair-bearing areas facilitates growth of microbes: clothing, plastic film, adhesive plaster, position (sitting occludes buttocks, lying in bed occludes back), prosthesis, natural occlusion in intertriginous sites (axillae, inframammary, anogenital). Tropical climate with high temperatures and high relative humidity. Topical corticosteroid preparations. Systemic antibiotic promotes growth of gram-negative bacteria in areas of acne. Diabetes mellitus. Immunosuppression.

History

Duration of Lesions Days. *S. aureus* and dermatophytic folliculitis can be chronic.

Skin Symptoms Usually nontender or slightly tender; may be pruritic.

Constitutional Symptoms Uncommonly, tender regional lymphadenitis

Physical Examination

Skin Lesions

TYPE   Papule or pustule confined to the ostium of the hair follicle, at times surrounded by an erythematous halo. Rupture of pustule leads to superficial erosions or crusts. Superficial infection heals without scarring, but in darkly pigmented individuals, postinflammatory hypo- and hyperpigmentation. Ex-

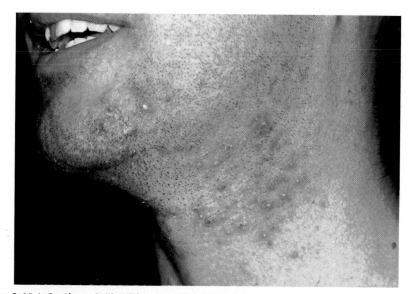

Figure 2-14 Infectious folliculitis, superficial: S. aureus *Numerous superficial erythematous papules and pustules in the ostia of hair follicles in the beard area. The condition was chronic, aggravated by shaving.*

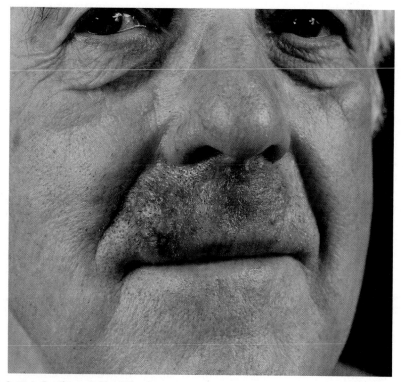

Figure 2-15 Infectious folliculitis, deep (sycosis): S. aureus *Confluent follicular pustules forming a tender, thick erythematous plaque on the upper lip. The differential diagnosis includes tinea barbae with kerion formation.*

tension of infection can progress to abscess or furuncle formation. In chronic folliculitis, a full range of lesions is noted. Pseudofolliculitis barbae caused by penetration of the skin by sharp tips of shaved hairs frequently is complicated by *S. aureus* secondary infection.

COLOR Erythema surrounding follicle. In darker skin types, postinflammatory hyperpigmentation.

ARRANGEMENT Scattered, discrete or, more frequently, grouped and clustered. Usually, only a small percentage of follicles in a region is infected.

DISTRIBUTION *Face* S. aureus. Gram-negative folliculitis resembles or may coexist with acne vulgaris.

Beard Area S. aureus folliculitis: folliculitis (sycosis) barbae most commonly of shaved beard area (Figure 2-15). Perifolliculitis barbae: especially in black men, perifolliculitis and follicular papules and pseudopustules (Figure 2-13). Dermatophytic folliculitis: tinea barbae; papulopustules may coalesce to deeply infiltrated kerion. *C. albicans.* Herpes simplex virus. Demodicidosis resembles rosacea.

Scalp S. aureus or dermatophytic

Neck S. aureus in shaved areas and nape of neck, occipital scalp (Figure 2-16). Pseudofolliculitis in shaved areas. Keloidal folliculitis in nape of neck (Figure 2-12); follicular keloids to large nodular, tumorous keloidal masses

Legs In Western nations, occurs in women who shave legs. In India, a chronic folliculitis occurs in young men, lasting for years. Pustular dermatitis atrophicans of the legs is reported commonly from West Africa, usually affecting the shins, sometimes the thighs and forearms.

Trunk S. aureus in axillae, especially in those who shave. *P. aeruginosa* ("hot tub") folliculitis (Figure 2-18). *Pityrosporum* folliculitis (Figure 2-17). *Candida* folliculitis on the back of hospitalized patients with fever who lie in a supine position. *S. aureus* folliculitis on trunk in diabetics.

Buttocks Common site for *S. aureus* folliculitis. Dermatophytic.

Variants

S. AUREUS FOLLICULITIS (Figures 2-14 to 2-16) Can be either superficial folliculitis (infundibular, follicular impetigo of Bockhart) or deep (sycosis, extension beneath infundibulum) with abscess formation (furuncle or boil and carbuncle). In the shaved beard area, also known as *sycosis vulgaris* or *barber's itch.* In severe cases (lupoid sycosis), the pilosebaceous units may be destroyed and replaced by fibrous scar tissue.

PITYROSPORUM FOLLICULITIS (Figure 2-17) (see page 39) More common in subtropical and tropical climates. Pruritic, monomorphic eruption characterized by follicular papules and pustules on the trunk, most often on the back and upper arms and less often on the neck and face; excoriated papules. Absence of comedones differentiates it from acne vulgaris.

P. AERUGINOSA FOLLICULITIS (Figure 2-18) Usually follows bathing in communal "hot tub".

GRAM-NEGATIVE FOLLICULITIS Occurs in individuals with acne vulgaris treated with oral antibiotics. "Acne" typically worsens, having been in good control. Characterized by small follicular pustules and/or larger abscesses on the cheeks and upper trunk.

DERMATOPHYTIC FOLLICULITIS Infection begins in the perifollicular stratum corneum and spreads into follicular ostia and hair shafts. Tinea capitis: "gray patch" (alopecia associated with scaling of the scalp), "black dot" (slight scaling and brittle hair breaking off at skin surface), and kerion (characterized by alopecia and an inflammatory boggy plaque); follicular involvement may not be apparent due to the more extensive involvement of the skin. Favus is characterized by suppurative and granulomatous folliculitis associated with scarring. In **Majocchi's or dermatophytic granuloma,** scattered papules and nodules, usually associated with tinea cruris or tinea corporis.

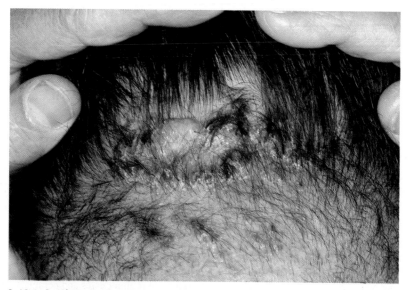

Figure 2-16 Infectious folliculitis: S. aureus *Follicular papules and pustules followed by keloidal scarring alopecia in a male with diabetes mellitus. The infection can extend more deeply with formation of furuncles or carbuncles.*

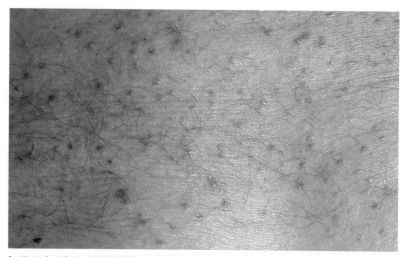

Figure 2-17 Infectious folliculitis: pityrosporum ovale *Multiple, discrete, follicular papulopustules on the lower back, mimicking acne vulgaris. Skin scrapings and biopsy showed yeast forms of P. ovale. The lesions resolved following treatment with oral itraconazole.*

C. ALBICANS FOLLICULITIS   Occurs in sites of occluded skin such as the back of a hospitalized febrile patient or under plastic dressing, especially if topical corticosteroid preparations are used. Large follicular pustules.

HERPETIC   FOLLICULITIS   Occurs predominantly in the beard area in men. Characterized by follicular vesicles and later crusts. (Figure 2-19)

MOLLUSCUM SYCOSIS   Presents as umbilicated skin-colored papules in a follicular and perifollicular distribution over the beard area.

SYPHILITIC FOLLICULITIS   Manifested by dull red papules; may be arranged in oval groups (corymbiform syphilis). Nonscarring alopecia of the scalp and beard.

DEMODICIDOSIS   Clinical presentation: perifollicular scaling (pityriasis folliculorum or rosacea-like erythematous follicular papules and pustules with a background of erythema on the face) (see Rosacea, p. 12).

Differential Diagnosis

Folliculitis ± Perifolliculitis   The differential diagnosis of follicular inflammatory disorders that may be confused with infectious folliculitis is extensive and includes the following: acneform disorders (acne vulgaris, rosacea, perioral dermatitis), HIV-associated eosinophilic folliculitis, chemical irritants (chloracne), adverse cutaneous drug reactions (halogens, corticosteroids, lithium), perforating folliculitis, follicular atopic dermatitis, keratosis pilaris, keratosis pilaris atrophicans, lichen planopilaris, pityriasis rubra pilaris, vitamin A deficiency, vitamin C deficiency, chronic cutaneous lupus erythematosus, keloidal folliculitis, pseudofolliculitis barbae.

Regional differential diagnosis of folliculitis ± perifolliculitis includes: *Face:* tinea barbae, acne, rosacea, perioral dermatitis, keratosis pilaris, pseudofolliculitis barbae (ingrowing hairs), miliaria. *Scalp:* acne necrotica. *Trunk:* acne vulgaris, pustular miliaria, transient acantholytic disease (Grover's disease), scurvy. *Extremities:* keratosis pilaris, scurvy. *Axillae and groins:* hidradenitis suppurativa.

Laboratory Findings

Gram's Stain   *S. aureus:* gram-positive cocci in grapelike clusters within polymorphonuclear leukocytes and extracellular organisms. Also visualizes fungi.

KOH Preparation   Dermatophytes: hyphae. *P. ovale:* multiple yeast forms of *Pityrosporum.* *Candida:* mycelial forms.

Culture   *Bacterial: S. aureus, P. aeruginosa;* gram-negative folliculitis: *Proteus, Klebsiella, Escherichia coli.* In cases of chronic relapsing folliculitis, culture nares and perianal region for *S. aureus* carriage. *Fungal:* dermatophytes, *C. albicans. Viral:* herpes simplex virus.

Dermatopathology   In the evaluation of a biopsy specimen of a follicular lesion, infectious folliculitis must be differentiated from noninfectious inflammatory follicular and perifollicular disorders. The following features should be evaluated: Are microorganisms present? Is the inflammatory infiltrate predominantly follicular or perifollicular? What region of the pilosebaceous structure is involved? Is the inflammatory process acute suppurative (neutrophilic), chronic lymphocytic, or granulomatous (foreign-body response to keratin subsequent to rupture of follicle)? Is any portion of the pilosebaceous structure destroyed?

Diagnosis

Clinical findings confirmed by laboratory findings

Course and Prognosis

S. aureus folliculitis can progress to deeper follicular and perifollicular infection with furuncle (abscess) formation. Infection of multiple

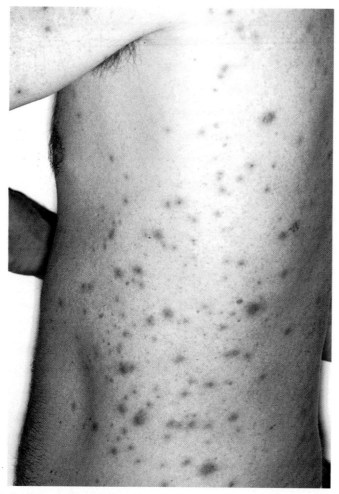

Figure 2-18 Infectious folliculitis: P. aeruginosa or "hot tub" *Multiple follicular pustules are present on the trunk appearing 3 days after bathing in a hot tub.* P. aeruginosa *was isolated on culture from a lesion. The lesions resolved spontaneously within a week.*

contiguous follicles results in a carbuncle. Many types of infectious folliculitis tend to recur or become chronic unless the predisposing conditions are corrected.

Management

Prophylaxis *Correct underlying predisposing condition.* Washing with antibacterial soap or benzoyl peroxide preparation.

Treatment

BACTERIAL FOLLICULITIS **S. aureus *Folliculitis*** Topical therapy: mupirocin ointment, applied b.i.d. to the involved skin as well as the nares, a common site of *S. aureus* carriage. Systemic therapy: dicloxacillin or cephalexin (adult dose, 1 to 2 g/day in 4 divided doses for 10 days). Alternatively and if *S. aureus* is sensitive, erythromycin (adult dose, 1 to 2 g/day in 4 divided doses for 10 days). For methicillin-resistant *S. aureus* (MRSA), minocycline, 100 mg b.i.d.

P. aeruginosa *Folliculitis* In most cases, "hot tub" folliculitis resolves spontaneously. In symptomatic cases, ciprofloxacin, 500 mg b.i.d.

Gram-Negative Folliculitis Associated with systemic antibiotic therapy of acne vulgaris. Discontinue current antibiotics. Wash with benzoyl peroxide. In some cases, ampicillin (250 mg q.i.d.) or sulfamethoxazole-trimethoprim (SMX-TMP) q.i.d. Isotretinoin.

FUNGAL FOLLICULITIS A variety of topical antifungal agents. Itraconazole 100 mg b.i.d. for 10 to 14 days for *Pityrosporum* or *Candida*. Terbinafine, 200 mg/day for dermatophytic infection. For *Candida* folliculitis, fluconazole 100 mg b.i.d. for 10 to 14 days.

HERPETIC FOLLICULITIS Acyclovir 400 mg t.i.d. for 7 days or one of the newer antiviral agents (see also therapy of herpes simplex)

DEMODICIDOSIS Permethrin cream

PSEUDOFOLLICULITIS BARBAE Treatment is unsatisfactory. The disorder will disappear if the patient grows a beard. Tretinoin solution (8 %) and benzoyl peroxide incorporated in shaving cream (Benzashave) have been recommended.

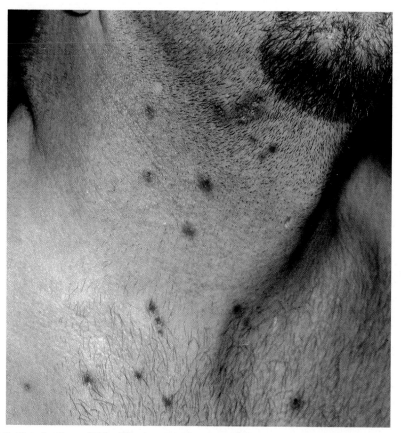

Figure 2-19 Infectious folliculitis: herpes simplex virus   *Discrete and grouped erosions in the beard area and chest in a male with advanced HIV disease. HSV was isolated on culture; lesional biopsy specimen showed multinucleated giant cells within the follicular epithelium.*

HIRSUTISM AND HYPERTRICHOSIS*

Hirsutism is excessive hair growth in androgen-dependent hair patterns (i.e., face, chest, areolae, linea alba, lower back, buttocks, inner thighs, and external genitalia) secondary to increased androgenic activity. Hypertrichosis is excessive hair growth also in areas that are not androgen-sensitive.

HIRSUTISM

Excessive hair growth secondary to increased androgenic activity.

Pathophysiology

- Androgens promote conversion of vellus hairs to terminal hairs in androgen-sensitive hair follicles (pubis, axillae, back, face, chest, abdomen).
- 5-α-Dihydrotestosterone, derived from conversion of testosterone by 5-α-reductase at the hair follicle, is the hormonal stimulus for hair growth.
- 50 % to 70 % of circulating testosterone in normal women is derived from precursors, androstenedione, and DHEA; the rest is secreted directly, mostly by the ovaries. In hyperandrogenic women, a greater percentage of androgens may be secreted directly.
- In women, adrenal glands secrete androstenedione, DHEA, DHEA sulfate, and testosterone; ovaries secrete mainly androstenedione and testosterone

Etiology

Adrenal Causes

ACTH-dependent Cushing's syndrome
Cushing's disease
Ectopic ACTH production
Androgen-producing adrenal tumors†
Congenital adrenal hyperplasia (CAH)
Classic†
Late-onset

Ovarian Causes

Ovarian hyperthecosis†
Ovarian neoplasms† (only 1 % of all ovarian tumors cause virilization)

Polycystic ovarian (PCO) syndrome
Acne, alopecia, acanthosis nigricans, obesity, menorrhagia, oligomenorrhea, amenorrhea, infertility
Elevated LH levels, increased LH/FSH ratio
Insulin resistance/obesity (triggers excess ovarian androgen production)

Exogenous Medications

Androgens
Anabolic steroids
Birth control pills (uncommon with current low-dose oral contraceptives)

Hyperprolactinemia/Prolactinoma (Galactorrhea, Amenorrhea)

GONADAL DYSGENESIS

Idiopathic

Epidemiology

- Familial, ethnic, and racial influences
- Hirsuteness: white > black > Asian
- College survey of women showed that 25 % had easily noticeable facial hair, 33 % had hair along the linea alba below the umbilicus, and 17 % had periareolar hair.
- Series of 100 patients: 15 % idiopathic, 3 % late-onset CAH (varies within ethnic group)

History

- Virilization symptoms: androgenic alopecia, acne, deepened voice, increased muscle mass, clitoromegaly, increased libido, personality change

---

*Angela Wong and Ann E. Taylor, M.D. were responsibile for the major portion of this précis.
†Associated virilization.

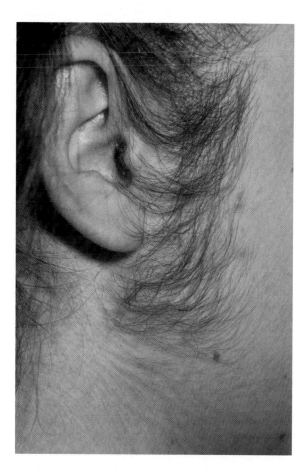

Figure 2-20 Hirsuitism *Increased hair grow in androgen-dependent hair follicles of the beard area in a female, associated with androgen excess.*

- Amenorrhea or changes in menstruation
- New-onset hypertension
- Family history
- Drug history
- Relatively recent or rapid onset of symptoms and signs *not* associated with puberty

Physical Examination

Careful documentation of the amount and all sites of hair is important in order to evaluate progression and therapy.

- Skin and hair changes: androgenic alopecia, acne, acanthosis nigricans, striae
- New growth of terminal hair (Figure 2-20), especially on chest (Figure 2-21), abdomen, upper back, shoulders
- Suspect Cushing's syndrome if centripetal obesity, muscle wasting (especially peripheral muscle weakness), and violaceous striae are found.
- If suspicious for PCO syndrome, perform pelvic examination.
- Ferriman-Gallwey scale rates hair growth in each of 11 androgen-sensitive areas (upper lip, chin, chest, upper back, lower back, upper abdomen, lower abdomen, arm, forearm, thigh, leg) from 0 (no hair growth) to 4. Score of 8 or more is considered hirsutism.

Laboratory Evaluation

Urinary 17-ketosteroid measurement helpful in evaluating the overall amount of androgen secretion. (The results should be checked against age-appropriate normal levels; peak levels occur at age 30, and there is a significant decline with age thereafter.)

- If menstrual dysfunction (oligomenorrhea or amenorrhea): minimal evaluation: prolactin, FSH, and total testosterone
- If (+) virilization:

    Serum testosterone: 200 ng/dl in women with ovarian or adrenal tumor
    Urinary 17-ketosteroids: elevated adrenal androgens
    Serum DHEA sulfate: most specific to adrenals (>90 % arising in adrenals); if >800 μg/day, suggestive of adrenal tumor

- If CAH (late onset) is suspected: refer patient to endocrinologist
- If Cushing's syndrome is suspected: refer patient to endocrinologist
- If tumor suspicion is high: refer patient to endocrinologist

---

Management

Cosmetic Shaving, waxing, electrolysis, hydrogen peroxide bleaching

Systemic Antiandrogen Therapy *Cyproterone Acetate (CPA)* Potent progestogen (not available in the United States)

Both antiandrogen and inhibitor of secretion of gonadotropin. Decreases androgen production. Increases testosterone clearance. Decreases 5-alpha-reductase activity. Administered with cyclical estrogens to maintain regular menstruation.
Regimen: 50 to 100 mg CPA for 10 days per cycle
Side effects: weight gain, fatigue, loss of libido, mastodynia, nausea, H/A, depression
Contraindications: smoking, obesity, hypertension

SPIRONOLACTONE An antihypertensive diuretic Decreases testosterone biosynthesis. Binds to androgen receptor. Decreases 5-alpha-reductase activity
Regimen: begin at 50 mg b.i.d. given from day 4 through day 22 of each menstrual cycle; can be given as high as 100 mg b.i.d.

CIMETIDINE Histamine-2 receptor antagonist; competes for target tissue binding with androgens; less effective than spironolactone

CORTICOSTEROID First-line therapy for classic CAH. *Regimen:* 1 mg dexamethasone q.h.s. For late-onset, nonclassic CAH, use antiandrogens or oral contraceptives.

ORAL CONTRACEPTIVES Suppress ovarian and adrenal androgen production by decreasing LH and FSH.

Recommend an oral contraceptive with the lowest tolerable dose of ethinyl estradiol (30 to 35 μg) and a low dose of a progestin with low androgenic potential (less than 1 mg of norethindrone, norgestimate, desogestrel, ethynodiol diacetate).

Avoid levonorgestrel, norgestrel, and high doses of norethindrone acetate.

HYPERTRICHOSIS

Hypertrichosis Lanuginosa

Congenital Hypertrichosis Lanuginosa Vellus and terminal hairs do not replace white, blond fetal pelage; fetal pelage grows excessively and may be >10 cm long.

Acquired Hypertrichosis Lanuginosa Production of lanugo hair in follicles previously producing vellus hair.

EPIDEMIOLOGY Usually harbinger of malignancy; of all cases of acquired hypertrichosis lanuginosa reported, 98 % had malignancy of the gastrointestinal tract, bronchus, breast, gallbladder, uterus, or bladder. Hypertrichosis can precede a neoplastic diagnosis by several years.

PHYSICAL EXAMINATION

- Hair may be >10 cm in length in nonscalp areas.

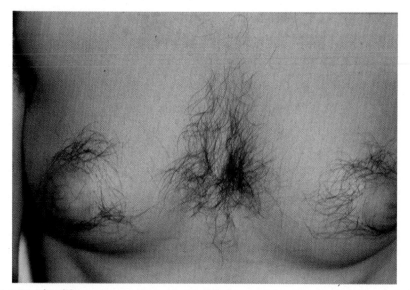

Figure 2-21 Hirsuitism *Increased constitutional hair growth in androgen-dependent hair follicles of the presternal and periareolar regions in a female. In this case, no androgen excess was detected, the finding occurring in other female relatives.*

- Can involve entire body, except for palms and soles.
- Fine, downy hair covers large areas of the body.
- In mild types, downy hair is limited to the face; hair on previously hairless areas such as the nose and eyelids is usually noticed first.
- Scalp, beard, and pubic hair may not be replaced.

Drug-Induced Hypertrichosis

History/Physical Examination Uniform growth of fine hair in a pattern unrelated to androgen sensitivity

Drugs

Diphenylhydantoin: after 2 to 3 months of treatment, affects extensor regions of limbs, face, trunk; clears by 1 year of drug cessation

Diazoxide: cosmetic problem in 50 %

Minoxidil

Cyclosporine: affects over 80 %

Benoxaprofen: after a few weeks of treatment, fine downy hair on face and exposed extremities

Streptomycin

Oral corticosteroids: forehead, temples, cheeks; sometimes back and extensor aspects of limbs

Penicillamine: lengthening and coarsening of hair on trunk and limbs

Psoralens: transient hypertrichosis of light-exposed areas

Other Conditions Associated with Hypertrichosis

Porphyria (variegate, cutanea tarda, congenital erythropoietic porphyria)

Epidermolysis bullosa

Hurler's syndrome and other mucopolysaccharidoses

Cornelia de Lange syndrome

Trisomy 18

Post-shock/head injuries

Fetal alcohol syndrome

Dermatomyositis

Malnutrition

Anorexia nervosa

At sites of trauma/scar/occupation-related sites of irritation

Section 3

ECZEMATOUS DERMATITIS

CONTACT DERMATITIS

*Contact dermatitis** is a generic term applied to acute or chronic inflammatory reactions to substances that come in contact with the skin. Contact dermatitis (nonallergic) is caused by a chemical irritant and contact (allergic) eczematous dermatitis by an antigen (allergen) that elicits a type IV (cell-mediated or delayed) hypersensitivity reaction.

Epidemiology

Age No influence on capacity for sensitization; however, allergic contact dermatitis is uncommon in young children.

Race Black skin is possibly less susceptible.

Occupation This is *the* important cause of disability in industry.

Etiology and Pathophysiology

Contact (nonallergic) dermatitis (Figure 3-1) may occur in normal skin or cause an exacerbation of preexisting dermatitis as a result of exposure to, for example, croton oil, kerosene,

Contact urticaria is a wheal and flare skin reaction that occurs following contact with antigens (immunologic) *or* as a reaction to urticariogenic agents that cause a nonallergic (nonimmunologic) urticaria. *Contact nonimmunologic urticaria,* which occurs on normal skin, can be caused, for example, by cinnamic acid, sorbic acid, benzoic acid, insect stings, and moths. *Contact immunologic urticaria* occurs on damaged (e.g., preexisting eczematous) skin and is caused by *topical antibiotics* (bacitracin, neomycin, gentamycin), *miscellaneous topical medications* (benzocaine, lindane, menthol, vitamin E oil), *vehicle ingredients* (polyethylene glycol, polysorbate 60, monomyalimine), *metals* (nickel, platinum), and many and various chemicals but also animal keratin (e.g., guinea pig hairs).

or detergents. *Contact (allergic) dermatitis,* more commonly called *contact eczematous dermatitis,* is a classic, delayed, cell-mediated hypersensitivity reaction. Exposure to a strong sensitizer such as poison ivy resin results in a sensitization in a week or so, while exposure to a weak allergen may take months to years for sensitization. The antigen is taken up by a specialized dendritic cell in the epidermis, the Langerhans cell, which processes the antigen, migrates from the epidermis to the draining lymph nodes where it presents the processed antigen in association with MHC class II molecules to T cells which then proliferate. Sensitized T cells then leave the lymph node and enter the blood circulation. Thus all the skin becomes hypersensitive to the contact allergen. The specially sensitized T-effector lymphocytes produce or mediate the release by other cells of a variety of cytokines after being presented with the same specific antigen.

History

Duration of Lesion(s) Acute contact—days, weeks; chronic contact—months, years

Skin Symptoms Pruritus

Constitutional Symptoms "Acute illness" syndrome (see page xxiv) (including fever) in severe allergic contact dermatitis (e.g., poison ivy)

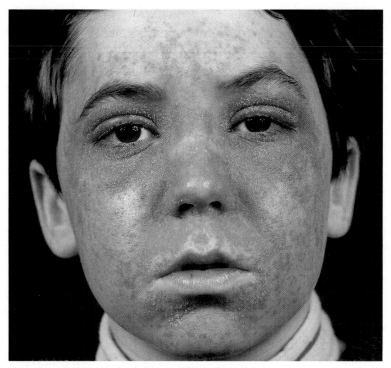

Figure 3-1 Acute allergic contact dermatitis: poison ivy *Acute eczematous dermatitis with erythematous papules and vesicles, which have become confluent, crusting, and facial edema, 5 days after exposure to poison ivy.*

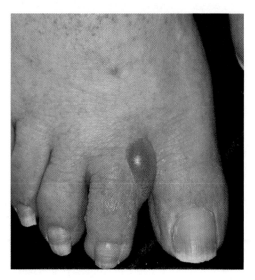

Figure 3-2 Acute allergic contact dermatitis: paraben *An acute eczematous dermatitis with erythema, vesicles, and a large bulla on the dorsum of the foot and toe-webs, recurred following the use of a paraben-containing foot cream.*

Physical Examination

Skin Lesions

TYPE *Acute* Well-demarcated plaques of erythema and edema on which are superimposed closely spaced, nonumbilicated vesicles (Figures 3-2 to 3-4), punctate erosions exuding serum, and crusts

Subacute Plaques of mild erythema showing small, dry scales or superficial desquamation, sometimes associated with small, red, pointed or rounded, firm papules (Figure 3-3)

Chronic Plaques of lichenification (thickening of the epidermis with deepening of the skin lines in parallel or rhomboidal pattern), with satellite, small, firm, rounded or flat-topped papules, excoriations, and pigmentation or mild erythema (Figure 3-4)

ARRANGEMENT Often linear, with artificial patterns, an "outside job". Plant contact often results in linear lesions.

DISTRIBUTION *Extent* Isolated, localized to one region (e.g., shoe dermatitis), or generalized (e.g., plant dermatitis)

Pattern Random or on exposed areas (as in airborne allergic contact dermatitis)

Laboratory and Special Examinations

Dermatopathology

SITE Epidermis and dermis

PROCESS Inflammation with intraepidermal intercellular edema (spongiosis) and monocyte and histiocyte infiltration in the dermis suggests allergic contact dermatitis, while more superficial vesicles containing polymorphonuclear leukocytes suggest a primary irritant dermatitis. In chronic contact dermatitis there is lichenification (hyperkeratosis, acanthosis, elongation of rete ridges, and elongation and broadening of papillae).

Patch Tests Sensitization is present on every part of the skin; therefore, application of the allergen to any area of normal skin will provoke inflammation. A positive patch test shows erythema *and* papules, as well as possibly vesicles confined to the test site. Patch tests should be delayed until the dermatitis has subsided at the selected site of application for at least 2 weeks. See Appendix B.

Course

Evolution of Contact Dermatitis Reaction

TOXIC IRRITANT CONTACT DERMATITIS *Acute* Erythema with a dull, nonglistening surface → vesiculation (or blister formation) → erosion → crusting–shedding of crusts and scaling

Chronic Inflammatory thickening of skin → scaling → fissures → crusting. Toxic irritant dermatitis heals spontaneously if exposures are not repeated, chronic toxic irritant contact dermatitis evolves when the noxious agent continues to come into contact with the skin. Chronic inflammation with thickening, fissuring, scaling, and crusting results. A previously sharp margination gives way to an ill-defined border, lichenification.

ALLERGIC CONTACT DERMATITIS *Acute* Erythema → papules → vesicles → erosions → crusts → scaling

Chronic Papules → scaling → lichenification → excoriations

NOTE: Contact dermatitis is always confined to the site of exposure to the allergen. Margination is originally sharp in allergic contact dermatitis; however, it spreads in the periphery beyond the actual site of exposure. If strong sensitization has occurred, spreading to other parts of the body and generalization occur. The main differences between toxic irritant and allergic contact dermatitis are summarized in Table 3-A.

NOTE: In the acute forms of contact dermatitis papules occur only in the allergic form.

GENERAL NOTES IN CONTACT DERMATITIS The acute form, which in severe cases may even lead to necrosis, occurs after a single exposure to the offending agent that is toxic to the

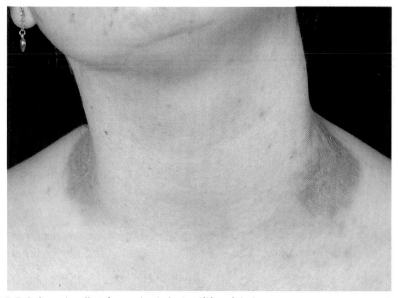

Figure 3-3 Subacute allergic contact dermatitis: nickel *Red/tan plaques consisting of tiny confluent papules with indistinct borders on the lateral base of the neck recurred whenever a necklace containing nickel was worn. The reaction also commonly occurs when nickel-containing jewelry is worn on the earlobes, wrists, and/or fingers of nickel-sensitized individuals.*

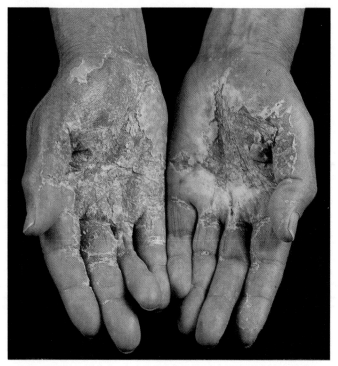

Figure 3-4 Chronic allergic contact dermatitis: chromate salts in cement *Papulosquamous dermatosis with hyperkeratosis, maceration, fissuring, and erosion on the hands of a concrete worker.*

skin (e.g., croton oil, phenols, kerosene, organic solvents, sodium and potassium hydroxide, lime acids). It is thus dependent on concentration of the offending agent and occurs in everyone, depending, of course, on the permeability and thickness of the stratum corneum. There is a threshold concentration for these substances above which they cause acute dermatitis and below which they do not. This sets it apart from acute allergic contact dermatitis which is dependent on sensitization and thus occurs only in sensitized individuals. Depending on the degree of sensitization, minute amounts of the offending agents may elicit a reaction but this of course is also dependent on the degree of sensitiv-

TABLE 3-A **DIFFERENCES BETWEEN TOXIC (IRRITANT) AND ALLERGIC CONTACT DERMATITIS**

		Toxic/Irritant CD	Allergic CD
Lesions	Acute	Erythema → vesicle → erosion → crust → scaling	Erythema → papules → vesicles → erosions → crusts → scaling
	Chronic	Papules, plaques, fissures, scaling, crusts	Papules, plaques, scaling, crusts
Margination and Site	Acute	Sharp, strictly confined to site of exposure	Sharp, confined to site of exposure but spreading in the periphery, usually tiny papules, may become generalized
	Chronic	Ill-defined	Ill-defined, spreads
Evolution	Acute	Rapid (few hours after exposure)	Not so rapid (12 to 74 hours after exposure)
	Chronic	Months to years of repeated exposure	Months or longer; exacerbation after every reexposure
Causative Agent		Dependent on concentration of agent; occurs only above threshold level	Relatively independent of amount applied; usually very low concentrations sufficient but depends on degree of sensitization
Incidence		May occur in practically everyone	Occurs only in the sensitized

ity. Since toxic irritant contact dermatitis is a toxic phenomenon it is confined to the area of exposure, and it is therefore always sharply marginated and never spreads. Allergic contact dermatitis is an immunologic reaction that tends to involve the surrounding skin (spreading phenomenon) and may even spread beyond affected sites. Generalization occurs.

CHRONIC TOXIC CONTACT DERMATITIS OF THE HANDS   This results from repeated exposures to toxic or subtoxic concentrations of offending agents and is usually associated with a chronic disturbance of the barrier function which allows even subtoxic concentrations of offending agents to penetrate into the skin and elicit a chronic inflammatory response. It is thus often the result of repeated exposure to alkaline detergents and organic solvents which in normal skin, if applied only once, do not elicit a reaction. Injury, (e.g., repeated rubbing of the skin), prolonged soaking in water, or chronic contact with corrosive agents fosters the evolution of chronic toxic contact dermatitis. A typical example is the hand eczema seen in bricklayers, me-

chanics, and painters. In these persons, hand eczema is usually a combination of chronic toxic contact dermatitis (alkaline medium of cement, sand, rubbing) and allergic contact dermatitis due to chromates that are present in cement.

Management

Acute

Identify and remove the etiologic agent.
Larger vesicles may be drained, but tops should *not* be removed.
Wet dressings using gauze soaked in Burow's solution changed every 2 to 3 hours
Topical class I corticosteroid preparations
In severe cases, systemic corticosteroids may be indicated.
Prednisone: two-week course, 70 mg initially, tapering by 5 mg daily

Subacute and Chronic   If the lesions are not bullous, it is possible to use a short course of one of the potent topical corticosteroid preparations, betamethasone dipropionate or clobetasol propionate.

TABLE 3-B   COMMON CONTACT ALLERGENS

Neomycin	Usually contained in creams, ointments
Procaine, benzocaine	Local anesthetics
Sulfonamides	
Terpentine	Solvents, shoe polish, printer's ink
Balsam of Peru	Topical
Thiuram	Rubber
Formalin	Disinfectant, curing agents, plastics
Mercury	Disinfectant, impregnation
Chromates	Cement, antioxidants, industrial oils, matches
Nickel sulfate	Metals, metals in clothing, jewelry, catalyzing agents
Cobalt sulfate	Cement, galvanization, industrial oils, cooling agents, eye shades
p-Phenylene diamine	Black or dark dyes of textiles, printer's ink
Parahydroxybenzoic acid ester	Conserving agent in foodstuffs

ATOPIC DERMATITIS

Atopic dermatitis (AD) is an acute, subacute, but usually chronic pruritic inflammation of the epidermis and dermis, often occurring in association with a personal or family history of hay fever, asthma, allergic rhinitis, or atopic dermatitis. *Definition of atopy:* literally, "no (without) place." A heritable clinical state associated with dermatitis, asthma, and allergic rhinitis.
Synonyms: "Eczema," atopic eczema, IgE dermatitis.

Epidemiology and Etiology

Age   Onset in first 2 months of life and by first year in 60 % of patients

Sex   Slightly more common in males than in females

Hereditary Predisposition   Over two-thirds of patients have a personal or family history of allergic rhinitis, hay fever, or asthma.

History

Onset   Most patients become afflicted between infancy and age 12, with 60 % by first year; 30 % are seen for the first time by age 5, and only 10 % develop AD between 6 and 20 years of age. Rarely atopic dermatitis has an adult onset.

Duration of Lesions   Untreated involved sites persist for months or years.

Skin Symptoms   Patients have dry skin. Pruritus is the *sine qua non* of atopic dermatitis— "Eczema is the itch that rashes." The constant scratching leads to a vicious cycle of itch → scratch → rash → itch (the rash being lichenification of the skin).

Other Symptoms of Atopy   Allergic rhinitis, characterized by sneezing, rhinorrhea, obstruction of nasal passages, conjunctival and pharyngeal itching, and lacrimation; may be seasonal when associated with lacrimation allergens such as pollen.

Exacerbating Factors   Allergies: contact allergens, food, inhalants (history or skin tests). Skin dehydration by frequent bathing and hand washing. Emotional stress. Hormonal: pregnancy, menstruation, thyroid. Infections: *Staphylococcus aureus,* group A streptococcus, fungus (dermatophytosis, candidiasis), herpes simplex virus. Season: in temperate climates, usually improves in summer, flares in winter. Clothing: pruritus flares *after* taking off clothing; wool clothing or blankets directly in contact with skin.

Skin Lesions

Acute   Poorly defined erythematous patches, papules, and plaques with or without scale. Edema with widespread involvement; skin appears "puffy" and edematous. Erosions: moist, crusted. Excoriations: occur as a result of scratching. Secondarily infected sites: *S. aureus.* Pustules (usually follicular). Crusts.

Chronic   Lichenification (thickening of the skin with accentuation of skin markings) that results from repeated rubbing or scratching; follicular lichenification (especially in brown and black persons). Fissures: painful, especially on palms, fingers, and soles. Alopecia: lateral one-third of the eyebrows as a result of rubbing the eyelids. Periorbital pigmentation: also as a result of compulsively rubbing the eyelids. Characteristic infraorbital fold in the eyelids (Dennie-Morgan sign).

Special Features Related to Ethnicity In blacks, so-called follicular eczema is common and is characterized by discrete follicular papules involving all hair follicles of the involved site.

Distribution of Lesions Predilection for the flexures, front and sides of the neck, eyelids, forehead, face, wrists, and dorsa of the feet and hands. Generalized in severe disease.

Associated Findings

Bilateral cataracts occur in up to 10 % in the more severe cases; the peak incidence is between 15 and 25 years of age.

"White" dermographism on stroking is a special and unique feature of involved skin; delayed blanch to cholinergic agents.

Ichthyosis vulgaris and keratosis pilaris occur in 10 % of patients.

Differential Diagnosis

Common Disorders Seborrheic dermatitis, contact dermatitis (allergic and irritant), psoriasis, nummular eczema, dermatophytosis, early stages mycosis fungoides

Rare Disorders Mimicking AD Acrodermatitis enteropathica, gluten-sensitive enteropathy, glucagonoma syndrome, histidinemia, phenylketonuria; also, some immunologic disorders including Wiskott-Aldrich syndrome, X-linked agammaglobulinemia, hyper-IgE syndrome, Letterer-Siwe disease, and selective IgA deficiency

Laboratory and Special Examinations

Bacterial Culture Colonization with *S. aureus* is very common in the nares and in the involved skin; almost 90 % of patients with severe AD are secondarily colonized/infected.

Viral Culture Rule out HSV infection in crusted lesions (eczema herpeticum).

Radioallergosorbent Testing (RAST) 90 % clinically relevant if negative, but only 20 % clinically relevant if positive

Dermatopathology

SITE   Epidermis and dermis

PROCESS   Varying degrees of acanthosis with rare intraepidermal intercellular edema (spongiosis). The dermal infiltrate is composed of lymphocytes, monocytes, and mast cells with few or no eosinophils.

Blood Studies Increased IgE in serum

Diagnosis

History in infancy, clinical findings (typical distribution sites, morphology of lesions, white dermographism)

Pathophysiology

Type I (IgE-mediated) hypersensitivity reaction occurring as a result of the release of vasoactive substances from both mast cells and basophils that have been sensitized by the interaction of the antigen with IgE (reaginic or skin-sensitizing antibody); however, the role of IgE in AD is still not fully clarified, but it has been shown that epidermal Langerhans cells possess high affinity IgE receptors through which an eczema-like reaction could be mediated.

Course and Prognosis

Spontaneous, more or less complete remission during childhood is the rule with occasional, more severe recurrences during adolescence. In most patients, the disease persists for 15 to 20 years. From 30 % to 50 % of patients develop asthma and/or hay fever. Adult-onset atopic dermatitis often runs a severe course.

Complications

Overriding *s. aureus* infection leads to extensive erosions and crusting, and herpes simplex infection to eczema herpeticum which may be life-threatening

Management

Education of the patient to avoid rubbing and scratching is most important. Topical preparations are valuable but are useless if the patient continues to scratch and rub the plaques.

An allergic workup is rarely helpful in uncovering an allergen; however, in patients who are hypersensitive to house dust, mites, various pollens, and animal hair proteins, exposure to the appropriate allergen may cause flares. Atopic dermatitis is considered by many to be related, at least in part, to emotional stress. Education of the patient to avoid rubbing and scratching is most important. Topical antipruritic (menthol/camphor) lotions are helpful in controlling the pruritus.

Warn patients of their special problems with herpes simplex and the frequency of superimposed staphylococcal infection, for which oral antibiotics are indicated. Acyclovir is indicated if HSV infection is suspected.

Acute

1. Wet dressings and topical corticosteroids; topical antibiotics (mupirocin ointment) when indicated
2. Oral H_1 antihistamines for pruritus
3. Oral antibiotics (cloxacillin, erythromycin) to eliminate staphylococci.

Subacute and Chronic

1. Oral H_1 antihistamines are useful in reducing itching.
2. Topical ointments containing H_1 and H_2 blockers (doxepin) are only rarely useful for pruritus.

3. Hydration (oilated baths or baths with oatmeal powder) followed by application of unscented emollients (e.g., hydrated petrolatum) is a basic daily treatment needed to prevent xerosis. Soap showers are permissible in order to wash the body folds, but soap seldom should be used on the other parts of the skin surface. 12 % ammonium lactate or 10 % alpha hydroxy acid lotion is very effective for the xerosis often seen in AD.

4. Topical anti-inflammatory agents such as corticosteroids, hydroxyquinoline preparations, and tar are the mainstays of treatment. Of these, corticosteroids are the most readily accepted by the patient.

5. Systemic corticosteroids should be avoided, except in rare instances for only short courses. For severe intractable disease, prednisone 70 mg tapered by 5 mg/day. Corticosteroids should be given with meals and in divided doses. AD patients tend to become dependent on oral corticosteroids. Often small doses (5 to 10 mg) will make the difference in control and can be reduced gradually, to even 2.5 mg daily.

6. Cyclic administration (e.g., every 2 or 3 weeks) for 5 to 6 days of erythromycin or other antibiotic to combat staphylococcal colonization.

7. Patients should learn and use stress management techniques.

8. UVA-UVB phototherapy and PUVA photochemotherapy are effective.

9. In severe cases of adult-onset AD, cyclosporin A (cyclosporine) treatment (starting dose 4 mg/kg/per day) is indicated when all other treatments fail but should be monitored closely.

INFANTILE ATOPIC DERMATITIS

Infantile atopic dermatitis is one of the most troublesome skin eruptions in children. There is an "atopic" background without a clearly defined immunologic pattern. Skin lesions seem to be a reaction to itching and rubbing. Since the advent of topical corticosteroids, the problem has lost much of its seriousness.

Physical Examination

Skin Lesions

TYPE   Red skin, tiny vesicles on "puffy" surface, scaling, exudation with wet crusts, and cracks (fissures) (Figures 3-5 and 3-6)

DISTRIBUTION   Regional, especially the face (sparing the mouth), the antecubital and popliteal fossae, wrists, and lateral aspects of the legs

Management

Influence of dietary measures is at best uncertain. Prompt response to potent corticosteroids; after improvement, use low-potency corticosteroids or emollients. For recurrence, return for a short period to the stronger corticosteroids. Beware of skin atrophy. With sensible use, no danger of suppression of pituitary-adrenal axis. For extra security, monitor growth curve. Tar baths, ointments, pastes, and gels are also effective. Reassurance of mother. (See Treatment, page 56.)

CHILDHOOD-TYPE ATOPIC DERMATITIS

Physical Examination

Skin Lesions

TYPE   Papular, lichenified plaques, erosions, crusts (Figures 3-7 and 3-8)

DISTRIBUTION   Especially on the antecubital and popliteal fossae.

Management
See above.

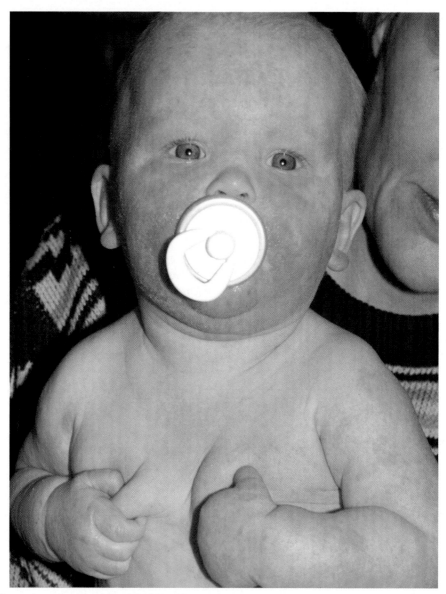

Figure 3-5 Atopic dermatitis: infantile *Confluent erythema, papules, microvesiculation, scaling, and crusting on the face, with similar involvement (to a lesser degree) on the trunk and arms. The facial involvement is more severe due to easier access to scratching; the baby is squeezing the breast skin to relieve the intense pruritus.*

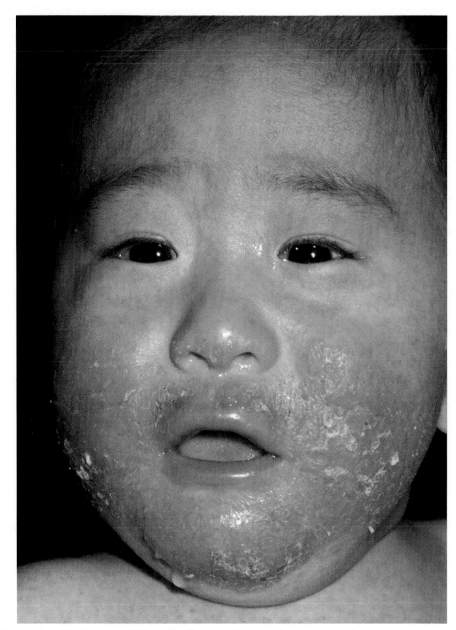

Figure 3-6 Atopic dermatitis: infantile *Confluent erythema, microvesiculation, papules, crust, and scale of a young Asian infant; the shoulders are relatively spared, being protected from scratching by clothing.*

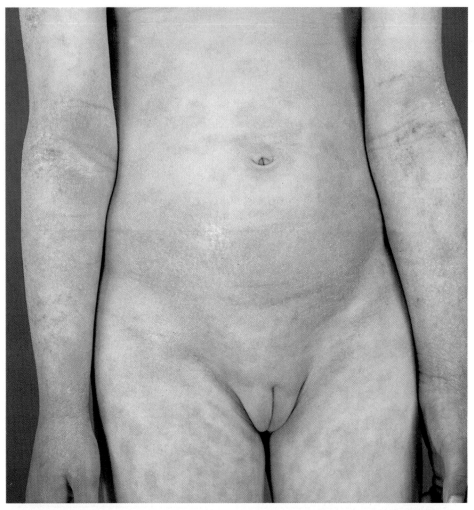

Figure 3-7 Atopic dermatitis: childhood-type *Ill-defined erythema, papules, excoriations, lichenification (thickening of the skin with accentuation of the skin lines) in the antecubital fossae, with less severe changes on the trunk and thighs.*

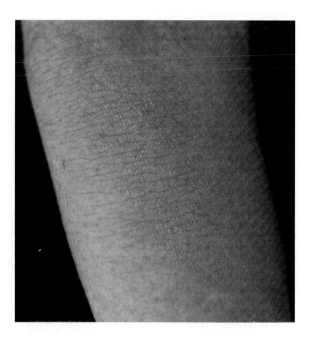

Figure 3-8 Atopic dermatitis
Confluent erythema and lichenification in the antecubital fossa occurs in juveniles, as well as adults, subsequent to rubbing the skin rather than excoriating.

ADULT-TYPE ATOPIC DERMATITIS

Adult-type dermatitis is a chronic recurrent disease in patients who have or have not had infantile or childhood atopic dermatitis or asthma. Exacerbations are often related to mental stress.

Physical Examination

Skin Lesions

TYPE *Acute* Poorly defined erythematous plaques, with or without scale (Figure 3-9). Excoriations occur as a consequence of scratching and rubbing. Secondarily infected sites: pustules (usually follicular), crusts.
Chronic Lichenification (Figure 3-10), a thickening of the skin with accentuation of skin markings, which results from repeated rubbing or scratching: diffusely lichenified areas; nodular lichenification (may be confused with prurigo nodularis)

Chronic Recurrent Papular and lichenified plaques, excoriations, pustules, erosions, dry and wet crusts, and cracks (fissures)

DISTRIBUTION Often generalized, with predilection for the flexures, front and sides of the neck, eyelids, forehead, face, wrists, and dorsa of feet and hands

Special Features Related to Ethnicity In blacks, so-called follicular eczema occurs and is characterized by discrete follicular papules involving all hair follicles of the involved site.

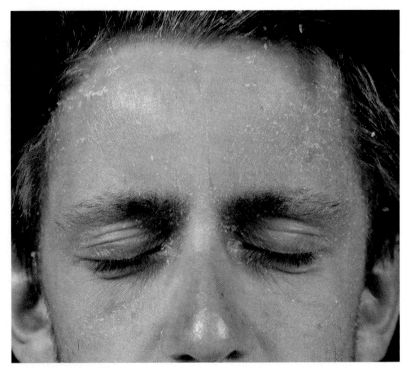

Figure 3-9 Atopic dermatitis *The facial skin shows confluent erythema, scale, and edema with more striking changes of the forehead and periorbital regions; the changes follow chronic rubbing of the skin, which has also caused thinning of the lateral eyebrows. These findings occur in juveniles and adults.*

Laboratory and Special Examinations

Culture Rule out secondary *Staphylococcus aureus* or herpes simplex virus (HSV) infection.

Radioallergosorbent Testing for IgE (PRIST) Usually elevated IgE levels

Radioallergosorbent Testing for Specific IgE Antibodies (RAST) 9sps0% clinically relevant if negative, but only 20% clinically relevant if positive

Patch Test Usually noncontributory. In patients who have IgE antibodies to house dust mites, pollens, or animal hair proteins, patch tests to these allergens may be positive

Management

General Considerations Education of the patient to avoid rubbing and scratching is most important. Topical treatments are valuable but are useless if the patient continues to scratch and rub the plaques. Warn patients of the special problems with HSV infection (eczema herpeticum) and *S. aureus* infection (impetiginization or secondarily infected AD); these complications require oral antiviral agents or antibiotics.

For details of management see page 56.

Dietary Treatment Not helpful in most cases. After RAST testing. For young children recalcitrant to therapy, the most common food allergens are eggs, fish milk, peanuts, soy, and wheat.

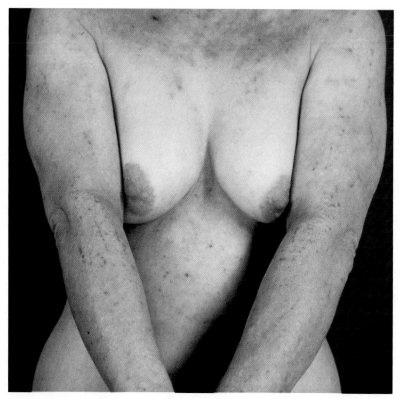

Figure 3-10 Atopic dermatitis *Chronic eczematous dermatitis with sparing under the bra; note lichenification and numerous long excoriations.*

LICHEN SIMPLEX CHRONICUS

Lichen simplex chronicus (LSC) is a special localized form of lichenification usually occurring in circumscribed plaques. Lichenification is a characteristic feature of atopic dermatitis, whether generalized or localized. Lichen simplex can last for decades unless the rubbing and scratching is stopped by treatment of the lichenified skin.

Epidemiology

Age Over 20 years

Sex More frequent in women

Race A possibly higher incidence in Asians and Native Americans

Factors Emotional stress in some cases

History

Duration of Lesion(s) Weeks to months to years

Skin Symptoms Pruritus, often in paroxysms. The lichenified skin is like an erogenous zone—it becomes a pleasure (orgiastic) to scratch. Often the areas on the feet are rubbed at night with the heel. The rubbing becomes automatic and reflexive and an unconscious habit.

Most patients with LSC give a history of itch attacks starting from minor stimuli: putting on clothes, removing ointments, clothes rubbing the skin, and when they go to bed, the skin becomes warmer and this precipitates itching.

Physical Examination

Skin Lesions

TYPE A solid plaque of lichenification, often with small papules on the margins (Figures 3-11 and 3-12) scaling is minimal except in nuchal lichen simplex. Lichenified skin is palpably thickened; skin markings (barely visible in normal skin) are accentuated and can be seen readily. Excoriations are often present. Lightly stroking the involved skin with a cotton swab generates a strong desire to scratch the skin; the same reflex is not present in uninvolved skin.

SPECIAL FEATURES RELATED TO ETHNICITY In black skin, lichenification may assume a special type of pattern—there is not a solid plaque, but the lichenification consists instead of a multitude of small (2- to 3-mm) lichenified papules.

COLOR Usually dull red, later brown or black hyperpigmentation, especially in skin phototypes IV, V, and VI

SHAPE Round, oval, linear (following path of scratching). Usually sharply defined

DISTRIBUTION Isolated single lesion or several randomly scattered plaques

CHARACTERISTIC SITES Nuchal area (female), scalp, ankles, lower legs, upper thighs, exterior forearms, vulva, pubis, anal area, scrotum, and groin

Differential Diagnosis

Chronic Pruritic Plaque

Psoriasis vulgaris, early stages of mycosis fungoides, contact dermatitis (irritant or allergic), epidermal dermatophytosis, Schamberg's disease

Laboratory and Special Examinations

KOH Preparation Rule out dermatophytosis.

Dermatopathology Hyperplasia of all components of epidermis: hyperkeratosis, acanthosis, and elongated and broad rete ridges. Spongiosis is infrequent. In the dermis there is a chronic inflammatory infiltrate.

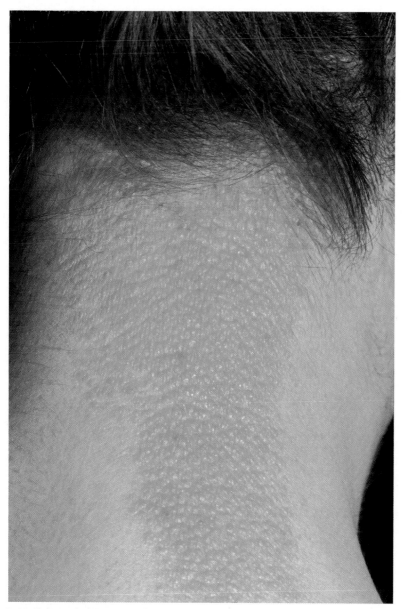

Figure 3-11 Lichen simplex chronicus *Confluent, papular, follicular eczema, creating a plaque of lichen simplex chronicus of the posterior neck and occipital scalp, has been present for many years, the result of chronic rubbing of the area.*

Diagnosis

Made on history and physical findings

Pathophysiology

A special predilection of the skin to respond to physical trauma by epidermal hyperplasia; skin becomes highly sensitive to touch, a fact probably related to proliferation of nerves in the epidermis. The very abnormal itching hyperexcitability of lichenified skin arises in response to minimal external stimuli that would not elicit an itch response in normal skin.

Management

Difficult! Repeatedly explain to the patient that the rubbing and scratching must be stopped. It is important to apply occlusive bandages at night to prevent rubbing and to facilitate penetration of topical corticosteroids.

Corticosteroids

TOPICAL CORTICOSTEROID PREPARATIONS Covered by continuous dry occlusive gauze dressings

INTRALESIONAL TRIAMCINOLONE Often highly effective (3 mg/ml; high concentrations may cause atrophy)

Tar Preparations Combinations of 5% crude coal tar in zinc oxide paste plus class II corticosteroids covered by occlusive cloth dry dressings are effective for body areas where this can be done (e.g., legs, arms).

Occlusive Dressings Corticosteroid preparations are usually applied first, followed by an occlusive dressing. The dressing alone, however, prevents the patient from scratching and is an effective treatment.

Occlusive Plastic Film

HYDROCOLLOID DRESSINGS Corticosteroids are applied first and are covered with hydrocolloid dressing, which can be left in place for up to 1 week.

CORTICOSTEROIDS INCORPORATED IN ADHESIVE PLASTIC TAPE (CORDRAN TAPE) Very effective and can be left on for 24 hours

UNNA BOOT A gauze roll dressing impregnated with zinc oxide paste is wrapped around a large lichenified area such as the calf. The dressing can be left on for up to 1 week.

Antihistamines

TOPICAL PREPARATIONS Doxepin 5 % ointment may be effective in some patients but may cause drowsiness.

ORAL Have little role in treatment of localized pruritus

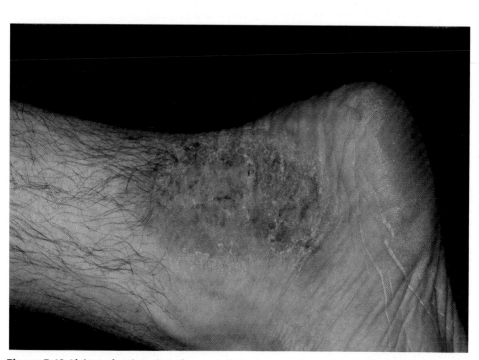

Figure 3-12 Lichen simplex chronicus *A thick plaque with crusted erosions and excoriations caused by years of rubbing the area with the opposite heel and fingernails*

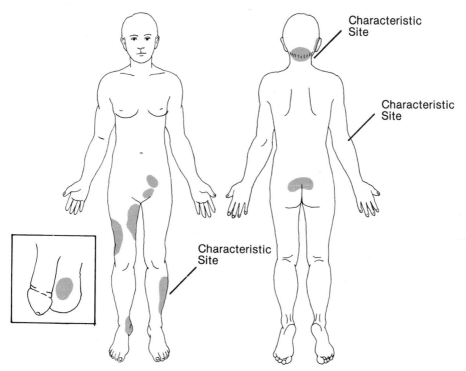

Characteristic Site

Characteristic Site

Characteristic Site

Figure I Lichen simplex

NUMMULAR ECZEMA

Nummular eczema is a chronic, pruritic, inflammatory dermatitis occurring in the form of coin-shaped plaques composed of grouped small papules and vesicles on an erythematous base, especially common on the lower legs of older males during winter months; often seen in atopic individuals. *Synonym:* Discoid eczema.

Epidemiology

Age Two peaks in incidence: young adults and old age

Season Fall and winter

History

Duration of Lesions Weeks to months

Skin Symptoms Pruritus, often intense

Physical Examination

Skin Lesions

TYPE

Closely grouped, small vesicles and papules that coalesce into plaques (Figure 3-13), often more than 4 to 5 cm in diameter, with an erythematous base with distinct borders. Plaques may become exudative and crust. Excoriations secondary to scratching.
Dry scaly plaques that may be lichenified

COLOR Pink to dull red

SHAPE Round or *coin-shaped,* hence the adjective *nummular* (Latin: *nummularis,* "like a coin"). Margins often more pronounced than center

DISTRIBUTION *Extent* Regional clusters of lesions (e.g., on legs) or generalized

Pattern Random

Sites of Predilection Lower legs (older men), trunk, hands and fingers (younger females)

Differential Diagnosis

Scaling Plaques Epidermal dermatophytosis, contact dermatitis (allergic or irritant), psoriasis vulgaris, early stages of mycosis fungoides, impetigo, familial pemphigus

Laboratory and Special Examinations

Bacterial Culture Rule out *Staphylococcus aureus* infection.

Dermatopathology Subacute inflammation with acanthosis and spongiosis

Pathophysiology

Unknown. Unrelated to atopic diathesis; IgE levels are normal. Incidence peaks in winter, when xerosis is maximal.

Course and Prognosis

Chronic. Often difficult to control even with potent topical corticosteroid preparations.

Management

Skin Hydration "Moisturize" involved skin after bath or shower with hydrated petrolatum or other moisturizing cream. (See Ichthyosis Vulgaris, page 96.)

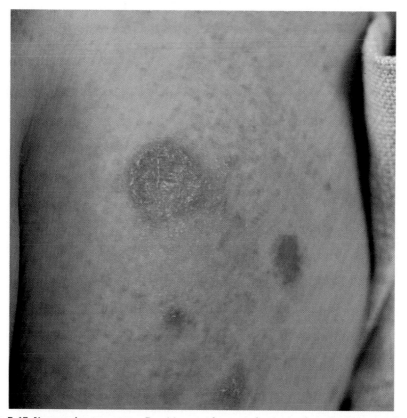

Figure 3-13 Nummular eczema *Pruritic, round, nummular (coin-shaped) plaques with erythema, scale, and crust with smaller satellite lesions of the buttocks.*

Corticosteroids

TOPICAL PREPARATIONS Potent ointment (classes I and II) applied b.i.d. until lesions have resolved. Steroid impregnated tape (Cordran tape)

INTRALESIONAL Triamcinolone 3 mg/ml is very effective.

Crude Coal Tar 2 % crude coal tar ointment daily. May be combined with corticosteroid preparation.

Systemic Therapy Systemic antibiotics if *Staphylococcus aureus* is present

PUVA Therapy Very effective but there are recurrences

DYSHIDROTIC ECZEMATOUS DERMATITIS

Dyshidrotic eczema is a special vesicular type of hand and foot dermatitis. It is an acute, chronic, or recurrent dermatosis of the fingers, palms, and soles, characterized by a sudden onset of many deep-seated pruritic, clear "tapioca-like" vesicles; later, scaling, fissures, and lichenification occur. Although implied by the name (*dyshidrosis*), there are no abnormalities of sweat gland function. *Synonyms:* Pompholyx, vesicular palmar eczema

Epidemiology

Age   Majority under 40 years (range 12 to 40 years)

Sex   Equal ratio

History

Duration of Lesions   Outbreaks usually last for several weeks.

Skin Symptoms   Pruritus at sites of new vesicles. Pain in fissures and secondarily infected lesions.

Physical Examination

Skin Lesions

TYPE   *Early*   Vesicles, usually small (1.0 mm), deep-seated, appearing like "tapioca" in clusters. Bullae, occasionally (Figure 3-14).
   Later   Papules, scaling, lichenification, painful fissures, and erosions which result from coalescing ruptured vesicles and may be quite extensive. Crusts. Secondarily infected lesions are characterized by pustules, crusts, cellulitis, lymphangitis, and painful lymphadenopathy

ARRANGEMENT   Vesicles grouped in clusters

DISTRIBUTION   Hands (80 %) and feet. Sites of predilection: initially, lateral aspects of fingers, palms, soles; later, dorsa of fingers.

Differential Diagnosis

Contact (allergic or irritant) dermatitis, atopic dermatitis of hands/feet, palmar/plantar pustulosis, bullous tinea pedis, "id" reaction (vesicular reaction to active dermatophytosis on the feet or stasis dermatitis), scabies

Laboratory and Special Examinations

Bacterial Culture   Rule out *Staphylococcus aureus* infection

KOH Preparation   Rule out epidermal dermatophytosis

Dermatopathology   Eczematous inflammation (spongiosis and intraepidermal edema) with intraepidermal vesicles

Pathophysiology

Despite the name *dyshidrotic eczema,* there is no evidence that sweating plays a role in the pathogenesis. About half the patients have an atopic background. Emotional stress is possibly a precipitating factor. Many patients claim the eruption recurs only in hot, humid weather.

Course and Prognosis

Recurrent attacks are the rule. Spontaneous remissions in 2 to 3 weeks. Interval between attacks is weeks to months. Secondary infection may complicate the course. Uncommonly, the disease may be disabling because of severe, frequently recurring outbreaks.

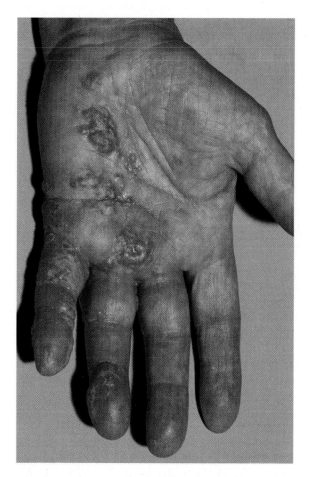

Figure 3-14 Dyshidrotic eczema
Confluent vesicles and bullae within the thick epidermis of the palms with underlying erythema and edema.

Management

A frustrating experience. Avoid systemic corticosteroids except in rare, short-term flare-ups; patients can become dependent on low-dose corticosteroids, and complications can occur.

Wet Dressing For early vesicular stage: Burow's wet dressings. Large bullae should be drained with a puncture but not unroofed.

Corticosteroids

TOPICAL High-potency corticosteroids with plastic occlusive dressings for 1 to 2 weeks to involved areas only

INTRALESIONAL INJECTION Very effective for small areas of involvement; 3 mg/ml triamcinalone

SYSTEMIC In severe cases, a short, tapered course can be given: prednisone 70 mg, tapering by 10 or 5 mg/day over 7 or 14 days.

Systemic Antibiotic For suspected (localized pain) or documented secondarily infected lesions (usually *S. aureus;* less commonly group A streptococcus) (See Impetigo, Section 23.)

PUVA Oral or topical as "soaks" is successful in many patients if given over prolonged periods of time and is worth trying, especially in severe cases.

SEBORRHEIC DERMATITIS

Seborrheic dermatitis (SD) is a very common chronic dermatosis characterized by redness and scaling occurring in regions where the sebaceous glands are most active, such as the face and scalp, and in the body folds. Mild scalp SD causes flaking, i.e., dandruff.
Synonyms: "Cradle cap" (infants), eczematoid seborrhea, pityriasis sicca (dandruff).

Epidemiology

Age Infancy (within the first months), puberty, majority between 20 and 50 years or older

Sex More common in males

Incidence 2 % to 5 % of the population

Predisposing Factors Often a genetic diathesis, the "seborrheic state," with marked seborrhea and marginal blepharitis. HIV-infected individuals have an increased incidence.

History

Duration of Lesions Gradual onset

Skin Symptoms Pruritus is variable, often increased by perspiration; worse during winter.

Physical Examination

Skin Lesions

TYPE Yellowish red, often greasy, or white dry scaling macules and papules of varying size (5 to 20 mm), rather sharply marginated (Figures 3-15 and 3-16). Sticky crusts and fissures are common when external ear, scalp, axillae, groin, and submammary areas are involved (weeping).

SHAPE Nummular, polycyclic, and even annular on the trunk

ARRANGEMENT Scattered, discrete on the face and trunk; diffuse involvement of scalp

Distribution and Major Types of Lesions (Based on Localization and Age)

HAIRY AREAS OF HEAD Scalp, eyebrows, eyelashes (blepharitis), beard (follicular orifices); cradle cap

FACE The flush ("butterfly") areas, behind ears, on forehead ("corona seborrheica"), nasolabial folds, eyebrows, glabella. Simulating lesions of tinea facialis. Ears: retroauricular, meatus.

TRUNK Simulating lesions of pityriasis rosea or pityriasis versicolor; yellowish brown patches over the sternum

BODY FOLDS Axillae, groins, anogenital area, submammary areas, umbilicus—presents as a diffuse, exudative, sharply marginated, brightly erythematous eruption; fissures are common.

GENITALIA Often with yellow crusts and psoriasiform lesions

Differential Diagnosis

Common Psoriasis vulgaris (the two diseases can be indistinguishable, i.e., "seborriasis"), impetigo, dermatophytosis (tinea capitis, tinea facialis, tinea corporis), pityriasis versicolor, candidiasis (intertriginous), subacute lupus erythematosus

Rare Langerhans cell histiocytosis (occurs in infants, usually associated with perifollicular purpura), acrodermatitis enteropathica, pemphigus foliaceus, glucagonoma syndrome

Laboratory Studies

Dermatopathology Focal parakeratosis, with few pyknotic neutrophils, moderate acanthosis, spongiosis (intercellular edema), nonspecific inflammation of the dermis. The most characteristic feature is neutrophils at the tips of the dilated follicular openings, which appear as crusts/scales.

Diagnosis

Usually made on clinical findings

Pathophysiology

Pityrosporon ovale is said to play a role in the pathogenesis. SD-like lesions are seen in nutritional deficiencies such as zinc deficiency (as a result of IV alimentation) and experimental niacin deficiency and in Parkinson's disease (including drug-induced).

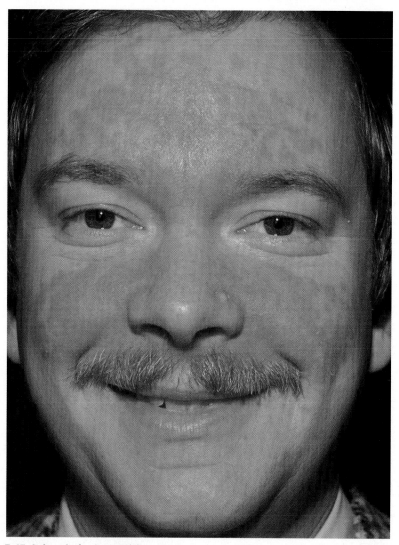

Figure 3-15 Seborrheic dermatitis *Erythema with yellow-orange and scale-forming plaques on the upper lip, cheeks, nasolabial fold, eyebrow area, glabella, and forehead; similar lesions were also present in the retroauricular areas and presternal chest.*

Course and Prognosis

SD is very common, affecting the majority of individuals at some time during life. UV radiation is beneficial for many individuals with SD; the condition improves in the summer and flares in the fall. Recurrences and remissions, especially on the scalp, may be associated with alopecia in severe cases. Infantile and adolescent SD disappear with age. Seborrheic eryth-roderma may occur. *Seborrheic erythroderma associated with diarrhea and failure to thrive and to generate C5a chemotactic factor is called* **Leiner's disease.**

Management

SD is a chronic disorder, which requires initial therapy followed by chronic maintenance ther-

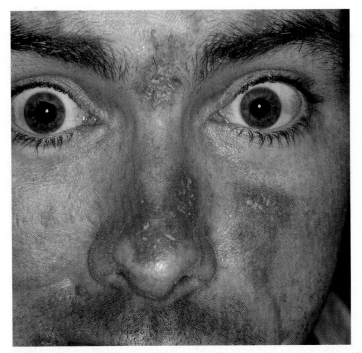

Figure 3-16 Seborrheic dermatitis in HIV disease *Erythema and scaling resembling psoriasis (sebopsoriasis) on the left cheek, nose, glabella, and eyebrows of an individual with advanced HIV disease. The patient has also suffered a stroke involving the left face, resulting in more severe seborrheic dermatitis in the involved side.*

apy. Topical corticosteroid preparations are effective but can cause atrophy (erythema, telangiectasia), especially on the face, or initiation/exacerbation of perioral dermatitis or rosacea. UV radiation is beneficial for many individuals with SD; the condition improves in the summer and flares in the fall.

Initial Topical Therapy

SCALP *Shampoo* Effective OTC shampoos containing selenium sulfide, zinc pyrithione, or "tar." By prescription (U.S.), 2 % ketoconazole shampoo, used initially to treat and subsequently to control the symptoms; lather can be used on face and chest during shower.
Corticosteroids Vioform-hydrocortisone lotion or low-potency fluorinated corticosteroid solution, lotion, or gel following a medicated shampoo for more severe cases

FACE AND TRUNK

Ketoconazole shampoo 2 %: lather face during shower.
Ketoconazole cream (approved for use in SD in the United States)

Corticosteroid cream: initially 1 % or 2.5 % hydrocortisone acetate cream b.i.d.

EYELIDS Seborrheic blepharitis is managed by gentle removal of the crusts in the morning using a baby shampoo (a cotton ball is dipped in a diluted shampoo); the scales are gently removed from the eyelids. Following this, the lids are covered with sodium sulfacetamide, 10 % in a suspension containing 0.2 % prednisolone and 0.12 % phenylephrine; this commercially available formulation should be used cautiously because it contains corticosteroids.

INTERTRIGINOUS AREAS Castellani's paint in oozing dermatitis of the body folds (often very effective)

Maintenance Therapy Ketoconazole 2 % shampoo. Ketoconazole cream or 3 % sulfur and 2 % salicylic acid in oil-in-water base. 1 % hydrocortisone cream q.d.; patients should be monitored to check for signs of atrophy.

ASTEATOTIC DERMATITIS

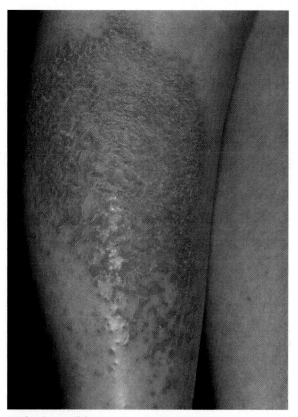

Figure 3-17 Asteatotic dermatitis (eczema craquelatum)* *Asteatotic dermatitis is a common pruritic dermatitis that occurs in the winter and in older persons (especially in males over age 60 years) on the legs, arms, and hands but also may be on the trunk. The eruption is characterized by dry, "cracked," fissured skin with slight scaling, and there are histologic changes similar to eczema (spongiosis) The disorder persists for weeks to months. Very often the eruption results from too frequent bathing in hot soapy baths or showers and in older persons living in rooms with a high environmental temperature and low relative humidity (as in heated rooms). The disorder is managed by avoiding overbathing with soap, especially tub baths, and increasing the ambient humidity, preferably above 50%; room humidifiers (in the bedroom) are very helpful; also, using tepid water baths containing bath oils followed by immediate liberal application of emollient ointments. Also helpful is the use of medium-potency corticosteroid ointments applied twice daily until the ezematous component has resolved.*

*A word meaning "marred with cracks," as in old china or ceramic tile.

Section 4

DISORDERS OF CELL KINETICS AND DIFFERENTIATION

PSORIASIS

Psoriasis, which affects 1.5 % to 2.0 % of the population in western countries, is a hereditary disorder of skin with several clinical expressions—but the most frequent type is *psoriasis vulgaris,* which occurs as chronic scaling papules and plaques in characteristic sites of the body, largely related to repeated minor trauma: scalp, elbows, forearms, lumbosacral region, knees, hands, and feet.

Psoriasis vulgaris is a challenge for the physician, because chronic generalized psoriasis is one of the "miseries that beset mankind," causing shame and embarrassment and a compromised lifestyle. The "heartbreak of psoriasis" is no joke. As the writer John Updike so poignantly said about a person with psoriasis, "Lusty, though we are loathsome to love. Keen-sighted, though we hate to look upon ourselves. The name of the disease, spiritually speaking, is Humiliation."

CLINICAL CLASSIFICATION OF PSORIASIS

Nonpustular	Pustular
Psoriasis vulgaris	Palmoplantar pustulosis
Early onset (type I)	Pustular psoriasis (annular type)
Late onset (type II)	von Zumbusch syndrome (acute febrile
Psoriatic erythroderma	generalized pustular psoriasis)

SOURCE: Modified from Christophers E, Sterry W, Psoriasis, in TB Fitzpatrick et al (eds), *Dermatology in General Medicine,* 4th ed. New York, McGraw-Hill, 1993, pp 489–514.

Epidemiology

Age

Type I: early onset (75 %) in females (16 years) and in males (22 years)

Type II: late onset (25 %) in males and females (56 years)

Sex Equal incidence in males and females

Race Low incidence in West Africans, Japanese, and Eskimos and a very low incidence or absence in North and South American Indians

Heredity Polygenic trait. When one parent has psoriasis, 8 % of offspring develop psoriasis, and when both parents have psoriasis, 41 % develop psoriasis. Class I antigens associated with psoriasis: HLA-B13, -B17, -Bw57, -CW6

Trigger Factors *Physical trauma* (Koebner's phenomenon) is a major factor in eliciting lesions; rubbing and scratching stimulates the psoriatic proliferative process. *Infections:* acute streptococcal infection precipitating guttate psoriasis. *Stress:* a factor in flares of psoriasis as high as 40 % in adults and higher in children. *Drugs:* systemic corticosteroids, Class I topical corticosteroids, oral lithium, antimalarial drugs, systemic interferon, and beta-adrenergic blockers can flare existing psoriasis and cause a psoriasiform drug eruption, alcohol ingestion(?).

History

Duration of Lesions Usually indolent lesions are present for months but may be of sudden onset, as in acute guttate psoriasis and generalized pustular psoriasis (von Zumbusch syndrome)

Skin Symptoms Pruritus is reasonably common, especially in scalp and anogenital psoriasis.

Constitutional Symptoms Joint pain in arthritis—a special type of arthritis, *psoriatic arthritis.* In von Zumbusch syndrome (acute onset of generalized pustular psoriasis), there is an "acute illness" syndrome with weakness, chills, and fever.

Physical Examination

Skin Lesions

TYPE

Papules and plaques, sharply marginated with marked silvery-white scale (see Figures 4-1 and 4-2); removal of scale results in the appearance of minute blood droplets (Auspitz phenomenon).
Pustules, erythroderma

COLOR "Salmon pink"

SHAPE Round, oval, polycyclic, annular, linear

ARRANGEMENT Zosteriform, arciform, serpiginous, scattered discrete lesions, erythroderma (involvement of almost the entire skin)

DISTRIBUTION *Extent* Single lesion or lesions localized to one area (e.g., penis, nails), regional involvement (scalp), generalized or universal (entire skin)

Pattern (1) Bilateral (see Figure 4-4) but rarely symmetrical; often spares exposed areas; favors elbows, knees, scalp, and intertriginous areas; facial region is uncommonly involved and is usually associated with refractory type of psoriasis. For characteristic patterns of distribution, see Figure II. (2) Disseminated small lesions without predilection of site (guttate psoriasis) (see page 82 and Figure 4-2)

Arthritis

Psoriatic arthritis is included among the seronegative spondyloarthropathies, which include ankylosing spondylitis and Reiter's syndrome. Incidence is 5 % to 8 %. Rare before age 20.
May be present (in 10 % of individuals) without any visible psoriasis; then search for a family history.
Two types: (1) "Distal"—seronegative, without subcutaneous nodules, and involving, asymmetrically, a few distal interphalangeal joints of the hands and feet: an asymmetrical oligoarthritis. (2) Mutilating psoriatic arthritis with bone erosion and osteolysis and, ultimately, ankylosis. Especially involving the sacroiliac, hip, and cervical areas with ankylosing spondylitis; seen especially in erythrodermic and pustular psoriasis. Type 2 arthritis associated with HLA-B28

Differential Diagnosis

Scaling Plaques *Seborrheic dermatitis*—may be indistinguishable in sites involved and morphology; sometimes this is termed *seborriasis; lichen simplex chronicus*—may complicate psoriasis due to pruritus; *candidiasis*—especially in intertriginous psoriasis; *psoriasiform drug eruptions*—especially beta blockers, gold, and methyldopa; *glucagonoma syndrome*—important differential because this is a serious disease (malignant tumor of the pancreatic islet cells).

Laboratory and Special Examinations

Dermatopathology There is (1) marked thickening and also thinning of the epidermis with elongation of the rete ridges, (2) increased mitosis of keratinocytes, fibroblasts, and endothelial cells, (3) parakeratotic hyperkeratosis (nuclei retained in the stratum corneum), and (4) inflammatory cells in the dermis (usually lymphocytes and monocytes) and in the epidermis (polymorphonuclear cells), forming microabscesses of Munro in the stratum corneum.

Serology Sudden onset of psoriasis may be associated with HIV infection. Determination of HIV serostatus is indicated in at-risk individuals.

Pathophysiology

Psoriasis probably refers to a cluster of diseases of differing pathogeneses. The principal abnormality in psoriasis is an alteration of the cell kinetics of keratinocytes. The major change is a shortening of the cell cycle from 311 to 36 hours; this results in 28 times the normal production of epidermal cells. The etiologic basis for this increased production is not known. The epidermis and dermis appear to respond as an integrated system: the changes in the germinative zone of the epidermis and the inflammatory changes in the dermis, which may "trigger" the epidermal changes. Immunologic phenomena recently have been proved to be a major factor in the pathogenesis of psoriasis inasmuch as immunosuppressive drugs such as

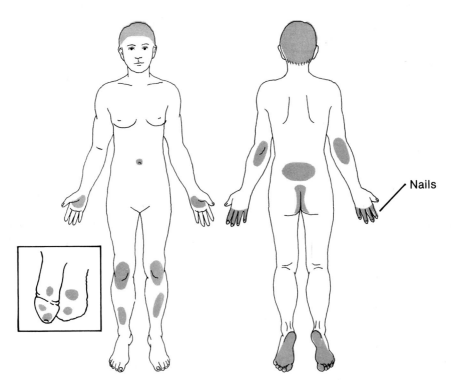

Nails

Figure II Psoriasis

cyclosporine are dramatically effective in causing a total remission of the disease. There are many T cells present in psoriatic lesions surrounding the upper dermal blood vessels and the cytokine spectrum is that of a Th 1 response. Maintenance of psoriatic lesions is considered by some as an ongoing autoreactive immune response.

Factors Influencing Selection of Management

1. Age: childhood, adolescence, young adulthood, middle age, >60 years

2. Type of psoriasis: guttate, plaque, palmar and pustular, generalized pustular psoriasis, erythrodermic psoriasis

3. Site and extent of involvement: *localized* to palms and soles, scalp, anogenital area, scattered plaques but less than 5 % involvement; *generalized* and greater than 30 % involvement

4. Previous treatment: ionizing radiation, systemic corticosteroids, PUVA, cyclosporine, arsenics, methotrexate

5. Associated medical disorders (e.g., HIV disease)

PSORIASIS VULGARIS: LIMITED TO THE ELBOWS, KNEES, AND ISOLATED PLAQUES (Figure 4-1)

Management

Instruct the patient never to rub or scratch the lesions because this trauma stimulates the psoriatic proliferative process (Koebner's phenomenon).

Treatment only with topical agents.

1. Topical fluorinated corticosteroids (betamethasone valerate, fluocinolone acetonide, betamethasone propionate, clobetasol propionate) in ointment base applied after removing the scales by soaking in water. The ointment is applied to the wet skin, covered with plastic wrap, and left on overnight. Corticosteroid impregnated tape (Cordran tape).

2. Use of hydrocolloid dressing left on for 24 to 48 hours is helpful and effective and prevents scratching. During the day, Classes I and II fluorinated corticosteroid creams can be used without occlusion. Patients will develop tolerance after long periods. *Caveat:* Prolonged application of the fluorinated corticosteroids leads to atrophy of the skin, striae, and unsightly telangiectasia. Clobetasol-17-propionate is stronger and active even without occlusion. To avoid systemic effects of this Class I corticosteroid: maximum of 50 g ointment per week.

3. For small plaques (≤ 4.0 cm), triamcinolone acetonide aqueous suspension is injected into the lesion 0.1 mg/mm^2. The injection should be intradermal rather than subcutaneous; *if the injection does not require some pressure to inject, it is not going into the dermis. Warning:* Hypopigmentation at the injection site can result; *this is more apparent in brown and black skin.*

4. Topical anthralin preparations are excellent when used properly. Follow directions on the package insert with attention to details.

5. Vitamin D analogues (calcipotriene 0.005 %) ointment and cream are good nonsteroidal antipsoriatic topical agents and are not associated with cutaneous atrophy. They are not as potent as Class I corticosteroids (e.g., clobetasol propionate) but can be combined with Class I corticosteroids, using the latter only on weekends, calcipotriene ointment or cream being used during the week. Calcipotriene should not be applied to more than 40 % of the body surface and not more than 100 g per week to avoid hypercalcemia.

6. Tazarotene (a new topical retinoid) is another alternative to topical corticosteroids or can be best combined with Class II (medium strength) topical corticosteroids, as tazarotene can cause some irritation. Also there is some indication but not proof that topical retinoids such as tazarotene may prevent cutaneous atrophy.

7. When there is more than 10 % (the palm of the hand = 1 %) involvement with psoriatic plaques, it is preferable to combine these topical treatments with phototherapy or PUVA photochemotherapy.

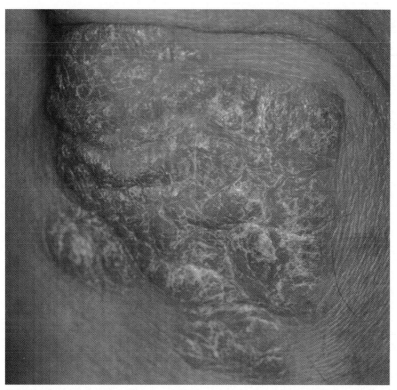

Figure 4-1 Psoriasis vulgaris: elbow *Well-demarcated, brightly erythematous plaque with a thick but loosely adherent silvery-white micaceous (mica-like) scale on the elbow, which has arisen from the coalescence of smaller papular lesions.*

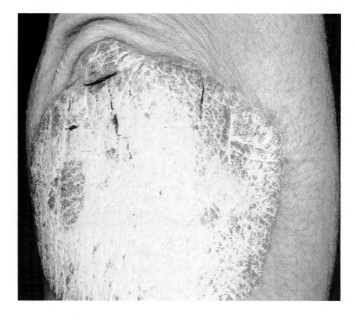

Figure 4-1A Psoriasis vulgaris: chronic stable type *This psoriatic plaque is completely covered by tightly adherent silvery-white scales that mimic asbestos.*

PSORIASIS VULGARIS: GUTTATE TYPE

This type of psoriasis, which is relatively rare (<2.0 % of all psoriasis), is like an exanthem: a shower of lesions appears rather rapidly in young adults, often following streptococcal pharyngitis. Guttate psoriasis may, however, be chronic and unrelated to streptococcal infection.

Physical Examination

Skin Lesions   (Figure 4-2)

TYPE   Papules 2.0 mm to 1.0 cm

COLOR   "Salmon pink"

SHAPE   Guttate (Latin: "spots that resemble drops")

ARRANGEMENT   Scattered discrete lesions

DISTRIBUTION   Generalized, usually sparing the palms and soles and concentrating on the trunk, less on the face, scalp, and nails

Differential Diagnosis

Multiple Small Scaling Plaques Psoriasiform drug eruption, secondary syphilis, pityriasis rosea

Laboratory Examinations

Serologic   An increased antistreptolysin titer in those patients with antecedent streptococcal infection

Culture   Throat culture for group A β-hemolytic streptococcus infection

Course and Prognosis

Sometimes this type of psoriasis disappears spontaneously in a few weeks without any treatment.

Management

The resolution of lesions can be accelerated by UVB phototherapy. For persistent lesions, treatment is the same as for generalized plaque psoriasis (see page 86). Penicillin VK or erythromycin if group A β-hemolytic streptococcus on throat culture.

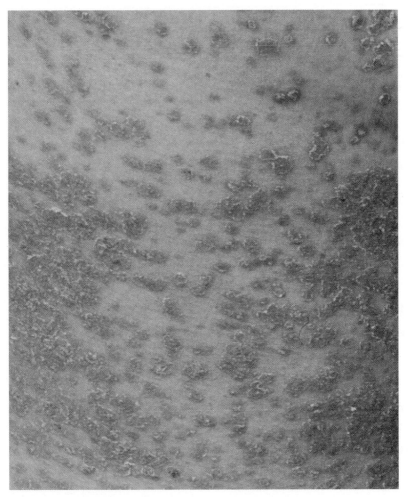

Figure 4-2 Psoriasis vulgaris: Guttate type *Confluent, erythematous, scaling, small papules and plaques on the trunk, arose following a group A beta-hemolytic streptococcal pharyngitis.*

PSORIASIS VULGARIS: SCALP

Psoriasis of the scalp presents a special therapeutic problem, similar to that of anogenital psoriasis. Both areas are inaccessible for phototherapy and are often pruritic, which results in lichenification and koebnerization.* Psoriasis of the scalp may be part of generalized plaque psoriasis, may coexist with isolated plaques, or may be the only site involved. It usually does not lead to hair loss.

History

Duration   Months to years

Relationship to Season   Does not go into remission with phototherapy or with sunlight exposure, as does the exposed psoriatic skin.

Skin Symptoms   Mild to severe pruritus, which often causes compulsive and subconscious scratching

Physical Examination

Skin Lesions

TYPE

Plaques, often with thick, adherent scales (Figure 4-3)
Lichenification (often superimposed on the basic psoriatic lesions and resulting from rubbing and scratching)
Exudation and fissures, especially behind the ears

ARRANGEMENT   Scattered discrete plaques or diffuse involvement of the entire scalp

(*Note:* Paradoxically, alopecia is an uncommon complication of psoriasis of the scalp, even after years of thick, plaque-type involvement. Thus the condition is not exposed to public view, and this may be one reason why patients learn to live with it and do not seek treatment.)

Differential Diagnosis

Red Scaling Plaques on Scalp   Seborrheic dermatitis of the scalp may be almost indistin-

*The phenomenon of induction of new lesions on "normal" skin by physical trauma, including rubbing and scratching.

guishable from psoriasis. Some have called this *seborriasis.* Tinea capitis, atopic dermatitis, lichen simplex chronicus

Management

Mild   Superficial scaling and lacking thick plaques:

- Tar or ketoconazole shampoos *followed by*
- Betamethasone valerate 0.1 % lotion 2 times weekly; if refractory, clobetasol propionate 0.05 % scalp application

Severe   Thick, adherent plaques:

- Vitamin D_3 analogues as lotion
- Removal of plaques before active treatment. Topical applications are virtually useless unless the thick scale is removed. This is accomplished by applications of 2 % to 10 % salicylic acid in mineral oil, covered with a plastic cap, and left on overnight.
- After scales have been removed (in one to three treatments), fluocinolone cream or lotion is applied, and the scalp is covered with plastic sheets or a shower cap, which is left on overnight.
- When the thickness of the plaques is reduced, scalp application of clobetasol propionate 0.05 % or calcipotriene lotion can be used for maintenance. *Compulsive subconscious scratching and rubbing will negate all attempts at maintenance treatment.* Hands off!

Course and Prognosis

The prognosis for control is good; following treatment as outlined above, the scalp lesions may undergo a remission for several months to years. Scratching and rubbing must be avoided to maintain the remission.

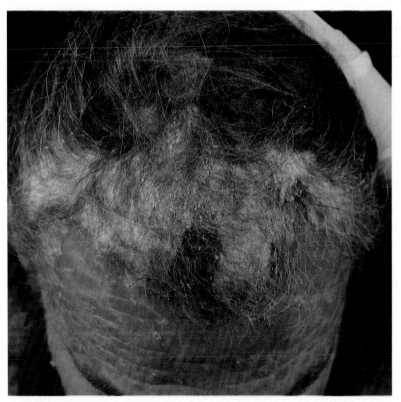

Figure 4-3 Psoriasis vulgaris: scalp *Cap-like, very thick scale covers the entire scalp, with erythematous plaques extending onto the forehead. Scalp psoriasis, even though severe as in this case, usually is not associated with hair loss.*

PSORIASIS VULGARIS: TRUNK

Management

The management of generalized plaque-type psoriasis (Figure 4-4) is the province of the dermatologist or of a psoriasis center where the major options are available: (1) UVB phototherapy with emollients, (2) PUVA photochemotherapy, (3) methotrexate (given weekly), (4) combination therapy using etretinate (or other retinoids such as acitretin or isotretinoin) or methotrexate with PUVA (such combinations are perhaps the ideal treatment available at the present time), or (5) cyclosporine.

Up to 50% of patients with thin-plaque psoriasis respond well to UVB plus emollients when given according to a published protocol. This is also true for topical calcipotriene as long as no more than 40 % of the body surface is involved and not more than 100 g/week is used. Response is slow. Those with thick plaques or who do not respond to UVB plus emollients are treated with oral PUVA photochemotherapy or ideally with a combination of retinoids plus PUVA. For males, combination treatment using etretinate and oral PUVA photochemotherapy (so-called Re-PUVA) is the most effective therapy. For females, isotretinoin can be used, but contraception is mandatory during and 2 months after treatment is completed. Methotrexate is used only in older patients ($>$50 years) or when combination phototherapy or photochemotherapy (retinoids plus PUVA or retinoids plus UVB plus emollients) has failed to bring about a remission.

Oral PUVA Photochemotherapy Treatment consists of oral ingestion of 8-methoxypsoralen (8-MOP) (0.3 to 0.6 mg 8-MOP per kilogram of body weight) and exposure to varying doses of UVA, depending on the sensitivity of the patient. Approximately 1 hour after ingestion of the psoralen, UVA is given, starting at a dose of 1 J/cm^2, adjusted upward for skin phototype. Alternatively, phototoxicity testing can be done, which

permits a better adjustment of the UVA dose to the individual's sensitivity to PUVA. The UVA dose is increased by 0.5 to 1.0 J/cm^2 each dose. Treatments are performed 2 or 3 times a week or, if employing a more intensive protocol, 4 times a week. The majority of patients clear after 19 to 25 treatments, and the amount of UVA needed ranges from 100 to 245 J/cm^2; long-term side effects: PUVA keratoses and squamous cell carcinomas in some cases.

In patients with recalcitrant plaque-type psoriasis, etretinate (in males) or isotretinoin (in females) may be combined with other antipsoriatic therapy, e.g., PUVA, UVB, topical corticosteroids, or anthralin. These combination modalities have been shown to reduce the length of treatment as well as the total amount of an antipsoriatic drug necessary for clearing. Topical corticosteroids, anthralin, methotrexate, and etretinate, combined with either PUVA or UVB, have all been shown to be effective in reducing the dose of one another.

Psoriasis Day-Care Centers These facilities have available UVB plus emollients *or* UVB plus tar (Goeckerman regimen) and PUVA. The patient remains in the phototherapy unit during the day and goes home at night. In these centers there is a camaraderie among the patients with psoriasis and the staff, which no doubt has a positive effect on the course of the disease and ensures compliance with the therapy.

Methotrexate Therapy Oral methotrexate (MTX) is one of the most effective treatments and certainly the most convenient treatment for generalized plaque-type psoriasis. Nevertheless, MTX is a potentially dangerous drug, principally because of liver toxicity that can occur following prolonged therapy. Hepatic toxicity occurs after cumulative doses in normal persons, but other risk factors include a history of alcohol intake, abnormal liver chemistries, and IV drug use; obesity is also a risk factor for he-

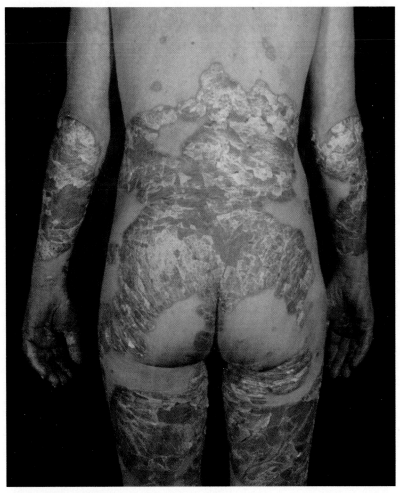

Figure 4-4 Psoriasis vulgaris: chronic plaque type *Very extensive erythematous plaques covered with thick membrane-like scale involving more than 50 percent of the posterior aspect of the trunk, arms, and legs.*

patic toxicity. Inasmuch as hepatic toxicity is related to total life dose, this therapy should, in general, *not* be given to young patients. There is some evidence that older patients can be controlled with lower doses of MTX because of slower excretion of the drug by the kidney.

SCHEDULE OF METHOTREXATE THERAPY USING THE TRIPLE-DOSE REGIMEN (preferred by most over the single-dose MTX once weekly). Begin with a test dose of 5.0 mg (2.5-mg tablet followed 24 hours later with a second 2.5-mg tablet). This will ascertain whether there is a special sensitivity to MTX. A complete blood count (CBC) is obtained after 1 week and every 1 to 4 weeks as the dose of MTX is increased. If the CBC is normal at 1 week, 2.5 mg (1 tablet) is given every 12 hours for a total of 3 doses of 7.5 mg (1/1/1 tablet schedule). Many patients will respond to this dose, but if not, the dose is increased after 2 weeks to four tablets (2/1/1) and in 2 weeks, if no improvement, to 2/2/2 or 15 mg = total dose; this is the highest dose recommended. This regimen achieves an 80 % improvement but not total clearing and higher doses increase the risk of toxicity. The dose of MTX can be reduced by one or two tablets periodically. Also, in the summer the dose of MTX may be decreased or the treatment discontinued during this period (Jeffes EWB, Weinstein GD. *Dermatol Clinics* 1995; 13:875-890).

MONITORING MTX AND PLATELET COUNT (at beginning of therapy and every 1 to 4 weeks; after on a stable dose, once monthly). Platelet count must be closely watched as it may decrease before the WBC.

RENAL AND LIVER FUNCTION Obtain LFTs just prior to MTX dose, at start and every 3 months; creatinine at start and every 2 to 4 months.

A pretreatment liver biopsy is required in all patients with a history of liver disease or in patients with abnormal liver chemistries. In patients with normal liver chemistries and in whom no risk factors are present, a liver biopsy should be done after a cumulative dose of approximately 1500 mg MTX; if the post-MTX liver biopsy is normal, repeat liver biopsy should be done after further therapy following an additional 1000 to 1500 mg MTX.* Be aware of various drug interactions with MTX.

Cyclosporin A (CyA) Therapy Still experimental in some countries, CyA treatment is highly effective at a dose of 4 to 5 mg/kg/day. As patient responds, the dose is tapered to the lowest effective maintenance dose. Monitoring blood pressure and serum creatinine is mandatory because of the known nephrotoxicity of the drug. CyA should be employed only in some psoriasis and only to patients without risk factors. (For details and drug interactions, see Mihatsch MJ, Wolff K: Consensus Conference on Cyclosporin A for Psoriasis. *Br J Dermatol* 1992; 126:621.)

*For details regarding MTX therapy of psoriasis, see Roenigk HH Jr, et al, Methotrexate in psoriasis: Revised guidelines. *J Am Acad Dermatol* 1988; 19:145.

PSORIASIS VULGARIS: NAILS

Psoriasis of the nails is quite common (25% of patients with psoriasis), varies in severity of involvement, and often disappears spontaneously or *pari passu* with treatment of psoriasis of the skin, especially with the three major treatments: UVB phototherapy, PUVA photochemotherapy, and methotrexate.

Physical Examination

Nail Findings

Fingernails and toenails frequently (25 %) involved, especially with concomitant arthritis. Nail changes include pitting, subungual hyperkeratosis, onycholysis (also nonspecific), and yellowish brown spots under the nail plate—the *oil spot* (pathognomonic). (Figures 4-5 and 4-6)

Management

Specially directed treatments of the fingernails (inasmuch as the nails are disfiguring and a nuisance) are unsatisfactory. Injection of the nail fold with intradermal triamcinolone acetonide (3 mg/ml) may be quite effective.

PUVA photochemotherapy is somewhat effective; the UVA is administered in special hand and foot lighting units providing high-intensity UVA. Long-term systemic retinoids (acitretin) 0.5 mg/kg are also effective as are systemic methotrexate and cyclosporin A (cyclosporine) therapy.

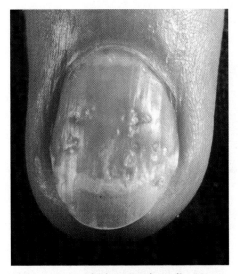

Figure 4-5 Psoriasis vulgaris: nail *Many depressions in the dorsum of the nail plate with mild distal onycholysis; small discrete pits are nearly pathognomonic of psoriasis. The differential diagnosis includes the "hammered brass" nail seen in alopecia areata. Distal onycholysis and minimal subungual hyperkeratosis is also seen.*

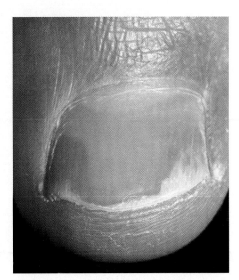

Figure 4-6 Psoriasis vulgaris: nail *An orange-brown discoloration of the distal lateral nail bed is pathognomonic of psoriasis; distal onycholysis is also present.*

PSORIASIS VULGARIS: PALMS AND SOLES (FIGURE 4-7)

This disease is a major therapeutic challenge. The palms and soles may be the only areas involved. Topical corticosteroids with plastic occlusion are quite ineffective. UVB phototherapy is not often effective.

Management

Effective treatments available are as follows:

1. PUVA photochemotherapy, administered in specially designed hand and foot lighting cabinets that deliver UVA, is effective.
2. Retinoids (etretinate) given alone orally are sometimes effective in clearing psoriasis vulgaris of the palms and soles.
3. Combinations of oral retinoids and PUVA improve the efficacy of each and permit a reduction of the dose and duration of each (see page 86).
4. In very severe cases MTX or CyA should be considered.

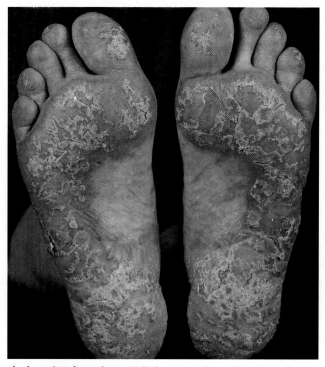

Figure 4-7 Psoriasis vulgaris: soles *Well-demarcated, erythematous plaques with thick, yellowish scale and desquamation on sites of pressure arising on the plantar feet; similar lesions were present on the palms.*

CHRONIC PSORIASIS OF THE PERIANAL AND GENITAL REGIONS AND OF THE BODY FOLDS

Psoriasis of the body folds (inguinal area (Figure 4-8), umbilicus, axillae, inframammary, intergluteal fold) and of the male and female genitalia is especially vulnerable to the development of steroid-induced skin atrophy; low-potency steroids are recommended but are not very effective. Anthralin and tar preparations are irritating in these areas. This poses a difficult problem in control. Castellani's paint is sometimes useful in genital and perianal psoriasis. The newer topical vitamin D_3 preparation, calcipotriene ointment, 50 μg/g, however, is effective in these areas, and there is no risk of skin atrophy or tachyphylaxis.

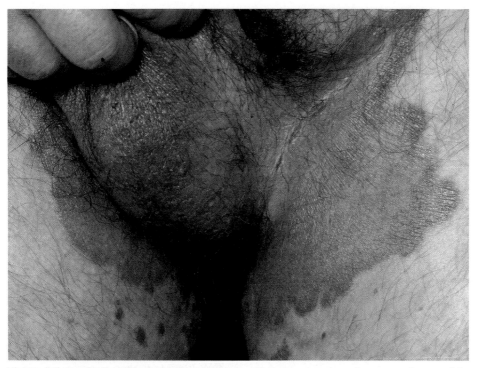

Figure 4-8 Psoriasis vulgaris: inverse pattern *Well-demarcated, erythematous plaques of the inguinal folds with maceration and fissuring, extending to the nonintertriginous skin of the thighs; the natural occlusion limits accumulation of scale. So-called inverse pattern psoriasis occurs in moist intertriginous sites (skin touching skin) in the axillae, inframammary region, umbilicus, and intergluteal/inguinal folds is commonly mistaken for candidiasis or tinea corporis, seborrheic and intertriginous dermatitis.*

PALMOPLANTAR PUSTULOSIS

Palmoplantar pustulosis is a chronic, relapsing eruption limited to the palms and soles and characterized by numerous sterile, yellow, deep-seated pustules that evolve into dusky-red macules.

Epidemiology and Etiology

Incidence Low

Age 50 to 60 years

Sex More common in females (4:1)

History

Duration of Lesions Months

Physical Examination

Skin Lesions

TYPE Pustules (Figure 4-9) in varying stages of evolution, 2.0 to 5.0 mm, deep-seated, develop into dusky-red macules and crusts; present in areas of erythema and scaling.

DISTRIBUTION Localized to palms and soles

SITES OF PREDILECTION Thenar and hypothenar, flexor aspects of fingers, heels, and insteps; acral portions of the fingers and toes usually spared.

Differential Diagnosis

Palmar/Plantar Dermatosis Epidermal dermatophytosis (tinea manus, tinea pedis), pustular psoriasis, dyshidrotic eczematous dermatitis, HSV infection

Laboratory and Special Examinations

KOH Preparations Rule out dermatophytosis.

Bacterial Culture Rule out *Staphylococcus aureus* infection if lesions are circumscribed and localized.

Viral Culture Rule out herpes simplex virus (HSV) infection.

Dermatopathology Edema and exocytosis of mononuclear cells form a vesicle and later many neutrophils, which form a unilocular spongiform pustule and some acanthosis. Mononuclear cells at first and later myriads of neutrophils.

Prognosis

Persistent for years and characterized by unexplained remissions and exacerbations; rarely psoriasis vulgaris may develop elsewhere.

Management

The condition is recalcitrant to treatment.

PUVA and Etretinate Alone or in combination and methotrexate are effective but not curative (see page 86 for details).

Topical Corticosteroids, Dithranol, and Coal Tar Ineffective. Strong corticosteroids under plastic occlusion (e.g., for the night) are often effective, but skin atrophy may limit prolonged use.

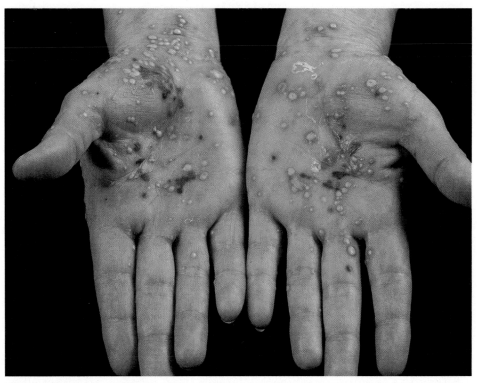

Figure 4-9 Palmar pustulosis *Deep-seated, dusky-red macules and creamy-yellow pustules progress to hyperkeratotic/crusted papules. Because of the pustules, the disorder is commonly mistaken for a bacterial or herpetic infection.*

GENERALIZED ACUTE PUSTULAR PSORIASIS (VON ZUMBUSCH)

This can be a life-threatening medical problem with an abrupt onset. The skin involvement is distinctive and starts with a burning erythema that spreads in hours to result in large areas of fiery-red skin. Pinpoint pustules then appear in clusters, peppering the red areas of skin; these pustules become confluent and form "lakes" filled with purulent fluid. Fever, generalized weakness, severe malaise, and a leukocytosis are prominent features in almost every patient. Impetigo herpetiformis is generalized acute pustular psoriasis with hypocalcemia occurring in pregnancy.

Epidemiology

Age   Adults, rarely children

Precipitating Factors   There are no known precipitating factors, and the patient may or may not have had a stable plaque-type psoriasis in the past.

History

Onset of Lesions   The constellation of fiery-red erythema followed by formation of pustules and "lakes" occurs over a period of less than 1 day. Waves of pustules may follow each other; as one set dries, another will appear.

Skin Symptoms   Marked burning, tenderness

Constitutional Symptoms

ACUTE   Headache, chills, feverishness, marked fatigue, severe malaise

Physical Examination

Appearance of Patient   Frightened, "toxic"

Vital Signs   Fast pulse, rapid breathing, fever that may be high

Skin Lesions

TYPE   There is a sequence of burning erythema followed by the appearance of clusters of tiny nonfollicular and very superficial pustules that usually become confluent, forming "lakes" of pus (Figure 4-10). Removal of the top yields superficial, oozing erosions, and there will be crusting.

ARRANGEMENT OF MULTIPLE LESIONS   Closely set small pustules, circinate lesions, isolated pustules; pustules are interfollicular.

DISTRIBUTION   Generalized, but especially involving the flexural areas and the anogenital regions

Hair and Nails   Nails become thickened, and there is onycholysis; subungual "lakes" of pus lead to shedding of nails; hair loss of the telogen defluvium type developing in 2 or 3 months may occur.

Differential Diagnosis

Widespread Erythema with Pustules   The abrupt onset and the typical evolution of erythema followed by pustulation are highly characteristic. Nevertheless, blood cultures always should be obtained because of possible superinfection, especially with staphylococcal bacteremia. Generalized herpes simplex has umbilicated pustules, and the Tzanck tests and viral cultures establish the diagnosis. Generalized pustular drug eruptions (e.g., after furosemide, amoxicillin/clavulanic acid, and other drugs) may be clinically indistinguishable and patients are less toxic.

Laboratory Examinations

Dermatopathology   Large spongiform pustules resulting from the migration of neutrophils from the capillaries in the dermal papilla to the upper stratum malpighii, where they aggregate within the interstices of the degenerated and thinned keratinocytes

BACTERIAL CULTURE OF TISSUE   Rule out *S. aureus* infection.

HEMATOLOGIC   Polymorphonuclear leukocytosis as high as 20,000 WBC

Pathogenesis

The fever and leukocytosis probably result from the marked increase in the number of polymorphonuclear cells that invade the dermis and release their chemical mediators. This causes inflammation and necrosis of cells (leukocytes and keratinocytes).

Significance

These patients are often brought to the emergency rooms of hospitals, and there is a serious question of overwhelming bacteremia until the blood cultures are shown to be negative.

Course and Prognosis

Relapses and remissions may occur over a period of years. May evolve into or be followed by psoriasis vulgaris.

Management

Acutely ill patients with generalized rash should be hospitalized and treated as a patient with extensive burns: bed rest, isolation, fluid replacement, and repeated blood cultures.

Systemic Therapy   Some patients undergo a rapid, spontaneous remission without any therapy, and if they have had a previous spontaneous remission and are having a recurrence, specific systemic treatment is often omitted. For new patients, most are started on IV antibiotics pend-

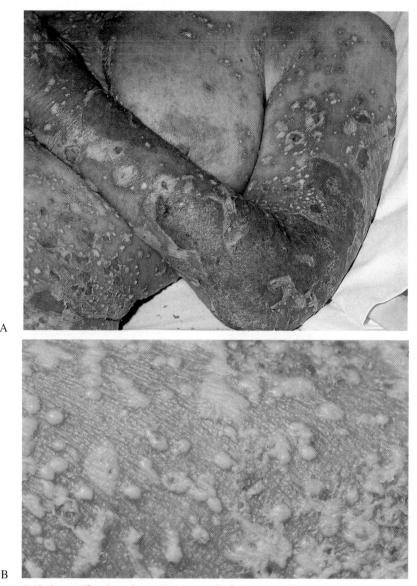

A

B

Figure 4-10 Generalized acute pustular psoriasis (von Zumbusch) *Multiple, creamy-white pustules on an erythematous base coalesce to form lakes of pus; these primary lesions rupture resulting in large areas of secondary erosion. Fever and neutrophilic leukocytosis were also present.*

ing the results of the blood culture. Systemic corticosteroids should be avoided and may be indicated only in the initial toxic phases of an eruption.

Retinoids First-line therapy of generalized pustular psoriasis is oral etretinate or acitretin, 0.5 to 1.0 mg/kg of body weight per day. It may result in rapid cessation of pustular eruptions

but will have to be continued for a considerable time to prevent recurrence.

PUVA Photochemotherapy Highly effective but is often difficult to perform in a toxic patient with fever. It is therefore added to etretinate once systemic symptoms have improved.

Parenteral Methotrexate 15.0 to 25.0 mg once a week. A second-line choice.

ICHTHYOSIFORM DERMATOSES

The ichthyosiform dermatoses are a group of hereditary disorders, characterized by an excess accumulation of cutaneous scale, whose severity varies from very mild and asymptomatic to life-threatening. A relatively large number of types of ichthyosis exist; most are extremely rare and often part of multiorgan syndromes. Only the four most common and important types are discussed below.

Classification

Dominant ichthyosis vulgaris (DIV)
X-linked ichthyosis (XLI)
Lamellar ichthyosis (LI)
Epidermolytic hyperkeratosis (EH)
(For XLI, LI, and EH, see Appendix I)

History

All four types of ichthyosis tend to be worse during the dry, cold winter months and improve during the hot, humid summer. Patients living in tropical climates may remain symptom-free but may experience appearance or worsening of symptoms on moving to a temperate climate.

Diagnosis

Usually made on clinical findings

Pathophysiology

In the various forms of ichthyosis, individual keratin genes may not be expressed or result in the formation of abnormal keratins. LI shows increased germinative cell hyperplasia and increased transit rate through the epidermis, and there is a transglutaminase K deficiency. In DIV and XLI, formation of thickened stratum corneum is caused by increased adhesiveness of the stratum corneum cells and/or failure of normal cell separation. Abnormal stratum corneum formation results in variable increases in transepidermal water loss. In XLI, there is a steroid sulfatase deficiency. In EH, disturbance of epidermal differentiation and expression of abnormal keratin genes result in vacuolization of the upper epidermal layers, blistering, and hyperkeratosis.

Management

Hydration of Stratum Corneum Pliability of stratum corneum is a function of its water content. Hydration is best accomplished by immersion in a bath followed by the application of petrolatum. Urea-containing creams may help bind water in the stratum corneum.

Keratolytic Agents Propylene glycol–glycerin–lactic acid mixtures are effective without occlusion. Another effective preparation is *6 % salicylic acid in propylene glycol and alcohol*; this is used under plastic occlusion. Alpha-hydroxy acids such as lactic acid or glycolic acid bind or control scaling. *Urea-containing preparations* (2 % to 20 %) are effective; some preparations contain both urea and lactic acid.

Systemic Retinoids Isotretinoin, acitretin, and *etretinate* are effective in all four types of ichthyosis, but careful monitoring for toxicity is required. Severe cases may require intermittent therapy over long periods of time.

ICHTHYOSIS VULGARIS

Ichthyosis vulgaris (IV) is characterized by mild generalized hyperkeratosis with xerosis most pronounced on the lower legs and by perifollicular hyperkeratosis (keratosis pilaris) and is frequently associated with atopy.

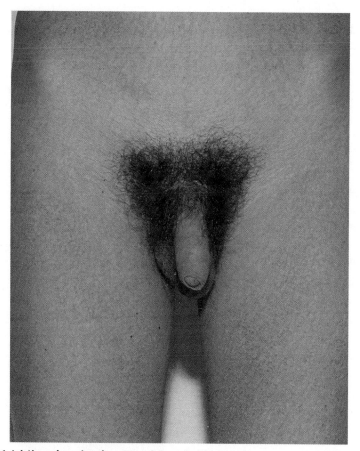

Figure 4-11 Ichthyosis vulgaris *Fine, fish scale-like hyperkeratosis and visible scaling on the thighs and the abdomen, with sparing of the inguinal regions.*

Epidemiology

Sex Equal incidence in males and in females

Mode of Inheritance Autosomal dominant

History

Age of Onset 3 to 12 months

Symptoms Very commonly associated with atopy, i.e., atopic dermatitis, allergic rhinitis, intrinsic asthma. Xerosis and pruritus worse in winter months. Keratosis pilaris and, less commonly, xerosis are of cosmetic concern to many patients. Occasionally, however, hyperkeratosis may be severe.

Physical Examination

Skin Lesions

TYPE Xerosis (dry skin) with fine "powdery" scaling (Figure 4-11). Follicular keratosis, i.e., keratosis pilaris. Hands/feet: palmoplantar markings more prominent (hyperlinear); keratoderma (uncommon). More than 50 % of individuals with IV also have atopic dermatitis (see Atopic Dermatitis, page 54).

COLOR Normal skin color (compare with X-linked ichthyosis)

SHAPE Fish-scale pattern most apparent on the shins (Figure 4-12)

DISTRIBUTION Diffuse involvement, accentuated on the shins, arms, and back. *Tends to spare the axillae and the fossae (antecubital and popliteal);* face usually spared, but cheeks and forehead may be involved (see Figure III), buttocks, lateral thighs; in childhood, keratosis pilaris (Figure 4-13) may be most prominent on the cheeks.

Eye Lesions Keratopathy (rare)

Differential Diagnosis

Xerosis/Hyperkeratosis Xerosis, acquired ichthyosis (may be a paraneoplastic syndrome; must be distinguished from IV), drug-induced ichthyosis (triparanol), X-linked ichthyosis, lamellar ichthyosis, widespread, epidermal dermatophytosis.

Laboratory and Special Examinations

Dermatopathology Compact hyperkeratosis; reduced or absent granular layer; germinative layer flattened. Electron microscopy: small, poorly formed keratohyalin granules.

Diagnosis

Usually by clinical findings; electron microscopic finding of abnormal keratohyalin granules makes the definitive diagnosis.

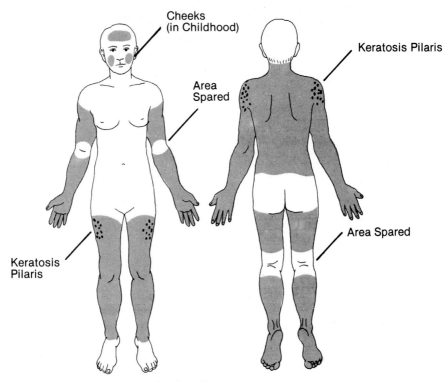

Figure III Ichthyosis vulgaris (dominant)

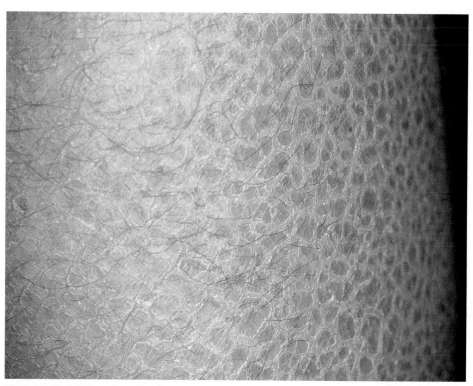

Figure 4-12 Ichthyosis vulgaris *Fine, fish scale-like pattern of adherent hyperkeratosis on the calf.*

Pathogenesis

Epidermis proliferates normally, but keratin is retained with a resultant thickened stratum corneum.

Course and Prognosis

May show improvement in the summer, in humid climates, and in adulthood. Keratosis pilaris occurring on the cheeks during childhood usually improves during adulthood.

Management

Support Group Foundation for Ichthyosis and Related Skin Types (FIRST), P. O. Box 20921, Raleigh, NC 27619; Tel: 800-545-3286; Fax: 919-781-0679.

Emollients There are many. Hydrated petrolatum.

Keratolytics

PROPYLENE GLYCOL 44 % to 60 % in water applied h.s. after bath and occluded with a plastic suit worn as pajamas. When excess scaling has been removed, repeat once weekly as necessary.

OTHER Salicylic acid, urea (10 % to 20 %), alpha-hydroxy acids such as glycolic acid and lactic acid in various vehicles

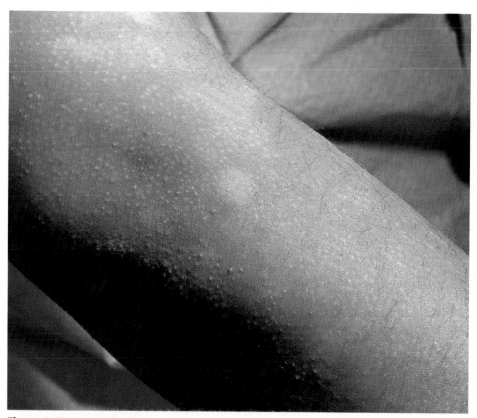

Figure 4-13 Keratosis pilaris *Small, follicular, horny spines occur as a manifestation of mild ichthyosis vulgaris, arising mostly on the shoulders, upper arms, and thighs.*

COLLODION BABY (ICHTHYOSIS IN THE NEWBORN)

Ichthyosis in the newborn presents most commonly as the collodion baby. Encasement in a transparent parchment-like membrane (Figure 4-14) may impair respiration and sucking. Breaking and shedding of the hyperkeratotic collodion membrane may lead initially to difficulties in thermoregulation and increased risk of infection. After healing, the skin will appear normal for some time until signs of ichthyosis develop. Collodion baby may be the initial presentation of lamellar ichthyosis or some less common forms of ichthyosis not discussed here. The collodion baby also may be a form of ichthyosis which, after shedding of the collodion membrane and clearing of the resultant erythema, will lead to normal skin for the rest of the child's life (Figure 4-15).

Harlequin Fetus

Harlequin fetus is a condition in which the child is born with very thick plates of stratum corneum separated by deep cracks and fissures. Eclabium, ectropion, absence of ears, or rudimentary ears give the newborn a grotesque appearance. These children usually die shortly after birth, but there are reports of survival for weeks to several months. This is a condition different from collodion baby and the other forms of ichthyosis with an unusual fibrous protein within the epidermis.

Management

Children should be kept in an incubator in which the air is saturated with water. Careful monitoring of the child's temperature and parenteral fluids and nutrient replacement may be necessary for some time. Infection of the skin and lungs is an important problem, and aggressive antibiotic therapy may be mandatory.

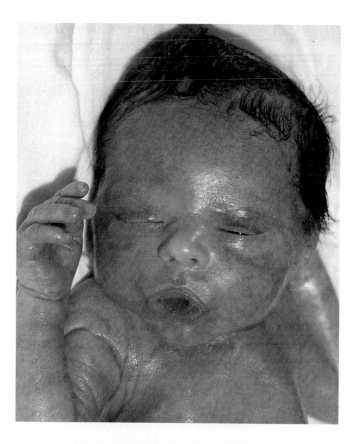

Figure 4-14 Ichthyosis in the newborn *A "collodion baby" shortly after birth with a parchment-like membrane covering the entire skin. The eyes and lips pucker outward, i.e., ectropion and eclabion.*

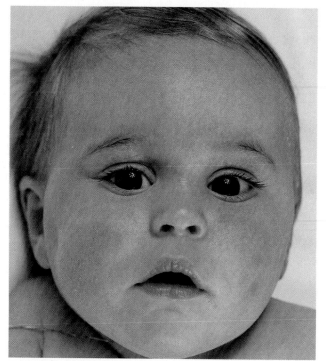

Figure 4-15 *At six months of age, the same infant is a beautiful baby with minimal residual scale and erythema on the cheeks.*

Section 5

MISCELLANEOUS INFLAMMATORY DISORDERS

PITYRIASIS ROSEA

Pityriasis rosea is an acute exanthematous eruption with a distinctive morphology and often with a characteristic course. First, a single (primary or "herald" plaque) lesion develops, usually on the trunk, and 1 or 2 weeks later a generalized secondary eruption develops in a typical distribution pattern; the entire process remits spontaneously in 6 weeks without any therapy.

Epidemiology

Age   10 to 35 years

Incidence   Common

Season   More common in the spring and fall in temperate climates.

History

Duration of Lesions   A single herald patch precedes the exanthematous phase. The exanthematous phase develops over a period of 1 to 2 weeks.

Skin Symptoms   Pruritus—absent (25 %), mild (50 %), or severe (25 %)

Physical Examination

Skin Lesions

TYPE   *Herald Patch*   (80 % of patients) oval, slightly raised plaque 2 to 5 cm, bright red, fine collarette scale at periphery, may be multiple

Exanthem   Fine scaling papules and plaques with typical marginal collarette (Figure 5-1)

COLOR   Dull pink or tawny (exanthem)

SHAPE   Oval lesions

ARRANGEMENT   Scattered discrete lesions (see Distribution, below)

DISTRIBUTION   Characteristic pattern of lesions—the long axes of the lesions follow the lines of cleavage in a "Christmas tree" distribution (see Figure IV). Lesions usually confined to trunk and proximal aspects of the arms and legs. Rarely on face.

Atypical Pityriasis Rosea

Lesions may be present only on the face and neck. The primary plaque may be absent or be the sole manifestation of the disease or be multiple. Most confusing are the examples of pityriasis rosea with vesicles, or purpura or pustules, or simulating erythema multiforme but occurring in the typical distribution of pityriasis rosea. This usually results from irritation and sweating, often as a consequence of inadequate treatment (pityriasis rosea irritata).

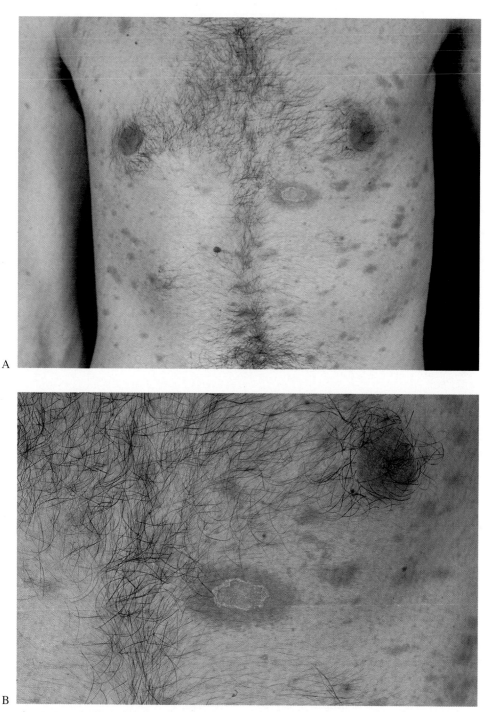

Figure 5-1 Pityriasis rosea: herald patch A *and* B, *An erythematous plaque with scale apparent in the central portion of the lesions. The scale forms a collarette on the trailing edge of the advancing border. Smaller lesions with morphology identical to the herald patch are also seen.*

Differential Diagnosis

Multiple Small Scaling Plaques   *Drug eruptions* (e.g., captopril, barbiturates), *secondary syphilis* (obtain serology, and it is always positive), *guttate psoriasis* (no marginal collarette), *erythema migrans* with secondary lesions

Dermatopathology

Site

EPIDERMIS

Patchy or diffuse parakeratosis
Absence of granular layer
Slight acanthosis
Focal spongiosis, microscopic vesicles
Dyskeratotic cells with an eosinophilic homogenous appearance

DERMIS

Edema
Homogenization of the collagen
Perivascular infiltrate by mononuclear cells

Course

Spontaneous remission in 6 to 12 weeks or less. If the eruption persists for over 6 weeks, a skin biopsy should be done to rule out parapsoriasis. Recurrences are uncommon but do occur.

Management

Pruritus may be controlled by UVB phototherapy or natural sunlight exposure if this is begun in the first week of eruption. The protocol is five consecutive exposures, starting with 80 % of the minimum erythema dose and increasing 20 % each exposure.

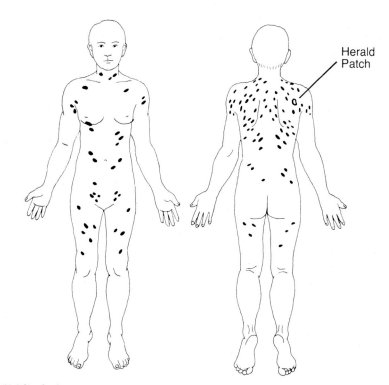

Figure IV Pityriasis rosea

Herald
Patch

GROVER'S DISEASE

Grover's disease (GD), or transient acantholytic dermatosis, is a pruritic dermatosis primarily affecting middle-aged men, located principally on the trunk, and occurring as crops of discrete papular and papulovesicular lesions. As the name implies, the principal histopathologic feature of the lesions is the presence of acantholysis. GD is self-limited but not transient, since the course may last for weeks to several months. The pruritus can be pesky and quite upsetting to work patterns, since the eruption tends to appear at the end of weekends following heavy exercise or in persons who work out during the weekend, especially in hot climates.

Epidemiology

Incidence   Uncommon

Age   Middle age and older, mean age 50 years

Sex   Males > females

Skin Phototype   I and II—so-called fair skin

Precipitating Factors   Heavy, sweat-inducing exercise, excessive solar exposure, persistent fever, exposure to heat or to ionizing radiation; also may occur in bedridden patients, with heat and sweating as factors.

History

Onset   Usually abrupt onset of crops of lesions, possibly correlated with heavy exercise, excessive sun exposure, or high fever

Skin Symptoms   Pruritus

Physical Examination

Skin Lesions

TYPE   Papules (small, 3 to 5 mm, some with slight scale or smooth) (Figure 5-2), papulovesicles, and erosions.

COLOR   Skin color or grayish pink

PALPATION   Smooth or warty

ARRANGEMENT   Scattered, discrete, no special grouping

DISTRIBUTION   Central trunk

Differential Diagnosis

The differential clinical diagnosis includes Darier-White disease, heat rash (miliaria rubra), papular urticaria, scabies, dermatitis herpetiformis (grouping is present and the lesions are symmetrical), *Pityrosporum* or eosinophilic folliculitis, insect bites, and drug eruptions.

Laboratory and Special Examinations

Dermatopathology

LIGHT MICROSCOPY   *Site*   Mainly the epidermis and papillary dermis
   Process   Acantholysis and spongiosis, focal acantholytic dyskeratosis with different patterns occurring at the same time and simulating Darier-White disease, pemphigus foliaceus, and Hailey-Hailey disease; in the dermis there is a superficial infiltrate of eosinophils, lymphocytes, and histiocytes.

Illumination (Side-Lighting in a Partially Darkened Room)   This permits the examiner to better see the eruption, since the contrast is accentuated. Allow for dark adaptation.

Diagnosis

The diagnosis of GD may be subtle, and a biopsy is required; the histology findings are diagnostic.

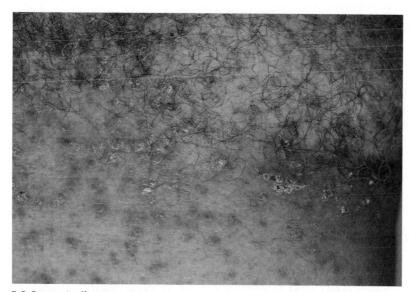

Figure 5-2 Grover's disease *Scaling papule with scales and crusts confluent on the central trunk of a male.*

Course and Prognosis

The disease is by no means always transient, and there appear to be two types: acute and chronic relapsing. The mean duration in one series was 47 weeks.

Management

Topical Class II topical corticosteroids under plastic (e.g., dry-cleaning plastic suit bags) are used for 4 hours or more.

Systemic Oral corticosteroids and dapsone have been used with success, but relapses occur following withdrawal.

Phototherapy UVB or PUVA photochemotherapy is useful for patients who do not respond to topical corticosteroids under plastic.

KYRLE'S DISEASE

Kyrle's disease (KD) is a disorder of keratinization first described by Joseph Kyrle (1916), characterized clinically by scattered or grouped keratotic papules on the extremities and trunk, occurring most commonly in the setting of diabetes mellitus and renal failure but also without associated disease, and characterized histologically by an invaginating epidermal keratotic plug that may perforate the dermal-epidermal junction into the underlying dermis.

Synonym: Hyperkeratosis follicularis et parafollicularis in cutem penetrans.

Epidemiology

Incidence   Uncommon

Age   Third to seventh decade; rarely in infancy or childhood

Sex   Females > males

Associated Diseases   Commonly, diabetes mellitus and renal failure. Other possibilities: hepatic insufficiency, congestive heart failure, hypothyroidism, hyperlipoproteinemia.

History

Onset   Insidious, asynchronous eruption and evolution of lesions

Skin Symptoms   Early lesions, asymptomatic to slightly pruritic. Older, larger lesions may be quite painful, especially with applied pressure. Traumatized lesions may become secondarily infected.

Systems Review   Those of associated disorders

Family History   First-degree relatives may be affected.

Physical Examination

Skin Lesions

TYPE   Initial lesion is a small, skin-colored, hyperkeratotic papule. Over time, lesions enlarge to form papules, nodules, and plaques surmounted by moderate to striking hyper-keratotic plugs (Figure 5-3). Removal of the plug leaves a crateriform depressed papule to nodule. Resolution of lesions, spontaneously or after therapy, usually leaves atrophic scars.

COLOR   Early lesions are skin-colored, but larger lesions are hyperpigmented, becoming dark brown to nearly black in individuals with darker skin pigmentation.

PALPATION   Firm; rough surface. Often larger lesions are tender.

ARRANGEMENT   Scattered, clustered, coalescence of enlarging lesions. Linear arrangement at sites of scratching.

DISTRIBUTION   Extensor surfaces of extremities, trunk, buttocks. Mucous membranes not involved.

General Examination   The majority of patients with KD have diabetes mellitus with renal failure.

Differential Diagnosis

Multiple Keratotic Papules/Nodules   Prurigo nodularis, multiple keratoacanthomas, perforating folliculitis, elastosis perforans serpiginosa, reactive perforating collagenosis, atypical mycobacterial infection, verruca vulgaris

Laboratory Examination

Dermatopathology

LIGHT MICROSCOPY   *Site*   Follicular and interfollicular epidermis and in the acrosyringium

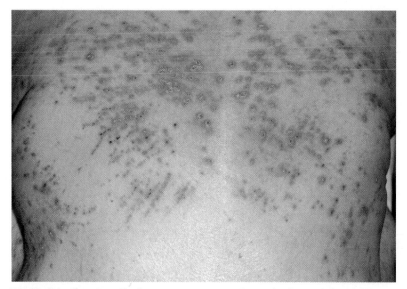

Figure 5-3 Kyrle's disease *Erythematous-to-tan papules and a few nodules with keratotic caps on the upper back, many with linear arrangement, at the sites of scratching, in an elderly female with diabetes mellitus.*

Process Central epidermal invagination forming a dilated keratotic plug with focal parakeratotic and basophilic debris; marked thinning or perforation of the epidermis; neutrophilic infiltrate at sites where the base of the keratotic plug contacts the dermis; lymphohistiocytic dermal infiltrate about the lesion

Chemistry Tests to check for diabetes mellitus

Diagnosis

Clinical findings confirmed by biopsy

Pathogenesis

Unknown; however, thought to represent an uncoupling of differentiation and keratinization leading to the migration of the level of keratinization toward the dermal-epidermal junction.

Course and Prognosis

This disease runs a chronic course. After spontaneous or traumatic excavation of the keratotic plug, the lesions may heal with atrophic, depressed scars with spotty pigmentary changes. Local recurrence is common.

Management

Destructive Modalities Destruction of individual lesions by cryo- , electro- , or CO_2 laser surgery with resultant scar formation may preclude recurrence of lesions at the treatment site.

Topical Agents Tretinoin gel or cream. Keratolytics such as salicylic acid also can flatten lesions.

Oral Retinoid High-dose etretinate may clear the lesions, but the need for chronic administration precludes the practicality of its use.

DISORDERS OF PSYCHIATRIC ETIOLOGY

Classification of Disorders of Psychiatric Etiology

Compulsive habits
  Neurotic excoriations
Delusions
  Delusions of parasitosis
  Dysmorphic syndrome
Factitious syndromes

NEUROTIC EXCORIATIONS

Neurotic excoriations present as an admixture of several types of lesions, principally excoriations, all produced by habitual picking of the skin with the fingernails; most often on the upper back, face, and extremities.

Epidemiology

Incidence Relatively common, although no prevalence data are available.

Age Third and fifth decades

Sex Females > males

History

Duration of Lesions Weeks to months

Relationship of Skin Lesions to Stress The patient may relate the onset to a specific event or to an ongoing stress. Patients often deny picking or scratching.

Skin Symptoms The patient often will volunteer that the pruritus disappears after the epidermis has been picked away.

Physical Examination

Skin Lesions

TYPES Excoriation with or without crust (Figures 6-1 and 6-2). Scars (macular and depressed)

COLOR Depigmented atrophic (scarred) macules, hyperpigmented macules

SHAPE Linear pattern not uncommon

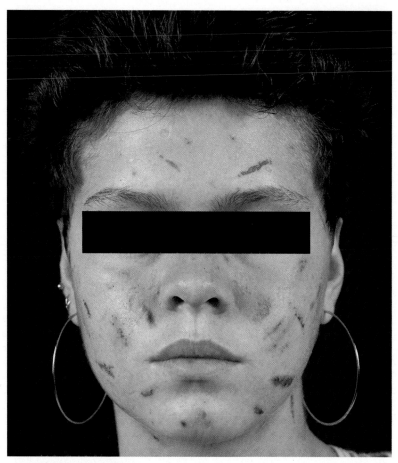

Figure 6-1 Neurotic excoriations   *Linear erosions (excoriations) on the face of a young woman with minimal acne vulgaris (acné excoriée des jeunes filles). Patients may be anxious or depressed and may intentionally or inadvertently excoriate small acne lesions, subsequently excoriating the crusts which they have created. When the behavior is discontinued, lesions may heal with hypopigmented macules or depressed scars. Patient admits doing this in front of a mirror.*

ARRANGEMENT OF MULTIPLE LESIONS   Scattered

DISTRIBUTION OF LESIONS   Trunk (only in areas the patient can reach and thus sparing the center of the back), extremities, face most common

Diagnosis

This may be difficult, and a careful workup for serious causes of pruritus is sometimes necessary unless the presentation is obvious.

Etiology and Pathogenesis

Psychiatric guidance is helpful; the patient may be obsessive-compulsive, rigid, perfectionistic, or depressed.

Significance

This is an important condition because it can be very disruptive not only to the patient but also to the family.

Course and Prognosis

Prolonged, unless life adjustments are made

Management

Topical   Menthol-camphor antipruritic lotions

Systemic   Pimozide (Orap) has been helpful in some patients. Pimozide blocks the receptors for opiates and dopamine and therefore may block the itch sensation. Also, antidepressant drugs: fluoxetine and clomipramine.

Psychotherapy   The patient should be evaluated at least once by a psychiatrist. Behavioral modification has been said to be effective.

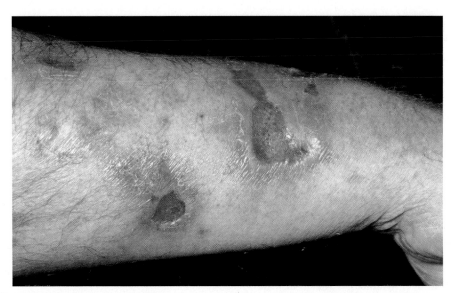

Figure 6-2 Neurotic excoriations *Large ulcerations with geographic shapes and old scars. The patient was very depressed, slept poorly, and admitted to creating the lesions in the early morning hours.*

DELUSIONS OF PARASITOSIS

This disorder is characterized by the presence of numerous skin lesions, mostly excoriations, which the patient truly believes are the result of a parasitic infestation.

Epidemiology

Incidence   Rare

Age   Adults

Precipitating Factors   The onset of the initial pruritus or paresthesia may be related to xerosis or, in fact, a previously treated infestation.

History

Duration of Symptoms   Months to years

Skin Symptoms   Pruritus, pain, paresthesia

Physical Examination

Skin Lesions

TYPES   Excoriations (Figure 6-3), scratch papules, or gouges

DISTRIBUTION   Generalized

Differential Diagnosis

It is important to rule out other causes of pruritus (see Appendix C).

Diagnosis

Patients usually have only one delusion; they will bring in fomites and other minute pieces of their own dried skin, believing that these are the actual parasites.

Significance

This is a serious problem; patients truly suffer and are opposed to seeking psychiatric help.

Course and Prognosis

Months, and patients may sell their houses to move away from the offending parasite.

Management

The patient should see a psychiatrist for at least one visit and for recommendations of drug therapy: pimozide plus an antidepressant. Treatment is often difficult.

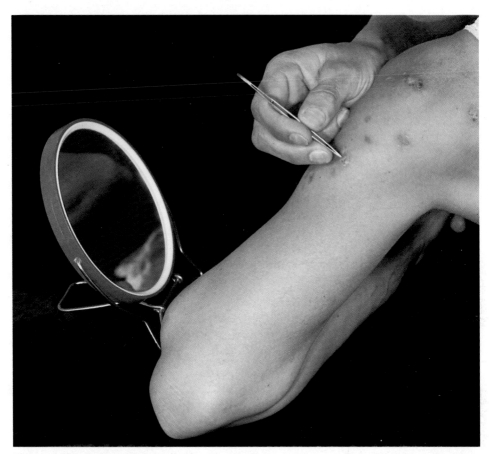

Figure 6-3 Delusions of parasitosis *Usually patients collect small pieces of debris from their skin by scratching with their nails and submit them to the doctor for examination for parasites. Occasionally this can progress to an aggressive behavior such as depicted in this case where the patient posed to demonstrate how she removes the "parasites" from her skin with a mirror and tweezers. "Objects" are then meticulously collected on a piece of paper that is submitted for examination. In the majority of cases, patients are not dissuaded from their monosymptomatic delusion unless treated with pimozide.*

FACTITIOUS SYNDROMES

The term *factitial* means "artificial," and in this condition there is a self-induced dermatologic lesion(s) which (1) the patient can claim no responsibility for or (2) it is determined that the patient is deliberately mutilating the skin.
Synonym: Munchhausen's syndrome.

Epidemiology

Age Adolescents and young adults

Sex Females >> males

History

The patient gives a vague history ("hollow history") of the evolution of the lesions.

Duration of Lesions Weeks, months, years

Physical Examination

Appearance of Patient May be normal looking and acting in every respect, although frequently there is a strange affect and bizarre personality.

Skin

TYPES OF LESIONS Scars, ulcers, sphacelus (dense adherent necrotic membrane) (Figure 6-4)

SHAPE OF INDIVIDUAL LESION Linear, bizarre shapes, geometric patterns

ARRANGEMENT OF LESIONS Single or multiple, bilateral or unilateral

DISTRIBUTION OF LESIONS Rarer on the face, but do occur there.

Differential Diagnosis

Large Ulcers/Scars Infections, granulomas, vasculitis

Diagnosis

The nature of the lesions (bizarre shapes) may immediately suggest an artificial etiology, but it is important to rule out every possible cause and perform a biopsy before assigning the diagnosis of *dermatosis artefacta*. This is for the benefit of the patient and because the physician may be at risk for malpractice if he or she fails to diagnose a true pathologic process. This makes it a difficult task.

Etiology and Pathogenesis

Serious personality and/or psychosocial stress

Significance

The condition demands the utmost tact on the part of the physician, who can avert a serious outcome (i.e., suicide) by attempting to gain enough empathy with the patient to ascertain the cause.

Course and Prognosis

This varies with the nature of the psychiatric problem. The condition may persist for years in a patient who has selected his or her skin as the target organ of his or her conflicts.

Management

Consultation and even management with a psychiatrist are mandatory in most patients.

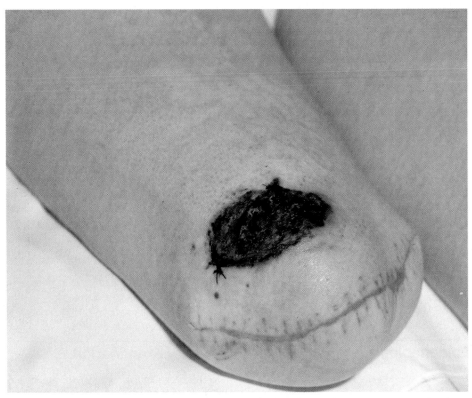

Figure 6-4 Factitious syndrome *This sharply demarcated necrosis was self-inflicted by the covert application of potassium hydroxide incorporated into soap and applied to the skin with a tightly fitting bandage. Similar ulcers had previously been present first on the toes and later on the lower extremities and have led to successive steps of amputation.*

DYSMORPHIC SYNDROME (DS)

Patients with dysmorphic syndrome (dysmorphia, Greek: "ugly") regard their image as distorted in the eyes of the public; this becomes almost an obsession. The patient with DS does not consult a psychiatrist, but a dermatologist or plastic surgeon. The typical patient with DS is a single, female, young adult who is an anxious and unhappy person. Common dermatologic complaints are facial (wrinkles, acne, scars, hypertrichosis, dry lips), scalp (incipient baldness, increased hair growth), genital (normal sebaceous glands on the penis, red scrotum, red vulva, vaginal odor), hyperhidrosis, and bromhidrosis. Management is a problem. One strategy is for the dermatologist to agree with the patient that there is a problem and thus establish rapport; in a few visits the complaint can be explored and further discussed. If the patient and physician do not agree that the complaint is a vastly exaggerated skin or hair change, then the patient should be referred to a psychiatrist; this latter plan is usually not accepted, in which case the problem may persist indefinitely.

Section 7

DISORDERS OF ORAL MUCOSA

DISORDERS OF THE TONGUE

HAIRY TONGUE

Hairy tongue is a disorder in which the hairlike filiform papillae that make up most of the dorsal surface of the tongue become increased in length and thickness as a result of the slowing of the normal removal of "squames" (i.e., scales) from the tips of the filiform papillae. Hairy tongue is also usually pigmented ("black") related to overgrowth of pigment-forming bacteria.

Epidemiology

Incidence Common

Age Adults. Children can have an off-white, "furred" tongue that occurs with fever.

Precipitating Factors Fever, dehydration, reduction in the normal salivary flow and the oral movements that promote desquamation; also, ingestion of antibiotics that can lead to an imbalance in the normal bacterial flora.

History

Relationship of Lesions to Medications (oral antibiotics); other factors (see Precipitating Factors, above)

Mucosal Symptoms None, but some patients note a bad taste or gagging with swallowing.

Physical Examination

The filiform papillae are hyperkeratotic and "coated" on the middorsal surface (Figure 7-1).

Management

When the precipitating factors are eliminated, the condition disappears. However, to speed the recovery, local measures can be used such as treatment with antimicrobial mouthwashes and using a toothbrush to dislodge the adherent material.

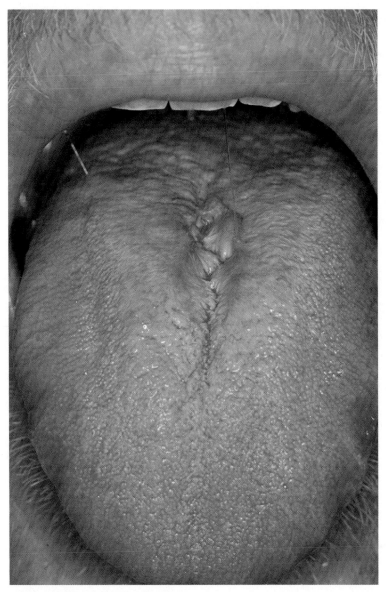

Figure 7-1 Hairy tongue *Note hairlike filiform hyperkeratoses of the papillae resulting in a brownish coating on the dorsum of the tongue.*

FISSURED TONGUE

A common benign, asymptomatic disorder in which there are changes in the surface morphology of the dorsum of the tongue; the tongue has numerous linear "valleys," resulting in a corrugated appearance.
Synonym: "Scrotal" tongue.

Epidemiology

Incidence   Estimated to be 5 % of the population

History

Common findings in otherwise healthy individuals.

Physical Examination

Dorsum of the Tongue

TYPE OF LESION   "Fissures" (Figure 7-2). The linear patterns are related to the deep valleys in the dorsal tongue that do not involve the mucosal epithelium and are therefore not painful.

COLOR   Normal red

PALPATION   Not indurated

General Examination   Nervous system: facial palsy when associated with Melkersson-Rosenthal syndrome; mental retardation (Down's syndrome)

Course

Persists and becomes more exaggerated throughout life

Management

Reassurance

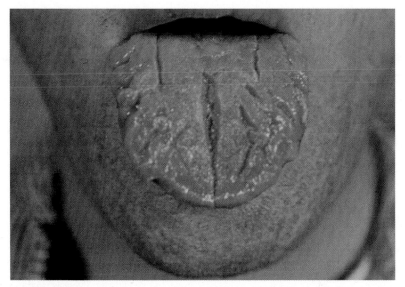

Figure 7-2 Fissured tongue *Deep furrows on the dorsum of the tongue are asymptomatic.*

MIGRATORY GLOSSITIS

Migratory glossitis is the most common of several conditions that have been termed *psoriasiform* lesions. These disorders present as reddish-white areas on the tongue. About 40 % of patients also have a fissured tongue.
Synonyms: Glossitis migrans, geographic tongue.

Epidemiology and Etiology

Incidence   2 % of the population

Age   Onset in young adults and persisting for life

Etiology   Unknown

History

Duration of Lesions   Wax and wane, sometimes over a period of hours

Mucosal Symptoms   None or minor irritation

Physical Examination

Lesions

TYPE   Sharply demarcated areas with a white rim and a depapillation of the tongue surface (Figure 7-3)

COLOR   Red

SHAPE   Irregular, "geographic," maplike

DISTRIBUTION   Dorsum of the tongue and rarely other areas of the mucosa and called *geographic stomatitis*

Differential Diagnosis

Hairy tongue, oral hairy leukoplakia, candidiasis, lichen planus

Laboratory and Special Examinations

Dermatopathology   Hyperkeratosis at the edge and spongiosis. There is migration in the epidermis of polymorphonuclear cells and lymphocytes, sometimes forming microabscesses. In the dermis, there may be nonspecific inflammatory infiltrates.

KOH Preparation   Rule out candidiasis.

Diagnosis

Clinical findings

Significance

Important to recognize and to reassure the patient of the benign nature of the condition; may be present in psoriasis

Course

Waxes and wanes over a lifetime; patients may be asymptomatic for years

Management

Reassure the patient as to the benign nature of the disorder.

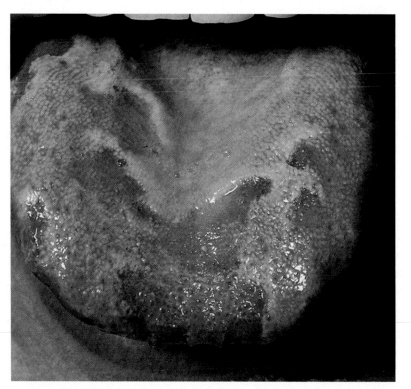

Figure 7-3 Geographic tongue (migratory glossitis) *Areas of hyperkeratosis alternate with areas of normal pink epithelium, creating a geographic pattern.*

MISCELLANEOUS DISORDERS OF BUCCAL AND GINGIVAL MUCOUS MEMBRANES

APHTHOUS ULCER

Aphthous ulcers (AU) are painful mucosal ulcerations of idiopathic etiology occurring commonly in the oropharynx and less commonly in the esophagus, upper and lower GI tracts, and anogenital epithelium, characterized clinically by pain and sharply marginated gray-based, red-rimmed ulcer(s). *Synonyms:* Aphthous (ancient Greek word for "ulcer") stomatitis, canker sores. Minor AU: recurrent aphthae of Mikulicz. Major AU: Sutton's disease, periadenitis mucosa necrotica recurrens.

Epidemiology and Etiology

Age Any age; often during second decade, persisting into adulthood, and becoming less frequent with advancing age

Sex Females > males

Etiology Unknown

Incidence Extremely common; the majority of adults experience AU at some time during their lives.

Risk Factors Local trauma, heredity

Associated Disorders Behçet's disease, cyclic neutropenia, HIV disease

Classification

Minor (MiAU), <1 cm in diameter. Major (MaAu) up to 3 cm
Herpetiform (HAU), up to 100 tiny erosions

History

AU may occur at the site of minor mucosal injury, such as a minor bite by teeth.

Symptoms Even though small, AU can be quite painful, which may impair nutrition. A burning or tingling sensation may be felt prior to ulceration. In persons with severe AU, malaise: weight loss associated with persistent, painful AU.

Physical Examination

Mucous Membranes

TYPE At times, small, painful red macule or papule prior to ulceration. More commonly, ulcer(s) (Figure 7-4), covered with fibrin (gray-white), with sharp, discrete, and at times edematous borders, MaAU may heal with white, depressed scars.

COLOR White-gray base with an erythematous rim

PALPATION Not indurated

SHAPE Round or oval

ARRANGEMENT Most commonly single; at times, multiple or numerous small, shallow, grouped—i.e., herpetiform

DISTRIBUTION Oropharyngeal, anogenital, any site in the GI tract. Oral lesions most commonly on the buccal and labial mucosae, less commonly on tongue, sulci, floor of mouth. MiAU rarely occur on the palate or gums. MaAU often occur on soft palate and pharynx.

NUMBER MiAU, 1 to 5; MaAU, 1 to 10; HAU up to 100

General Findings With MaAU, occasionally tender cervical lymphadenopathy. Findings of Behçet's disease, cyclic neutropenia, HIV disease

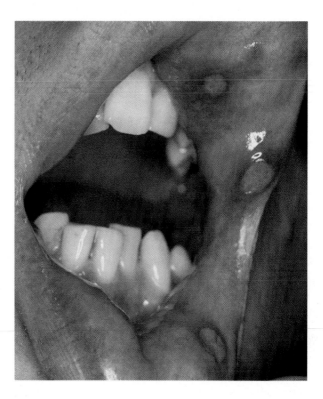

Figure 7-4 Aphthous ulcers
Multiple, very painful, gray-based ulcers with erythematous halos on the labial mucosa. Ulcers usually occur singly but can be multiple. In this case, the patient also had genital aphthous ulcers with a diagnosis of Behçet's disease.

Differential Diagnosis

Oropharyngeal Ulcer(s) Primary herpetic gingivostomatitis, herpangina, hand-foot-and-mouth disease, bullous diseases (erythema multiforme, pemphigus vulgaris, bullous pemphigoid, cicatricial pemphigoid), lichen planus, Reiter's syndrome, adverse drug reaction (fixed eruption, systemic chemotherapy, gold), squamous cell carcinoma, Behçet's disease

Dermatopathology

The findings are not diagnostic, showing varying degrees of epithelial ulceration and inflammatory response; specific causes of epithelial ulceration can be ruled out by histologic findings, including infection (syphilitic chancre, histoplasmosis), inflammatory disorders (lichen planus), or cancers (squamous cell carcinoma).

Diagnosis

Usually by clinical findings

Pathophysiology

Unknown; probably immune-mediated tissue damage

Course and Prognosis

In many persons, MiAU tend to recur during adulthood. Uncommonly, may be almost constant in the oropharynx or anogenitalia, referred to as *complex aphthosis*. MiAU heal spontaneously in 1 to 2 weeks. MaAU may persist for 6 weeks or more, healing with scarring. HAU usually heal in 1 to 2 weeks. Behçet's disease should be considered in patients with persistent oropharyngeal AU, with or without anogenital AU, associated with systemic findings.

Management

Topical Modalities Tetracycline retention "enema" (the contents of one capsule suspended in water and held in the mouth for 15 minutes), topical corticosteroids (Kenalog in Orabase, Diprolene ointment), topical anesthetics (diphenhydramine elixir, EMLA, viscous lidocaine). Cauterization with $AgNO_3$ stick will alleviate pain and accelerate healing in individual lesions.

Intralesional Corticosteroid Injection Triamcinolone, 3 to 10 mg/ml

Systemic Therapy In persons with large, persistent, painful AU interfering with nutrition, a brief course of oral corticosteroids is effective. Thalidomide particularly has been used in persons with HIV disease and large, painful AU.

MUCOCELE

This is a painless, translucent, blister-like swelling of the mucous membrane that is easily ruptured and drains a clear fluid and then refills. It develops at sites where minor salivary glands are easily traumatized: mucous membranes of the lip and floor of the mouth. May be chronic, recurrent, and then it presents as a firm, inflamed nodule.
Synonym: Ranula.

Epidemiology

Incidence Common

Age More frequent in younger persons

Sex Males > females

Precipitating Factors Physical trauma to minor salivary glands

History

Duration of Lesions Weeks, but may recur in same site for months, and chronic lesions may be present for a year or longer.

Physical Examination

Lesions

TYPE Mucus-filled cavity, with a thick roof (Figure 7-5); chronic lesions are firm, inflamed, poorly circumscribed nodules.

COLOR Bluish, translucent

PALPATION Fluctuant

SITE Areas in the mouth where salivary glands are exposed to trauma, i.e., floor of the mouth, lower lip

epidermal site of the basement membrane; in other words, they are intraepidermal.

2. *Compound melanocytic NCN:* Nevus cells invade the papillary dermis, and nevus cell nests are now found both intraepidermally and dermally.

3. *Dermal melanocytic NCN:* These represent the last stage of the evolution of NCN. "Dropping off" (*Abtropfung*) into the dermis is now completed, and the nevus grows or rests intradermally. With progressive age, there will be gradual fibrosis.

Since common melanocytic NCN lose their capacity for melanization, the further the nevus cells penetrate into the dermis, the lesser is the intensity of pigmentation with the increase in the dermal proportion of the nevus. Purely dermal NCN are therefore almost always without pigment.

Junctional Melanocytic Nevocellular Nevi

Skin Lesions

TYPE Macule, or only very slightly raised (Figure 8-1)

SIZE If >1.0 cm, the mole is a congenital nevomelanocytic nevus or a dysplastic melanocytic nevus.

COLOR Uniform tan, brown, or dark brown

SHAPE Round or oval with smooth, regular borders

ARRANGEMENT Scattered discrete lesions

DISTRIBUTION Random

SITES OF PREDILECTION Trunk, upper extremities, face, lower extremities, occasionally palmar and plantar

Differential Diagnosis

Tan/Brown/Black Macule Solar lentigo, lentigo maligna

Compound Melanocytic Nevocellular Nevi

Compound melanocytic nevocellular nevi represent a combination of junctional and dermal NCN and are usually darkly pigmented (junctional component of NCN), elevated, and often papillomatous due to their dermal component.

Skin Lesions

TYPE Papules or nodules (Figure 8-2)

COLOR Dark brown, sometimes even black; color may become mottled as progressive conversion into dermal NCN occurs

SHAPE Round, dome-shaped, smooth, occasionally papillomatous or hyperkeratotic, often associated with bristle-like terminal hairs

DISTRIBUTION Face, scalp, trunk, extremities

Differential Diagnosis

Tan/Brown/Black Papule Seborrheic keratosis, dermatofibroma, dysplastic nevus, Spitz nevus, blue nevus, and nodular melanoma must be considered.

Figure 8-1 Junctional nevomelanocytic nevus *Two uniformly brown small macules, round in shape with smooth regular borders.*

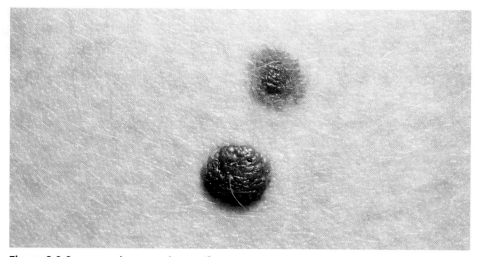

Figure 8-2 Compound nevomelanocytic nevus *Uniformly pigmented, papule and domed nodule, tan (with a more elevated, darker center) and chocolate brown, dark brown to sometimes black papules. The larger lesion is older; the smaller is younger and has a predominantly junctional component at the periphery.*

Dermal Melanocytic Nevocellular Nevi

Skin Lesions

TYPE   Papule or Nodule

COLOR   Skin-colored, tan, brown, or flecks of brown, often with telangiectasia

SHAPE   Round, dome-shaped (Figure 8-3)

DISTRIBUTION   More common on the face and neck but can occur on the trunk or extremities

OTHER FEATURES   Usually present in the second or third decade. Older lesions, mostly on the trunk, may become papillomatous or pedunculated and do not disappear spontaneously

Differential Diagnosis

Skin-Colored Papule   Basal cell carcinoma, neurofibroma, trichoepithelioma, sebaceous hyperplasia, dermatofibroma

Management of Melanocytic NCN

Indications for removal of acquired melanocytic NCN are

1. Site—lesions on the scalp, soles, all mucous membranes, anogenital area
2. Color—if color is or becomes variegated
3. Border—if irregular borders are present or develop
4. Symptoms—if lesion begins to persistently itch, hurt, or bleed
5. If criteria for malignancy are detected by epiluminescence microscopy

Melanocytic NCN never become malignant because of manipulation or trauma. If there is an indication for the removal of an NCN, the nevus always should be excised for histologic diagnosis and for definite treatment (this particularly applies to and is decisive in ruling out congenital, dysplastic, or blue nevi).

Removal of papillomatous, compound, or dermal NCN for cosmetic reasons by electrocautery requires that a nevus be unequivocally diagnosed as benign NCN and histology be performed. If an early melanoma cannot be excluded with certainty, an excision for histologic examination is obligatory but can be performed with narrow margins.

The criteria listed above are based on anatomic sites at risk for change of acquired nevi to malignant melanoma or changes in individual lesions (color, border) that indicate the development of a focus of cells with dysplasia, the precursor of malignant melanoma. Clark's dysplastic melanocytic nevi are usually >6.0 mm, with distinctive variegation of color (tan, brown) and irregular borders. These lesions occur over the trunk and upper extremities but also on the buttocks, groin, scalp, and female breasts and may arise *de novo* during adulthood.

See also Recommendations for the Management of Pigmented Lesions to Facilitate Early Diagnosis of Malignant Melanoma in Appendix E.

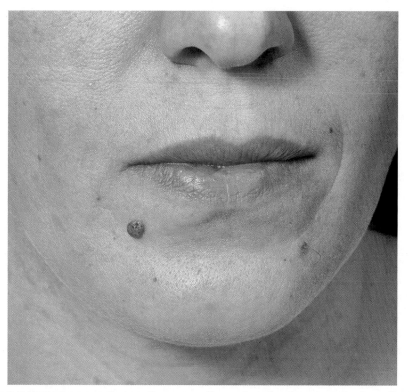

Figure 8-3 Dermal nevomelanocytic nevus *Dome-shaped, soft, tan papule. A smaller dermal nevus is seen on the opposite side.*

HALO NEVOMELANOCYTIC NEVUS

This lesion is a nevomelanocytic nevus that is encircled by a halo of leukoderma or depigmentation. The leukoderma is based on a decrease of melanin in melanocytes or disappearance of melanocytes at the dermal-epidermal junction. Halo nevi often undergo spontaneous involution and often with regression of the centrally located pigmented nevus.
Synonym: Sutton's leukoderma acquisitum centrifugum.

Epidemiology and Etiology

Age   First three decades

Race and Sex   All races, both sexes

Incidence   Occurs in patients with vitiligo, 18 % to 26 %. May herald vitiligo

Family History   Halo nevi occur in siblings and with history of vitiligo in family.

Associated Disorders   Vitiligo, metastatic melanoma (around lesions and around nevus cell nevi)

History

Three Stages

1. Development (in months) of halo around preexisting nevus cell nevus. Halo may be preceded by faint erythema
2. Disappearance (months to years) of nevus cell nevus
3. Repigmentation (months to years) of halo

Physical Examination

Skin Lesions

TYPE   Papular brown nevus cell nevus (5.0 mm) with halo of sharply marginated hy-pomelanosis (Figure 8-4). The nevus is centrally located.

SHAPE   Oval or round hypomelanosis

ARRANGEMENT   Scattered discrete lesions (1 to 90)

DISTRIBUTION   Trunk (same as distribution of nevus cell nevus)

Differential Diagnosis

"Halo" Depigmentation around Other Lesions   Can occur around blue nevus, congenital garment nevus cell nevus, Spitz's juvenile nevus, verruca plana, primary melanoma, dermatofibroma, and neurofibroma.

Dermatopathology

Nevus Cell Nevus   Junctional dermal or compound nevus surrounded by lymphocytic infiltrate (lymphocytes and histiocytes) around and between nevus cells. Nevus cells develop evidence of cell damage and disappear.

Halo (Epidermis)   Decrease or total absence of melanin and melanocytes (as shown by electron microscopy

Diagnosis

If clinical findings atypical, confirm histologically

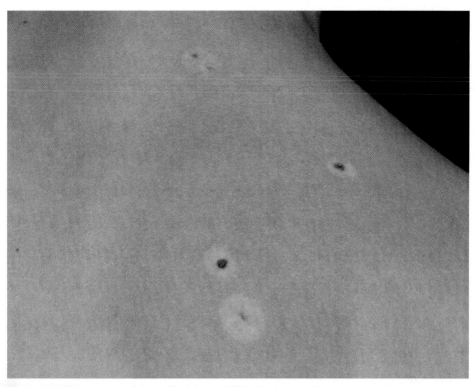

Figure 8-4 Halo nevomelanocytic nevus *White depigmented halos surround several compound nevomelanocytic nevi on the upper back; in time, the nevus may disappear leaving only the white macular portion.*

Pathophysiology

Immunologic phenomena are responsible for the dynamic changes through the action of circulating cytotoxic antibodies and/or cytotoxic lymphocytes. This disease awaits a reevaluation using newer techniques.

Course

The lesions undergo spontaneous resolution. Nevus cell nevi within the halo always must be evaluated for clinical criteria of malignancy (variegation of pigment and irregular borders) because a halo can and does occasionally develop around primary malignant melanoma.

Management

Reassurance

Excision If clinical findings are atypical, diagnosis uncertain, lesion should be excised.

BLUE NEVUS

A blue nevus is an acquired, benign, firm, dark-blue to gray-to-black, sharply defined papule or nodule representing a localized proliferation of melanin-producing dermal melanocytes. *Synonyms:* Blue neuronevus, dermal melanocytoma.

Epidemiology and Etiology

Age Onset in late adolescence

Sex Equal distribution

Variants Cellular blue nevus, combined blue nevus–nevomelanocytic nevus

History

Nearly always asymptomatic, occasionally of cosmetic concern. Appearance gradual and often not observed by patient or parents.

Physical Examination

Skin Lesions

TYPE Papules to nodules usually <10.0 mm in diameter (Figure 8-5)

COLOR Blue, blue-gray, blue-black. Occasionally has target-like pattern of pigmentation

SHAPE Usually round to oval

PALPATION Firm

SITES OF PREDILECTION Most common on dorsa of hands or feet; may occur at any site.

Differential Diagnosis

Blue/Gray Papule Dermatofibroma, glomus tumor, primary (nodular) or metastatic melanoma, pigmented spindle cell (Spitz) nevus, traumatic tattoo

Dermatopathology

Melanin-containing fibroblast-like dermal melanocytes grouped in irregular bundles admixed with melanin-containing macrophages; excessive fibrous tissue production in upper reticular dermis. Epidermis normal.

Diagnosis

Usually made on clinical findings including epiluminescence microscopy, at times confirmed by excision and dermatopathologic examination to rule out nodular melanoma

Pathogenesis

Probably represents ectopic accumulations of melanin-producing melanocytes in the dermis during their migration from neural crest to sites in the skin.

Course and Prognosis

Most remain unchanged. Malignant melanoma rarely develops in blue nevi.

Management

Blue nevi smaller than 10.0 mm in diameter and stable for many years usually do not need excision. Sudden appearance or change of an apparent blue nevus warrants surgical excision and dermatopathologic examination.

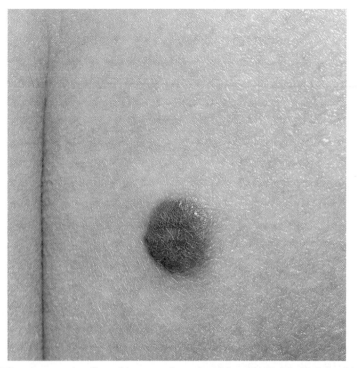

Figure 8-5 Blue nevus *A solitary blue-gray dermal nodule with slightly ill-defined borders on the posterior arm.*

SPITZ NEVUS

Spitz nevus is a benign, dome-shaped, hairless, small (<1.0 cm in diameter) nodule, most often pink or tan. About half the patients are children. The clinical presentation is distinctive, and there is often a history of recent rapid growth. However, the pathology of Spitz nevus is misleading, consisting of spindle and epithelioid nevus cells, some of which may be atypical. Differentiation from nodular malignant melanoma may require the help of an experienced dermatopathologist.
Synonyms: Spitz tumor, formerly also juvenile melanoma, epithelioid cell–spindle cell nevomelanocytic nevus.

Epidemiology

Incidence   1.4:100,000 (Australia)

Age   Occurs at all ages. A third of the patients are children under 10 years of age, a third are 10 to 20 years old, and a third are older than 20; rarely seen in persons 40 years of age or older.

History

Onset of Lesions   Recent (within months). The large majority of the lesions (>90 %) are acquired.

Skin Symptoms   None

Family History   None

Physical Examination

Skin Lesions

TYPE   Papule or nodule, smooth-topped, hairless

COLOR   Uniform pink (Figure 8-6), tan (Figure 8-7), brown, dark brown

PALPATION   Form: nodule

SHAPE OF INDIVIDUAL LESION   Round, dome-shaped, well-circumscribed

DISTRIBUTION   Head and neck

Differential Diagnosis

Pink or Tan Papule   Pigmented spindle cell nevus of Reed is considered by many to be a variant of Spitz nevus. The tumor is dome-shaped, deeply pigmented, and often surrounded by a lighter brown regular rim; epiluminescence is particularly helpful; the tumor

cells are not "diffusely infiltrating," as in the Spitz nevus, but grow in a compact nodular pattern. Other lesions in the differential diagnosis are pyogenic granuloma, hemangioma, molluscum contagiosum, juvenile xanthogranuloma, mastocytoma, dermatofibroma, atypical melanocytic nevi, nodular melanoma, and dermal melanocytic nevus.

Dermatopathology

LIGHT MICROSCOPY   *Site*   Reticular dermis and epidermis
  Process   Hyperplasia of epidermis, neoplasm of melanocytes, dilatation of capillaries
  Cell Types   Admixed large epithelioid cells, large spindle cells with abundant cytoplasm, occasional mitotic figures; there are sometimes bizarre cytologic patterns; nests of large cells extend from the epidermis ("raining down") into the reticular dermis as fascicles of cells form an "inverted triangle," with the base lying at the dermal-epidermal junction and the apex in the reticular dermis.

Diagnosis

Although the clinical appearance and recent growth are characteristic of a Spitz nevus, histologic examination must be done to confirm the clinical diagnosis.

Significance

Excision in its entirety is important because the condition recurs in 10 % to 15 % of all cases in lesions that have not been excised completely. This tumor poses some special problems in cytologic diagnosis. Atypical lesions are worri-

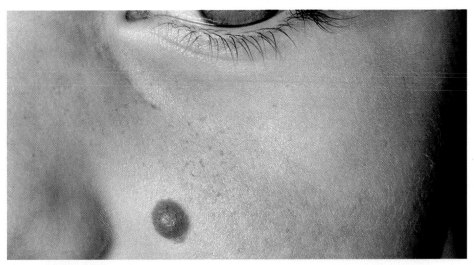

Figure 8-6 Spitz nevus *Bright red dome-shaped nodule on the cheek of a child, developing abruptly within the previous few months; the lesion is easily mistaken for a hemangioma.*

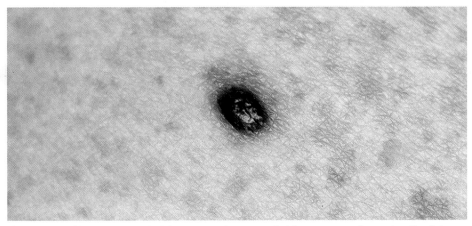

Figure 8-7 Spitz nevus *A dark brown papule surrounded by a tan macular region (lentiginous) developed within a few months on the back of a young female; the lesion was excised and the diagnosis confirmed histologically. The differential diagnosis includes superficial spreading and nodular melanoma.*

some. While the majority of Spitz nevi are benign, there can be a histologic similarity between Spitz nevi and melanoma. Also, atypical Spitz nevi can occur and even have occasional "metastases" from such lesions. Melanoma has been reported to arise rarely in Spitz nevi.

Course and Prognosis

Spitz tumors probably do not involute, as do common acquired nevomelanocytic nevi. However, some lesions have been observed to transform into common compound NMC, some undergo fibrosis and in late stages may resemble dermatofibromas.

Management

Excision with a border of 5 mm. Follow-up in 6 to 12 months is advised, especially for atypical lesions.

LENTIGO SIMPLEX

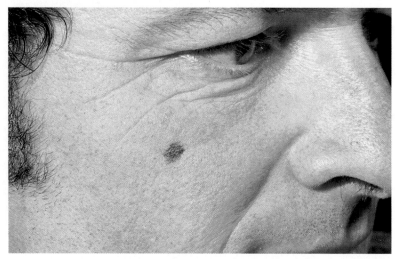

Figure 8-8 Lentigo simplex

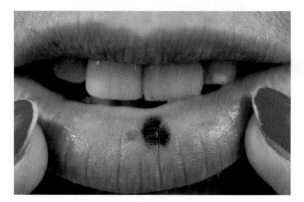

Figure 8-9 Lentigo simplex:
pigmented labial macule

Lentigo simplex *The adjective* simplex *is necessary to distinguish this small, dark pigmented lesion from several other lentigines that are distinctively different from lentigo simplex. All lentigines are brown to dark brown macules.* Solar lentigo *may be brown in color, but most other lentigines are dark brown or black. Lentigo simplex (LS) is a small round or oval lesion, usually <5 mm, brown or dark brown, and occurring anywhere on the skin without relation to sun-exposed areas. LS is clinically identical in size and color to a junctional nevus; both lesions have an increased number of melanocytes. However, in the junctional nevus, while there is an increased number of melanocytes, the melanocytes are arranged in "nests." LS can occur as a single lesion: in black persons in the nail bed, giving rise to linear streaks in the nail plate, or on the lip, lower lip especially, where it is termed* pigmented labial macules *(9). There may be a single or many lesions. The term* lentiginosis *refers to a collection of lesions simulating LS clinically and histologically, but their number and distribution are distinctive; this may occur as multiple lesions in the vulvar mucous membrane or as isolated lesions on the lips, on the buccal mucosa, or on the fingers and toes; in these locations it is associated with small bowel polyposis (see Peutz-Jeghers Syndrome, page 516) and rarely carcinoma of the small intestine. When LS occurs on the penis (especially on the glans), it has the same significance as in other areas. There is no concern for development of malignant melanoma.*

NEVUS SPILUS

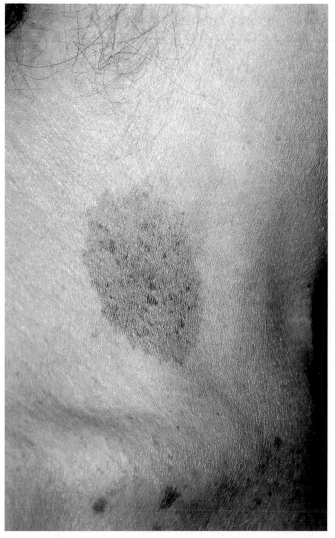

Figure 8-10 Nevus spilus   *This is a rather common disorder of melanocyte morphology that consists of a varying-sized, light brown pigmented macule from a few centimeters to a very large area (>15 cm); the distinctive feature of this lesion is the many dark brown small macules (2 to 3 mm) or papules scattered throughout the pigmented background. The term* spilus *(Latin: "spot") refers to these spots. These can be either flat (macules) or slightly raised (papules). The pathology of the background of the macular pigmented lesion is the same as lentigo simplex, i.e., increased numbers of melanocytes, while the flat or raised lesions scattered throughout are either junctional or compound nevi. Rarely, these are dysplastic melanocytic junctional or compound nevi. The lesions are not as common as junctional or compound nevi but are not at all rare. In one series in a large dermatology practice, the nevus spilus was present in 3 % of white patients. Malignant melanoma very rarely arises in these lesions.*

MONGOLIAN SPOT

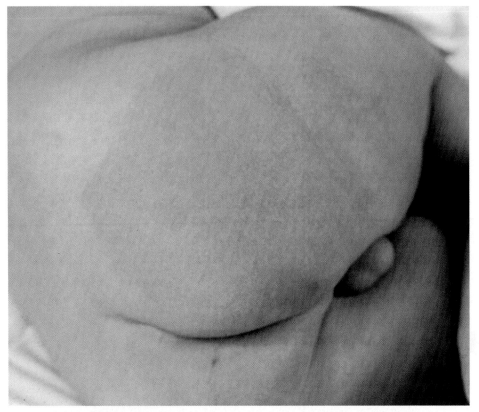

Figure 8-11 Mongolian spot *These* congenital *gray-blue macular lesions, which are characteristically located on the lumbosacral area, also can occur on the scalp or anywhere on the skin. There is usually a single lesion, but rarely, several truncal lesions can be present at birth. Melanocytes are not normally present in the dermis, and it is believed that these ectopic melanocytes represent pigment cells that have been interrupted in their migration from the neural crest to the epidermis. Mongolian spots disappear in early childhood (see Nevus of Ota, Figure 8-12). As the term* Mongolian *implies, these lesions are found almost always (99 % to 100 %) in infants of Asiatic and Amerindian origin; however, they have been reported in black and, rarely, in white infants. No melanomas have been reported to occur in these lesions.*

NEVUS OF OTA

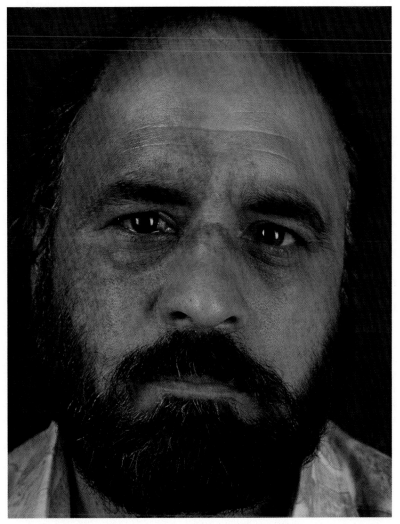

Figure 8-12 Nevus of Ota *This pigmentary disorder is very common in Asiatic populations and is said to occur in 1 % of outpatient visits in Japan. It has been reported in East Indians, blacks, and, rarely, whites. The pigmentation, which can be quite subtle or markedly disfiguring, consists of a mottled, dusky admixture of blue and brown hyperpigmentation of the skin. The pigmentation mostly involves the skin and mucous membranes innervated by the first and second branches of the trigeminal nerve. The blue hue results from the presence of ectopic melanocytes in the dermis, in the hard palate, and in the conjunctivae, sclerae, and tympanic membranes. It may be congenital but is not hereditary; more often it appears in early childhood or during puberty and remains for life, in contrast to the Mongolian spot, which disappears in early childhood. Treatment with lasers has been a very effective new modality for this disfiguring disorder. Malignant melanoma can occur but is rare.*

DISORDERS OF BLOOD VESSELS

CLASSIFICATION OF VASCULAR "BIRTHMARKS"*

Hemangiomas of Infancy (Strawberry Nevus, Angiomatous Nevus)

Benign vascular proliferations of endothelial lining that undergo spontaneous involution

Vascular Malformations

Capillary Malformations (Nevus Flammeus or Port-Wine Stain) Capillary malformations that do not undergo spontaneous involution

Venous Malformations (Cavernous Hemangioma) Venous malformations *without* endothelial proliferation, and may be combinations of capillaries, veins, arteries, lymphatics; these disorders do not undergo spontaneous involution

*This classification was proposed by Mulliken and Glowacki as a more rational basis for these disorders (Mulliken JB, Glowacki J. Hemangioma and vascular malformation in infants and children: A clarification based on endothelial characteristics. *Plast Reconstr Surg* 1982; 69:412–420).

CAPILLARY HEMANGIOMA OF INFANCY

A capillary hemangioma of infancy (CHI) is a soft, bright-red to deep-purple, vascular nodule-to-plaque that develops at birth or soon after birth and disappears spontaneously by the fifth year. *Synonyms:* Nevus or mark, angiomatous nevus.

Epidemiology

Incidence   1 % to 2 %

Race   White

Other Factors   Low birth weight

History

Duration of Lesions   Lesion appears as a pale patch within the first month of life in the majority of patients and always by the ninth month. There is a rapid enlargement during the first year.

Physical Examination

Skin Lesions

TYPE   Nodule, plaque, 1.0 to 8.0 cm (Figure 8-13A). With the onset of spontaneous regression, a white-to-gray area appears on the surface of the central part of the lesion. Ulceration may occur with rapid regression. Ulcerated lesions may become secondarily infected. Multiple CHI may be associated with hemangiomas of CNS, GI tract, and/or liver. Often resolve with minimal scarring

COLOR   The superficial CHI is bright red (Figure 8-13A); the deeper CHI is purple and lobulated.

PALPATION   Soft or moderately firm, depending on the proportionate amount of vascular and fibrous elements. On diascopy, does not blanch completely

DISTRIBUTION   Localized or extending over an entire region. Head and neck 50 %, trunk 25 %

SITES OF PREDILECTION   Face, trunk, legs, oral mucous membrane

Differential Diagnosis

Red/Purple Nodule/Tumor/Plaque   The distinction between a *CHI* and a *cavernous angioma* is based on color and depth. Mixed angiomas (both superficial and deep) may occur.

Dermatopathology

Proliferation of endothelial cells in varying amounts in the dermis and/or subcutaneous tissue; there is more endothelial proliferation in the superficial type, and in the deep angiomas there is little or no endothelial proliferation.

Pathophysiology

CHI is a localized proliferation of angioblastic mesenchyme.

Diagnosis

Made on clinical findings and MRI

Course and Prognosis

CHI spontaneously involutes by the fifth year, with some few percent disappearing only by age 10 (Figure 8-13A and 13B). There is virtually no residual skin change at the site in most lesions (80 %), in the rest there is residual atrophy, depigmentation, and infiltration. Deeper lesions, especially those involving mucous membranes, may not involute completely. Synovial involvement may be associated with hemophilia-like arthropathy. Large CHI, usually associated with cavernous hemangiomas, may have platelet entrapment and thrombocytopenia (Kasabach-Merritt syndrome; see page 154).

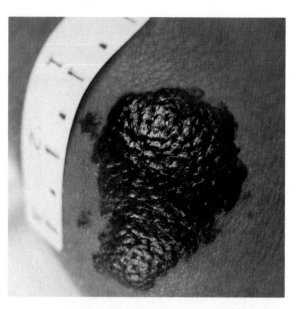

Figure 8-13A Capillary hemangioma of infancy *A purple dermal nodular lesion near the elbow of a newborn.*

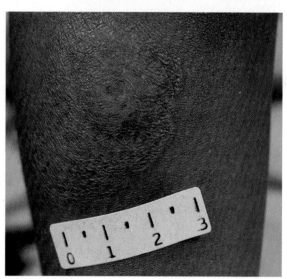

Figure 8-13B *By 6 years of age, the vascular lesion has undergone spontaneous resolution with minimal residual scarring.*

Rarely, morbidity associated with CHI occurs secondary to hemorrhage or high-output heart failure.

Management

Each lesion must be judged individually re-

garding the decision to treat or not to treat and the selection of a treatment mode. Surgical or medical interventions include either continuous wave or pulsed dye laser, cryosurgery, or systemic corticosteroids. When possible, treatment should be avoided because spontaneous resolution gives the best cosmetic results.

PORT-WINE STAIN

A port-wine stain (PWS) is an irregularly shaped, red or violaceous, macular, vascular malformation of dermal blood vessels that is present at birth and never disappears spontaneously except for the salmon patch (see below); the malformation is usually confined to the skin but may be associated with vascular malformations in the eye and leptomeninges (Sturge-Weber syndrome).
Synonym: Nevus flammeus.

Epidemiology

Age   Congenital

Incidence   0.3 %

Clinical Variants

Nevus flammeus nuchae (stork bite, erythema nuchae, salmon patch) occurs in approximately one-third of infants on the nape of the neck and tends to regress spontaneously. Similar lesions occur on eyelids and glabella.

Sturge-Weber syndrome (SWS) is the association of PWS with vascular malformations in the eye (glaucoma) and leptomeninges and superficial calcifications of the brain.

Klippel-Trénaunay-Weber syndrome may have an associated PWS overlying the deeper vascular malformation of soft tissue and bone.

PWS on the midline back may be associated with an underlying arteriovenous malformation of the spinal cord.

History

Skin Symptoms   None

Systemic Symptoms   SWS may be associated with contralateral hemiparesis, muscular hemiatrophy, epilepsy, mental retardation; glaucoma and ocular palsy may occur.

Physical Examination

Skin Lesions

TYPE   In infancy and childhood, PWS are macular (Figure 8-14). With increasing age of the patient, papules or nodules (Figure 8-15) often develop, leading to significant disfigurement.

COLOR   Varying hues of pink to purple (Figures 8-14 and 8-15)

SHAPE   Irregular. Large lesions follow a dermatomal distribution and rarely cross the midline.

DISTRIBUTION   Unilateral (85 %). Most commonly involve the face but may occur at any cutaneus site. In SWS, PWS occurs in the distribution of the trigeminal nerve, usually the superior and middle branches; mucosal involvement of conjunctiva and mouth may occur. PWS intrigeminal distribution is common and does not necessarily indicate the presence of SWS.

PATTERN   Dermatomal in SWS

Diagnosis

Made on clinical findings. All patients should be screened for glaucoma and for CNS involvement.

Laboratory and Special Examinations

Dermatopathology   Developmental defect leading to ectasia of capillaries. No proliferation of endothelial cells

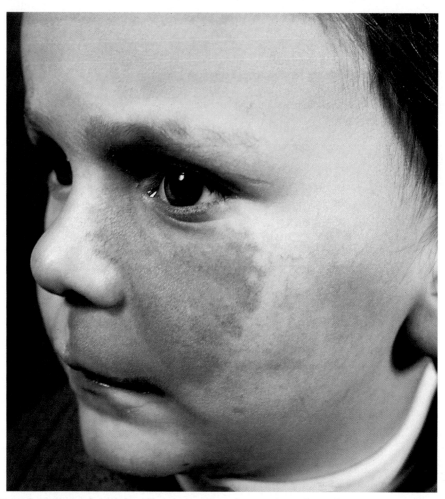

Figure 8-14 Port-wine stain *Sharply marginated, port-wine-red macule occurring in a distribution of the second branch (maxillary) of the trigeminal nerve in a young child.*

Imaging In SWS, skull x-rays show characteristic calcifications of angiomas or localized linear calcification along cerebral convolutions. CT scan should be done.

Course and Prognosis

PWSs do not regress spontaneously. The area of involvement tends to increase in proportion to the size of the child. In adulthood, PWSs usu-ally become raised with papular and nodular areas and are the cause of significant progressive cosmetic disfigurement (Figure 8-15).

Management

During the macular phase, PWS can be covered with makeup such as Covermark. Treatment with tunable dye or copper vapor lasers is very effective.

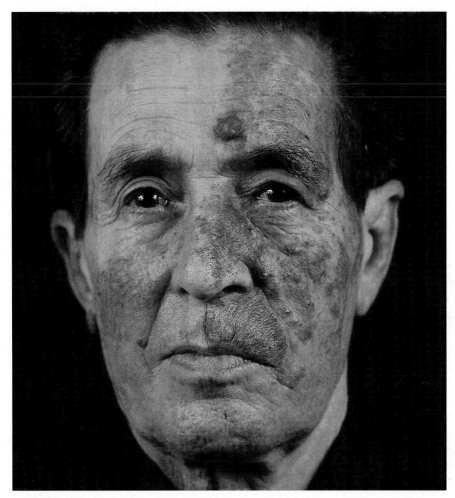

Figure 8-15 Port-wine stain   *With increasing age, the color deepens and papular and nodular hemangiomas develop within the previously macular lesion causing progressively increasing disfigurement.*

CAPILLARY/VENOUS/LYMPHATIC (CVL) MALFORMATIONS

CVL malformations are deep vascular malformations, characterized by soft compressible deep-tissue swelling, which, at times, is associated with varicosities, arteriovenous shunts and nevus flammeus-like changes.

Synonym: Cavernous hemangioma.

Epidemiology

Age Lesions are not apparent at birth but become so during childhood.

History

Lesions usually asymptomatic except for cosmetic appearance. Limb hypertrophy may interfere with function

Physical Examination

Skin Lesions

TYPE Soft tissue swelling, dome-shaped or multinodular (Figure 8-16). When vascular malformation extends to the epidermis, surface may be verrucous. Borders poorly defined. Considerable variation in size.

COLOR Often, normal skin color. Nodular portion blue to purple

PALPATION Easily compressed, fills promptly when pressure released. Some types may be tender.

Variants

VASCULAR HAMARTOMAS CVL with deep soft-tissue involvement and resultant swelling or diffuse enlargement of extremity. May involve skeletal muscle with muscle atrophy. Cutaneous changes include dilated tortuous veins and arteriovenous fistulas.

KLIPPEL-TRÉNAUNAY-WEBER SYNDROME Local overgrowth of soft tissue and bone with resultant enlargement of an extremity. Associated cutaneous changes include phlebectasia, arteriovenous aneurysms, and nevus flammeus-like cutaneous telangiectasia. Associated developmental abnormalities: nevus unius lateris, syndactylism, polydactylism.

BLUE RUBBER BLEB NEVUS Spontaneously painful and/or tender, compressible, soft, blue swelling in dermis and subcutaneous tissue. Size ranges from a few millimeters to several centimeters. May exhibit localized hyperhidrosis over CVL. Occur, often multiply, on trunk and upper arms. Similar vascular lesions can occur in GI tract and may be a source of hemorrhage.

MARFUCCI'S SYNDROME CVL associated with dyschondroplasia, manifested as hard nodules on fingers or toes, bony deformities. Some CVL may be blue rubber bleb variant.

Diagnosis

Clinical diagnosis, at times confirmed by arteriography

Laboratory and Special Examinations

Dermatopathology Dilated, blood-filled vascular spaces lined with flattened endothelial cells. Vessels may be of cavernous, capillary, venous, and lymphatic types.

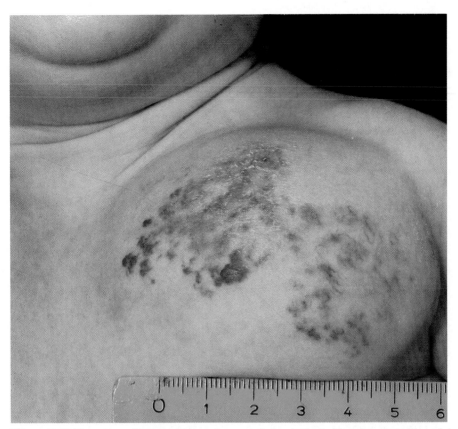

Figure 8-16 Cavernous hemangioma *Large, soft, hemispheric blue-tinged swelling of the dermis and subcutaneous tissue; superficial telangiectases are pesent in the upper dermis.*

Course and Prognosis

CVL may be complicated by ulceration and bleeding, scarring, secondary infection, and high-output heart failure in large lesions. Platelet sequestration and destruction may result in thrombocytopenia (Kasabach-Merritt syndrome) located in mucous membranes of mouth, pharynx, and larynx. May interfere with food intake or breathing; if located on eyelids or vicinity of eyes, in an instant it will obstruct vision and may lead to blindness.

Management

There is no satisfactory treatment except compression. In larger lesions and, if organ function is compromised, surgical procedures, intravascular coagulation. High-dose systemic corticosteroids, interferon alpha

CHERRY ANGIOMA

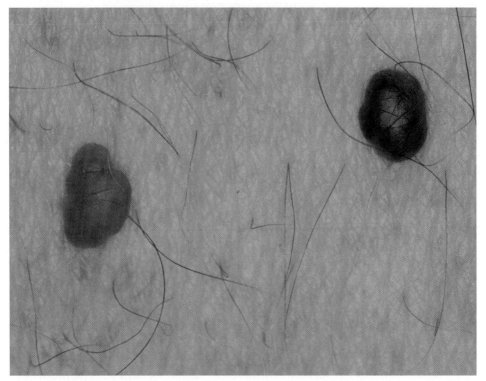

Figure 8-17 Cherry angioma Synonyms: *Campbell de Morgan spots, senile (hem)angioma. Cherry angiomas are exceedingly common, asymptomatic, bright-red to violaceous, domed vascular lesions, or they can occur as myriads of tiny red spots simulating petechiae. They are found principally on the trunk. The differential diagnosis includes angiokeratoma (especially on genital skin), venous lake, pyogenic granuloma, nodular melanoma, and metastatic carcinoma (especially hypernephroma) to skin. The lesions appear first at about 30 and increase in number over the years. The histology consists of numerous moderately dilated capillaries lined by flattened endothelial cells; stroma is edematous with homogenization of collagen. They are of no consequence other than their cosmetic appearance. Management is electro- or laser coagulation if indicated cosmetically for small lesions, excision for larger lesions. Cryosurgery is not effective.*

VENOUS LAKE

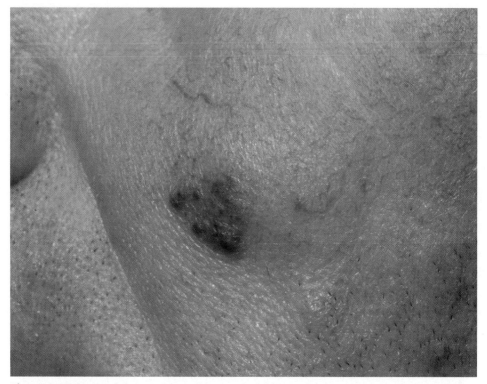

Figure 8-18 Venous lake   *A venous lake is a dark blue to violaceous, asymptomatic, soft papule resulting from a dilated venule, occurring on the face, lips, and ears of patients over 50 years of age. The etiology is unknown, although it has been thought to be related to solar exposure. These lesions are few in number and remain for years. The lesion results from a dilated cavity lined with a single layer of flattened endothelial cells and a thin wall of fibrous tissue filled with red blood cells. The lesion may be confused with nodular melanoma or pyogenic granuloma. The use of epiluminescence microscopy permits an easy diagnosis as a vascular lesion and not a pigment cell neoplasm such as a melanoma. The management is for cosmetic reason and can be accomplished with electrosurgery or laser or, rarely, with surgical excision.*

SPIDER ANGIOMA

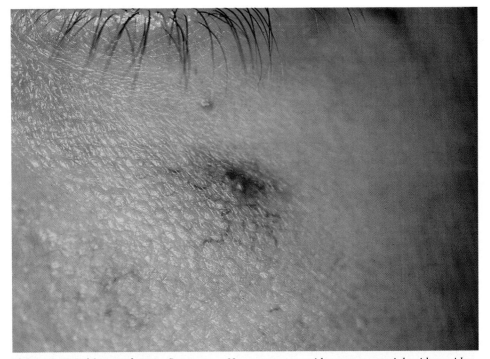

Figure 8-19 Spider angioma Synonyms: *Nevus araneus, spider nevus, arterial spider, spider telangiectasia, vascular spider. A spider angioma is red and is a focal telangiectatic network of dilated capillaries radiating from a cental arteriole (punctum). The central papular punctum is the site of the feeding arteriole with macular radiating telangiectatic vessels. Up to 1.5 cm in diameter. Usually solitary. On diascopy, the radiating telangiectasia blanches and the central arteriole may pulsate. Most commonly occurs on the face, forearms, and hands. It not infrequently occurs in normal persons and is more common in females. It may be associated with hyperestrogenic states, such as pregnancy (one or more in two-thirds of pregnant women) or in patients receiving estrogen therapy, e.g., oral contraceptive use, or in hepatocellular disease such as subacute and chronic viral hepatitis and alcoholic cirrhosis. The lesion can occur in young children without any significance. Spider angioma arising in childhood and pregnancy may regress spontaneously. The lesion may be confused with hereditary hemorrhagic telangiectasia, ataxia-telangiectasia, or systemic scleroderma. Lesions may be treated easily with electro- or laser surgery.*

ANGIOKERATOMA

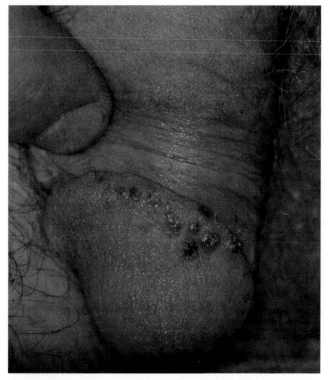

Figure 8-20 Angiokeratoma   *The term* angio *("blood vessel")* keratoma *would imply a vascular tumor with keratotic elements. In fact, this term has been used to describe several quite distinctive conditions, each with its own characteristic features. The most common is* angiokeratoma of Fordyce; *this disease involves the scrotum and vulva; the lesions are dilated venules 4 mm in size and dark red in color, present in quite large numbers;* Angiokeratoma of Mibelli *comprises pink to dark red papules that occur on the elbows, knees, and dorsa of the hands. This autosomal dominant disease is rare and occurs in young females.* Angiokeratoma corporis diffusum *(Fabry's disease), an X-linked recessive (virtually only occurring in males) disease, is an inborn error of metabolism in which there is a deficiency of alpha-galactosidase A leading to an accumulation of neutral glycosphingolipid ceramide trihexoside in endothelial cells, fibrocytes, and pericytes in the dermis, heart, kidneys, and autonomic nervous system. The lesions of Fabry's disease are numerous dark red, punctate, and tiny (<1.0 mm), located on the lower half of the body: lower abdomen, genitalia, and buttocks, although lesions also may occur on the lips. The homozygous males have not only the skin lesions but also symptoms related to involvement of other organ systems: acroparesthesias, excruciating pain, transient ischemic attacks, and myocardial infarction. Heterozygous females may have corneal opacities.*

PYOGENIC GRANULOMA

Pyogenic granuloma is a rapidly developing hemangioma, at times arising at sites of minor trauma, characterized by a solitary eroded vascular nodule that bleeds spontaneously or following minor trauma. *Synonym:* Granuloma telangiectaticum.

Epidemiology

Age Usually children; <30 years old

Sex Equal

History

Duration of Lesions Months

Skin Symptoms Recurrent bleeding from the lesion occurs frequently.

Physical Examination

Skin Lesions

TYPE Nodule with smooth surface, with or without crusts, with or without erosion (see Figure 8-21)

COLOR Bright red, dusky red, violaceous, brown-black

SIZE AND SHAPE Less than 1.5 cm in diameter. Dome-shaped, sessile, or pedunculated.

On palmar and soles: epidermal collarette at base

DISTRIBUTION Isolated single lesion

SITES OF PREDILECTION Fingers, lips, mouth, trunk, toes

Differential Diagnosis

Red Nodule Nodular malignant melanoma (especially amelanotic), squamous cell carcinoma, glomus tumor, nodular basal cell carcinoma, metastatic carcinoma, bacillary angiomatosis

Laboratory and Special Examinations

Dermatopathology Proliferation of capillaries with prominent endothelial cells embedded in edematous, gelatinous stroma; epidermis commonly eroded. Dense infiltrate of neutrophilia common

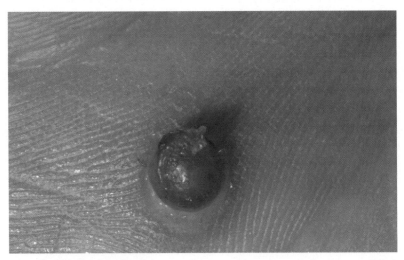

Figure 8-21 Pyogenic granuloma

GLOMUS TUMOR

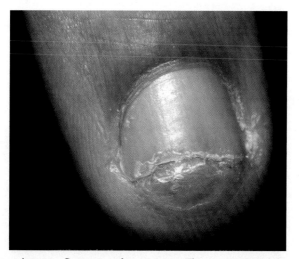

Figure 8-22 Glomus tumor Synonym: *glomangioma. This is a tumor of the* glomus body. *The* glomus body *is an anatomic and functional unit composed of specialized smooth muscle, the* glomus cells, *that surround thin-walled endothelial spaces; this anatomic unit functions as an A-V shunt linking arterioles and venules. The glomus cells surround the narrow lumen of the Sucquet-Hoyer canal that branches from the arteriole and leads to the collecting venule segment that acts as a reservoir. Glomus bodies are present on the pads and nail beds of the fingers and toes and also on the volar aspect of hands and feet, in the skin of the ears, and in the center of the face. The glomus tumor presents as an exquisitely tender subungual papule or nodule. Glomus tumors are characterized by paroxysmal painful attacks, especially elicited by exposure to cold. They are most often present as solitary* solid *subungual tumors but may rarely occur as multiple papules or nodules, then called glomangiomas. These do not occur under the nail but are noted, especially in children, as discrete papules or sometimes plaques anywhere on the skin surface. They are mostly vascular and not solid as are the solitary glomus tumor.*

Diagnosis

Clinical findings confirmed by histologic findings

Course and Prognosis

Lesions persist for many months, bleeding frequently. A significant percentage of lesions treated with removal and ablation of the base recur, requiring additional therapy. Recurrence following surgical excision is uncommon.

Management

In that pyogenic granuloma cannot be distinguished from primary or secondary (metastatic) carcinoma or melanoma, the lesion should be sent for histologic examination.

Surgical Excision The lesion can be excised surgically; the cosmetic results are usually excellent.

Ablation of the Base Following removal of the major portion of the lesion by curettage, parallel-plane, or scissors excision (for histopathologic examination), the base of the lesion can be destroyed by electrodesiccation or (pulse-dye) laser surgery. Cosmetic results are excellent.

MUCOCUTANEOUS CYSTS AND PSEUDOCYSTS

A true mucocutaneous cyst is a closed sac lined by epidermally or adnexally derived epithelium and filled with a liquid or semisolid material derived from that epithelium; various pseudocysts occur within the dermis and are not epithelial-lined.

EPIDERMOID CYST

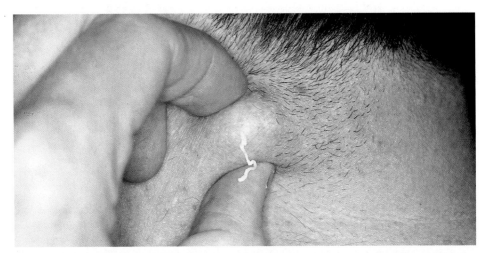

A

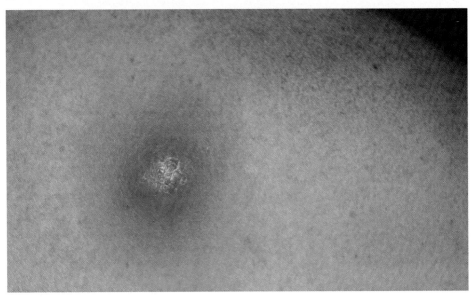

B

Figure 8-23 Epidermoid cyst

TRICHILEMMAL CYST

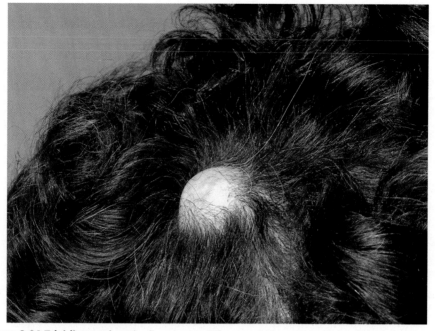

Figure 8-24 Trichilemmal cyst Synonyms: *Pilar cyst, isthmus catagen cyst.* Archaic terms: *Wen, sebaceous cyst.* A trichilemmal cyst is the second most common type of cutaneous cyst (the most common being the epidermoid cyst) and is seen most often on the scalp and, in middle age, more frequently in females. It is often familial. Occurs frequently as multiple lesions. These are smooth, firm, dome-shaped, 0.5- to 5.0-cm nodules to tumors (lacks the central punctum seen in epidermoid cysts). Over 90 % occur on the scalp, and the overlying scalp hair is usually normal but may be thinned if cyst is large. Not connected to epidermis. The cyst wall is usually thick; it can be removed intact. The wall is a stratified squamous epithelium with a palisaded outer layer resembling that of outer root sheath of hair follicle. The inner layer is corrugated without a granular layer. The cyst contains keratin, very dense, pink, homogeneous. Often calcified, cholesterol clefts. If cyst ruptures, may be inflamed and very painful.

Figure 8-23 Epidermoid cyst Synonyms: *Wen, sebaceous cyst, infundibular cyst, epidermal cyst.* An epidermoid cyst is the most common cutaneous cyst, derived from epidermis or the epithelium of the hair follicle, and is formed by cystic enclosure of epithelium within the dermis that becomes filled with keratin and lipid-rich debris (A); because of their thin walls, rupture is common and accompanied by a painful inflammatory mass. It occurs in young to middle-aged adults. The lesions occur on the face, neck, upper trunk, and scrotum. The lesion, which is usually solitary but may be multiple, is a dermal-to-subcutaneous nodule, 0.5 to 5.0 cm, which often connects with the surface by keratin-filled pores. The cyst has an epidermal-like wall (stratified squamous epithelium with well-formed granular layer); the content of the cyst is keratinaceous material—cream-colored with a pasty consistency and the odor of rancid cheese. Scrotal lesions may calcify. The cyst wall is relatively thin. Following rupture of the wall, the irritating cyst contents initiate an inflammatory reaction, enlarging the lesion manyfold; the lesion is now associated with a great deal of pain. Ruptured cysts (B) are often misdiagnosed as being infected rather than ruptured. (See opposite page.)

EPIDERMAL INCLUSION CYST

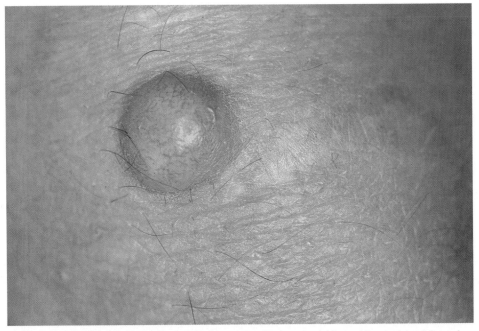

Figure 8-25 Epidermal inclusion cyst Synonym: *Traumatic epidermoid cyst. An epidermal inclusion cyst occurs secondary to traumatic implantation of epidermis within the dermis. Traumatically grafted epidermis grows in the dermis, with accumulation of keratin within the cyst cavity, enclosed in a stratified squamous epithelium with a well-formed granular layer. The lesion appears as a dermal nodule and most commonly occurs on the palms and soles. It should be excised.*

DIGITAL MYXOID CYST

Figure 8-27 Digital myxoid cyst Synonyms: *Mucous cyst, synovial cyst, myxoid pseudocyst. A digital myxoid cyst is a pseudocyst occurring over the distal interphalangeal joint and the base of the nail of the finger or toe, often associated with Heberden's (osteophytic) node. The lesion occurs in older patients, usually >60 years of age. It is usually a solitary cyst, rubbery, translucent, and occurs on the dorsal aspect of the distal interphalangeal joint of the finger, less commonly of the toe. A clear gelatinous viscous fluid may be extruded from the opening (A). (B) When the myxoid cyst is over the nail matrix, a nail plate dystrophy occurs in the form of a 1- to 2-mm groove that extends to the length of the nail. The lesion is easy to recognize, but many physicians are not acquainted with the entity. Various methods of management have been advocated, including surgical excision, incision and drainage, injection of sclerosing material, and injection of a triamcinolone suspension. A simple and most effective method is to use firm compression (daily) of the lesion over a period of weeks. (Figures 8-27A and 8-27B on opposite page.)*

MILIUM

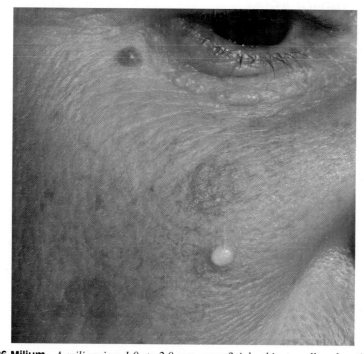

Figure 8-26 Milium *A milium is a 1.0- to 2.0-mm, superficial, white to yellow, keratin-containing epidermal cyst, occurring multiply, located on the eyelids, cheeks, and forehead in pilosebaceous follicles and at sites of trauma. The lesions can occur at any age, even in infants. Milia arise from pluripotential cells in epidermal or adnexal epithelium either* de novo, *especially around the eye, or in association with various dermatoses with subepidermal bullae or vesicles (pemphigoid, porphyria cutanea tarda, bullous lichen planus, epidermolysis bullosa) and skin trauma (abrasion, burns, dermabrasion, radiation therapy). Incision and expression of contents are the method of treatment.*

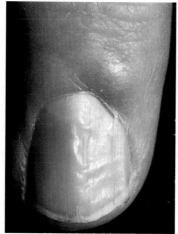
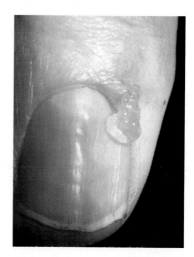

A   B

Figure 8-27 Digital myxoid cyst

MISCELLANEOUS BENIGN NEOPLASMS AND HYPERPLASIAS

SEBORRHEIC KERATOSIS

The seborrheic keratosis is perhaps the most common of the benign epithelial tumors. These lesions, which are hereditary, do not appear until age 30 and continue to occur over a lifetime, varying in extent from a few scattered lesions to literally thousands in some very elderly patients.

Epidemiology and Etiology

Age   Rarely before 30 years of age

Sex   Slightly more common and more extensive involvement in males

Other Features   Probably autosomal dominant inheritance

History

Duration of Lesions   Usually months to years

Skin Symptoms   Rarely pruritic; tender if secondarily infected

Physical Examination

Development   The lesion starts as a *macule,* a skin-colored or light tan lesion, and in the course of time becomes more pigmented; at this time the lesion has a "stuck on" appearance in the form of a *plaque;* further on in their course, the surface appears "warty," and there are multiple plugged follicles or "horn cysts" that are very characteristic of seborrheic keratosis and are virtually pathognomonic of this lesion.

Skin Lesions

TYPE   *Early*   Small, 1.0- to 3.0-mm, barely elevated papule (Figure 8-28) or plaque with or without pigment. The surface often shows, with 7× to 10× magnification, fine stippling like the surface of a thimble.
  Late   Plaque with warty surface and "stuck on" appearance (Figure 8-29), "greasy"; with a hand lens (7× to 10×), horn cysts often can be seen. Size from 1.0 to 6.0 cm. Nodule.

COLOR   Brown, gray, black, skin-colored

SHAPE   Round, oval

ARRANGEMENT   Scattered, discrete lesions

DISTRIBUTION   Isolated lesion or generalized

SITES OF PREDILECTION   Face, trunk, upper extremities

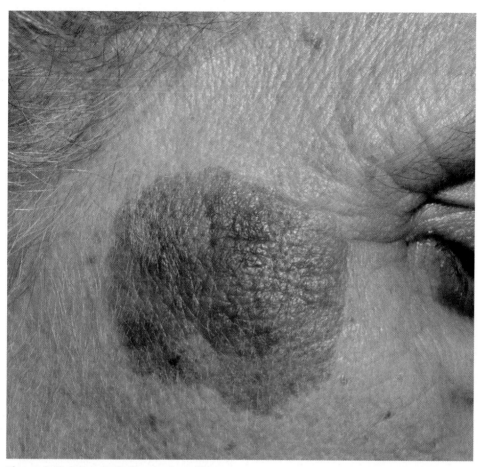

Figure 8-28 Seborrheic keratosis, solitary *A very large, slightly raised, keratotic, brown, flat plaque on the temple in an older female. The differential diagnosis includes lentigo maligna and lentigo maligna melanoma.*

Differential Diagnosis

Tan Macules Early "flat" lesions confused with solar lentigo or spreading pigmented actinic keratosis (surface of seborrheic keratosis is more verrucous; also, horn cysts are present)

Skin-Colored/Tan/Black Verrucous Papules/Plaques Larger pigmented lesions are easily mistaken for pigmented basal cell carcinoma or malignant melanoma (only biopsy will settle this); verruca vulgaris

Dermatopathology

Site Epidermis

Process Proliferation of keratinocytes (with marked papillomatosis) and melanocytes, formation of horn cysts. Some lesions can exhibit atypia of keratinocytes, mimicking Bowen's disease or squamous cell carcinoma, and these should be excised.

Management

Light electrocautery will permit the whole lesion to appear to be easily rubbed off. Then the base can be lightly cauterized to prevent recurrence. This, however, precludes histopathologic verification of diagnosis and should be done only by an experienced diagnostician. Cryosurgery with liquid nitrogen spray is excellent, but recurrences are possibly more frequent. Best approach is curettage after slight freezing with cryosurgery; this also permits histopathologic examination.

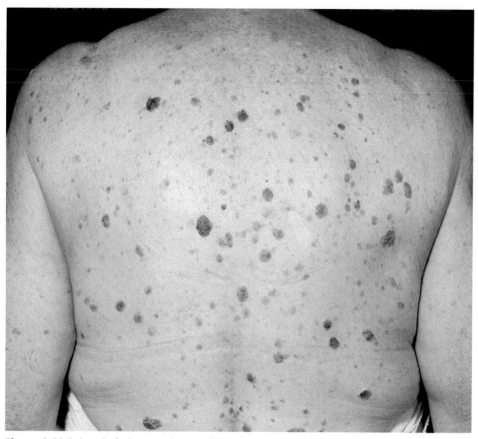

Figure 8-29 Seborrheic keratoses, multiple *Multiple brown, warty papules and nodules on the back, having a "stuck on" appearance.*

KERATOACANTHOMA

Keratoacanthoma (KA) is a special lesion, occurring as an isolated nodule, usually on the face. It presents as a dome-shaped nodule with a central keratinous crater that mimics squamous cell carcinoma. Unique features are its rapid growth rate, much faster than a squamous cell carcinoma, and also its spontaneous remission over a period of several months. Still, in every solitary KA, tissue must be obtained to rule out squamous cell carcinoma.

Epidemiology

Age   Over 50 years; rare below 20 years

Sex   Male : female ratio, 2:1

Race   Caucasians; rare in Asians, blacks

History

Onset   Rapid growth, achieving a size of 2.5 cm within a few weeks

Duration of Lesions   Untreated, months to years

Skin Symptoms   Usually none. Cosmetic disfigurement. Occasional tenderness.

Physical Examination

Skin Lesions

TYPE   Nodule, dome-shaped often with a central keratotic plug (Figures 8-30 and 8-31)

COLOR   Skin-colored or slightly red, tan/brown

PALPATION   Firm but not hard

SIZE AND SHAPE   2.5 cm (range 1.0 to 10.0 cm), round

DISTRIBUTION   Isolated single lesion. Uncommonly, may be multiple, eruptive.

SITES OF PREDILECTION   On exposed skin: cheeks, nose, ears, hands (dorsa)

Differential Diagnosis

Solitary KA   Squamous cell carcinoma (SCC), hypertrophic actinic keratosis, verruca vulgaris

Laboratory and Special Examinations

Dermatopathology   A representative biopsy that extends through the entire lesion to present the architecture of the nodule is required. Central, large, irregularly shaped crater filled with keratin. The surrounding epidermis extends in a liplike manner over the sides of the crater. The keratinocytes are atypical and many are dyskeratotic. Differentiation of KA from SCC may not be possible, in which case the lesion is best regarded and treated as an SCC.

Diagnosis

Clinical findings confirmed by dermatopathologic findings

Pathophysiology

HPV-9, -16, -19, -25, and -37 have been identified in keratoacanthomas. Other possible etiologic factors include ultraviolet radiation and chemical carcinogens (industrial: pitch and tar).

Course and Prognosis

Spontaneous regression in 2 to 6 months or sometimes more than 1 year

Management

Surgery   Surgical excision is recommended in that KAs cannot always be distinguished from SCCs.

Multiple KAs   Systemic retinoids and methotrexate have been used and the former are hardly effective. If resolution does not occur lesion is SCC and must be excised.

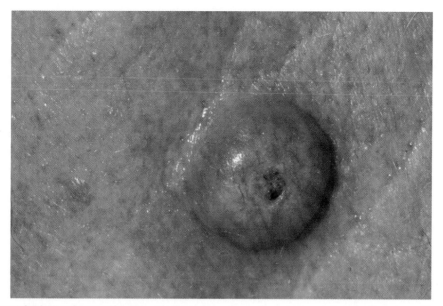

Figure 8-30 Keratoacanthoma *Erythematous, dome-shaped, tumor, 1 cm in diameter with a central keratinaceous plug in the center, developing on facial skin exhibiting moderate dermatoheliosis.*

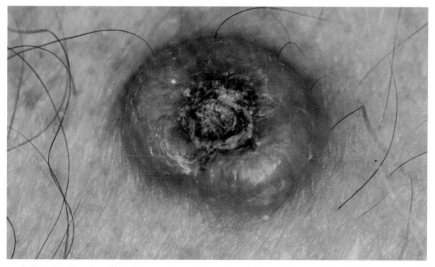

Figure 8-31 Keratoacanthoma *Erythematous, dome-shaped, tumor with a large, central, keratotic plug arising on the upper trunk and of 6-weeks duration. The lesion cannot be distinguished clinically from squamous cell carcinoma.*

DERMATOFIBROMA

A dermatofibroma is a very common, button-like dermal nodule, usually occurring on the extremities, important only because of its cosmetic appearance or its being mistaken for other lesions, such as malignant melanoma. The lesion may be tender.
Synonyms: Solitary histiocytoma, sclerosing hemangioma.

Epidemiology and Etiology

Age   Adults

Sex   Females > males

Etiology   Unknown

History

Symptoms   May be tender

Physical Examination

Skin Lesions

TYPE   Papule or nodule (Figure 8-32), 3.0 to 10.0 mm in diameter. Surface variably domed but may be depressed below plane of surrounding skin. Texture of surface may be dull, shiny, or scaling. Top may be crusted or scarred secondary to excoriation or shaving. Borders ill-defined, fading to normal skin.

COLOR   Variable: skin color, pink, brown, tan, dark chocolate brown. Usually darker at center, fading to normal skin color at margin. Often center shows postinflammatory hypo- or hyperpigmentation secondary to repeated trauma.

PALPATION   Firm dermal button- or pealike papule or nodule. *Dimple sign:* lateral compression with thumb and index finger produces a depression or "dimple."

DISTRIBUTION   Legs > arms > trunk. Uncommonly occurs on head, palms, soles. Usually solitary, may be multiple, and are randomly scattered.

Differential Diagnosis

Firm Dermal Papule/Nodule   Primary malignant melanoma, scar, blue nevus, pilar cyst, metastatic carcinoma, Kaposi's sarcoma, dermatofibrosarcoma protuberans

Dermatopathology

Whorling fascicles of spindle cells with small amounts of pale blue cytoplasm and elongate nuclei. Variable increase in vascular spaces. Overlying epidermis frequently hyperplastic.

Diagnosis

Clinical findings, "dimple" sign (Figure 8-32B)

Course and Prognosis

Lesions appear gradually over several months, may persist without increase in size for years to decades, and may regress spontaneously.

Management

Surgical removal is not usually indicated, in that the resulting scar is often less cosmetically acceptable than the dermatofibroma. Indications for excision include repeated trauma, unacceptable cosmetic appearance, or uncertainty of clinical diagnosis.

Cryosurgery   Cryosurgery with liquid nitrogen spray is often effective and produces a cosmetically acceptable scar in most patients.

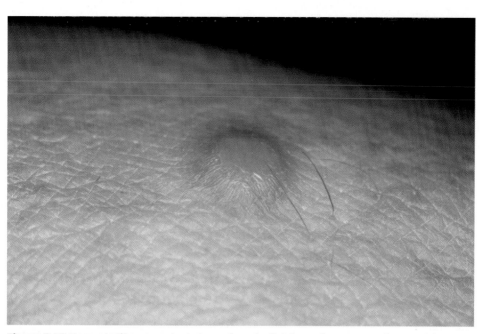

Figure 8-32 Dermatofibroma A. *A dome-shaped, slightly erythematous and tan nodule with a button-like, firm consistency.*

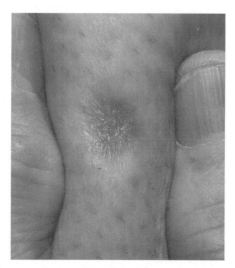

Figure 8-32 Dermatofibroma B. *Dimpling of the lesion is seen when pinched between two fingers.*

HYPERTROPHIC SCARS AND KELOIDS

Hypertrophic scars and keloids are exuberant fibrous repair tissues following a cutaneous injury. A *hypertrophic scar* remains confined to the site of original injury; a *keloid,* however, extends beyond this site, often with clawlike extensions.

Epidemiology and Etiology

Age   Third decade, but range from early first decade to senescence

Sex   Equal incidence in males and in females

Race   Much more common in blacks than in whites

Etiology   Unknown. Usually follow injury to skin, i.e., surgical scar, laceration, abrasion, cryosurgery, electrocoagulation, as well as vaccination, acne, etc. May also arise spontaneously, without history of injury, usually in presternal site.

History

Skin Symptoms   Usually asymptomatic. May be pruritic or painful if touched. May be cosmetically very unsightly.

Physical Examination

Skin Lesions

TYPE   Papules to nodules (Figure 8-33) to tumors to large tuberous lesions

COLOR   Red or usually color of the normal skin

SHAPE   May be linear following traumatic or surgical injury. Hypertrophic scars tend to be dome-shaped and are confined to approximately the site of the original injury. Keloids, however, may extend in a clawlike fashion far beyond any slight original injury.

PALPATION   Firm to hard; surface smooth

SITES OF PREDILECTION   Earlobes, shoulders, upper back, chest

Differential Diagnosis

Scar, dermatofibroma, dermatofibrosarcoma protuberans, desmoid tumor, scar with sarcoidosis, foreign-body granuloma

Laboratory and Special Examinations

Dermatopathology

HYPERTROPHIC SCAR   Whorls of young fibrous tissue and fibroblasts in haphazard arrangement

KELOID   Features of hypertrophic scar with added feature of thick, eosinophilic, acellular bands of collagen

Diagnosis

Clinical diagnosis; biopsy not warranted unless there is clinical doubt, because another biopsy may induce new hypertrophic scarring.

Course and Prognosis

Hypertrophic scars tend to regress, in time becoming flatter and softer. Keloids, however, may continue to expand in size for decades.

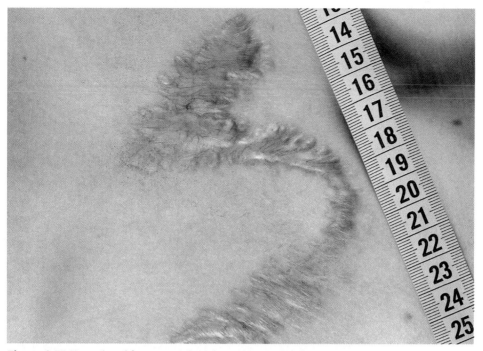

Figure 8-33 Hypertrophic scar *A broad, raised scar developing at the site of surgical incision with large telangiectatic blood vessels and a shiny atrophic epidermis.*

Management

Prevention Individuals prone to hypertrophic scars or keloids should be advised to avoid cosmetic procedures such as ear piercing. Prior to surgery in individuals at risk of formation of hypertrophic scars or keloids, triamcinolone acetonide (5 mg/ml) injected in the incision site may reduce risk of development of hypertrophic scars or keloids.

Cryotherapy Liquid nitrogen spray to lesions, freezing the entire volume of the lesion, is effective in reducing the bulk of some lesions.

Intralesional Corticosteroids Intralesional injection of triamcinolone acetonide (10 to 40 mg/ml) every month may reduce pruritus or sensitivity of lesion, as well as reduce its volume and flatten it. Previously untreated lesions are difficult to inject because of the density of collagen.

Combined Cryotherapy and Intralesional Triamcinolone The lesion is initially frozen with liquid nitrogen spray, allowed to thaw for 15 minutes, and then injected with triamcinolone acetonide (10 to 40 mg/ml). Subsequent to freezing, the lesion becomes edematous and is much easier to inject.

Surgical Excision Lesions that are excised surgically often recur larger than the original lesion. Excision with immediate postsurgical irradiation with iridium has been reported beneficial.

SKIN TAG

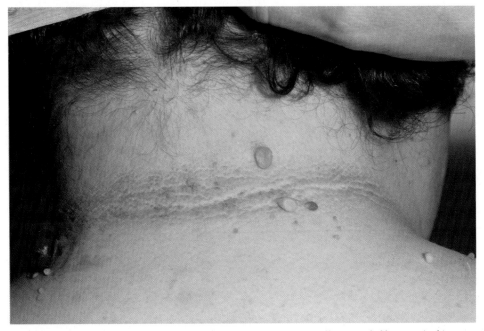

Figure 8-34 Skin tag Synonyms: *Acrochordon, cutaneous papilloma, soft fibroma. A skin tag is a very common, soft, skin-colored or tan or brown, round or oval, pedunculated papilloma (polyp); it is usually constricted at the base and may vary in size from <1.0 mm to as large as 10 mm. Histologic findings include an epidermis that is thinned and which contains a loose fibrous tissue stroma. It occurs more often in the middle aged and in the elderly. The lesion is asymptomatic but occasionally may become tender following trauma or torsion and may become crusted or hemorrhagic. The lesion is more common in females and in obese patients. It is most often noted in intertriginous areas (axillae, inframammary, groin) but is common on the neck and the eyelids. It may be confused with a pedunculated seborrheic keratosis, dermal or compound melanocytic nevus, solitary neurofibroma, or molluscum contagiosum. Lesions tend to become larger and more numerous over time, especially during pregnancy. Following spontaneous torsion, autoamputation can occur. Management is accomplished with simple snipping with a scissors or with electrodesiccation.*

TRICHOEPITHELIOMA

Figure 8-36 Trichoepithelioma *Trichoepitheliomas are benign appendage tumors with hair differentiation. The lesions, which appear at puberty, occur on the face and less often on the scalp, neck, and upper trunk. The lesions, which may be only a few small pink or skin-colored papules at first, gradually increase in number and may become quite large and be confused with basal cell carcinoma. Trichoepithelioma can also appear as solitary tumor, which may be nodular, or appear as ill-defined plaques of sclerodermiform BCC (see page 214). (Figure 8-36 on opposite page.)*

SYRINGOMA

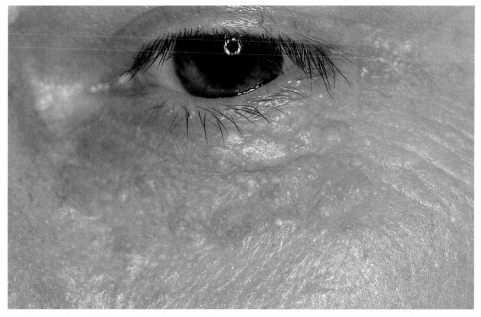

Figure 8-35 Syringoma *Syringoma is a benign adenoma of the intraepidermal eccrine ducts. They are 1- to 2-mm, skin-colored or yellow, firm papules that occur mostly in women beginning at puberty and may be familial. The lesions, most often multiple rather than solitary, occur most frequently around the eyelids and on the face, axillae, umbilicus, upper chest, and vulva. The lesions have a specific histologic pattern: many small ducts in the dermis with comma-like tails with the appearance of "tadpoles." The lesions are considered to be disfiguring, and most patients want them removed; this can be done easily with electrosurgery, using lidocaine-prilocaine topical anesthesia when there are large numbers of lesions.*

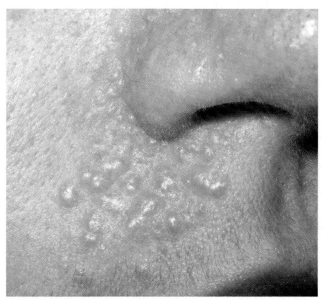

Figure 8-36   Trichoepithelioma

SEBACEOUS HYPERPLASIA

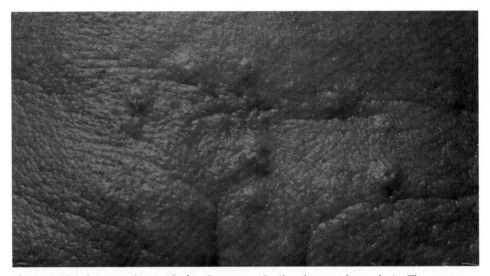

Figure 8-37 Sebaceous hyperplasia Synonym: *Senile sebaceous hyperplasia. These are very common lesions in older persons and are confused with basal cell carcinomas (BCC). The lesions are 1 to 3 mm in diameter and have both telangiectasia and central umbilication. Two distinguishing features from BCC: sebaceous hyperplasia is* soft *to palpation, not firm as in BCC, and second, with firm lateral compression it is often possible to elicit a very small globule of sebum in the valley of the umbilicated portion of the lesion. Sebaceous hyperplasias can be destroyed with light electrocautery.*

LIPOMA

Figure 8-39 Lipoma *Lipomas are single or multiple, benign subcutaneous tumors that are easily recognized because they are soft, rounded, or lobulated and movable against the overlying skin. Many lipomas are small but also may enlarge to > 6.0 cm. They occur especially on the neck and trunk but also may be found on the extremities. Lipomas are composed of fat cells that have the same morphology as normal fat cells. There may, however, in some lesions, be a connective tissue framework in many lipomas. Single and/or few lipomas should be excised when they are small as they can reach a very large size, as large as 12 cm, and then are much more difficult to excise.* Familial lipoma syndrome, *an autosomal dominant trait appearing in early adulthood consists of hundreds of slowly growing nontender lesions. Multiple tender lipomas may arise in adult life and this is then called* adipositas dolorosa *or* Dercum's disease *and occurs in women in middle age; they consist of multiple tender circumscribed or even diffuse fatty deposits. Benign symmetric* lipomatosis, *which affects middle-aged men consists of several large nontender, coalescent poorly circumscribed lipomas mostly on the trunk; coalescence on the neck may lead to a "horse-collar" appearance.* (Figure 8-39 on opposite page.)

NEVUS SEBACEOUS

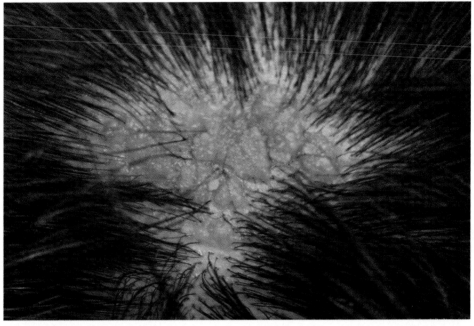

Figure 8-38 Nevus sebaceous   Synonym: *Organoid nevus. This congenital malformation of sebaceous differentiation occurs on the scalp or rarely on the face. The lesion appears on the scalp and has a distinctive morphology: a hairless, thin, elevated, 1- to 2-cm plaque with a characteristic orange color. About 10 % of patients can be expected to develop basal cell carcinoma in the lesion. Excision is recommended at around puberty for cosmetic reasons and also to prevent the occurrence of basal cell carcinoma.*

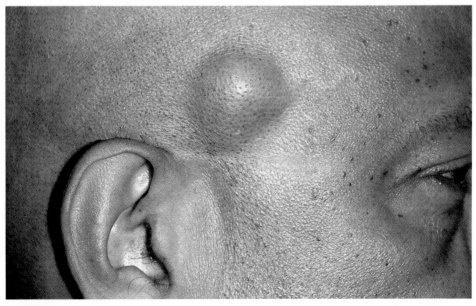

Figure 8-39 Lipoma

MELANOMA PRECURSORS AND PRIMARY CUTANEOUS MELANOMA

CUTANEOUS MELANOMA AND PRECURSORS

Cancer education programs in the 1970s stressed the "danger signs of cancer"; the markers of a dangerous pigmented lesion were "bleeding or ulcer" in a mole. These are now regarded as features of advanced disease, the melanoma being incurable 50 % of the time by excision surgery. Cutaneous melanoma education in the 1990s stresses the detection of early melanoma, with high cure rates following surgical excision.

Of all the cancers, melanoma of the skin represents the greatest challenge in what we have called *preventive detection*, finding early curable primary tumors, thereby preventing metastatic disease and death. Melanoma of the skin in white persons is now not a rare tumor in the United States— 38,300 new primary melanomas will develop in 1996, and 7300 deaths will occur in the United States. By year 2000, it is projected that 1 in 90 individuals will develop melanoma.

In males aged 30 to 49, melanoma is the second most prevalent cancer (the first being cancer of the testis), and in slightly older males (aged 50 to 59), melanoma is the fourth most prevalent cancer, exceeded only by bladder, lung, and rectal cancer (in that order). Primary melanoma of the skin is therefore a disease affecting the young and middle-aged. Mortality rates of primary melanoma for single years from 1976 to 1987 rose at the rate of 3 % per year for men and 1 % per year for women. Early accessibility to physicians is especially important in primary melanoma because curability is directly related to the size and depth of invasion of the tumor.

Even with a rising mortality, there has been an encouraging increase in the detection of early melanoma, with very high 5-year survival rates (approaching 98 %) for thin (<0.75 mm) primary melanoma and an 83 % rate for all stages. The trend over the past three decades illustrates the dramatic increased survival of melanoma patients: In 1960–1963 the overall 5-year survival for melanoma was 60 %, and by 1977–1983 this had increased to 80 %. This is paradoxically high for a tumor malignant as malignant melanoma and is almost solely to be ascribed to early detection of this tumor. At the present time, the most critical tool for conquering this disease is therefore the identification of early "thin" melanomas by clinical examination. In most instances, early melanoma can be recognized by three physical characteristics: *color, contour,* and *size* of the lesion.

Total skin examination for melanoma and its precursors should be done routinely. Special attention should be given to the back above the waist; the legs, between the knees and ankles in women; the scalp; the toes and soles of black- and brown-skinned persons; and the skin around body orifices (mouth, anus, vulva).

About 30 % of melanomas arise in a preexisting melanocytic lesion; 70 % arise in normal skin. Most all melanomas show an initial radial growth phase and followed by a subsequent vertical growth phase. Radial growth phase refers to a mostly intraepidermal, preinvasive, or minimally invasive growth pattern; vertical growth refers to growth into the dermis and thus into the vicinity of vessels that serve as avenues for metastasis. Since melanomas represent proliferating malignant melanocytes that in most melanomas produce melanin pigment, even preinvasive melanomas in their radial growth phase are clinically detectable by their color. The prognostic difference between the clinical types relates mainly to the duration of the radial growth phase, which may last from years to decades in lentigo maligna melanoma, from months to 2 years in superficial spreading melanoma, and may be very short (6 months or less) in nodular melanoma. Since metastasis occurs only infrequently (or some believe not ever) during the radial growth phase, detection of melanoma (i.e., "thin" melanomas) during this phase is essential.

CLASSIFICATION OF CUTANEOUS MALIGNANT MELANOMA AND PRECURSORS

Malignant Melanoma
- A. *Most Common*
  1. Superficial spreading melanoma
  2. Nodular melanoma
  3. Lentigo maligna melanoma
- B. *Less Common*
  4. Acral lentiginous melanoma
  5. Melanoma of the mucous membrane
  6. Melanoma arising in congenital melanocytic nevus
  7. Melanoma arising in dysplastic melanocytic nevus
- C. *Rare*
  8. Desmoplastic melanoma

Precursors of Cutaneous Melanoma
1. Congenital nevomelanocytic nevus (giant *or* small)
2. Clark's (dysplastic) melanocytic nevus
3. Lentigo maligna

THE CLARK MELANOCYTIC NEVUS (DYSPLASTIC MELANOCYTIC NEVUS)

Clark melanocytic nevi (CMN) are a special type of acquired, circumscribed, pigmented lesions that represent disordered proliferations of variably atypical melanocytes. CMN arise *de novo* or as part of a compound melanocytic nevus. CMN differ from common acquired nevi, are clinically distinctive, and have characteristic histologic features. CMN are regarded as potential precursors of superficial spreading melanoma and also as markers of persons at risk for developing primary malignant melanoma of the skin.

Epidemiology

Prevalence CMN occur in almost every patient with familial cutaneous melanoma and in 30 % to 50 % of patients with sporadic nonfamilial primary melanomas of the skin. CMN are, moreover, present in 5.0 % of the general white population.

Race White persons. Data on persons with brown or black skin are not available; CMN are rarely seen in the Japanese population.

Age Children and adults

Sex Equal in males and in females

Transmission Autosomal dominant

History

Duration of Lesions CMN usually arise later in childhood than common acquired nevomelanocytic nevi, appearing first in late childhood, just before puberty. New lesions continue to develop over many years in affected persons; in contrast, common acquired nevomelanocytic nevi do not appear after middle age and disappear entirely in older persons. CMN are thought not to undergo spontaneous regression at all or at least much less than common acquired nevomelanocytic nevi.

Precipitating Factors Exposure to sunlight is regarded by some as an inducing agent for CMN; nevertheless, CMN are not infrequently observed in completely covered areas such as the scalp and anogenital areas.

Skin Symptoms Asymptomatic

Family History In the familial setting, family members can develop melanoma without the presence of CMN.

Physical Examination

See Comparative Clinical Features of Three Pigmented Neoplasms, Table 9-A (Figures 9-1 to 9-3). Melanoma arising in a CMN appears initially as a small papule (often of a different color) within the precursor lesion (Figures 9-3 and 9-4).

Differential Diagnosis

Congenital nevomelanocytic nevi, common acquired nevomelanocytic nevi, superficial spreading malignant melanoma, melanoma *in situ,* lentigo maligna, Spitz nevus, pigmented basal cell carcinoma

Laboratory and Special Examinations

Dermatopathology Hyperplasia and proliferation of melanocytes in a single-file, "lentiginous" pattern in the basal cell layer either as spindle cells or as epithelioid cells and as irregular and dyshesive nests.

1. Melanocytes are "atypical," larger than normal size, exhibiting both pleomorphism of nuclei and cell bodies and hyperchromasia of nuclei.
2. Increased number of melanocytes with a tendency for dyshesive and irregular nesting; "bridging" between rete ridges by

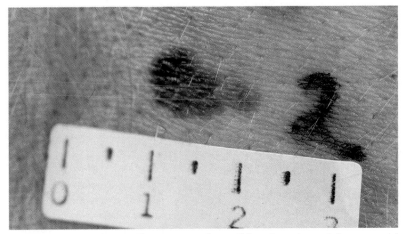

Figure 9-1 Dysplastic melanocytic nevus *A large (1.2 cm), variegated, brown macule with a slight raised area (10 o'clock), fuzzy margins, and oval shape.*

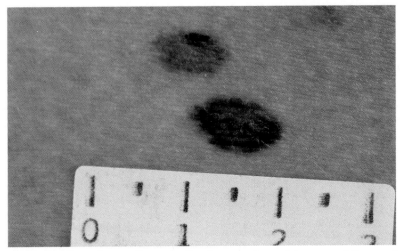

Figure 9-2 Dysplastic melanocytic nevi *Two large, variegated, brown oval flat papules.*

melanocytic nests; spindle-shaped melanocytes are oriented parallel to skin surface.

3. Lamellar fibroplasia and concentric eosinophilic fibrosis (not a constant feature)
4. Proliferation of blood vessels (not a constant feature)
5. Sparse or dense lymphocytic infiltrate (not
   a constant feature)

Association Most CMN arise in contiguity
with a compound melanocytic nevus (rarely, a
junctional nevus) that is centrally located; i.e.,
CMN often have extension of intraepidermal
melanocytic hyperplasia beyond the shoulder of
the dermal nevus component; some CMN may
not have a dermal nevus component.

Wood's Lamp Examination This will
markedly accentuate the epidermal hyperpigmentation of the individual lesions.

Epiluminescence Microscopy This noninvasive technique allows for a clinical improvement of diagnostic accuracy in CMN by 25 to
30 %.

Diagnosis

The diagnosis of CMN is made by clinical
recognition of typical distinctive lesions and diagnostic accuracy is considerably improved by
epiluminescence microscopy; one of these lesions should be excised for histologic confirmation of the diagnosis of CMN. The clinico-
pathologic correlations are now well
documented. Siblings, children, and parents
also should be examined for CMN once the diagnosis is established in one family member.

Etiology and Pathogenesis

Multiple loci, including 1p36 and 9p21, have
been implicated in familial melanoma/dysplas-
tic nevus syndrome. The abnormal clone of
melanocytes can be activated by exposure to
sunlight. Immunosuppressed patients (renal
transplantation) with dysplastic nevi have a
higher incidence of melanoma.

Significance

Anatomic association (in contiguity) of dysplastic nevi has been observed in 36 % of sporadic primary melanomas, in about 70 % of familial primary melanomas, and in 94 % of
melanomas with familial melanoma and dysplastic nevi. The lifetime risks of developing
primary malignant melanoma are estimated to be:

General population	0.8 %
Familial dysplastic nevus syndrome with two blood relatives with melanoma	100.0 %
All other patients who have dysplastic nevi	18.0 %

Management and Follow-Up

Surgical excision of lesions with minimal margins. Laser or other types of physical destruction should never be used because they do not
permit histopathologic verification of diagnosis.
The following guidelines for selection of lesions
to be excised are suggested:

• Lesions that are changing (increase in size,
  change in pigmentation pattern, changes in
  shape and/or border)
• Lesions that cannot be closely followed by
  the patient by self-examination (on the scalp,
  genitalia, upper back)

Patients with dysplastic nevi in the familial
melanoma setting need to be followed carefully:
in the familial dysplastic nevi, every 3 months;
in sporadic dysplastic nevi, every 6 months to
one year. Search for changes in existing dysplastic nevi and development of new nevi. Photographic follow-up is important with Polaroid
prints of the trunk and extremities; also 1:1 Polaroid prints of larger lesions (>7.0 mm) and
lesions that have some variegation. Patients
should be given color-illustrated pamphlets that
depict the clinical appearance of CMN, malignant melanoma, and common acquired nevomelanocytic nevi. Patients with dysplastic nevi (familial and nonfamilial) should not sunbathe and
should use sunscreens when outdoors. They
should not use tanning parlors. Family members
of the patient should also be examined regularly.

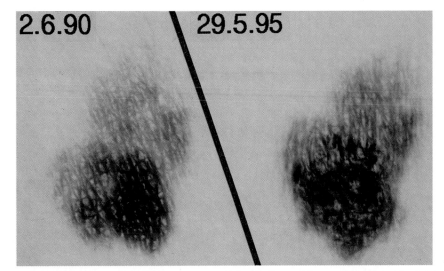

Figure 9-3 Dysplastic melanocytic nevus evolving into a melanoma in situ *The left image (2 June 1990) variegation of pigmentation and irregular borders. Five years later (29 May 1995), the lesion (right) shows darkening of melanin pigmentation, more irregularity in shape, and elevation in the most darkly pigmented region. Histologically, the lesion showed dysplastic nevus evolving into melanoma in situ. Evolution of dysplastic nevi into in situ and/or invasive melanoma can occur in a period of months or many years.*

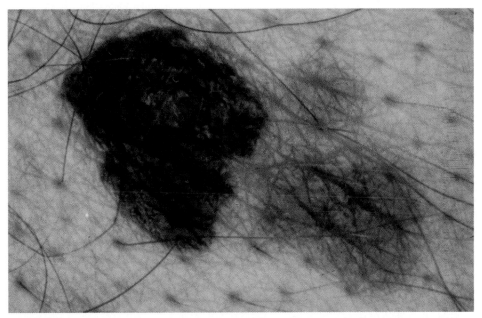

Figure 9-4 Superficial spreading melanoma arising with a dysplastic nevus *The lighter macular portion of this lesion is a dysplastic lesion on the upper back; the blue-black plaque is a superficial spreading melanoma (1.2 mm thickness) arising with the dysplastic nevus. The patient was a 34-year-old internist who died 36 months following detection and excision of this lesion.*

TABLE 9-A COMPARATIVE CLINICAL FEATURES OF THREE PIGMENTED NEOPLASMS (IN WHITES)

Lesion	Common Acquired Nevomelanocytic Nevus	Dysplastic (Clark) Melanocytic Nevus	Malignant Melanoma (Early)
Number	One or many, average in white males is 12 to 15; 10 %–30 % have no nevi	One or many, especially in familial melanoma	Single lesion (1 %–2 %) have multiple primaries
Distribution	Predominate anywhere on trunk and extremities	Mostly on the trunk, arms, legs; rarely on the face. Exposed and covered areas, including scalp. Dorsa of feet and buttocks are often involved.	Anywhere, but predominant on upper back, legs (females), trunk, arms (see Figure E-4 in Appendix E)
Types	Small lesions (junctional nevi) are macules; compound and dermal nevi are uniformly elevated papules or plaques.	Macules (Figures 9-1 to 9-3) with only slightly elevated portions, especially in the center	Macule (*in situ*) and lentigo maligna Plaque [superficial spreading melanoma (SSM) or lentigo maligna melanoma (LMM)] Nodule (SSM, LMM, and nodular)
Size	Most lesions, despite elevation, are rarely >10 mm in diameter, usually <5 mm. 10 % of whites have one or two nevi ≥5 mm	Usually ≥5 mm, but may be smaller. May be up to 15 mm or larger. Pigmented nevi or lesions >15 mm are dysplastic melanocytic or congenital nevomelanocytic nevi or melanoma	Most ≥5 mm. 30 % <6 mm
Shape	Round, oval, papillomatous Regular	Round, oval, ellipsoid Irregular	Round, oval, ellipsoid, asymetrical Irregular
Border	Sharply demarcated	May have distinct margin when target-like. Usually indistinct margin, "fuzzy" margins	Distinct border in nodular melanomas, SSM, and some other varieties
Color	Brown (medium or dark), tan	Brown (dark, light, or medium), tan, pink, or red	Brown (dark, light), black, red, gray, blue, white
Pattern	Uniform or orderly pattern	Irregular display (variegation) of color	Marked variegation

SOURCE: Thomas B. Fitzpatrick and Arthur R. Rhodes, 1996.

CONGENITAL NEVOMELANOCYTIC NEVUS

Congenital nevomelanocytic nevi (CNN) are pigmented lesions of the skin usually present at birth; rare varieties of CNN can develop and become clinically apparent during infancy. CNN may be any size from very small to very large. CNN are benign neoplasms composed of cells called *nevomelanocytes,* which are derived from melanoblasts. All CNN, regardless of size, may be precursors of malignant melanoma.

Epidemiology

Age Present at birth (congenital). Some CNN become visible after birth (*tardive*), "fading in" as a relatively large lesion over a period of weeks. Large nevomelanocytic nevi (i.e., >1.5 cm) that are historically "acquired" should be regarded as tardive CNN.

Sex Equal prevalence in males and females

Race All races

Prevalence Present in 1.0 % of white newborns—majority <3.0 cm in diameter. Larger varieties of CNN are present in 1:2000 to 1:20,000 newborns. Lesions ≥9.9 cm in diameter have a prevalence of 1:20,000, and giant CNN (occupying a major portion of a major anatomic site) occur in 1:500,000 newborns.

Physical Examination

Small and Large CNN CNN have a rather wide range of clinical features, but the following are typical:

TYPE OF LESION CNN usually distort the skin surface to some degree and are therefore a plaque with or without coarse terminal hairs.

BORDERS Sharply demarcated or merging imperceptibly with surrounding skin; regular or irregular contours

PALPATION Large lesions may be "wormy" or soft but are not normally firm except in desmoplastic types of CNN (rare).

SURFACE May or may not have altered skin surface ("pebbly," mamillated, rugose, cerebriform, bulbous, tuberous, or lobular). These surface changes are observed more frequently in lesions that extend into the reticular dermis (so-called deep CNN).

COLOR Light or dark brown. When examined with a 10× magnification lens (under oil), a fine speckling of a darker hue with a lighter surrounding brown hue is seen; often the pigmentation is follicular. A "halo" similar to the type that is observed in leukoderma acquisitum centrifugum (so-called halo nevus) may occur rarely.

SIZE Small (Figure 9-5) or large (Figure 9-6). Nevomelanocytic nevi >1.5 cm in diameter should be regarded as probably CNN when a history is not available; dysplastic melanocytic nevi must, however, be excluded.

SHAPE Oval or round

DISTRIBUTION OF LESIONS Isolated, discrete lesion in any site. Fewer than 5 % of CNN are multiple. Multiple lesions are more common in association with large CNN. Numerous small CNN are uncommon, except in patients with giant CNN, in whom there may be numerous small CNN on the trunk and extremities away from the site of the giant CNN.

Very Large ("Giant") CNN (Figure 9-7) Giant CNN of the head and neck may be associated with involvement of the leptomeninges with the same pathologic process; this presentation may be asymptomatic or be manifested by seizures, focal neurologic defects, or obstructive hydrocephalus.

NUMBER OF LESIONS While small CNN usually occur as single lesions (95 %), giant CNN often present as a single very large lesion and multiple smaller lesions (Figure 9-7).

TYPE OF LESION Usually a plaque with at least some surface distortion, often with focal nodules and papules on a background of a raised plaque, often with coarse, usually dark hair.

SIZE Entire segments of the trunk, extremities, head, or neck

SHAPE Oval or round, bizarre shapes. Borders may be regular or irregular.

DISTRIBUTION OF LESIONS Present on any region of the body and localized or widespread

Differential Diagnosis

Common acquired nevomelanocytic nevi, dysplastic melanocytic nevi, congenital blue nevus, nevus spilus, Becker's nevus, pigmented epidermal nevi, and café-au-lait macules should be considered in the differential diagnosis of CNN. Small CNN are virtually indistinguishable clinically from common acquired nevomelanocytic nevi except for size, and lesions >1.5 cm may be presumed to be either CNN or dysplastic melanocytic nevi. Without a good history or photographs, it may not be possible to ascertain the age of onset of a nevomelanocytic nevus <1.5 cm in diameter.

Laboratory and Special Examinations

Histopathology

Nevomelanocytes occur as well-ordered clusters (*theques*) in the epidermis and in the dermis as sheets, nests, or cords. *A diffuse infiltration of strands of nevomelanocytes in the lower one-third of the reticular dermis and subcutis is, when present, quite specific for CNN.*

Small and large CNN: Unlike the common acquired nevomelanocytic nevus, the nevomelanocytes in CNN tend to occur in the skin appendages (eccrine ducts, hair follicles, sebaceous glands) and in nerve fascicles and/or arrectores pilorum muscles, blood vessels (especially veins), and lymphatic vessels and extend into the lower two-thirds of the reticular dermis and deeper.

Very large or giant CNN: A similar histopathology to small and large CNN, but the nevomelanocytes may extend into the muscle, bone, dura mater, and cranium.

Etiology and Pathogenesis

Congenital and acquired nevomelanocytic nevi are presumed to occur as the result of a developmental defect in neural crest–derived melanoblasts. This defect probably occurs after 10 weeks in utero but before the sixth uterine month; the occurrence of the "split" nevus of the eyelid is an indication that nevomelanocytes migrating from the neural crest were in place in this site before the eyelids split (24 weeks).

Course and Prognosis

By definition, CNN appear at birth, but varieties of CNN may arise during infancy (so-called tardive CNN). The life history of CNN is not documented, but CNN have been observed in elderly persons, an age when acquired nevomelanocytic nevi have disappeared.

Very large or giant CNN: The lifetime risk for development of melanoma in large CNN has been estimated to be at least 6.3 %; in 50 % of patients who develop melanoma in large CNN, the diagnosis is

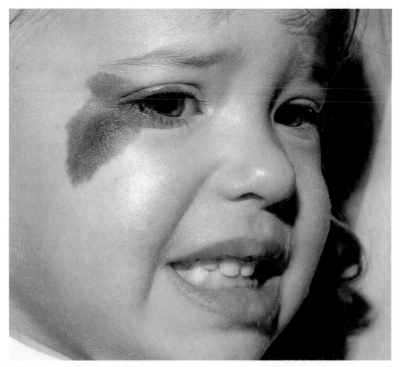

Figure 9-5 Congenital nevomelanocytic nevus *A sharply demarcated, tan-brown plaque, involving the upper and lower eyelids and the right cheek.*

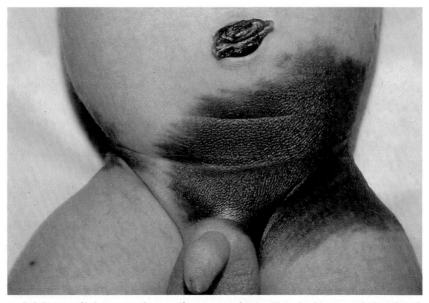

Figure 9-6 Congenital nevomelanocytic nevus, giant *Sharply demarcated chocolate-brown hairless plaque with smudged borders in a newborn. With increasing age, lesions usually become elevated and hairy.*

made between the ages of 3 and 5 years. Melanoma that develops in a large CNN has a poor prognosis.

Small CNN: The lifetime risk of developing malignant melanoma is 1 % to 5 %.

Management

Small Nevi Nevi <1.5 cm that are not known to be present at birth should be assumed to be acquired and be managed according to the appearance and growth pattern. Atypical-appearing CNN should be removed. Small CNN should be removed before age 12 years.

Large Nevi Nevi >1.5 cm that are not obviously dysplastic melanocytic nevi should be managed as CNN when the history is not available.

Alternatives

Prophylactic excision
Periodic follow-up for life, *or*

Patient's parents or patient advised to see physician only if a change (color, pattern, size) in the lesion.

Surgical Excision Surgical excision is the only acceptable method.

Small and large CNN:
Excision, with full-thickness skin graft, if required
Swing flaps, tissue expanders for large lesions

Giant CNN: Risk of development of melanoma is significant even in the first 3 to 5 years of age, and therefore, giant CNN should be removed as soon as possible. Individual considerations are necessary (size, location, degree of loss of function, or amount of mutilation). New surgical techniques utilizing the patient's own normal skin grown in tissue culture can now be used to facilitate removal of very large CNN. Also, tissue expanders can be utilized.

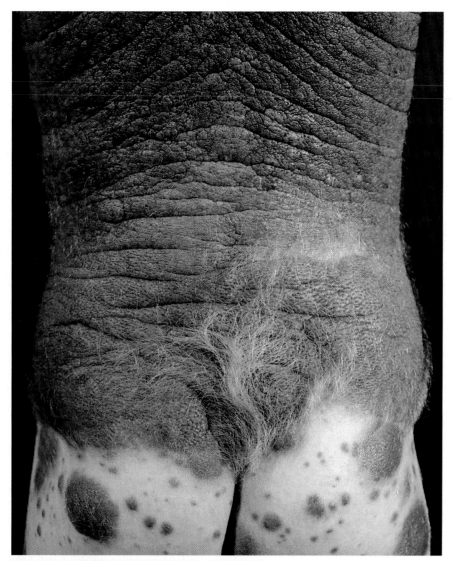

Figure 9-7 Congenital nevomelanocytic nevus, giant *The lesion involves the majority of the skin, with complete replacement of normal skin of the back and multiple smaller CNN on the buttocks and thighs. Note hypertrichosis of the sacral area.*

LENTIGO MALIGNA AND LENTIGO MALIGNA MELANOMA

Lentigo maligna melanoma is the least common (5 %) of the three principal melanomas of white persons [superficial spreading melanoma (SSM), nodular melanoma (NM), and lentigo maligna melanoma (LMM)] and occurs in older persons on the most sun-exposed areas, the face and forearms. While there is still some debate about the role of sunlight in the pathogenesis of malignant melanoma, few will question the role of sunlight in the pathogenesis of LMM; the tumor was first noted on the faces of women working outdoors in the vineyards of France by Dubreuilh, who called it *melanosis circumscripta preblastomatosa*. Lentigo maligna (LM) is a flat (macular) intraepidermal neoplasm and the precursor or evolving lesion of LMM. Focal papular and nodular areas signal invasion into the dermis; the lesion is then called LMM.

Epidemiology and Etiology

Age   Median age is 65 for LMM.

Sex   Incidence in males and in females is equal.

Race   Rare in brown- (e.g., Asiatics, East Indians) or black-skinned (African Americans) peoples. Highest incidence in whites and skin phototypes I, II, and III.

Incidence   5 % to 10 % of primary cutaneous melanomas

Predisposing Factors   Same factors as in sun-induced nonmelanoma skin cancer (squamous cell carcinoma and basal cell carcinoma): older population, outdoor occupations (farmers, sailors, construction workers)

History

LMM very slowly evolves from LM over a period of several years, sometimes 20 years.

Physical Examination

Skin Lesions

TYPE   *Lentigo Maligna*   Uniformly flat, macule (Figure 9-8, on right side of photo)
Lentigo Maligna Melanoma   Flat with focal areas of papules (Figure 9-9, on left side of photo) and nodules (Figure 9-9, center)

COLOR   *Lentigo Maligna*   Striking variations in hues of brown and black, appears like a "stain," haphazard network of black on a background of brown. The clinical change that indicates the development of LMM is a very dark brown or black pigmentation within the background of LM or appearance of papules or plaques.
Lentigo Maligna Melanoma   Same as LM plus gray areas (indicates focal regression), and blue areas indicate dermal pigment (melanocytes or melanin). Papules or nodules may be blue, black, or pink. Rarely LMM may be nonpigmented.

SIZE   *Lentigo Maligna*   3.0 to 20.0 cm or larger
Lentigo Maligna Melanoma   Same as LM

SHAPE   *Lentigo Maligna and Lentigo Maligna Melanoma*   Irregular borders, often with a notch, "geographic" shape with inlets and peninsulas. Sharply defined

DISTRIBUTION   *Lentigo Maligna and Lentigo Maligna Melanoma*   Single isolated lesion on the sun-exposed areas: forehead, nose, cheeks, neck, forearms, and dorsa of hands, rarely on lower legs

OTHER SKIN CHANGES IN AREAS OF TUMOR   Sun-induced changes: solar keratosis, freckling, telangiectasia, thinning of the skin, i.e., dermatoheliosis

General Medical Examination   Check for regional lymphadenopathy.

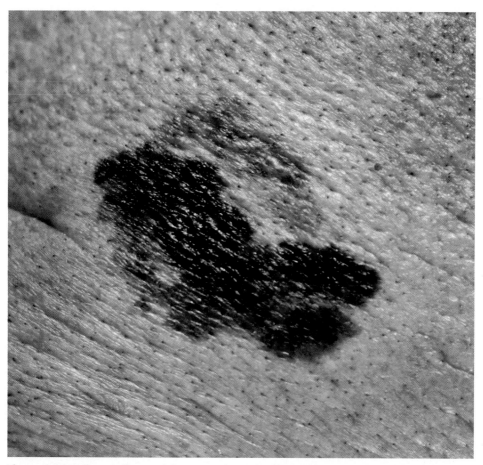

Figure 9-8 Lentigo maligna *A large macule on the cheek with irregular borders and striking variegation of melanin pigment (white, tan, brown, dark brown, black).*

Differential Diagnosis

Variegate Tan-Brown Macule LMM and LM are quite unique dark flat lesions, with focal elevations (papules and nodules) in LMM. *Seborrheic keratoses* may be dark but are exclusively papules or plaques and have a characteristic stippled surface often with a verrucous component, i.e., a "warty" surface which, when scratched, exhibits fine scales; also "horn cysts" often can be seen. *Solar lentigo,* although macular, does not exhibit the intensity or variegation of brown, dark brown, and black hues seen in LM.

Laboratory and Special Examinations

Dermatopathology

See Figure E-1 in Appendix E. LM may and does extend into the hair follicles and may thus reach the mid-dermis even in the preinvasive stage. This is the reason why such lesions should be excised (see Management, below).

Pathophysiology

In contrast to SSM and NM, which appear to be related to intermittent high-intensity sun exposure and occur on the intermittently exposed areas (back and legs) and in young or middle-aged adults, LM and LMM occur on the face and neck and dorsa of the forearms or hands; furthermore, LM and LMM occur almost always in persons with evidence of heavily sun-damaged skin (telangiectasia, marked freckling, atrophy and solar keratosis, basal cell carcinoma).

Prognosis

Summarized in Table E-1 in Appendix E.

Management

1. Excise with 1.0-cm or greater margin beyond the clinically visible lesion, provided the flat component does not involve a major organ. Use of Wood's lamp will help in defining borders.
2. Excise down to the fascia. Graft may be needed. Margin width greater than 1.0 cm is determined by location; a greater margin should be obtained if technically possible.
3. No node dissection recommended unless nodes are clinically palpable.

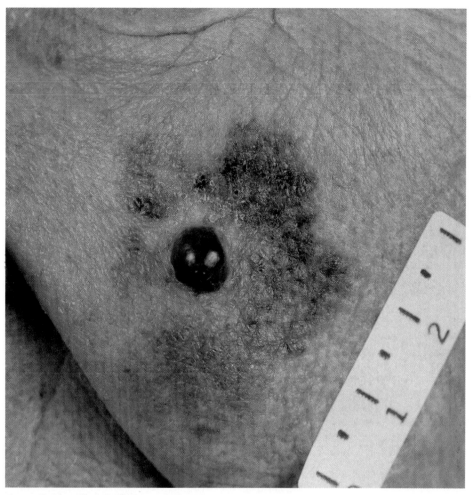

Figure 9-9 Lentigo maligna melanoma *A typical large lentigo maligna (in situ melanoma) on the left cheek with a black nodule of invasive melanoma arising within it.*

DESMOPLASTIC MELANOMA

The term *desmoplasia* refers to connective tissue proliferation and when applied to malignant melanoma describes different clinical presentations; however, each has a similar microscopic pathology, characterized by (1) a dermal fibroblastic component with only minimal or absent melanocytic proliferation at the dermal-epidermal junction or (2) nerve-centered superficial malignant tumors with or without an atypical intraepidermal melanocytic component or (3) other lesions in which the tumor appears to arise in lentigo maligna or, rarely, in acral lentiginous melanoma or superficial spreading melanoma. Also, desmoplastic melanoma (DM) growth patterns have been noted in recurrent malignant melanoma. The primary tumors occur on the head and neck, most commonly on the face, but may be first noted on the trunk or extremities. Desmoplastic melanoma occurs more frequently in women and in persons with dermatoheliosis ("photoaging"). The diagnosis requires an experienced dermatopathologist; S-100 immunoperoxidase positive spindle cells need to be identified in the matrix collagen. HMB-45 staining may be negative.

Epidemiology

Age Median age at diagnosis 56 years (range, fourth to ninth decades)

Sex More common in women

Race Skin phototypes I to III

Incidence Rare

Etiology Since most, but not all, lesions are seen on the sun-damaged skin of the head and neck, ultraviolet radiation exposure has been implicated in its pathogenesis, just as it has in superficial spreading melanoma, lentigo maligna melanoma, and nodular melanoma.

Predisposing and Risk Factors DM occurs most frequently on the head and neck, in a distribution similar to lentigo maligna and lentigo maligna melanoma.

History

Duration of Lesion Months to many years. DM is commonly misdiagnosed clinically as a dermatofibroma or neurofibroma because of the absence of color.

Skin Symptoms Asymptomatic. Early and slowly growing lesions are often overlooked by the patient, even though visible on the face and neck.

Physical Examination

Skin Lesions

TYPE *Macule* Early lesions may appear as a variegated lentiginous macule, at times with small blue-gray dermal nodules. The lesions actually may arise in lentigo maligna melanoma.
Papule/Nodule (Figure 9-10) May appear as a dermal nodule, with or without any epidermal involvement

COLOR Tumors commonly lack any melanin pigmentation. When melanin is principally contained in malignant melanocytes in the dermis, DM may be gray to blue.

SIZE Because of delay in correct diagnosis, DM may be large.

PALPATION Early lesions often cannot be palpated. Older nodular lesions are firm, like a dermal scar or dermatofibroma.

SHAPE Borders are irregular when epidermal involvement is present, as in lesions arising in lentigo maligna melanoma.

DISTRIBUTION 85 % of DM occurs on the head and neck, and the majority of these on the face (Figure 9-10), but lesions also occur rarely on the trunk and in acral areas.

Differential Diagnosis

Blue/Gray Nodule Basal cell carcinoma, blue nevus, cellular blue nevus, Spitz (spindle cell) nevus, metastatic melanoma to skin, LM, LMM

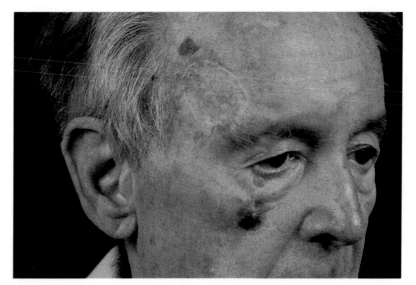

Figure 9-10 Desmoplastic melanoma *A large nodule with bluish-red and brown portion in an elderly male; lesions often are surrounded by a macular portion resembling lentigo maligna. A nonmelanoma skin cancer had been previously excised from the temple.*

Laboratory and Special Examinations

Dermatopathology

EPIDERMIS Atypical junctional melanocytic proliferation, either individual or focal nests, occurs, resembling lentigo maligna.

DERMIS S-100–positive spindle-shaped cells embedded in matrix collagen that widely separates the spindle cell nuclei. Spindle cells may have non-membrane-bound melanosomes and premelanosomes. Small aggregates of lymphocytes are commonly seen at periphery of DM. Neurotropism is characteristic, i.e., fibroblast-like tumor cells around or within endoneurium of small nerves. DM often has a thickness of >2.0 mm. Often, DM is seen with a background of severe solar damage to the dermis.

Histologic Differential Diagnosis Pigmented malignant schwannoma, blue nevus, malignant melanoma arising in a blue nevus, cellular blue nevus, dermatofibroma, neurofibroma, scar, desmoplastic Spitz nevus, lentigo maligna melanoma

Diagnosis

It is essential to obtain an adequate biopsy; punch biopsies can be misleading.

Pathophysiology

DM may be a variant of lentigo maligna melanoma in that most lesions occur on the head and neck in patients with sun-damaged skin. DM is more likely to recur locally and metastasize than lentigo maligna melanoma, however.

Course and Prognosis

Diagnosis of DM is often delayed because of the bland clinical appearance and ill-defined margins. There are mixed views about the prognosis of DM. In one series following primary excision of DM, approximately 50 % of patients experienced local recurrence, usually within 3 years of excision; some patients experienced multiple recurrences. Lymph node metastasis occurs less often than local recurrence. In one series, 20 % developed metastases, and DM was regarded as a more aggressive tumor than lentigo maligna melanoma.

Management

Aggressive surgical treatment.

SUPERFICIAL SPREADING MELANOMA

Superficial spreading melanoma (SSM) is one of two major cancers [SSM and nodular melanoma (NM)] that arise in melanocytes of persons with white skin. It arises most frequently on the upper back and occurs as a moderately slow-growing lesion over a period of years. SSM has a distinctive morphology: a uniformly elevated, flattened lesion (plaque). The pigment variegation of SSM is similar to but often less striking than the variety of color present in most lentigo maligna melanomas. The color display is a mixture of brown, dark brown, blue, black, and red, with slate-gray or gray regions in areas of tumor regression.

Epidemiology

Age   30 to 50 (median, 37) years

Sex   Slightly higher incidence in females

Race   In world surveys, white-skinned persons overwhelmingly predominate. Only 2 % were brown- or black-skinned. Furthermore, brown and black persons have melanomas usually occurring on the extremities; half of brown or black persons have primary melanomas arising on the sole of the foot.

Incidence   SSM constitutes 70 % of all melanomas arising in white persons. Melanoma accounts for about 5 % of all skin cancers, but new cases increase each year by 7 %.

Predisposing and Risk Factors   Four important risk factors are, in order of importance:

1. Presence of precursor lesions (Clark's dysplastic melanocytic nevus, congenital melanocytic nevus; see pages 182 and 187)
2. Family history of melanoma in parents, children, or siblings
3. Light skin color with inability to tan with ease (skin phototypes I and II)
4. Excessive sun exposure, especially during preadolescence.

Especially increased incidence in young urban professionals, with a frequent pattern of intermittent, intense sun exposure ("weekenders") or winter holidays near the equator.

History   Evolves over a period of 1 to 2 years

Physical Examination

Skin Lesions (Figures 9-11 to 9-15)

TYPE   Flattened papule, becoming a plaque, and then developing one or more nodules

COLOR   Dark brown, black, with admixture of pink, gray, and blue-gray hues—with marked variegation and a haphazard pattern. White areas indicate regressed portions.

SIZE   Mean diameter 8.0 to 12.0 mm. Early lesions, 5.0 to 8.0 mm; late lesions, 10.0 to 25.0 mm.

SHAPE   Asymmetrical (one half unlike the other), oval with irregular borders and often with one or more indentations (notches). Sharply defined

DISTRIBUTION   Isolated, single lesions; multiple primaries are rare.

Sites of Origin
Back (males and females)
Legs (females, between knees and ankles)
Anterior trunk and legs in males
Relatively fewer lesions on covered areas, e.g., swim suit, bra

General Examination   Always search for regional nodes.

Laboratory and Special Examinations

Biopsy

Total excisional biopsy with narrow margins—optimal biopsy procedure, where possible (see Appendix E)

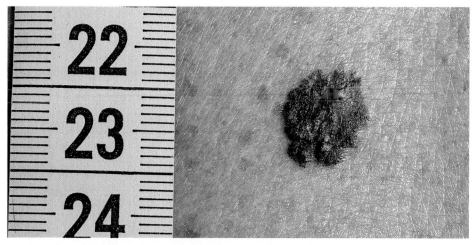

Figure 9-11 Superficial spreading melanoma arising de novo *A flat-topped, elevated, plaque on the trunk with sharply demarcated and irregular margins exhibiting variegation of melanin pigmentation, which ranges from light brown to dark brown and black as well as hues of red. The surface is irregular with a cobblestoned pattern.*

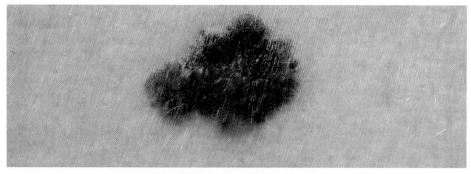

Figure 9-12 Superficial spreading melanoma arising de novo *An asymmetrical, flat plaque with irregular and sharply defined margins. The melanin pigmentation ranges from light brown to pink, dark brown, black, and blue. A dark red-black nodule represents vertical growth and invasion of this SSM.*

Incisional or punch acceptable when total excisional biopsy cannot be performed or when lesion is large, requiring extensive surgery to remove the entire lesion

Wood's Lamp Examination Useful for defining borders

Epiluminescence Microscopy Increases diagnostic accuracy by 30 %.

Dermatopathology See Figure E-2 in Appendix E. Malignant melanocytes are S100 and usually also HMB-45 positive.

Diagnosis (ABCDE)

The five cardinal features of SSM are

A, for asymmetry
B, border is irregular and scalloped
C, color is mottled, haphazard display of

brown, black, gray, pink

D, diameter is large—greater than a pencil eraser (6.0 mm)

E, (1) *enlargement,* growth in size, very important sign of evolving melanoma, and (2) *elevation* is almost always present with surface distortion, subtle or obvious, and assessed by side-lighting of lesion

Pathophysiology

In the early stages of growth there is an intraepidermal or "radial growth" phase, during which tumorigenic pigment cells are confined to the epidermis and thus cannot metastasize (this is called *melanoma in situ*)—or "thin" SSM, in which the tumor cells are confined to the epidermis and upper dermis. This "grace period" of the radial growth phase, with potential for cure, is followed by the invasive "vertical growth" phase, in which malignant cells consist of a tumorigenic nodule that invades the dermis with potential for metastasis (see Figure E-2 in Appendix E).

The pathophysiology of SSM is not yet understood. Certainly, in some considerable number of SSM, sunlight exposure is a factor, and both SSM and NM are related to occasional bursts of recreational sun exposure during a susceptible period (<14 years). About 10 % of the 32,000 new melanomas each year occur in high-risk families. The rest of the cases may occur sporadically among people without a specific genetic risk. Persons at high risk inherit the gene in a mutated form of a normal gene that controls melanocytic proliferation.

Course and Prognosis

Left untreated, SSM develops deep invasion (vertical growth) over months to years. Prognosis is summarized in Table E-1 in Appendix E. Melanoma will be responsible for about 7300 deaths in 1996; this is three times the number of deaths from other skin cancers.

Management and Follow-Up

See Appendix E.

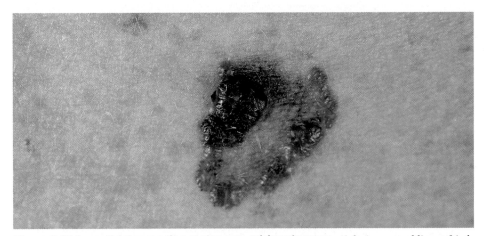

Figure 9-13 Superficial spreading melanoma arising de novo *A lesion resembling a fried egg with a flat portion with color variegation (horizontal growth phase) with a black nodule arising within it (vertical invasive growth phase). The central, whitish-bluish area represents inflammatory regression of the melanoma.*

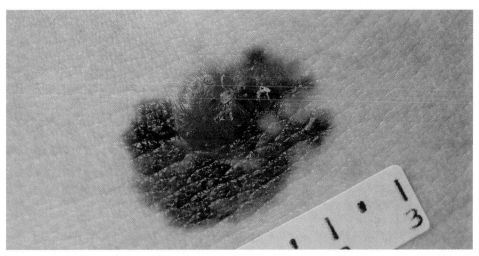

Figure 9-14 Superficial spreading melanoma arising within dysplastic nevus *A macule with a red-brown nodule arising within it: the macular portion (a preexisting dysplastic nevus) shows variegation of melanin pigmentation; the nodule shows slight erosion and crusting and represents the invasive vertical growth phase.*

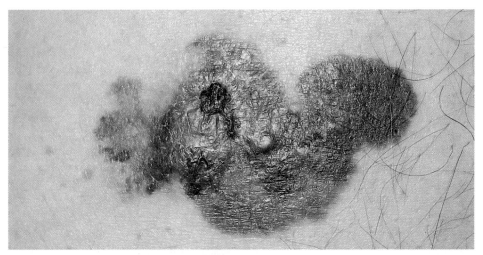

Figure 9-15 Superficial spreading melanoma *A highly characteristic lesion with all features of SSM: Asymmetry, Borders which are highly irregular, Colors that are widely variegated, Diameter much greater than 1-cm, and Elevation of the central portion. Note also ulceration in the central portion of the lesion.*

NODULAR MELANOMA

Nodular melanoma (NM) is second in frequency (14 %) after superficial spreading melanoma (SSM) in most series, occurring largely in middle life in persons with white skin and, as in SSM, on the less commonly exposed areas. The tumor from the beginning is in the "vertical growth" phase and could appropriately be called a *deeply penetrating melanoma* (as opposed to SSM). NM is uniformly elevated and presents as a thick plaque or an exophytic, polypoid lesion (a *nodule* is defined as a palpably round lesion). The color pattern is usually not variegated, and the lesion is uniformly blue or blue-black or, less commonly, can be very lightly pigmented or nonpigmented (amelanotic melanoma) and confused with a pyogenic granuloma or other nonpigmented tumors. NM is the one type of primary melanoma that arises quite rapidly (4 months to 2 years) from normal skin or from a melanotic nevus as a nodular (vertical) growth without an adjacent epidermal component, as is always present in SSM and LMM.

Epidemiology and Etiology

Age   Median age is 50 years.

Sex   Equal incidence in males and in females

Race   NM occurs in all races, but in the Japanese it occurs eight times more frequently (27 %) than SSM (3 %).

Incidence   NM constitutes 15 % to 30 % of the melanomas in the United States.

Predisposing Risk Factors   Four important risk factors, in order of importance, are *presence of precursor lesions* (Clark's dysplastic melanocytic nevus, congenital nevomelanocytic nevus); *family history* of melanoma in parents, children, or siblings; *light skin color* with inability to tan with ease; and *excessive sun exposure,* especially during preadolescence. Especially increased incidence in young urban professionals with a frequent pattern of intermittent intense sun exposure ("weekenders" or winter holidays near the equator).

History

Evolution over 6 to 18 months

Physical Examination

Skin Lesions

TYPE   Uniformly elevated "blueberry-like" nodule (Figures 9-16 and 9-17 and E-3) or ulcerated or "thick" plaque; may become polypoid.

COLOR   Uniformly dark blue, black, or "thundercloud" gray; polypoid lesions may appear pink (amelanotic) with trace of brown.

SIZE   1.0 to 3.0 cm (early lesions) but may grow much larger if undetected

SHAPE   Oval or round, usually with smooth, not irregular, borders, as in all other types of melanoma. Sharply defined

DISTRIBUTION   Same as SSM. In the Japanese, NM occurs on the extremities (arms and legs).

General Medical Examination   Always search for nodes.

Differential Diagnosis

Blue/Black Papule/Nodule   NM can be confused with *hemangioma* (long history) and *pyogenic granuloma* (short history—weeks) and is sometimes almost indistinguishable from *pigmented basal cell carcinoma* although it is usually softer (only biopsy settles this) and blue nevus (present for life). A "blueberry-like" nodule of recent origin (6 months to 1 year) should be excised or, if large, an incisional biopsy is mandatory for histologic diagnosis.

Laboratory Examinations

Biopsy

Total excisional biopsy with narrow margins—optimal biopsy procedure, where possible (see Appendix E)

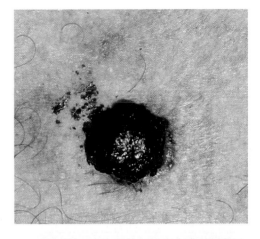

Figure 9-16 Nodular melanoma arising de novo *An eroded, bleeding, black nodule with an eccentric, gray-black, noneroded, cresent-shaped portion, having a mushroom-like configuration. Such lesions can be mistaken for a vascular lesion such as a pyogenic granuloma and should be excised, and the diagnosis confirmed histologically.*

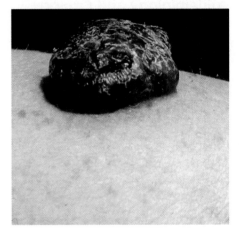

Figure 9-17 Nodular melanoma arising de novo *A mushroom cap-shaped, blue-black nodule, which is slightly hyperkeratotic, soft, and friable, arising on the shoulder.*

Incisional or punch acceptable when total excisional biopsy cannot be performed or when lesion is large, requiring extensive surgery to remove the entire lesion.

Dermatopathology See Figure E-3 in Appendix E. Tumor is S100 and HMB-45 positive.

Pathophysiology

Both SSM and NM occur in approximately the same sites (upper back in males, lower legs in females), and presumably the same pathogenetic factors are operating in NM as were described in SSM (page 200). The reason for the high frequency of NM in the Japanese is not known.

Prognosis

Summarized in Table E-1 in Appendix E.

Management and Follow-Up

See Appendix E.

ACRAL LENTIGINOUS MELANOMA

Acral lentiginous melanoma (ALM) is a special presentation of cutaneous melanoma arising on the sole, palm, fingernail or toenail bed, or the mucocutaneous skin of the mouth, genitalia, or anus. ALM occurs most often in Asians, sub-Saharan Africans, and African-Americans, comprising 50 % to 70 % of the melanomas of the skin found in these populations. It occurs most often in older males (>60 years) and often grows slowly over a period of years. The delay in development of the tumor is the reason these tumors are often discovered only when nodules appear or in case of nail involvement, the nail is shed; therefore, the prognosis is poor. The tumor may be misdiagnosed as a verruca plantaris, subungual hematoma, or an onychomycosis of the fingernail or the nail of the large toe. Subungual melanoma most often occurs on the nail bed of the thumb or large toe. The clinical features are less striking than in other melanomas, appearing in the radial growth phase as macules: dark brown, blue-black, or black, with little variegation and often ill-defined.

Epidemiology and Etiology

Age   Median age is 65.

Sex   Male : female ratio 3:1

Race   The best data are on American blacks and Japanese brown-skinned persons, and the incidence of melanoma is about one-seventh that of white persons. ALM is the principal melanoma in the Japanese and in American and sub-Saharan African blacks. ALM accounts for 50 % to 70 % of melanomas in Japanese.

Incidence   7 % to 9 % of all melanomas; in whites, 2 % to 8 %

Predisposing Factors   There are pigmented lesions on the soles of African blacks that are regarded by some as precursor lesions. Subungual melanoma is the most frequent type of ALM in white persons, but trauma has not been proved to be a factor.

History

ALM is slow growing (about 2.5 years from appearance to diagnosis). The tumors occur on the volar surface (palm or sole) and in their radial growth phase may appear as a gradually enlarging "stain"; brown-black or bluish and occupying relatively large areas (8.0 to 12.0 cm) of the sole especially. ALM subungual (thumb or great toe) melanoma appears first in the nail bed and involves, over a period of 1 to 2 years, the nail matrix, eponychium, and nail plate. In the vertical growth phase nodules appear; often there are areas of ulceration, and nail deformity may occur.

Physical Examination

Skin Lesions

PALM OR SOLE   *Type*   Macular lesion in the radial growth phase with focal papules and nodules developing during the vertical growth phase
   Color   Marked variegation of color including brown, black, blue, depigmented pale areas
   Size   3.0 to 12.0 cm
   Shape   Irregular borders like lentigo maligna melanoma; usually well-defined but not infrequently ill-defined.
   Distribution   Soles, palms, fingers, and toes

SUBUNGUAL   *Type*   Subungual macule beginning at the nail matrix and extending to involve the nail bed and nail plate (Figure 9-18). Papules, nodules, and destruction of the nail plate may occur in the vertical growth phase (Figure 9-19).
   Color   Dark brown or black pigmentation that may involve the entire nail. Often the nodules or papules are unpigmented. Amelanotic melanoma is often overlooked for weeks to months.
   Distribution   Thumb or great toe

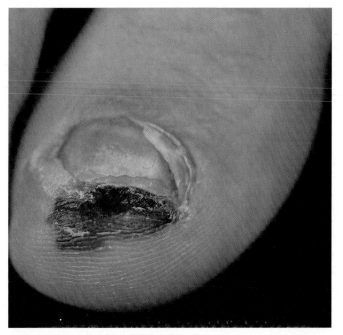

Figure 9-18 Acral lentiginous melanoma, early *A variegated, well-demarcated macule arising in the distal nail bed of the great toe and enlarging distally. The toe had been traumatized and the nail is regrowing. The ALM might be mistaken for a subungual ecchymosis or hematoma and diagnosis should be confirmed histologically.*

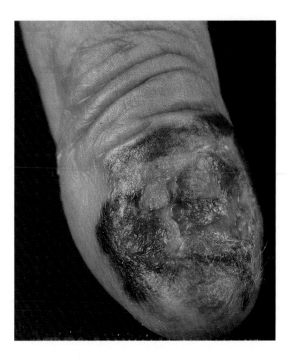

Figure 9-19 Acral lentiginous melanoma *The tumor has replaced the entire nail bed and surrounding skin; the most peripheral parts are macular and resemble a lentigo maligna. The central portion is amelanotic and eroded.*

Differential Diagnosis

Variegated Macule/Nodule (Volar) ALM (plantar type) is not infrequently regarded as a "plantar wart" and treated as such. Examination with Wood's lamp may reveal extensive, barely visible pigmentation far beyond what appears to be the borders when viewed with normal light.

Subungual Discoloration ALM (subungual) is usually considered to be traumatic bleeding under the nail and, in fact, subungual hematomas may persist for over 1 year, but usually the whole pigmented area moves gradually forward. Distinction of ALM from subungual hemorrhage can be made by epiluminescence microscopy (>95 %). With the destruction of the nail plate, the lesions are most often regarded as "fungal infection." When nonpigmented tumor nodules appear, these are diagnosed as a pyogenic granuloma.

Laboratory and Special Examinations

Dermatopathology The histologic diagnosis of the radial growth phase of the volar type of ALM may be difficult and may require large incisional biopsies to provide for multiple sections. There is usually an intense lymphocytic inflammation at the dermal-epidermal junction. Characteristic large melanocytes with prominent dendrites along the basal cell layer may extend as large nests into the dermis, as along eccrine ducts. Invasive malignant melanocytes are often spindle shaped so that ALM frequently has a desmoplastic appearance histologically.

Pathophysiology

Relatively rare compared to SSM in whites. Probably same incidence in Asians/Blacks who have fewer melanoma in general. The pigmented macules that are frequently seen on the soles of African blacks could be comparable with Clark's dysplastic melanocytic nevi.

Prognosis

The volar type of ALM can be deceptive in its clinical appearance, and "flat" lesions may be quite deeply invasive. Survival rates (5 years) are less than 50 %.

The subungual type of ALM has a better 5-year survival rate, 80 %, than does ALM (volar type). There are so few patients that the data are probably not accurate. Poor prognosis of ALM (volar type) may be related to inordinate delay in the diagnosis.

Management

In considering surgical excision, it is important that the extent of the lesion be ascertained by viewing the lesion with a Wood's lamp and epiluminescence microscopy. The borders of the tumor are indistinct or blurred. There may be a spread of pigment around the nail and onto the nail fold. Subungual ALM and volar type ALM: amputation [toe(s), finger(s)] and regional node dissection and/or regional perfusion with chemotherapeutic agents such as melphalan L-phenylalanine mustard).

MALIGNANT MELANOMA ARISING IN A CONGENITAL NEVOCELLULAR NEVUS

The lifetime risk of developing a malignant melanoma in a *giant* congenital nevocellular nevus (GCNN; so-called garment nevus or bathing-trunk nevus) (Figure 9-20) is at least 6.3 %, and these melanomas often appear before the age of 5 years. GCNN are lesions that cover large areas of the body.

Based on the detection of congenital nevi in association with melanoma using histology and a careful history, there is a significantly increased risk for developing melanoma in persons with small congenital nevus cell nevi (SCNN). This risk is as high as 21-fold based on history and 3- to 10-fold based on histology. Fifteen percent of 134 patients with primary cutaneous melanoma stated that the melanoma arose in a congenital nevus. Of 234 primary melanomas, 8.1 % had nevus cell nevi with congenital features. The expected association of SCNN and melanoma is less than 1:171,000 based on chance alone. Nonetheless, all SCNN should be considered for prophylactic excision at puberty if there are no atypical features (variegated color and irregular borders); SCNN with atypical features should be excised immediately.

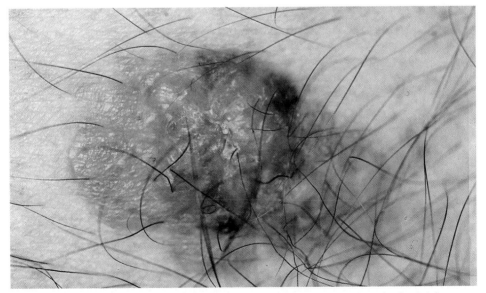

Figure 9-20 Melanoma in congenital nevus *A nodule with variegation of color (pink, tan, brown, gray) arising in a tan, 2-cm congenital nevomelanocytic nevus on the anterior pectoral region of a 40-year-old white male.*

PRECANCEROUS LESIONS AND CUTANEOUS CARCINOMAS

CUTANEOUS NONMELANOMA CANCERS (SQUAMOUS CELL CARCINOMA AND BASAL CELL CARCINOMA)

The two principal serious nonmelanoma cancers are squamous cell carcinoma (SCC) and basal cell carcinoma (BCC). Both are invasive into the dermis, and SCC can metastasize. Certain types (e.g., SCC induced by ionizing radiation or by inorganic trivalent arsenic) can be aggressive and are probably responsible for the mortality from this cancer. BCC in certain locations (nasolabial areas, around the eyes, and in the posterior auricular sulcus) can become deeply invasive and pose a major therapeutic challenge. Invasive SCC of the anogenital skin is induced by human papillomavirus (HPV); it is an increasingly common disorder in women under 40 years of age and, while not a highly aggressive tumor, HPV can be associated with carcinoma of the anogenital area, with cancer of the cervix, and with cancer of the bladder.

ORAL LEUKOPLAKIA

The term *leukoplakia* is a clinical, not a histologic, designation and describes (in the mouth) a sharply defined, white, macular or slightly raised area that cannot be rubbed off and which remains after the irritation (e.g., tobacco smoking) has been stopped for several weeks. *Candida* infection may be a secondary invader. Oral leukoplakia should be classified as a premalignant lesion because it is caused by exposure to the same agents that induce squamous cell carcinoma (SCC): smoking, alcohol, irritation from dentures or a jagged tooth, and occurrence (30 %) adjacent to SCC. The clinical assessment of dysplasia is deceptive because while dysplasia or early SCC can be present in white lesions, the most important to biopsy are red lesions (erythroplasia) or "speckled" ulceration within the white plaques because these are clinical indicators of dysplasia. Speckled white papules on an atrophic red background constitute a site that needs to be biopsied because these are usually sites of malignant transformation. Histologic hyperplastic leukoplakia seldom becomes transformed into SCC (<5 %), and these lesions have a high rate of spontaneous regression. Leukoplakia with histologic evidence of dysplasia (<10 % of lesions) is associated with a 10-fold higher rate of transformation into SCC.

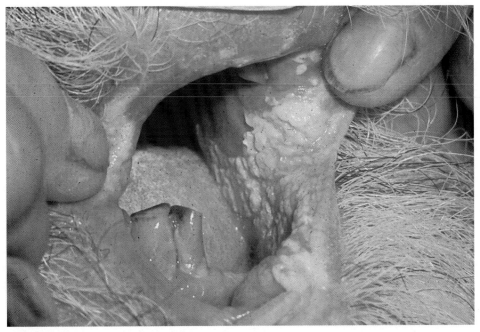

Figure 10-1 Oral leukoplakia *A white, thick plaque of firm consistency and irregular margins on the inner side of the cheek and on the vermilion border of the lips. The surface is rough and the lesion firmly adherent. The lesion, in a heavy pipe smoker, progressed to a verrucous carcinoma.*

Epidemiology

Age 40 to 70 years

Sex Males : females: 2:1

Etiology or Predisposing Factors Smoking (cigar, pipe, and cigarette), oral snuff (smokeless tobacco), alcohol, and human papillomavirus (HPV-11 and HPV-16). Syphilis may be the etiology of leukoplakia of the tongue and may complicate atrophic glossitis of tertiary syphilis.

History

Duration of Lesions Years

Skin Symptoms None

Physical Examination

Mucous Membrane Lesions

TYPE   Small or large plaque; homogeneous or "speckled"; ulceration may be present.

COLOR   Gray-white, red areas (erythroplakia)

PALPATION   Moderately rough or leathery

SHAPE AND SIZE   Angular. Size varies from a small (2.0 cm) to very large (4.0 cm) plaque.

SITES OF PREDILECTION   Buccal mucosa (Figure 10-1), retrocommissural mucosa, tongue, hard palate, sublingual region, and gingiva

Differential Diagnosis

Lichen planus, oral lesion of chronic cutaneous lupus erythematosus, oral hairy leukoplakia, condyloma acuminatum, bite "callus," leukoderma, nicotine stomatitis

Dermatopathology

Site Epidermis

Process Neoplastic. Dysplasia of keratinocytes with keratinization of single cells, abnormal mitoses, increased nuclear/cytoplastic ratio, cell and nuclear pleomorphism, enlarged and/or multiple nucleoli.

Pathophysiology

A premalignant lesion arising from chronic irritation or inflammation. Certain types carry a high risk for developing malignancy: (1) leukoplakia that is speckled (with gray and white patches) rather than homogeneous and (2) leukoplakia in certain sites—floor of the mouth and central surface of the tongue. Pipe and cigar smoking can produce *leukokeratosis nicotina palati,* which rarely becomes malignant and regresses with cessation of smoking. It is confined to the palate and appears as diffuse whitish thickening of the mucous membranes studded with multiple red dots (openings of salivary gland ducts).

Prognosis

About 10 % of leukoplakic lesions can progress to malignancy, and the frequency of this event is related to the site of occurrence. Leukoplakia on the buccal mucosa is almost always found to be benign. On the other hand, leukoplakia on the floor of the mouth is serious, with over 60 % showing either carcinoma *in situ* or invasive squamous cell carcinoma; these patients must be followed carefully. Also, clinically speckled gray and white patches are more likely to develop carcinoma. Oral cancer is clearly related to smoking, alcohol, and oral snuff.

Management

Careful follow-up is important, and lesions should be biopsied to exclude dysplasia or frank carcinoma. Lesions with dysplasia can be treated with cryosurgery. Recent studies have shown that oral beta-carotene may cause a partial regression of leukoplakia. Chemopreventative trials with synthetic retinoids look promising. Leukoplakia that shows *in situ* carcinoma or invasive carcinoma must be excised surgically.

RADIATION DERMATITIS*

Radiation dermatitis is defined as skin changes resulting from exposure to ionizing radiation. There are *reversible effects,* i.e., erythema, epilation, suppression of sebaceous glands, and pigmentation that lasts for weeks to months to years, and *irreversible effects,* i.e., acute and chronic radiation dermatitis and radiation-induced cancers.

Type of Exposure

Result of therapy (for cancer, formerly used for acne and psoriasis), accidental, or occupational (e.g., formerly in physicians, dentists). The radiation causing radiodermatitis includes superficial and deep x-ray radiation, electron-beam therapy, and grenz-ray therapy. It is a prevailing myth among some dermatologists that grenz rays are "soft" and not carcinogenic; it has been

estimated that SCC can appear from more than 5000 cGy of grenz rays.

Types of Reactions

Acute Temporary erythema that lasts 3 days and then the main erythema, which reaches a peak in 2 weeks (Figure 10-2); pigmentation appears about day 20; a late erythema also can occur beginning on day 35 to 40, and this lasts 2 to 3 weeks. Massive reactions lead to blistering and ulceration. Permanent scarring may result.

*We acknowledge the contribution of Prof. F. Urbach and Prof. A. Wiskemann.

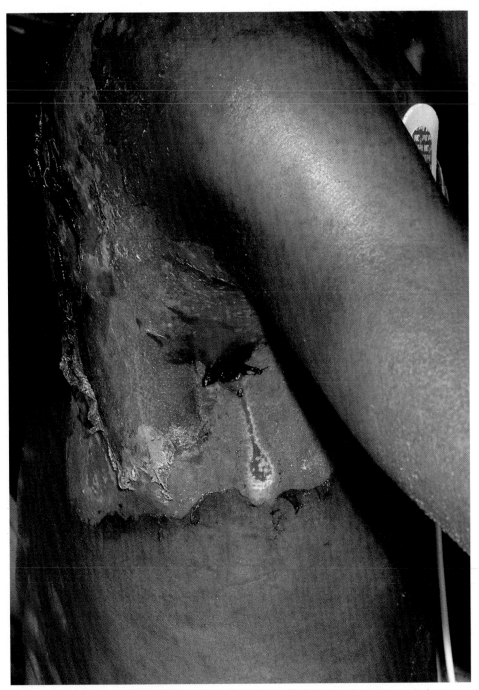

Figure 10-2 Radiation dermatitis: acute *Extensive, well-demarcated erosions and ulcerations at the site of radiotherapy given for rhabdomycosarcoma. The necrosis had rapidly worsened after a course of chemotherapy, so-called radiation recall.*

Chronic Following *fractional* but relatively intensive therapy with total doses of 3000 to 6000 rad, there develops an epidermolytic reaction in 3 weeks. This is repaired in 3 to 6 weeks, and scars and hypopigmentation develop; there is loss of all skin appendages and atrophy of the epidermis and dermis. During the next 2 to 5 years, the atrophy increases; there is hyper- and hypopigmentation telangiectasia, and superficial venules become ectatic. There are hyperkeratoses (x-ray keratoses) but necroses and ulceration are rare except by accidental exposure or error in doses: *very small doses at frequent intervals (monthly or weekly).* When necrosis occurs, it is leathery, yellow, and adherent and the base and surrounding skin are extremely painful. Ulcerations have a very poor tendency to heal and usually require surgical intervention (Figure 10-3). Accidental exposure occurs mostly in occupational exposure and affects the hands, feet, and face. There is a destruction of the fingerprint pattern, xerosis, scanty hair, atrophy of sebaceous and sweat glands, and development of keratoses. Persistent painful ulcers may appear.

Generalized Exanthems These occur beyond the irradiated area and usually follow deep x-ray therapy for internal cancers given through multiple ports. There may be fever and a dermatosis mimicking erythema multiforme or urticaria.

Physical Examination

Skin Lesions See Figure 10-3.

TYPE See preceding descriptions of acute and chronic radiation dermatitis

SHAPE

Sharp borders, rectangular, square (when result of therapy)

Diffuse involvement (when the result of prolonged, repeated exposures, as on the hands)

DISTRIBUTION

Hands and fingers (in professional personnel, in dentists, or in physicians using fluoroscopy)

Any site of previous therapy with ionizing radiation

Nails Longitudinal striations (in chronic radiodermatitis—following repeated exposures). Thickening, dystrophy

Dermatopathology (Chronic Radiation Dermatitis)

Site Epidermis and dermis

Atrophy of epidermis, with loss of hair follicles, sebaceous glands, and alteration of sweat glands

Hyalinization, loss of nuclei, fusion of collagen and elastic tissue

Vessel changes, including telangiectatic dilatation and fibrous thickening of the arterial wall

Course, Prognosis, and Management

Chronic radiation dermatitis is permanent, progressive, and irreversible. Squamous cell carcinoma (SCC) may develop in 4 to 39 years, with a median of 7 to 12 years, almost exclusively from the chronic repeated types of exposures. SCC always develops within the area of radiodermatitis, never in normal skin. The tumors are often multiple and metastasize late in about 25 %; despite extensive surgery (excision, grafts, etc.), the prognosis is poor, and recurrences are common. In recent years there has been about an equal incidence of SCC and basal cell carcinoma (BCC). BCC appears mostly in patients formerly treated with x-rays for acne vulgaris and acne cystica or epilation (tinea capitis). The tumors may appear 40 to 50 years after exposure. Excision and grafting is often possible before SCC develops.

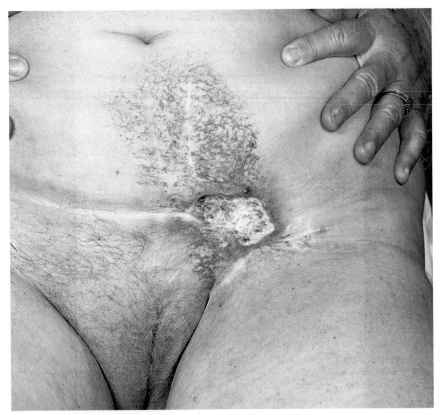

Figure 10-3 Radiation dermatitis: chronic *Atrophy, poikiloderma, telangiectasia, and ulceration with firm, adhering necrosis of yellow color on the lower abdomen at a portal of radiotherapy given 5 years previously. Ulceration arising in a site of chronic radiation dermatitis may represent progression to invasive squamous cell carcinoma.*

BASAL CELL CARCINOMA

Basal cell carcinoma (BCC) is the most common type of skin cancer. This malignant tumor is locally invasive, aggressive, and destructive, but there is a limited capacity to metastasize. The reason for this is the tumor's growth dependency on its stroma, which upon invasion of tumor cells into the vessels is not disseminated with the tumor cells. When tumor cells lodge at distant sites, they do not multiply and grow because of the absence of growth factors derived from the stroma of the tumor. Exceptions occur when a BCC shows signs of dedifferentiation, for instance, after inadequate radiotherapy. BCC usually arises only from epidermis that has a capacity to develop (hair) follicles. Therefore, BCCs rarely occur on the vermilion border of the lips or on the genital mucous membranes.

The majority of lesions are readily controlled by various surgical techniques or cryotherapy. Serious problems, however, may occur with BCC arising in certain locations on the face: around the eyes, in the nasolabial folds, around the ear canal, or in the posterior auricular sulcus. In these sites the tumor may invade deeply, cause extensive destruction of muscle and bone, and even invade to the dura mater. In such cases, death may result from hemorrhage of eroded large vessels or infection (meningitis).

Epidemiology and Etiology

Incidence United States: 500 to 1000 per 100,000, higher in the sunbelt; >400,000 new patients annually

Age Over 40 years

Sex Males more than females

Race Rare in brown- and black-skinned persons

Predisposing Factors White-skinned persons with poor tanning capacity (skin phototypes I and II) and albinos are highly susceptible to develop BCC with prolonged sun exposure. Previous therapy with x-rays for facial acne greatly increases the risk of BCC, even in those persons with a good ability to tan (skin phototypes III and IV). Superficial multicentric BCC occurs 30 to 40 years after ingestion of arsenic but also without apparent cause. Recent evidence of a history of heavy sun exposure in youth predisposing the skin to the development of BCC later in life puts BCC in the same category as malignant melanoma, in which sun exposure before age 14 sets a pattern for development of melanoma 30 to 40 years later.

Physical Examination

Skin Lesions

TYPE Papule or nodule, translucent or "pearly" (Figures 10-4 and 10-5). Ulcer (often covered with a crust) with a rolled border (rodent ulcer) (Figure 10-6). Cicatricial BCCs appear as scars (Figure 10-7). Superficial multicentric BCC appear as thin plaques (Figure 10-8).

COLOR Pink or red; characteristic fine thread-like telangiectasia can be seen with the aid of a hand lens. Pigmented BCC may be brown to blue or black (Figure 10-9).

SURFACE Smooth, glistening

PALPATION Hard, firm; cystic lesions may occur, however.

SHAPE Round, oval, depressed center ("umbilicated")

DISTRIBUTION Isolated single lesion; multiple lesions are not infrequent. Search carefully for danger sites: medial and lateral canthi, nasolabial fold.

Variants

SCLEROSING (SCLERODERMIFORM OR MORPHEA-LIKE) BCC (Figure 10-7) In this infiltrating type of BCC there is an excessive amount of fibrous stroma. The lesion therefore appears as a whitish, sclerotic patch with ill-defined borders and only occasional pearly papules at the periphery. Histologi-

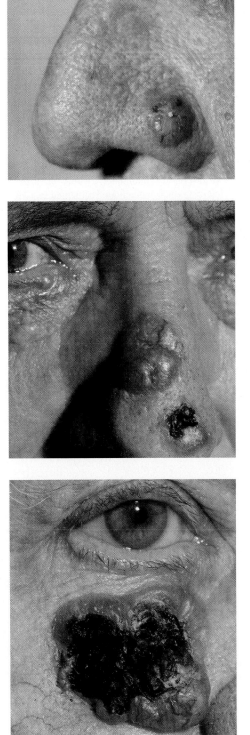

Figure 10-4 Basal cell carcinoma: nodular type *A solitary, shiny, red nodule with large telangiectatic vessels on the ala nasi, arising on skin with dermatoheliosis (solar elastosis).*

Figure 10-5 Basal cell carcinoma: nodular and ulcerative types *Two lesions are seen on the nose: a large, shiny, red nodule with a cobblestoned surface and an ulcerated nodule near the tip, arising in the setting of dermatoheliosis.*

Figure 10-6 Basal cell carcinoma: rodent-ulcer type *Large ulcer with well-demarcated borders that have the typical nodules of a BCC (a translucency, telangiectasia) and with a large crusted central necrotic area in the cheek; note setting of dermatoheliosis on the face (telangiectasias).*

cally, finger-like strands of tumor extend far into the surrounding tissue, and excision therefore requires wide margins.

SUPERFICIAL BCC (Figure 10-8) These superficial lesions are usually multiple, occur on the trunk, and often have no relation to sun exposure. They appear as erythematous, slightly scaly plaques, often but not always with a fine, rolled, pearly border. These lesions can mimic psoriasis, seborrheic keratosis, Bowen's disease, and tinea corporis.

PIGMENTED BCC These may occur in skin phototypes IV and V and are easily confused with primary malignant melanoma, especially nodular melanoma. Pigmented BCC is usually hard, whereas NM is soft. Epiluminescence microscopy permits a clinical diagnosis of BCC versus malignant melanoma.

Dermatopathology

Site Epidermis and dermis

Process Proliferating atypical basal cells (large, oval, deep-blue staining on H&E, but with little anaplasia and infrequent mitoses); variable amounts of mucinous stroma

Diagnosis

Serious BCCs occurring in the danger sites are readily detectable by careful examination with good lighting, a hand lens, and careful palpation.

Management

Excision with primary closure, skin flaps, or grafts. Cryosurgery and electrosurgery are options, but not in the danger sites. For lesions in the danger sites (nasolabial area, around the eyes, in the ear canal, in the posterior auricular sulcus, in sclerosing BCC, and on the scalp) microscopically controlled surgery (Mohs' surgery) is the best approach. Radiation therapy is an acceptable alternative but should be given only when disfigurement may be a problem with surgical excision (e.g., eyelids or large lesions in the nasolabial area).

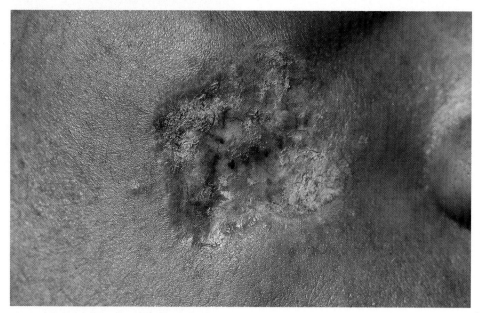

Figure 10-7 Basal cell carcinoma: sclerosing type *A large depressed area resembling a scar or morphea; many small areas of pigmentation typical of BCC and telangiectasia are seen with the lesion; the lateral margin is slightly raised.*

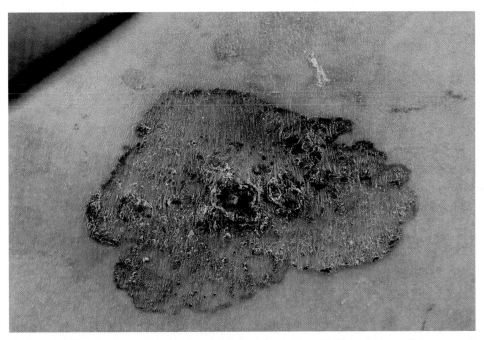

Figure 10-8 Basal cell carcinoma: superficial *A large (6-cm × 10 cm), flat, well-demarcated plaque on the trunk. The margin is sharply defined by a slightly rolled border. The lesion also contains a pigmented BCC with multiple blue-black dots giving a stippled pattern. These lesions usually bleed when lightly scratched with a fingernail; trauma has induced several superficial crusted erosions.*

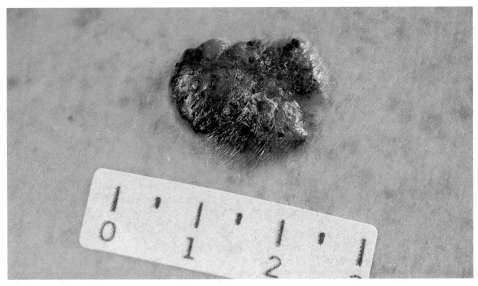

Figure 10-9 Basal cell carcinoma: pigmented *A nodule with irregular borders and variegation of melanin hues, easily confused with a malignant melanoma. Features indicating BCC are the areas of translucency and surface telangiectasia.*

BASAL CELL NEVUS SYNDROME

This autosomal dominant disorder affects skin [multiple basal cell carcinomas (BCCs) and palmoplantar pits] and has a variable expression of abnormalities in a number of systems, including skeletal malformations (mandibular "keratocysts"), soft tissue, eyes, CNS, and endocrine organs.

Epidemiology

Incidence   Frequency not known, but the condition is not rare.

Age   The BCCs may begin in late childhood, although several abnormalities are congenital.

Heredity   Autosomal dominant

Race   Mostly white but also occurs in African-Americans and Asians

Sex   Equal incidence

Precipitating Factors   There appear to be more BCCs on the sun-exposed areas of the skin, but they can occur in covered areas also.

History

Duration of Lesions   The BCCs begin to appear singly in childhood or early adolescence and continue to appear throughout life.

Systems Review   Congenital anomalies include undescended testes, hydrocephalus, blindness from coloboma, cataracts, and glaucoma.

Family History   Autosomal dominant with variable penetrance

Physical Examination

Appearance of Patient   There may be hundreds of lesions. Characteristic facies, with frontal bossing, broad nasal root, and hypertelorism

Skin Lesions

PRINCIPAL LESIONS   Basal cell carcinomas (translucent, 1.0- to 10.0-cm papules and nodules with and without ulcers) that are skin-colored or pigmented. Invasive tumors are uncommon but do occur. Tumors on the eyelids, axillae, and neck tend to be pedunculated.

ARRANGEMENT   Bilateral, often symmetrical

DISTRIBUTION   Face (Figure 10-10), neck, upper trunk, axillae, usually sparing scalp and extremities

PALMOPLANTAR LESIONS (see Figure 10-11) Present in 50 %, and these pits are pinpoint to several millimeters in size and 1.0 mm deep. There may be hundreds, especially on the lateral surfaces of the palms, soles, and fingers. The pits are the result of premature shedding of the horny layer. There may rarely be a BCC and there are almost always telangiectases at the bottom of the pit.

EXTRACUTANEOUS LESIONS   *Bone*   Mandibular jaw odontogenic keratocysts, which are multiple and may be unilateral or bilateral. Other bone lesions include defective dentition, bifid or splayed ribs, pectus excavatum, short fourth metacarpals, scoliosis, and kyphosis.
Eye   Strabismus, hypertelorism, dystopia canthorum, and congenital blindness
Central Nervous System   Agenesis of the corpus callosum, medulloblastoma; mental retardation is rare. Calcification of the lamellar falx.
Internal Neoplasms   Fibrosarcoma of the jaw, ovarian fibromas, teratomas, and cystadenomas

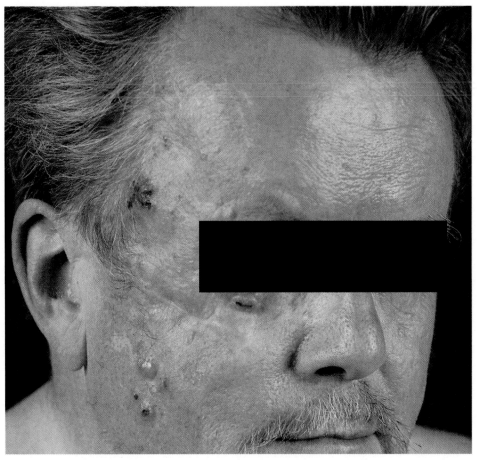

Figure 10-10 Basal cell nevus syndrome: basal cell carcinomas *Multiple nodular BCCs on the right side of the face, frontal bossing, and a large scar on the right cheek at the site of excision of an odontogenic cyst.*

Laboratory Examinations

Dermatopathology All types of basal cell carcinomas: solid, adenoid, cystic, ulcerating, superficial, and sclerodermiform

Imaging Lamellar calcification of the falx is a useful diagnostic sign.

Diagnosis

The disease is often discovered by oral surgeons or dentists because of the mandibular bone cysts, and the patient is referred to a dermatologist, who detects the palmar pits and observes the characteristic facies; confirmed histologically.

Etiology and Pathogenesis

The gene for the basal cell nevus syndrome has been identified and is located in chromosome 9q22.

Significance

The large number of skin cancers create a lifetime problem of vigilance on the part of the patient and the physician. The multiple excisions can cause considerable scarring.

Course and Prognosis

The tumors continue throughout life, and the patient must be followed carefully to detect early lesions in order to prevent disfiguring scars.

Management

Surgical excision and Mohs' surgery for cancers in certain locations such as the central areas of the face and behind, in, and around ears. Small lesions on the trunk or extremities can be treated with electrocautery or with combined topical tretinoin and 5 % fluorouracil for 25 to 30 days.

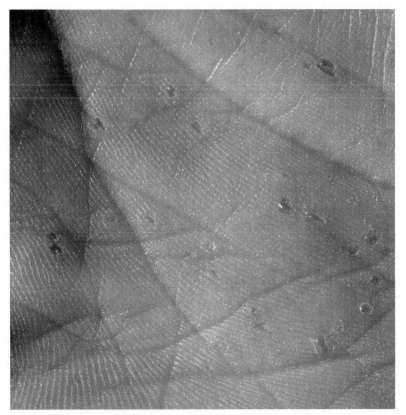

Figure 10-11 Basal cell nevus syndrome: palmar pits *Palmar surface of hand showing 1- to 2-mm, sharply marginated, depressed red lesions, i.e., palmar pits.*

SQUAMOUS CELL CARCINOMA OF SKIN AND MUCOUS MEMBRANES

Squamous cell carcinoma (SCC) is a malignant tumor of epithelial keratinocytes (skin and mucous membrane). SCC arises as a result of exogenous carcinogens [sunlight exposure, ingestion of arsenic, exposure to ionizing radiation (x-rays and gamma rays), and other etiologies].

Epidemiology

Incidence Continental United States: 12 per 100,000 white males; 7 per 100,000 white females; 1 per 100,000 blacks. Hawaii: 62 per 100,000 whites.

Race Persons with white skin and poor tanning capacity (skin phototypes I and II). Brown- or black-skinned persons can develop SCC from numerous etiologic agents other than sunlight exposure.

Age Over 55 years in the United States; in Australia, in the 20s and 30s

Sex Males > females, but SCC can occur more frequently on the legs of females.

Geography SCC induced by sunlight exposure is most common in geographic areas that have many days of sunshine annually and are inhabited by fair-skinned individuals. Penile SCC accounts for approximately 20 % of SCC in developing countries, but in the United States, for only 1 %. SCC of the oral mucosa is a special problem in the province of the oral surgeons (see Oral Leukoplakia, Section 33). Its incidence varies according to the country of origin, being higher in India, Southeast Asia, and Puerto Rico and low in Japan, Israel, and Scandinavia. This may be due to the use of the betel nut in India and Southeast Asia.

Occupation Persons (usually male) working outdoors—farmers, sailors, telephone linemen, construction workers, dock workers. Industrial workers exposed to chemical carcinogens (nitrosureas, polycyclic aromatic hydrocarbons)

Etiology

Human papillomavirus (induction of carcinoma of the anogenital area and periungual skin); the types of HPV linked to carcinomas in these areas are HPV-16, -18, -31, -33, -35, and -45. *Immunosuppression* (a major factor in rapidly promoting SCC and BCC in the sun-exposed sites of the skin of renal transplant patients on immunosuppressive drugs; *topical nitrogen mustards* (for the treatment of mycosis fungoides) can induce cutaneous SCC; *oral PUVA photochemotherapy* can lead to promotion of SCC in patients who are skin phototypes I and II and those patients with psoriasis who have had previous exposure to ionizing radiation, including electron beam and grenz rays; *discoid lupus erythematosus* (a rare event); *industrial carcinogens* (pitch, tar, crude paraffin oil, fuel oil, creosote, lubricating oil); and *arsenic* (inorganic trivalent arsenic as a medication in the past, as Fowler's solution used as a tonic and for the treatment of psoriasis; nowadays arsenic can still be present in the drinking water in some regions).

History

Slowly evolving—any isolated keratotic or eroded papule or plaque in a suspect patient that persists for over a month is considered a carcinoma until proved otherwise. Potential carcinogens often can be detected only after detailed interrogation of the patient.

INTRAEPITHELIAL *(IN SITU)* SQUAMOUS CELL CARCINOMA

Classification

PRECANCEROUS INTRAEPITHELIAL LESIONS

1. Solar (actinic) keratosis (see page 238)
2. Ionizing radiation–induced keratoses
3. Arsenical keratoses
4. Tar keratosis

IN SITU SCC

1. Bowen's disease
2. Erythroplasia (Queyrat)
3. HPV-induced SCC *in situ:* oropharynx, larynx, anus/perineum, vulva, cervix, penis

BOWEN'S DISEASE AND EFRYTHROPLASIA OF QUEYRAT

Bowen's disease is a solitary lesion (Figure 10-12) on the exposed (induced by solar radiation) and on the unexposed (related to ingestion of inorganic trivalent arsenic) skin. The lesion appears as a slowly enlarging erythematous plaque with a sharp border and little infiltration. There is usually slight scaling and some crusting. There is not a fine threadlike border as is seen in superficial basal cell carcinoma.

When this lesion occurs, usually in uncircumcised men, on the glans penis (Figure 10-13), coronal sulcus, or inner surface of the prepuce, or rarely on the vulva, it is known as *erythroplasia of Queyrat,* although it is identical clinically and histologically to Bowen's disease. The lesions of erythroplasia of Queyrat, however, are believed to metastasize more frequently (up to 30 % in one series) than in Bowen's disease on the glabrous skin. Invasive (three-dimensional) growth leads to fleshy, granulating, easily vulnerable, bleeding, and crusted nodules of rather soft consistency (Figure 10-14).

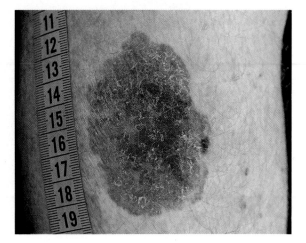

Figure 10-12 Squamous cell carcinoma in situ: Bowen's disease *A large, sharply demarcated, scaly, erythematous plaque simulating a psoriatic lesion on the calf.*

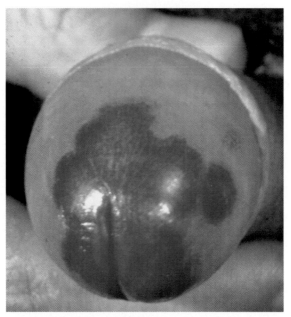

Figure 10-13 Squamous cell carcinoma in situ: erythroplasia of Queyrat *A well-demarcated, erythematous, glistening plaque on the glans.*

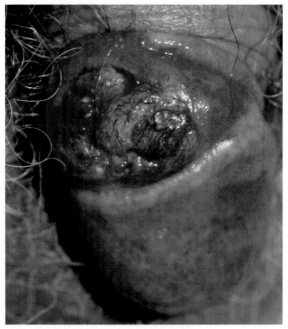

Figure 10-14 Squamous cell carcinoma arising from erythroplasia of Queyrat *A large, ulcerated, fungating nodule arising within an area of SCC in situ (erythroplasia of Queyrat) of the preputial sac.*

INVASIVE SQUAMOUS CELL CARCINOMA

Squamous cell carcinoma usually develops from a precancerous condition or a carcinoma *in situ,* often on the lips and other sun-exposed sites, and has the capacity to metastasize. For didactic reasons, two types can be distinguished:

1. Highly differentiated SCCs, which practically always show signs of keratinization either within or on the surface of the tumor. These are firm or hard upon palpation.
2. Poorly differentiated SCCs, which do not show signs of keratinization and clinically appear fleshy, granulomatous, and consequently are soft upon palpation.

Physical Examination

TYPE   Indurated papule, plaque, or nodule (Figure 10-16); adherent thick keratotic scale or hyperkeratosis; when eroded or ulcerated, the lesion may have a crust in the center and a firm, hyperkeratotic, elevated margin. Horny material may be expressed from the margin or the center of the lesion.

COLOR   Erythematous, yellowish, skin color

PALPATION   Hard

SHAPE   Polygonal, oval, round, or umbilicated

DISTRIBUTION   Usually isolated but may be multiple. Exposed areas. Sun-induced keratotic and/or ulcerated lesions especially on the face (cheeks, nose, lips), tips of ears, preauricular areas, scalp (in bald men), dorsa of the hands, and forearms, trunk, and shins (females)

MISCELLANEOUS OTHER SKIN CHANGES   Evidence of chronic sun exposure, termed *dermatoheliosis*: telangiectasia, freckling, dry scaly atrophic skin, small hypopigmented macules

OTHER PHYSICAL FINDINGS   Regional lymphadenopathy due to metastases

SPECIAL FEATURES   SCCs of the lips develop from leukoplakia or actinic cheilitis; in 90 % of cases they are found on the lower lip (Figure 10-15). In chronic radiodermatitis they arise from radiation-induced keratoses; in individuals with a history of chronic intake of arsenic from arsenical keratoses. SCCs in scars from burns or in chronic stasis ulcers of long duration are often difficult to identify. Suspicion is indicated when nodular lesions are hard and show signs of keratinization.

HISTOPATHOLOGY   SCCs with various grades of anaplasia and keratinization within the parenchyma or on its surface

Undifferentiated SCC

TYPE   Fleshy, granulating, easily vulnerable, erosive papules and nodules and papillomatous vegetations. Ulceration with a necrotic base and soft, fleshy margin. Hemorrhage, crusting (Figure 10-17).

COLOR   Red

PALPATION   Soft

SHAPE   Polygonal, irregular, often cauliflower-like

DISTRIBUTION   Isolated but also multiple, particularly on the genitalia, where they arise from erythroplasia (Figures 10-13 and 10-14), and on the trunk or face (rare), where they arise from Bowen's disease

MISCELLANEOUS OTHER SKIN CHANGES   Lymphadenopathy as evidence of regional metastases is more common than with differentiated, hyperkeratotic SCCs.

HISTOPATHOLOGY   Anaplastic SCC with multiple mitoses and little evidence of differentiation and keratinization

Differential Diagnosis

As stated previously, any persistent nodule, plaque, or ulcer, but especially when these occur in sun-damaged skin, on the lower lips, in areas of radiodermatitis, in old burn scars, or on the genitalia, must be examined for SCC. *In situ* SCC: nummular eczema, psoriasis, Paget's disease, superficial multicentric BCC.

Management

Surgery: depending on localization and extent of lesion, excision with primary closure, skin flaps, or grafting

Microscopically controlled surgery in difficult sites

Radiotherapy should be performed only if surgery is not feasible.

Carcinoma *in situ*: cryotherapy, 5-fluorouracil topically

Prognosis

SCC has an overall remission rate after therapy of 90 %. Those tumors which are induced by ionizing radiation, or following inorganic trivalent arsenic, or in an old burn scar, or on the lip or genitalia, are more likely to metastasize. SCC in patients with arsenical ingestion can also have primary SCC of the lung and the bladder. SCC in the skin has an overall metastatic rate of 3 % to 4 %, with those lesions arising in solar keratoses having the lowest potential for metastasis; cancers arising in chronic osteomyelitis sinus tracts and in burn scars and sites of radiation dermatitis have a much higher metastatic rate (31 %, 20 %, and 18 %, respectively).

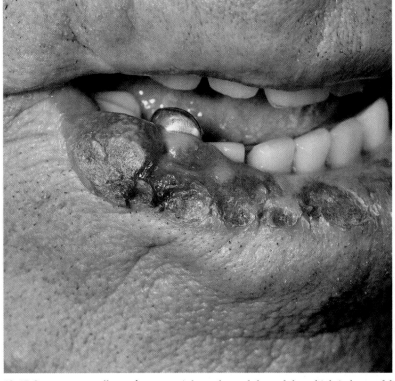

Figure 10-15 Squamous cell carcinoma *A large but subtle nodule, which is better felt than seen, on the vermilion border of the lower lip with areas of hyperkeratosis and erosion, arising in the setting of dermatoheliosis.*

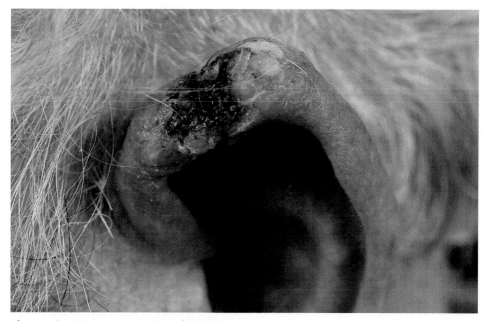

Figure 10-16 Squamous cell carcinoma *A large notch on the superior aspect of the helix, a nodule of SCC with hyperkeratosis and ulceration.*

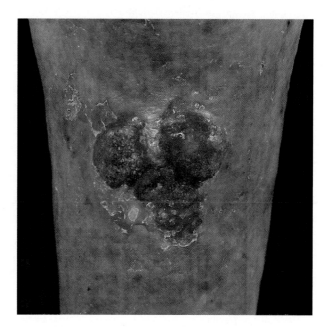

Figure 10-17 Squamous cell carcinoma: undifferentiated
Large, eroded, friable, red nodules arising within an old leg scar resemble granulation tissue, lacking the hyperkeratotic surface of a more well-differentiated SCC.

Section 11

PHOTOSENSITIVITY AND PHOTOINDUCED DISORDERS

SKIN REACTION TO SUNLIGHT EXPOSURE

Classification of Photosensitivity

Acute

Sunburn
Phototoxicity
    Drug-induced
    Plant-induced (phytophotodermatitis)
Photoallergy
    Drug-induced
    Solar urticaria
Idiopathic
    Polymorphic light eruption
    Actinic prurigo
    Hydroa vacciniforme

Chronic

Dermatoheliosis ("photoaging")
Chronic actinic dermatitis
Solar lentigo
Solar keratosis
Skin cancer
    Basal cell carcinoma
    Squamous cell carcinoma
    Malignant melanoma

Acute and/or Chronic

Porphyria cutanea tarda
Variegate porphyria
Erythropoietic protoporphyria
Xeroderma pigmentosum
Pellagra

Clinicians are always excited when, in a confusing eruption, they discover a clue to the eti-ology—this narrows the differential diagnostic list. Once the etiologic role of light is established, there is, moreover, a possibility of control of the disorder by discontinuing drugs or by topical or systemic treatment. The term *photosensitivity* describes an abnormal response to light, usually sunlight, occurring within minutes, hours, or days of exposure and lasting up to weeks and months.

Two broad types of *acute* photosensitivity are

1. A *sunburn*-type response with the development of morphologic skin changes simulating a normal sunburn: erythema, edema, vesicles, bullae. Examples are phototoxic reactions to drugs and phytophotodermatitis.
2. A *rash* response to light exposure with development of varied morphologic expressions: macules, papules, plaques, eczematous dermatitis, urticaria. Examples are polymorphous light eruption, eczematous drug reaction to sulfonamides.

Chronic repeated sun exposures over time result in degenerative polymorphic skin changes that have been termed *dermatoheliosis* (see page 232).

Diagnosis of Photosensitivity Disorders

This is presented in Appendix H in the form of several tables and drawings.

ACUTE SUN DAMAGE (SUNBURN)

Sunburn is an acute, delayed, and transient inflammatory response of the skin following exposure to ultraviolet radiation (UVR) obtained from sunlight or artificial sources. Sunburn is characterized by erythema and, if severe, by vesicles and bullae, edema, tenderness, and pain; in normal sunburn there are never "rashes," i.e., scarlatiniform macules, papules, or plaques that occur in abnormal reactions to UVR. UVR in photomedicine is divided into two principal types: UVB (290 to 320 nm), the "sunburn spectrum," and UVA (320 to 400 nm); UVA has recently been subdivided into UVA-1 (340–400 nm) and UVA-2 (320–340 nm). The unit of measurement of sunburn is the *minimum erythema dose* (MED), which is the minimum ultraviolet exposure that produces a clearly marginated erythema in the irradiated site following a single exposure. The MED is expressed in the amount of energy per unit area: mJ/cm^2 (UVB) or J/cm^2 (UVA). The MED for UVB in Caucasians is 20 to 40 mJ/cm^2 (about 20 minutes in northern latitudes at noon in June) and for UVA is 15 to 20 J/cm^2 (about 120 minutes in northern latitudes at noon in June). UVB erythema develops in 12 to 24 hours and fades within 72 to 120 hours. UVA erythema peaks between 4 and 16 hours and fades within 48 to 120 hours.

Epidemiology

Incidence and Skin Phototypes Sunburn is seen most frequently in individuals who have white skin and a limited capacity to develop *facultative* or inducible melanin pigmentation (tanning) following exposure to UVR. Skin color (*constitutive* melanin pigmentation) is divided into white, brown, and black. Not all persons with white skin have the same capacity to develop tanning, and this is the principal basis for the classification of individuals into four *skin phototypes* (SPT). The SPT is based on a *person's own estimate* of sunburning and tanning. One question will permit the identification of the SPT: "Do you tan easily?" Persons with SPT I or II will say immediately, "No," and those with SPT III or IV will say, "Yes." Persons with SPT I or II are regarded as "melanocompromised" and those with SPT III or IV as "melanocompetent." Regardless of their phenotype (hair and eye color), SPT I persons sunburn easily with short exposures (30 minutes) and *never* tan. SPT IV persons tan with ease and do not sunburn with short exposures. SPT II persons are a subgroup of SPT I and sunburn easily but *tan with difficulty,* while SPT III persons have some sunburn with short exposures but can develop, over time, marked tanning. It is estimated that about 25 % of white-skinned persons in the United States are SPT I and II. Persons with constitutive brown skin are termed SPT V and with black skin SPT VI.

Race Persons with brown and black skin color can, in fact, sunburn following long exposures. The SPT of various races has not yet been determined, but it is known that some Asiatics and Hispanics have SPT I and II.

Age Very young children and elderly persons appear to have a reduced capacity to sunburn.

Geography Sunburn can occur at any latitude and may be observed less frequently in the indigenous populations near the equator who respect the sun; sunburn is seen more often in people who frequent beaches or who travel to sunny vacation areas and obtain severe sunburns.

History

Relationship of Sunburn to Medications An "exaggerated" sunburn response can occur in persons who are taking phototoxic drugs: sulfonamides (chlorothiazides, furosemide), tetracyclines (doxycycline), phenothiazines, nalidixic acid, amiodarone, naproxen, psoralens.

Skin Symptoms Pruritus may be severe even in mild sunburn; pain and tenderness with severe sunburn.

Constitutional Symptoms Headache, chills, feverishness, and weakness are not infrequent in severe sunburn; some SPT I and II persons develop headache and malaise even following short exposures.

Family History Skin phototypes are genetically determined.

Physical Examination

Appearance of Patient In severe sunburn, the patient is "toxic"—with fever, weakness, and lassitude.

Vital Signs In severe sunburn, pulse rate is rapid.

Skin Lesions

TYPES Confluent erythema (Figure 11-1), edema, vesicles, and bullae confined to areas of exposure; no "rash"

COLOR Bright red

PALPATION Edematous areas are raised and tender.

DISTRIBUTION Strictly confined to areas of exposure; sunburn can occur in areas covered with clothing, depending on the degree of UV transmission through clothing, the degree of exposure and the SPT of the person.

Mucous Membranes Sunburn of the tongue can occur rarely in mountain climbers who hold their mouth open "panting"; is frequent on the vermilion border of the lips.

Differential Diagnosis

Sunburn Obtain history of *medications* that can induce phototoxic erythema; *systemic lupus erythematosus* (SLE) can cause a sunburn-type erythema. *Erythropoietic protoporphyria* causes erythema, vesicles, edema, purpura and, only rarely, urticarial wheals.

Laboratory and Special Examinations

Dermatopathology

LIGHT MICROSCOPY *Site* Epidermis, dermis, and subcutis
Process Inflammation

Cell Types Epidermis: "sunburn" cells (damaged keratinocytes); also, exocytosis of lymphocytes, vacuolization of melanocytes and Langerhans cells. Dermis: endothelial cell swelling of superficial blood vessels and in the subcutaneous fat. Dermal changes are more prominent with UVA erythema with a denser mononuclear infiltrate and more severe vascular changes.

SEROLOGY ANA To rule out SLE

HEMATOLOGY Leukopenia may be present in SLE.

Diagnosis

History of UVR exposure and sites of reaction on exposed areas

Pathogenesis

The chromophores (molecules that absorb UVR) for UVB sunburn erythema are not known, but damage to DNA possibly may be the initiating event. The mediators that cause the erythema include histamines for both UVA and UVB. Also, in UVB erythema, other mediators include serotonin, prostaglandins, lysosomal enzymes, and kinins.

Significance

History of "blistering" sunburns in youth is definitely a risk factor for development of malignant melanoma of the skin in later years. Repeated sunburns result in dermatoheliosis, or "photoaging," over time.

Course

Sunburn, unlike thermal burns, cannot be classified on the basis of depth into first degree, second degree, or third degree, and scarring rarely, if ever, is seen following sunburn. At most, there can be a permanent hypomelanosis, probably related to destruction of melanocytes.

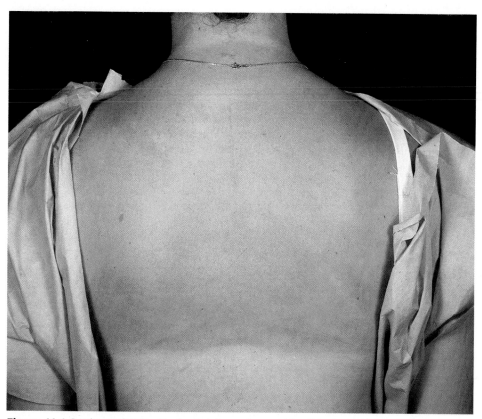

Figure 11-1 Acute sunburn *Tender, bright erythema with mild edema of the upper back and arms with sharp demarcation between sun-exposed and sun-protected white areas (neck, lower back).*

Management

Prevention There are many highly effective topical chemical filters (sunscreens) in lotion, gel, and cream formulations. Persons with SPT I or II should avoid sunbathing, especially between 1100 and 1400 hours.

Moderate Sunburn

TOPICAL   Cool wet dressings, topical corticosteroids

SYSTEMIC   Acetylsalicylic acid, indomethacin

Severe Sunburn Bed rest. If very severe, a "toxic" patient is best managed in a specialized "burn unit" for fluid replacement, prophylaxis of infection, etc.

TOPICAL   Cool wet dressings, topical corticosteroids

SYSTEMIC   Oral corticosteroids are often given but have not been established to be efficacious by controlled studies.

DERMATOHELIOSIS ("PHOTOAGING")

Repeated solar injuries over many years ultimately can result in the development of a skin syndrome, *dermatoheliosis*. Dermatoheliosis (DHe) results from excessive and/or prolonged exposure of the skin to ultraviolet radiation (UVR). The syndrome results from the cumulative effects of sun exposure following the first exposures in early life. DHe describes a polymorphic response of various components of the skin, especially cells in the epidermis, the vascular system, and the dermal connective tissue, to prolonged and/or excessive sun exposure. The severity of DHe depends principally on the duration and intensity of sun exposure and on the indigenous (constitutive) skin color and the capacity to tan (facultative melanin pigmentation). It is observed almost exclusively in persons with white skin but especially in skin phototypes I and II (SPT; see page 229).

Epidemiology

Incidence   In persons of SPT I to IV who have had *prolonged* exposure to sunlight or UVR from artificial sources. The population susceptible to development of DHe consists of persons with SPT I and II, who comprise about 25 % of the white population in the United States.

Age   DHe is observed most often in persons over 40 years; young white children (age 10) living in southern Borneo (cool climate with high UVR) have been observed to have DHe.

Skin Phototype   Persons with SPT I and II are most susceptible, but persons with SPT III and IV and even V (brown skin color) can develop DHe.

Sex   Higher incidence in males

Occupation   Farmers ("farmer's skin"), telephone linemen, sea workers ("sailor's skin"), construction workers, lifeguards, swimming instructors, sportspersons, and "beach bums"; affluent women who spend considerable time of the year in mountain or sea resorts.

Geography   DHe is more severe in the white population living in areas with high solar UVR (at high altitudes, in low latitudes)

HISTORY

Personal History   There is a history of intensive exposure to sun in youth (before 35 years); sun exposure may have been limited in later years.

Family History   Skin phototypes are genetically determined, and therefore, there is often a family history of DHe.

Physical Examination

Appearance of Patient   Wrinkled, wizened, leathery, "prematurely aged," or "looks old but is young." Persons with brown and black skin color are deceptively young looking because of the virtual absence of DHe. Persons with black skin who are albinos can develop DHe and sun-induced skin cancers.

Skin Findings

EPIDERMIS   *Keratinocytes*   Atrophy: increased translucence. Solar keratosis (see Figure 11-2). Xerosis (dryness).
   Melanocytes   Solar lentigo (see Figure 11-3). Ephelides (freckles) of "old age" (less seasonal dependency than juvenile ephelides). Guttate hypomelanosis.

DERMIS   *Vascular System*   Permanent dilatation of vessels (telangiectasia). Purpura, easy bruising.
   Connective Tissue   Wrinkling (fine surface, deep furrows), roughness, and elastosis (fine nodularity and inelasticity), yellow dermal papules and plaques (Figure 11-2).
   Pilosebaceous Unit   Comedones (especially periorbital) (Favre-Racouchot disease).

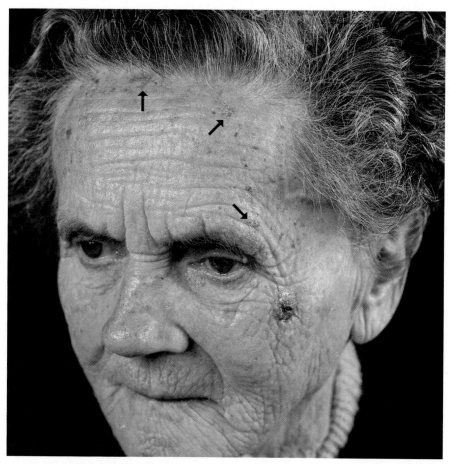

Figure 11-2 Advanced dermatoheliosis *Severe wrinkling, solar elastosis, solar lentigines, solar keratoses (upper forehead)* (arrows), *and a nodular basal cell carcinoma (cheek). Dermal elastosis results in a leathery appearance of the skin.*

Exposed areas. Scalp (bald males). Nuchal area: cutis rhomboidalis ("red neck") with rhomboidal furrows. Periorbital areas: wrinkling.

Dermatopathology

Epidermis Acanthosis of epidermis, increased horny layer. Flattening of the dermal-epidermal junction. Atypia of the keratinocytes.

Dermis Marked alteration in microcirculation with loss of small vessels in the papillary dermis. Elastosis: degraded elastic tissue with formation of coarse amorphous masses and increase in glycosaminoglycans. Increase in fibroblasts but a decrease in collagen and increase in elastin.

Differential Diagnosis

Wrinkled/Freckled Dry Skin *Xeroderma pigmentosum* exhibits severe DHe in addition to skin cancers (squamous cell and basal cell carcinoma, melanoma, fibrosarcoma, angiosarcoma); however, the disorder is present at a very young age. In *progeria* there is little or no wrinkling, but atrophy of skin and subcutis with marked increase in translucency of the epidermis. There are no pigmentary changes and no xerosis of the skin or solar keratoses.

Pathogenesis

While UVB is the most obvious damaging UVR, it is now known that UVA can, in high doses, produce connective tissue changes in mice. In addition, visible (400 to 700 nm) and infrared (1000 to 1,000,000 nm) radiations have been implicated, e.g., infrared has been shown to augment the action of UVB on induction of elastosis in guinea pigs. The action spectrum for DHe is not known for certain; there is some experimental evidence in mice that infrared radiation is implicated, in addition to UVB and UVA.

Significance

There is evidence based on case-control studies that severe sunburns in youth can lead to the development of malignant melanoma two or three decades later in life. This may result from sun-induced mutations in the gene regulating melanocytes present in common acquired nevomelanocytic and in dysplastic melanocytic nevi. The appearance of DHe marks a relatively young person as "old," a state that everyone tries to put off. There is a current wave to prevent skin cancers and to prevent the development of DHe by the use of protective sunblocks, by change of behavior in the sun, and by the use of topical chemotherapy (tretinoin) that reverses some of the changes that occur in DHe (solar keratoses, solar lentigo, vascular and connective tissue changes).

Course and Prognosis

DHe is inexorably progressive and irreversible, but some repair of connective tissue effects can occur if the skin is protected. Some processes leading to DHe continue to progress, however, even when sun exposures are severely restricted in later life; solar keratoses and lentigo develop in the sun-damaged skin that is now being protected by avoidance and sunblocks. Yet there are documented examples of spontaneous reversal of solar keratoses.

Management and Prevention

Topical Treatment

Tretinoin in lotions, gels, and creams in varying concentrations has been demonstrated in controlled studies to effect a reversal (clinical and histologic) of some aspects of DHe, especially the connective tissue and vascular changes. There is a current notion that topical tretinoin can alter the progression of incipient epithelial skin cancers.

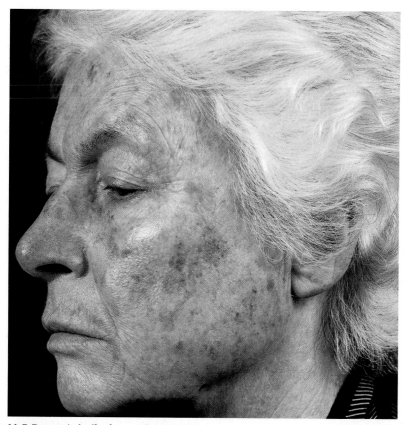

Figure 11-3 Dermatoheliosis: moderate *Moderate wrinkling, solar elastosis (creamy yellowing), and dyschromia (solar lentigines) with multiple, variegated, tan-to-dark-brown macules on the malar and frontal area in the face.*

5-Fluorouracil in lotions and creams is highly effective in causing a disappearance of solar keratoses.

Prevention Persons of SPT I and II should be identified early in life and advised that they are susceptible to the development of DHe and skin cancers, including melanoma. These persons should never sunbathe and should, from an early age, adopt a daily program of self-protection using substantive and effective topical sun-protective solutions, gels, or lotions that can filter DNA-damaging UVB; UVA filters are less ef-fective. SPT I and II persons should avoid the peak hours of UVB intensity, which are the 2 hours before and after solar noon (1200 GMT). CAUTION: There is now experimental evidence that while sunscreens protect from sunburn they do not protect from UV-induced local immuno-suppression. Prevention of sunburn may lure in-dividuals into exposing themselves to the sun for prolonged periods which may abrogate im-munosurveillance mechanisms in the skin. This has been linked to the rising incidence of melanoma.

SOLAR LENTIGO

Solar lentigo is a circumscribed 1.0- to 3.0-cm brown macule resulting from a localized proliferation of melanocytes due to chronic exposure to sunlight.

Epidemiology and Etiology

Age Usually over 40 years but may occur at 30 years in sunny climates

Sex No data available, probably equal incidence

Race Most common in Caucasians but seen also in Asians

Predisposing Factors Generally correlated with skin phototypes I to III and duration and intensity of solar exposure

Physical Examination

Skin Lesions

TYPE Strictly macular (Figures 11-3 and 11-4), 1.0 to 3.0 cm, as large as 5.0 cm

COLOR Light yellow, light brown or dark brown; variegated mix of brown and not uniform color, as in café-au-lait macules

SHAPE Round, oval, with slightly irregular border

ARRANGEMENT Often scattered, discrete lesions

DISTRIBUTION Exclusively exposed areas: forehead, cheeks, nose, dorsa of hands and forearms, upper back, chest

Dermatopathology

Site Epidermis

Process Proliferative. Club-shaped elongated rete ridges that show hypermelanosis and an increased number of melanocytes in the basal layer.

Differential Diagnosis and Management

Brown Macules "Flat," acquired, brown lesions of the exposed skin of the face, which may on cursory examination appear to be similar, have distinctive features: solar lentigo, seborrheic keratosis (see page 238), pigmented solar keratosis (see SPAK, page 239) lentigo maligna (see page 192).

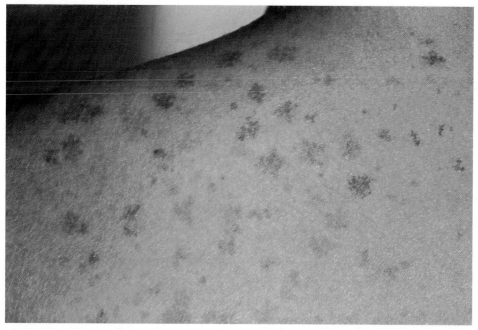

Figure 11-4 Solar lentigos *Multiple, stellate, sharply demarcated macules on the sun-exposed shoulders, usually result from repeated sunburns in individuals with skin phototypes 1 or 2.*

SOLAR KERATOSIS

These single or multiple, discrete, dry, rough, adherent scaly lesions occur on the habitually sun-exposed skin of adults.

Synonym: Actinic keratosis.

Epidemiology and Etiology

Age   Middle age, although in Australia and southwestern United States solar keratoses may occur in persons under age 30.

Sex   More common in males

Incidence   Sun is an etiologic agent. It has been estimated to occur in Australia in 1 : 1000 persons.

Race   Skin phototypes (SPT) I, II, and III, rare in SPT IV, and almost never in blacks or East Indians

Occupation   Outdoor workers (especially farmers, ranchers, sailors) and outdoor sports persons (tennis, golf, mountain climbing, deep-sea fishing)

History

Duration of Lesions   Months

Skin Symptoms   Some lesions may be tender.

Physical Examination

Skin Lesions

TYPE   Adherent hyperkeratotic scale (Figure 11-5), which is removed with difficulty and pain. May be papular.

COLOR   Skin-colored, yellow-brown, or brown; often there is a reddish tinge (Figure 11-5).

PALPATION   Rough, like coarse sandpaper

SIZE AND SHAPE   Most commonly <1.0 cm, oval or round

DISTRIBUTION   Isolated single lesion or scattered discrete lesions (Figures 11-5 and 11-6)

SITES OF PREDILECTION   Face (forehead, nose, cheeks, temples, vermilion border of lower lip), ears (in males), neck (sides), forearms, and hands (dorsa), shins

Differential Diagnosis

Small Keratotic Pink Macules in Sun-Exposed Sites   Flat solar keratoses, especially red, may be confused with *discoid lupus erythematosus.* Biopsy is necessary.

Dermatopathology

Site   Epidermis

Process   Proliferative and neoplastic. Large bright-staining keratinocytes, with mild to moderate pleomorphism in the basal layer, parakeratosis, and atypical (dyskeratotic) keratinocytes.

Pathophysiology

Prolonged and repeated solar exposure in susceptible persons (SPT I, II, and III) leads to cumulative damage to keratinocytes by the action of ultraviolet radiant energy, principally, if not exclusively, UVB (290 to 320 nm).

Course and Prognosis

Solar keratoses may disappear spontaneously, but in general they remain for years. The actual incidence of squamous cell carcinoma in preexisting solar keratoses is unknown but has been estimated at 1 squamous cell carcinoma developing annually in each 1000 solar keratoses.

Management and Prevention

Prevention is afforded by use of highly effective UVB/UVA sunscreens, which should be applied daily to the face and ears during the summer in northern latitudes for SPT I and SPT II persons and for those SPT III persons who sustain prolonged sunlight exposures.

Most solar keratoses react to local application to the lesion of 5 % 5-fluorouracil cream over a period of several days to weeks and then erode and disappear. Short exposure to liquid nitrogen alone or followed in 3 days by topical application of 5 % 5-fluorouracil cream is most effective; the latter avoids depigmented areas that occur when therapeutic exposures of liquid nitrogen are used alone.

Nodular lesions should be excised.

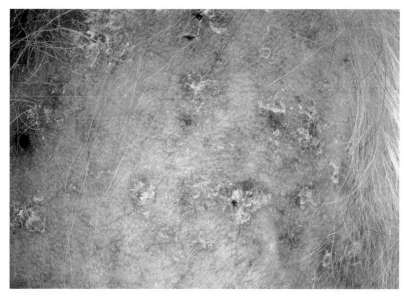

Figure 11-5 Solar keratosis *Erythematous macules and papules with coarse, adherent scale becoming confluent on the forehead, arising in a background of dermatoheliosis. Gently abrading lesions with a fingernail usually induces pain, even in early subtle lesions, a helpful diagnostic finding.*

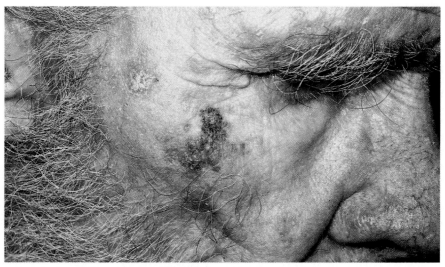

Figure 11-6 Spreading pigmented actinic keratosis (SPAK) *This is a rather uncommon variant of actinic keratosis. The distinctive features of SPAK include* size *(1.5 cm or larger),* pigmentation *(brown to black and variegated), and* history of lateral spreading, *especially the verrucous surface. The lesion is important because it can mimic lentigo maligna (LM). It is, however, easily distinguished from LM because LM is completely flat without evidence of verrucous change. The epidermal change in SPAK may appear as a slightly verrucous surface perceptible only with a hand lens and oblique lighting. Biopsy is necessary to confirm the clinical diagnosis. The lesion responds to a combination of cryosurgery (a very light freeze) followed by application of 5 % 5-fluorouracil ointment for 10 to 12 days; the application of the ointment is begun 3 days* after *the cryosurgery, after the scale falls off.*

PHYTOPHOTODERMATITIS (PLANT + LIGHT = DERMATITIS)

Phytophotodermatitis (PPD) is an inflammation of the skin caused by contact with certain plants during, and subsequent to, recreational or occupational exposure to sunlight. The inflammatory response is a phototoxic reaction to photosensitizing chemicals present in several plant families; a common type of PPD is due to exposure to limes.

Synonyms: Berloque dermatitis, lime dermatitis

Epidemiology and Etiology

Age   PPD can occur at any age; in children, exposure to plants in the grassy meadows near beaches may occur.

Race   All skin colors; brown- and black-skinned peoples may develop only marked spotty dark pigmentation without erythema or bullous lesions.

Occupation   Celery pickers, carrot processors, gardeners [exposed to carrot greens or to "gas plant" (*Dictamnus albus*)], and bartenders (lime juice)

Etiology   The phototoxic reaction is caused by the presence of photoactive chemicals, mostly psoralens contained in the plants.

History

The patient gives a history of exposure to certain plants (lime, lemon, wild parsley, celery, giant hogweed, parsnips, carrot greens, figs). Lime juice is a frequent cause: making lime drinks, hair rinses with lime juice. Women who use perfumes containing oil of bergamot (which contains bergapten, 5-methoxypsoralen) may develop only streaks of pigmentation in areas where the perfume was applied, especially the sides of the neck, upper anterior chest, and wrists. This is called *berloque dermatitis* (*berloque,* French: "pendant"). Persons walking on beaches containing meadow grass will develop phytophotodermatitis on the legs; meadow grass contains agrimony.

Relationship of Skin Lesions to Season
Seen most often during the summer months in northern latitudes or all year in tropical climates

Skin Symptoms   Marked pruritus

Physical Examination

Skin Lesions

TYPES   Acute: erythema, vesicles, and bullae (Figure 11-7), but not an eczematous dermatitis as seen in *Rhus* dermatitis. Residual dark hyperpigmentation in bizarre streaks (Figure 11-8).

SHAPE   Bizarre streaks, artificial patterns that indicate an "outside job"

DISTRIBUTION AND ARRANGEMENT   Scattered areas on the sites of contact, especially the arms and legs

Special Examinations

Wood's Lamp Examination   The sites of involvement can be detected by the enhancement of the erythema and pigmentation.

Diagnosis

This is easily made if the pattern is recognized and a careful history is taken.

Significance

May be an important occupational problem, as in celery pickers.

Course

The acute eruption fades spontaneously, but the pigmentation may last for weeks.

Management

Wet dressings may be indicated in the acute vesicular stage. Topical costicosteroids

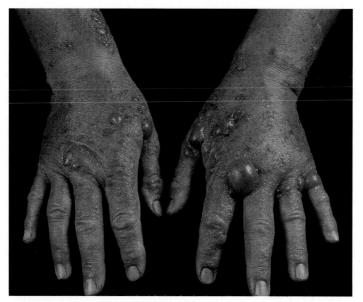

Figure 11-7 Acute phytophotodermatitis *Erythema, edema, vesicles, and bullae following skin contact with Umbiliferae weed containing furocoumarins while being exposed to solar UVA radiation.*

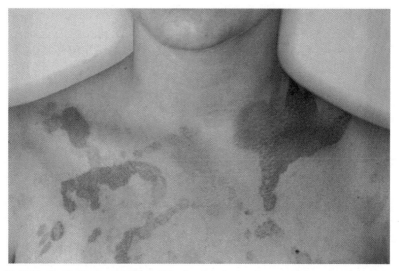

Figure 11-8 Phytophotodermatitis *Whorls of melanin pigmentation occurring at sites where an oil of bergamot (5-methoxypsoralen from orange rind)-containing perfume had been applied while exposed to solar UVA radiation. This enhanced tanning response can persist for many months causing significant cosmetic disfigurement.*

DRUG-INDUCED PHOTOSENSITIVITY

Drug-induced photosensitivity describes an adverse reaction of the skin that results from simultaneous exposure to certain drugs (via ingestion, injection, or topical application) and to ultraviolet radiation (UVR) or visible light. The chemicals may be therapeutic, cosmetic, industrial, or agricultural. There are two types of reaction: (1) *phototoxic,* which *can* occur in all individuals and is essentially an exaggerated sunburn response (erythema, edema, vesicles, etc.), and (2) *photoallergic,* which involves an immunologic response and in which the eruption is papular, vesicular, eczema-like and occurs only in the previously sensitized.

PHOTOTOXIC DRUG-INDUCED PHOTOSENSITIVITY

Epidemiology and Etiology

Incidence   Phototoxic drug reactions are more frequent than photoallergic drug sensitivity.

Age   Can occur at any age

Race   All types of skin color: black, white, and brown

Etiology   Amiodarone, thiazides, coal tar and derivatives, doxycycline, furosemide, nalidixic acid, demethylchlortetracycline, oxytetracycline, phenothiazines, piroxicam, psoralens (furocoumarins), sulfonamides

History

There are three patterns of phototoxic reaction: (1) immediate erythema and urticaria, (2) delayed sunburn-type pattern developing within 16 to 24 hours or later (48 to 72 hours in psoralen-related phototoxic reactions), or (3) delayed (72 to 96 hours) melanin hyperpigmentation.

Skin Symptoms   Pruritus or burning or stinging

Physical Examination

Skin   The skin lesions are those of an "exaggerated sunburn." In phototoxic drug reactions there is erythema, edema (Figure 11-9), and vesicle and bulla formation (e.g., pseudoporphyria). An eczematous reaction pattern is not seen in phototoxic reactions. Marked brown epidermal melanin pigmentation may occur in the course of the eruption, and especially with certain drugs (chlorpromazine and amiodarone), a gray dermal melanin pigmentation develops. After repeated exposure, some scaling and lichenification can develop.

DISTRIBUTION OF LESIONS   Confined exclusively to areas exposed to light (see distribution pattern of light eruption; Figure VA and VB).

Nails   Photoonycholysis can occur with certain drugs (psoralens, demethylchlortetracycline, and benoxaprofen).

Differential Diagnosis

Acute Photosensitivity   Phototoxic reactions due to excess of endogenous porphyrins (see Porphyrias, page 254); photosensitivity due to other diseases, e.g., systemic lupus erythematosus.

Laboratory Examinations

Dermatopathology   Inflammation, "sunburn cells" in the epidermis, epidermal necrobiosis, intraepidermal and subepidermal vesiculation. Absence of eczematous changes.

Diagnosis

History of exposure to drugs is most important as well as the types of morphologic changes in the skin characteristic of photo-

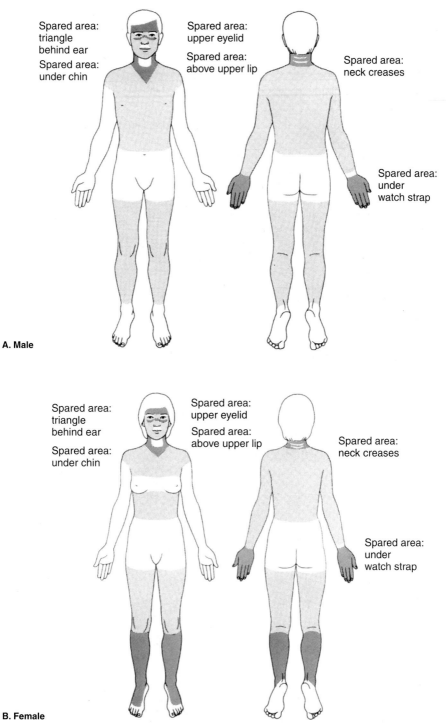

Figure V *Variations in solar exposure on different body areas:* ☐, *Rarely or never exposed (including doubly covered areas);* ▨, *often exposed;* ▮, *habitually exposed*

toxic drug eruptions: confluent erythema, edema, vesicles, bullae.

Phototesting

For verification of incriminated agent, template test sites are exposed to increasing doses of UVA (phototoxic reactions are almost always due to UVA) *while patient is on incriminated drug.* The UVA minimum erythema dose (MED) will be much lower than in normal individuals of the same skin phototype (SPT). After drug is excreted and then eliminated from the skin, a repeat UVA phototest will reveal an *increase* in the UVA MED. This test may be important if patient was on multiple potentially phototoxic drugs.

Pathogenesis

Formation of toxic photoproducts such as free radicals or reactive oxygen species such as singlet oxygen. The principal sites of damage are nuclear DNA or cell membranes (plasma, lysosomal, mitochondrial, microsomal). The action spectrum is UVA.

Significance

Phototoxic drug sensitivity is a major problem, since the abnormal reactions seriously limit or exclude the use of important drugs: diuretics, antihypertensive agents, drugs used in psychiatry. It is not known why some individuals show phototoxic reactions to a particular drug and others do not.

Course and Prognosis

Phototoxic drug reactions disappear following cessation of drug.

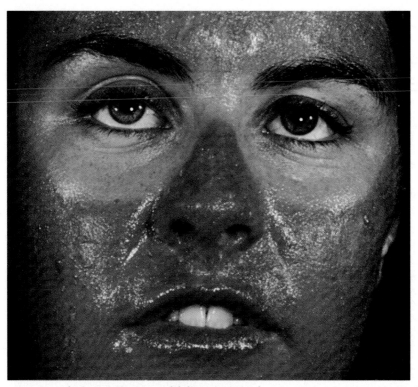

Figure 11-9 Drug-induced photosensitivity: phototoxic *An acute, severe, exaggerated sunburn in individual being treated with demethylchlortetracycline for acne. The sun exposure occurred when snow skiing for three hours; goggles protected the periorbital area.*

PHOTOALLERGIC DRUG-INDUCED PHOTOSENSITIVITY

In photoallergic drug photosensitivity, the chemical agent (drug) present in the skin absorbs photons and forms a photoproduct; this photoproduct then binds to a soluble or membrane-bound protein to form an antigen. Since photoallergy depends on individual immunologic reactivity, it develops in only a small percentage of persons exposed to drugs and light.

Epidemiology and Etiology

Incidence   Photoallergic drug reactions occur much less frequently than do phototoxic drug reactions.

Age   Probably more common in adults

Race   All types of skin color: black, white, and brown

Etiology   Halogenated salicylanilides, phenothiazines, sulfonamides; PABA esters, benzocaine, neomycin, benzophenones, and 6-methylcoumarin in sunscreens; musk ambrette in aftershave lotions; and stilbenes in whiteners

History

The history may be more difficult in that initial exposure induces sensitization to delayed-type hypersensitivity reactions, and the eruption occurs on subsequent exposure. Topically applied photosensitizers are the most frequent cause of photoallergic eruptions, e.g., halogenated salicylanilides, benzocaine (in soaps and other household products used to inhibit bacterial overgrowth), or musk ambrette used in aftershave lotions; photoallergy also results from the systemic administration of a drug.

Skin Symptoms   Pruritus

Physical Examination

Skin   The morphology of the skin reaction is much different from that in phototoxic drug sensitivity. Acute photoallergic reaction patterns resemble (1) allergic contact eczematous dermatitis (Figure 11-10) similar to allergic contact dermatitis or (2) lichen planus–like eruptions. In chronic drug photoallergy, there is scaling, lichenification, and marked pruritus mimicking atopic eczematous dermatitis or chronic contact eczematous dermatitis.

Distribution of Lesions   Confined primarily to areas exposed to light (see distribution pattern of photosensitivity; Figure VA and VB; Figure 11-10), but there may be spreading onto adjacent nonexposed skin; therefore, not so well circumscribed as in phototoxic reactions.

Laboratory Examinations

Dermatopathology   Acute and chronic delayed-type hypersensitivity reaction: epidermal spongiosis with lymphocytic infiltration

Diagnosis

History of exposure to drug is most important, as well as the types of morphologic changes in the skin that are characteristic of photoallergic drug reactions; this is essentially a contact eczematous pattern, while phototoxic drug eruptions mimic an exaggerated sunburn.

In essence, the differential diagnosis between phototoxic and photoallergic is identical to that described for toxic/irritant and allergic contact dermatitis (see Table 3-A in Section 3).

Pathogenesis

Formation of photoproduct that conjugates with protein producing an antigen. The action spectrum involved is UVA.

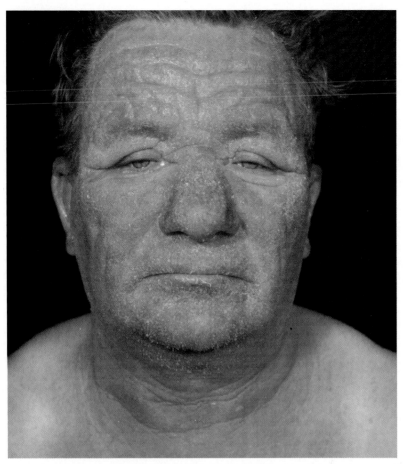

Figure 11-10 Drug-induced photosensitivity: photoallergic *Erythema, edema, and honey-colored crusting on the face, neck, and upper chest in a hydrochlorthiazide-treated individual. The rash had waxed and waned for months following minimal sun-exposure.*

Significance

Photoallergic drug reactions are difficult to diagnose and require the use of patch and photopatch tests. Photopatch tests are done in duplicate because photoallergens also can cause contact hypersensitivity. As in patch tests for contact hypersensitivity, photoallergens are applied to the skin and covered. After 24 hours, one set of the duplicate test sites is exposed to UVA while the other remains covered, and test sites are read for reactions after 48 to 96 hours. An eczematous reaction in the irradiated site but not in the nonirradiated site confirms photoallergy to the particular agent tested.

Course and Prognosis

Photoallergic dermatitis can persist for months to years. This is known as *persistent light reaction (chronic actinic dermatitis)* and was first observed in soldiers in World War II in whom topical sulfonamides were used and in patients with chronic chlorpromazine photoallergy. The classic generalized persistent light reactions were caused by exposure to topical salicylanilides. In the persistent light reactor, the action spectrum usually broadens to involve UVB, and the condition persists despite discontinuation of the causative photoallergen with each new UV exposure aggravating the condition. Chronic eczema-like lichenified and itching confluent plaques result (Figure 11-11), which lead to gross disfigurement and a distressing situation for the patient. As the condition is now independent from the original photoallergen and is aggravated by each new solar exposure, avoidance of photoallergen will not cure the disease; in severe cases, immunosuppression (Imuran plus corticosteroids or oral cyclosporine) is required.

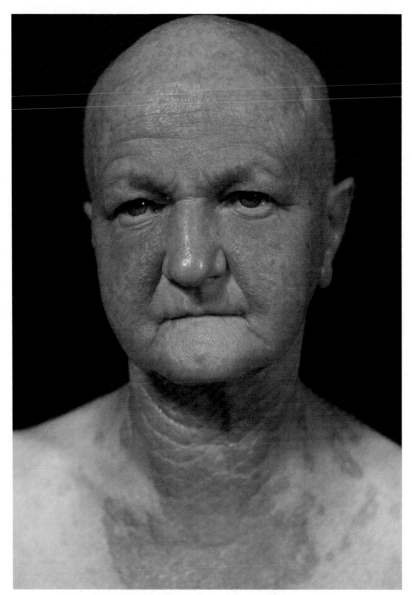

Figure 11-11 Drug-induced photosensitivity: persistent light eruption *Thick erythema-tous plaques confined to the scalp, face, and exposed chest, sparing areas shaded by the nose.*

POLYMORPHOUS LIGHT ERUPTION

Polymorphous light eruption (PMLE) is a term that describes a group of heterogeneous, idiopathic, acquired, acute recurrent photodermatoses characterized by delayed abnormal reactions to ultraviolet radiation (UVR) and manifested by varied lesions. The various morphologic types include erythematous macules, papules, plaques, and vesicles. However, in each patient the eruption is consistently monomorphous. By far the most frequent morphologic types are the papular and papulovesicular eruptions.

Epidemiology

Incidence Most common of the photodermatoses

Age Average age of onset is 23 years.

Race All races, including brown and black peoples. In American Indians (North and South America) there is a hereditary type of PMLE that is also called *actinic prurigo.*

Skin Phototype (SPT) More often seen in SPT I, II, III, and IV

Sex Much more common in females

Geography PMLE is less frequently observed in areas that have high solar intensity throughout the year. PMLE often occurs for the first time in persons traveling for short vacations to tropical areas in winter from northern latitudes.

History

Onset and Duration of Lesions PMLE appears in spring or early summer, and not infrequently the eruption does not recur by the end of summer, suggesting a "hardening." The rash comes on suddenly, following hours to days of sun exposure. PMLE most often appears within 18 to 24 hours of exposure and, once established, persists for 7 to 10 days, thereby limiting the vacationer's subsequent time in the sun.

Special Features The eruption is elicited most frequently by exposure to UVA but also can be caused by UVB or by both; since UVA is transmitted through window glass, PMLE can be precipitated while riding in a car. In patients who travel to sunny vacation areas such as the Caribbean, the eruption will occur but is not noted even during the summer months in the northern latitudes; presumably the "threshold" for elicitation occurs with higher solar intensities. Also, areas of the skin habitually exposed (face and neck) are often spared, despite severe involvement of the arms, trunk, and legs.

Skin Symptoms Pruritus (may precede the onset of the rash) and paresthesia (tingling)

Systems Review Negative

Family History PMLE in American Indians is hereditary (actinic prurigo) and is characterized by papules, plaques, and nodules mostly on the face that can cause disfigurement.

Physical Examination

Types of Lesions The papular and papulovesicular types (Figures 11-12 and 11-13) are the most frequent. Less common are plaques or urticarial plaques. The lesions are pink to red. It is of note that in the individual patient, lesions are quite monomorphous, i.e., either papulovesicular or urticarial or plaques. Recurrences follow the original pattern.

Distribution of Lesions The eruption often spares the face and is seen most frequently on

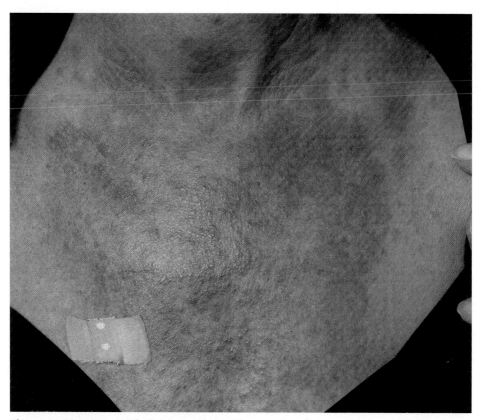

Figure 11-12 Polymorphic light eruption *Clusters of confluent, extemely pruritic papules and vesicles on the exposed chest, occurred the day following the first sun exposure of the season. The eruption involved the dorsum of the arms, but spared the face and dorsal hands.*

the forearms, V area of the neck and arms. The lesions may also occur on the trunk if there has not been previous exposure.

Differential Diagnosis

Rashes in Light-Exposed Areas Lupus erythematosus is the most important disease to exclude, as is discussed under Diagnosis below. Serologic study of antinuclear antibodies (ANA) and anti-Ro and anti-La antibodies is necessary in plaque-type PMLE. Photosensitivity eruptions caused by systemic or topical drugs and cosmetics can be ruled out by history.

Laboratory and Special Examinations

Dermatopathology (Characteristic but not diagnostic)

LIGHT MICROSCOPY In papular and eczematous lesions there is edema of the epidermis, spongiosis, vesicle formation, and mild liquefaction degeneration of the basal layer but no atrophy or thickening of the basement membrane. A dense lymphocytic infiltrate is present in the dermis, with occasional neutrophils. There is edema of the papillary dermis and endothelial swelling.

IMMUNOFLUORESCENCE (DIRECT) Negative

SPECIAL TECHNIQUES Monoclonal antibody immunopathology techniques reveal that the mononuclear cells are predominantly T cells.

SEROLOGY ANA is negative.

HEMATOLOGY There is no leukopenia.

Diagnosis

The diagnosis is not difficult: delayed onset of eruption, characteristic morphology, histopathologic changes that rule out lupus erythematosus, and the history of disappearance of the eruption in days. In plaque-type PMLE, a biopsy and immunofluorescence studies are mandatory to rule out lupus erythematosus. *Phototesting* is done with both UVB and UVA. Test sites are exposed daily, starting with 2 MEDs of UVB and UVA, respectively, for 1 week to 10 days, using increments of the UV dose. In 50 % of patients, a PMLE-like eruption will occur in the test sites, confirming the diagnosis. This also helps to determine whether the action spectrum is UVB, UVA, or both.

Pathogenesis

A delayed-type hypersensitivity reaction to an antigen induced by UVR is possible because of morphology of the lesions and the histologic pattern, which shows an infiltration of T cells. Immunologic studies thus far have not been rewarding.

Significance

This is a pesky problem that severely limits recreational or occupational exposure to the sun.

Course and Prognosis

The course is chronic and recurrent and may, in fact, become worse each season. Although some patients may develop "tolerance" by the end of the summer, the eruption usually recurs again the following spring and/or when the person travels to tropical areas in the winter. However, spontaneous improvement or even cessation of eruptions occurs after years.

Management

Prevention Sunblocks, even the potent UVA-UVB sunscreens, are rarely effective but should be tried first in every patient. Even when systemic drugs or photochemotherapy is used, potent topical UVA-UVB sunblocks should be used in addition.

Systemic Beta-carotene has not been very effective but can be tried before antimalarials. Antimalarials (hydroxychloroquine 200 mg b.i.d. one day before and daily while on vacation or on weekends) are the effective drugs for the treatment of PMLE in some patients and should be used in selected patients not helped by topical sunblocks or oral beta-carotene.

PUVA Photochemotherapy This treatment given in early spring induces "tolerance" for the following summer. It is highly effective. PUVA treatments are given 3 times weekly for 4 weeks. It is not known whether their effectiveness is based on the production of an increase in the "filtering" capacity of the epidermis (increase in the stratum corneum and in melanin content of the epidermis) or to an effect of PUVA on T cells. PUVA treatments will have to be repeated each spring but are usually not necessary for more than 3 or 4 years.

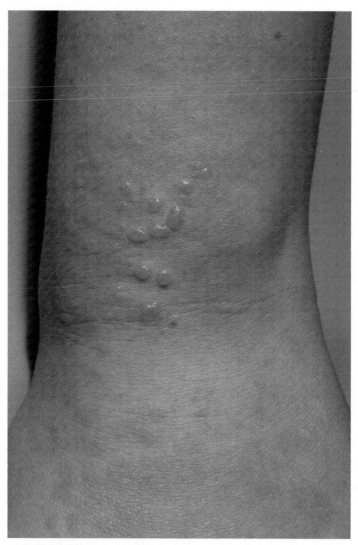

Figure 11-13 Polymorphic light eruption *Clusters of pruritic papules and vesicles on the dorsal wrist and arm, and an erythematous plaque on the dorsum of the hand following first sun exposure of the season. The face and dorsal hand are typically spared.*

TABLE 11-A CLASSIFICATION OF PORPHYRIA

	Erythropoietic Porphyrias		Hepatic Porphyria		
	Congenital Erythropoietic Porphyria	Erythropoietic Protoporphyria	Porphyria Cutanea Tarda	Variegate Porphyria	Intermittent Acute Porphyria
Inheritance	Autosomal recessive	Autosomal dominant	Autosomal dominant (familial form)	Autosomal dominant	Autosomal dominant
Signs and symptoms					
Photosensitive	Yes	Yes	Yes	Yes	No
Cutaneous lesions	Yes	Yes	Yes	Yes	No
Attacks of abdominal pain	No	No	No	Yes	Yes
Neuropsychiatric syndrome	No	No	No	Yes	Yes
Laboratory abnormalities					
Red blood cells:					
Uroporphyrin	+++	N	N	N	N
Coproporphyrin	++	+	N	N	N
Protoporphyrin	(+)	+++	N	N	N
Urine					
Porphobilinogen	N	N	N	(+++)	(+++)
Uroporphyrin	+++	N	+++	+++	+++
Feces					
Protoporphyrin	+	++	N	+++	N

NOTE: N, normal; +, above normal; ++, moderately increased; +++, markedly increased; (+++), frequently increased—depends on whether patient has an attack or is in remission; (+), increased in some patients.

PORPHYRIA CUTANEA TARDA

Porphyria cutanea tarda (PCT), as the name implies, occurs mostly in adults rather than children. *Patients do not present with photosensitivity* but with complaints of "fragile skin," vesicles, and bullae, particularly on the dorsa of the hands, especially following minor trauma; the diagnosis is confirmed by the presence of an orange-red fluorescence in the urine when examined with a Wood's lamp. PCT is distinct from variegate porphyria (VP) and acute intermittent porphyria (AIP) in that patients with PCT do not have acute life-threatening attacks (abdominal pain, peripheral autonomic neuropathy, and respiratory failure). Furthermore, the drugs that induce PCT (ethanol, estrogens, and chloroquine) are fewer than the drugs that induce VP and AIP (see Variegate Porphyria, page 260).

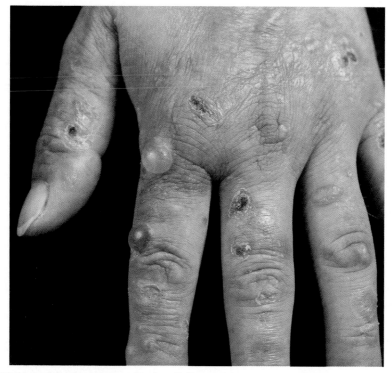

Figure 11-14 Porphyria cutanea tarda *Bullae, erosions, crusts, milium, atrophic scars on the dorsal hand.*

Epidemiology and Etiology

Age 30 to 50 years, rarely in children; females on oral contraceptives (18 to 30 years of age); males on estrogen therapy for prostate cancer (>60 years of age)

Sex Equal in males and in females

Heredity Most PCT patients have *PCT-symptomatic* (not hereditary) induced by drugs, especially alcohol, or chemicals (e.g., hexachlorobenzene fungicide). *PCT-hereditary*— possibly these patients actually have VP, but this is not yet resolved.

Chemicals and Drugs That Induce PCT Ethanol, estrogen, hexachlorobenzene (fungicide), chlorinated phenols, iron, tetrachloro-dibenzo-*p*-dioxin. High doses of chloroquine may lead to clinical manifestations in "latent" cases (low doses are used as treatment).

Other Predisposing Factors Diabetes mellitus (25 %), hepatitis C virus, AIDFS

History

Duration of Lesions No *acute* skin changes but gradual onset, and patients may present with bullae on the hands and feet based on a photosensitivity reaction to sun and yet will have a suntan.

Symptoms Pain from erosions in easily traumatized skin ("fragile skin")

Systems Review In VP there is autonomic neuropathy with acute abdominal pain and peripheral neuropathy. In erythropoietic protoporphyria and PCT there can be hepatic disease. Associated diseases may lead to multisystem alterations (see Differential Diagnosis, below).

Physical Examination

Skin Lesions

TYPE

Bullae: tense bullae on normal-appearing skin (Figure 11-14)
Erosions: in the sites of the vesicles and bullae; erosions slowly heal to form pink atrophic scars at sites of erosions.

Milia (Figure 11-14), 1.0 to 5.0 mm
Hypertrichosis of the face (may be presenting complaint)
Scleroderma-like induration
Purple-red suffusion ("heliotrope") of central facial skin (Figure 11-15), especially periorbital areas
Brown hypermelanosis, diffuse, on exposed areas (uncommon)

DISTRIBUTION (See Figure VI)

Dorsa of hands and feet (toes), nose (vesicles, bullae, and erosions)
Scleroderma-like changes, diffuse or circumscribed, waxy yellowish white areas on exposed areas of face, neck, and trunk, sparing the doubly clothed area of the breast in females
Hypertrichosis: dark brown or black hair on the temples and cheeks and, in severe disease, on the trunk and extremities

DIAGNOSIS

By clinical features, red fluorescence of urine and elevated urinary porphyrins

---

Differential Diagnosis

Bullae on Dorsa of Hands and Feet

Pseudo-PCT: (Figure 11-16) A distinctive syndrome with blisters and erosions indistinguishable from PCT. Drugs (naproxen, ibuprofen, tetracyclines, nalidixic acid, dapsone, amiodarone, bumetanide, cyclosporine, etretinate, furosemide, chlortalidone, diazide, pyridoxine). Chronic renal failure with hemodialysis. Tanning salon radiation (visible and UVA). Other associated conditions: hepatoma, SLE, sarcoidosis, Sjögren's syndrome, hepatitis C. May occasionally resemble dyshidrotic eczema but is on the dorsa! *Epidermolysis bullosa acquisita:* has the same clinical picture (increased skin fragility, easy bruising, and light-provoked bullae) and some of the histology (subepidermal bullae with little or no dermal inflammation).
Variegate porphyria (VP): See page 260.

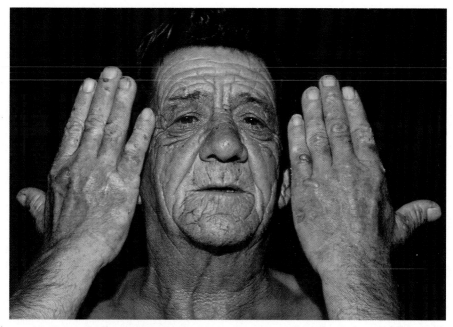

Figure 11-15 Porphyria cutanea tarda *Periorbital and malar violaceous coloration, hyper-pigmentation, and hypertrichosis on the face; bullae, crust, and scars on the dorsa of the hands.*

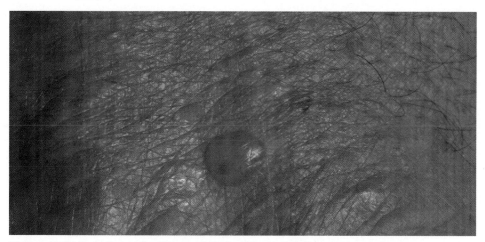

Figure 11-16 Pseudoporphyria associated with renal failure *Tense bulla on a nonin-flamed base on the dorsal hand in an individual on chronic hemodialysis, indistinguishable from those seen in porphyria cutanea tarda.*

Laboratory Examination

Dermatopathology

SITE Epidermis and papillary dermis, blood vessels

PROCESS Bullae, subepidermal with "festooned" (undulating) base. PAS reveals thickened vascular walls.

IMMUNOFLUORESCENCE IgG and other immunoglobulins at the dermal-epidermal junction and in and around blood vessels, in the sun-exposed areas of the skin. Thickening of vessel walls is due to multiple reduplications of vascular basement membrane and deposits of immunoglobulins and fibrin.

CELLS Paucity of an inflammatory infiltrate

Laboratory Examinations of Blood, Stool, and Urine

Blood Chemistry

Increased plasma iron (33 % to 50 %) (there is increased hepatic iron in Kupffer cells and hepatocytes)

Blood glucose increased in those patients with diabetes mellitus (25 % of patients)

Porphyrin Studies in PCT (See Table 11-B)

Increased uroporphyrin (I isomer, 60 %) in urine and plasma

Increased isocoproporphyrin (type III) and 7-carboxylporphyrin in the feces

No increase in δ-aminolevulinic acid or porphobilinogen in the urine

Wood's lamp examination of the urine. To enhance the orange-red fluorescence, add a few drops of 10 % hydrochloric acid.

It is important to obtain levels of porphyrins in the stool to rule out VP, which has markedly elevated fecal protoporphyrin as the diagnostic hallmark.

Liver Biopsy Reveals porphyrin fluorescence and more often fatty liver

Pathophysiology

In some patients there is a reduction in the liver enzyme uroporphyrin decarboxylase, which catalyzes decarboxylation of the four acetate groups to methyl groups. This reduction of enzyme may occur in familial or nonfamilial PCT.

Management

1. Avoid ethanol, stop drugs that could be inducing PCT, such as estrogen, and eliminate exposure to chemicals (chlorinated phenols, tetrachlorodibenzo-*p*-dioxin). In some patients, complete avoidance of ethanol ingestion will result in a clinical and biochemical remission and in depletion of the high level of iron stores in the liver.

2. Phlebotomy is done by removing 500 ml of blood at weekly or biweekly intervals until the hemoglobin is decreased to 10 g. Clinical and biochemical remission occurs within 5 to 12 months after regular phlebotomy. Relapse within a year is uncommon (5 % to 10 %).

3. Chloroquine is used to induce remission of PCT in patients in whom phlebotomy is contraindicated because of anemia. Since chloroquine can exacerbate the disease and, in higher doses, may even induce hepatic failure in these patients, this treatment requires considerable experience. However, long-lasting remissions and, in a portion of patients, clinical and biochemical "cure" can be achieved.

4. Presently, the most efficient therapeutic approach to the treatment of PCT is a combination of phlebotomy (three to four sessions) followed by low-dose chloroquine therapy.

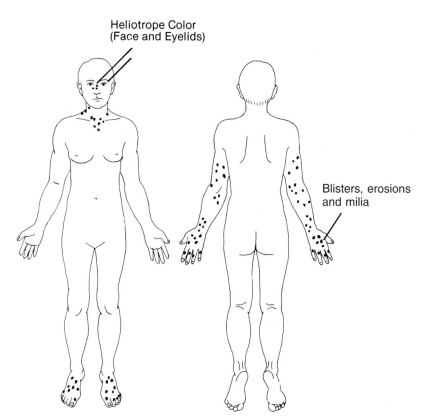

Heliotrope Color (Face and Eyelids)

Blisters, erosions and milia

Figure VI Porphyria cutanea tarda

TABLE 11-B   LABORATORY DIFFERENTIAL DIAGNOSIS OF HEPATIC PORPHYRIAS

	Porphyria Cutanea Tarda	Variegate Porphyria
Urine tests		
During acute attacks		
PBG	N	+ +
URO	+ +	+ +
COPRO	+	+ +
Between acute attacks		
PBG	N	N
URO	+ +	N
COPRO	+	N
Ratio URO/COPRO	> 1	< +
Stool tests		
COPRO	+ +	+ +
PROTO	+	+ +
URO	+	N

ABBREVIATIONS: N, normal; +, mild elevation; + +, marked elevation.

VARIEGATE PORPHYRIA

Variegate porphyria is a serious autosomal dominant disorder of heme biosynthesis characterized by skin lesions which are identical to those of PCT (vesicles and bullae, skin fragility, milia, and scarring of the dorsa of the hands and fingers), acute attacks of abdominal pain and neuropsychiatric manifestations, and increased excretion of porphyrins; especially characteristic are high levels of protoporphyrin in the feces.
Synonym: Porphyria variegata.

Epidemiology

Race   All races; especially common in white South Africans (3:1000) (a large proportion of the present white population was descended from early Dutch settlers who emigrated to South Africa from Holland in 1680). It is increasingly recognized in Europe (Finland) and the United States.

Age   Second to fourth decades

Heredity   Autosomal dominant

Precipitating Factors   See Table 11-C

History

Change with Seasons   Skin lesions occur during the summer season but may persist throughout the winter; lesions result from exposure to sunlight.

Skin Symptoms   Painful erosions, skin fragility

Constitutional Symptoms   None

Systems Review   Acute attacks of abdominal pain, constipation, nausea and vomiting, muscle weakness, seizures, confusional state, psychiatric symptoms (depression, coma); rarely, cranial nerve involvement, bulbar paralysis, sensory loss, and paresthesias

Drug Exposure   See Table 11-C

Physical Examination

Skin Lesions

TYPE

Vesicles or, more commonly, bullae (Figure 11-17)
Erosions, milia
Sclerosis (scleroderma-like changes)
Scars (pink, atrophic)

COLOR

Periorbital heliotrope hue
Diffuse melanoderma on exposed areas

ARRANGEMENT   Scattered, discrete lesions

DISTRIBUTION   Localization to dorsa of hands, fingers, and feet (exposed areas)

Hair   Hypertrichosis (especially in sunny climates)

Miscellaneous Findings   Neurologic, especially peripheral neuropathy

Laboratory and Special Examinations

Dermatopathology

SITE   Dermal-epidermal interface and dermis

PROCESS   Subepidermal bullae formation (festooning); PAS-positive, diastase-resistant depositions in and around blood vessels of the upper dermis

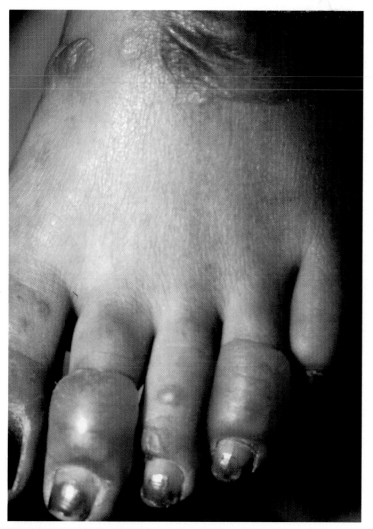

Figure 11-17 Variegate porphyria *Large bullae on the sunexposed dorsal foot and toes; the spared area was protected by a sandal.*

General Laboratory Examination

PORPHYRINS   See Table 11-B
  Plasma   Distinctive plasma fluorescence with emission maximum at 626 nm
  Urine   Increased porphobilinogen during acute attacks
  Stools   High protoporphyrin

Pathophysiology

The basic metabolic defect is accentuated by ingestion of certain drugs (sulfonamides, barbiturates, phenytoin, estrogens, alcohol, and others) (see Table 11-C), with the resultant precipitation of acute attacks of abdominal pain and neuropsychiatric disorders (delirium, seizures, personality changes). There is an enzyme defect resulting in a reduction of protoporphyrin oxidase, with accumulation of protoporphyrinogen in the liver, which is excreted in the bile and is nonenzymatically converted to protoporphyrin; this accounts for the high fecal protoporphyrin.

Course

Lifetime disease with onset after puberty and peak incidence in the second to fourth decades; skin manifestations not provoked by drugs that precipitate abdominal and neuropsychiatric symptoms, except for estrogens, which provoke cholestatic hepatitis, diverting porphyrin from the bile to the blood, with resulting increased porphyrin deposition in the skin.

Prognosis

Good, if exacerbating factors are avoided (certain drugs, alcohol, infection). Rarely, death can occur following ingestion or injection of drugs (e.g., barbiturates, general anesthesia) that induce increased amounts of cytochrome P450 and create a demand for increased synthesis of heme.

Management

None; oral beta-carotene may or may not control the skin manifestations but has no effect on porphyrin metabolism or the important systemic manifestations.

TABLE 11-C   DRUGS HAZARDOUS TO PATIENTS WITH VARIEGATE PORPHYRIA

Anesthetics: barbiturates and halothane
Anticonvulsants: hydantoins, carbamazepine, ethosuximide, methsuximide, phensuximide, primidone
Antimicrobial agents: chloramphenicol, griseofulvin, novobiocin, pyrazinamide, sulfonamides
Ergot preparations
Ethyl alcohol
Hormones: estrogens, progestins, oral contraceptive preparations

Imipramine
Methyldopa
Minor tranquilizers: chlordiazepoxide, diazepam, oxazepam, flurazepam, meprobamate
Pentazocine
Phenylbutazone
Sulfonylureas: chlorpropamide, tolbutamide
Theophyline

ERYTHROPOIETIC PROTOPORPHYRIA

This hereditary metabolic disorder of porphyrin metabolism is unique among the porphyrias in that porphyrins or porphyrin precursors are not excreted in the urine. Also, erythropoietic protoporphyria (EPP) is characterized by an acute sunburn-like photosensitivity, in contrast to the other common porphyrias (porphyria cutanea tarda or variegate porphyria), in which obvious acute photosensitivity is *not* a presenting complaint.

Synonym: Erythrohepatic protoporphyria.

Epidemiology and Etiology

Age Acute photosensitivity begins early in childhood; rarely, late onset in early adulthood.

Sex Equal in males and in females

Race All ethnic groups, including blacks

Heredity Autosomal dominant

Incidence Not uncommon; series reported from Europe (in The Netherlands, 1:100,000, Austria, United Kingdom), and the United States.

History

Duration of Onset of Lesions Stinging and itching may occur within a few minutes of sunlight exposure; later, erythema and edema appear after 1 to 8 hours.

Seasonal Changes Photosensitivity is less common in the winter months in temperate areas.

Symptoms Burning or "stinging" sensation within minutes may be the only abnormality. Children may choose not to go out in the direct sunlight after a few painful episodes, which may cause serious sociopsychologic problems. Symptoms occur when exposed to sunlight through window glass.

Systems Review Biliary colic, even in children

Physical Examination

Skin Changes in Acute Reactions to Sunlight Exposure Bright red erythema, later edema (swelling of hands especially), urticaria (less common), purpura [especially on the nose (Figure 11-18) and tips of ears]. Vesicles or bullae rarely occur. These changes appear within 1 to 8 hours and subside after several hours or days without obvious scarring.

Skin Changes Following Chronic Recurrent Exposures Shallow, often linear scars, especially on the nose and dorsa of the hands ("aged knuckles"). Diffuse wrinkling of the skin of the face (nose, around the lips, cheeks) with obvious thickening of the skin and a waxy color (Figure 11-19). Crusted, erosive lesions may occur on the nose and lips. Absence of sclerodermoid changes, hypertrichosis, or hyperpigmentation.

General Medical Findings

Hemolytic anemia with hypersplenism (rare) Cholelithiasis (12 %), even in children. Stones contain large amounts of protoporphyrin.

Liver disease may result from massive deposition of protoporphyrin in the hepatocytes; fatal hepatic cirrhosis is rare.

Laboratory and Special Examinations

Porphyrin Studies Increased protoporphyrin in red blood cells (RBCs), plasma, and stools but no excretion in the urine except in the rare cases with fatal hepatic cirrhosis. Decreased activity of the enzyme, ferrochelatase, in the bone marrow, liver, and skin fibroblasts

Liver Function Tests for liver function are indicated. Liver biopsy has demonstrated portal and periportal fibrosis and deposits of brown pigment and birefringent granules in hepato-cytes and Kupffer cells. With electron microscopy, needle-like crystals have been observed. About 20 patients have been reported with cirrhosis and portal hypertension.

Special Examination for Fluorescent Erythrocytes   RBCs in a blood smear exhibit a characteristic *transient* fluorescence when examined with a fluorescent microscope with a mercury or tungsten-iodide lamp that emits 400-nm radiation.

Dermatopathology

SITE   Upper dermis

PROCESS   Marked eosinophilic homogenization and thickening of the blood vessels in the papillary dermis; there is an accumulation of an amorphous, hyaline-like eosinophilic substance in and around blood vessels.

Radiography   Gallstones may be present.

Pathophysiology

The specific enzyme defect occurs at the step in porphyrin metabolism in which protoporphyrin is converted to heme by the enzyme ferrochelatase. This leads to an accumulation of protoporphyrin that is highly photosensitizing.

Diagnosis

In EPP there is photosensitivity but no "rash," only an exaggerated sunburn response that appears much earlier than ordinary sunburn erythema. Also, the skin changes occur behind window glass. Finally, there are virtually no photosensitivity disorders in which the symptoms appear so rapidly (minutes after exposure to sunlight). Porphyrin examination establishes the diagnosis with elevated free protoporphyrin levels in the RBCs and in the stool. The fecal protoporphyrin is most consistently elevated. The urinary porphyrins are not elevated.

Course and Prognosis

EPP persists throughout life, but the photosensitivity may become less apparent in late adulthood. Liver cirrhosis may become manifest in adults. Rarely, fatal outcome due to hepatic failure.

Management

There is no treatment for the basic metabolic abnormality, but symptomatic relief of the photosensitivity can be achieved in many patients with oral beta-carotene in divided doses of 180 mg daily. Therapeutic levels of carotenoids are achieved in 1 to 2 months. This treatment brings about an amelioration of the photosensitivity but does not completely eliminate the problem of photosensitivity. Patients on beta-carotene can remain outdoors longer by a factor of 8 to 10 but still burn if exposures are too long. Nevertheless, many patients can participate in outdoor sports for the first time. There is no toxicity with prolonged treatment with beta-carotene. Protection by beta-carotene can be considerably enhanced by PUVA photochemotherapy-induced tanning.

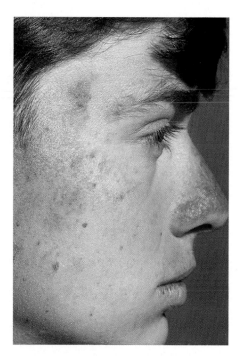

Figure 11-18 Erythropoietic protoporphyria
Diffuse erythematous infiltration of the nose with edema, petechial hemorrhage, and scattered atrophic scars on the side of the face with telangiectasia.

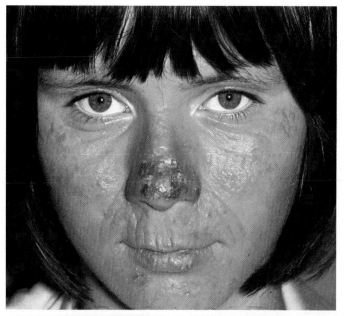

Figure 11-19 Erythropoietic protoporphyria   *Erythema, edema, erosion, crusting of the nose with less severe changes on the chin of a 15-year-old female. Deep wrinkling and a peculiar waxy thickening on the upper lip and cheeks similar to dermatoheliosis in photoaged skin.*

Section 12

NONINFECTIOUS INFLAMMATORY SKIN DISORDERS

LICHEN PLANUS

Lichen planus (LP) is an acute or chronic inflammatory dermatosis involving skin and/or mucous membranes, characterized by flat-topped (Latin: *planus,* "flat"), violaceous, shiny, pruritic papules on the skin and milky white papules in the mouth.

Epidemiology and Etiology

Age   30 to 60 years

Sex   Females > males

Race   Hypertrophic LP more common in blacks

Etiology   Unknown. Drugs may induce a lichen planus-like eruption.

History

Onset   Acute (days) or insidious onset over weeks

Duration of Lesions   Months to years

Symptoms

SKIN   Asymptomatic or pruritic, which may be severe.

MUCOUS MEMBRANE   Painful, especially when ulcers are present.

Physical Examination

Skin Lesions

TYPE   Papules, flat-topped, 1.0 to 10.0 mm, sharply defined, shiny (Figures 12-1 and 12-2). Bullae, rarely. Hypertrophic plaques, often with postinflammatory hyperpigmentation.

COLOR   Violaceous, with white lines (Wickham's striae), seen best with hand lens after application of mineral oil. In dark-skinned individuals, postinflammatory hyperpigmentation is common.

SHAPE   Polygonal or oval

ARRANGEMENT   Grouped, linear (isomorphic phenomenon), annular, or disseminated scattered discrete lesions

DISTRIBUTION   Wrists (flexor), lumbar region, eyelids, shins (thicker, hyperkeratotic lesions), scalp, and glans penis. Lichen planus actinicus occurs in sun-exposed sites.

Mucous Membranes   40 % to 60 % of individuals with LP have oropharyngeal involvement.

TYPES OF LESIONS   *Reticular LP:* reticulate (netlike) pattern of lacy white hyperkeratosis on buccal mucosa (Figure 12-3), lips, tongue, gingiva; the most common pattern of oral LP. *Plaque-type LP:* leukoplakia with Wickham's striae; arises on buccal mucosa. *Atrophic LP:* shiny red plaque, often with Wickham's striae in surrounding mucosa.

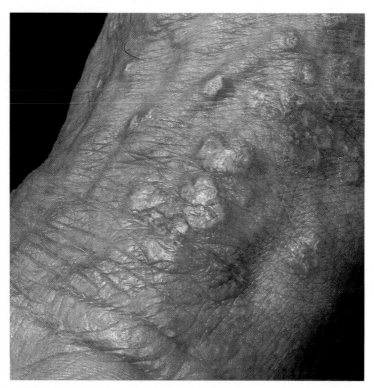

Figure 12-1 Lichen planus *Flat-topped, grouped, violaceous papules; the surface is shiny and has a lacy white pattern (Wickham's striae).*

Erosive or ulcerative LP: superficial erosion with overlying fibrin clot; occurs on tongue and buccal mucosa; shiny red painful erosion of gingiva (desquamative gingivitis) (Figure 12-4). *Bullous LP:* intact blisters up to several centimeters in diameter; rupture results in erosive LP. Milky-white papules, with white lacework on the buccal mucosa. May become erosive and painful. Carcinoma may very rarely develop in mouth lesions.

SITES OF PREDILECTION Buccal mucosa, gingiva (Figure 12-4), tongue, lips, esophagus

Genitalia Papular, annular, or erosive lesions arise on penis (especially glans), scrotum, labia majora, labia minora, vagina.

Hair and Nails

SCALP Atrophic scalp skin with scarring alopecia

NAILS Destruction of nail fold and nail bed, especially in the large toe

Variants

HYPERTROPHIC Large thick plaques arise on the shins; more common in black males.

FOLLICULAR Individual keratotic-follicular papules and plaques that lead to cicatricial alopecia (see page 32). Spinous follicular lesions, typical skin and mucous membrane lichen planus, and cicatricial alopecia of the scalp are called *Graham Little syndrome.*

VESICULAR Vesicular or bullous lesions may develop within lichen planus patches or independent of these within normal-appearing skin. In the latter there are direct immunofluorescence findings consistent with bullous pemphigoid (see page 406), and the sera of these patients contain bullous pemphigoid IgG autoantibodies.

ACTINICUS Papular LP lesions arise in sun-exposed sites, especially the dorsum of hands and arms.

ULCERATIVE Lichen planus may become bulbous and lead to therapy-resistant ulcers, particularly on the soles, requiring skin grafting.

Lichen Planus-Like Eruptions Lichen planus-like eruptions closely mimic typical lichen planus, both clinically and histologically. They occur as a clinical manifestation of chronic graft-versus-host disease, in dermatomyositis, and as cutaneous manifestations of malignant lymphoma but also may develop as the result of therapy with certain drugs and following industrial use of certain compounds (see Table 12-A).

TABLE 12-A AGENTS REPORTED TO INDUCE CUTANEOUS DISORDERS THAT VERY CLOSELY RESEMBLE TYPICAL LICHEN PLANUS

Types of Agents	Specific Agents
Angiotensin-converting enzyme inhibitors	Captopril
	Enlapril
Antiarthritic	Gold
Antibiotic	Streptomycin
	Tetracycline
Antimalarial	Quinacrine
	Chloroquine
	Quinine isomer, quinidine
Antitubercular	*p*-Amino salicylic acid
Ataractic	Phenothiazine derivatives
	Metopromazine
	Levomepromazine
Chelator	Penicillamine
Color film developer	*p*-Phenylenediamine salts
	2-Amino-5-diethylaminotoluene monochloride (CD2)
	4-Amino-*N*-diethyl-aniline sulfate (TTS)
	Antimony trioxide
Diuretic	Chlorothiazide
	Hydrochlorothiazide
Hypoglycemic agents	Chlorpropamide
	Tolazamide

SOURCE: From Arndt KA.: Lichen planus, in TB Fitzpatrick et al (eds): *Dermatology in General Medicine,* 4th ed. New York, McGraw-Hill, 1993, pp 1134–1144.

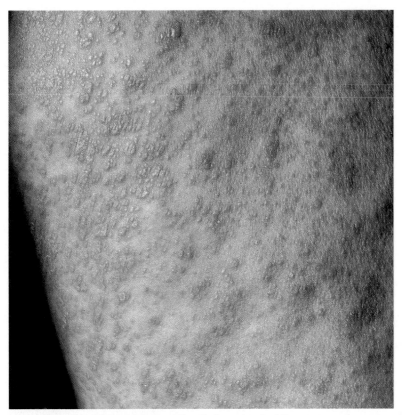

Figure 12-2 Generalized lichen planus *Small, flat-topped, violaceous papules, some groups and some with a follicular pattern, becoming confluent on the trunk.*

Differential Diagnosis

Skin

PAPULAR LP   Chronic cutaneous lupus erythematosus, psoriasis, pityriasis rosea, eczematous dermatitis, lichenoid graft-versus-host disease, superficial BCC, Bowen's disease (*in situ* SCC)

HYPERTROPHIC LP   Psoriasis vulgaris, lichen simplex chronicus, prurigo nodularis, stasis dermatitis, Kaposi's sarcoma

DRUG-INDUCED LP   See Table 12-A.

Mucous Membrane   Leukoplakia, pseudomembranous candidiasis (thrush), HIV-associated hairy leukoplakia, lupus erythematosus, bite trauma, mucous patches of secondary syphilis, pemphigus vulgaris, bullous pemphigoid

Laboratory and Special Examinations

Dermatopathology   Inflammation with hyperkeratosis, increased granular layer, irregular acanthosis, liquefaction degeneration of the basal cell layer, and bandlike mononuclear infiltrate that hugs the epidermis. Lymphocytes are predominantly CD4+ helper inducer cells. Degenerate keratinocytes (colloid, Civatte bodies) are found at the dermal-epidermal junction. Direct immunofluorescence reveals heavy deposits of fibrin at the junction and IgM and less frequently IgA, IgG, and C3 in the colloid bodies.

Diagnosis

Clinical findings confirmed by histologic findings

Course

Duration of LP: Cutaneous LP usually persists for months, but in some cases, for years; hypertrophic LP on the shins often persists for decades; oral LP often persists for decades. The incidence of oral cancer in individuals with oral LP is increased by 50-fold; patients should be followed at regular intervals.

Management

Local

CORTICOSTEROIDS   Topical corticosteroids with occlusion for cutaneous lesions. Intralesional triamcinolone (3 mg/ml) is helpful for symptomatic cutaneous or oral mucosal lesions.

CYCLOSPORINE   The solution can be used as a retention "mouthwash" for severely symptomatic oral LP.

Systemic

CORTICOSTEROIDS   Oral prednisone is effective for individuals with symptomatic pruritus, painful erosions, dysphagia, or cosmetic disfigurement. A short, tapered course is preferred: 70 mg initially, tapered by 5 mg daily.

SYSTEMIC RETINOIDS (ACITRETIN OR ETRETINATE)   1 mg/kg per day is helpful as adjunctive measure in severe cases but usually requires additional topical treatment.

CYCLOSPORINE   In very resistant and generalized cases, 5 mg/kg per day will induce rapid remission, quite often not followed by recurrence.

PUVA Photochemotherapy   Indicated in symptomatic individuals with generalized LP or cases resistant to topical therapy.

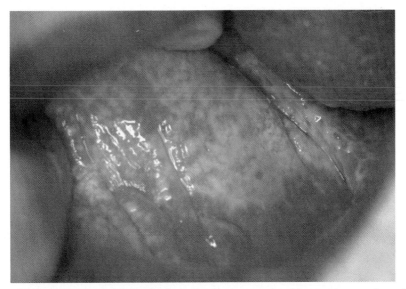

Figure 12-3 Oral lichen planus: reticular *Confluent, smooth, white papules creating a lacy pattern on the buccal mucosa.*

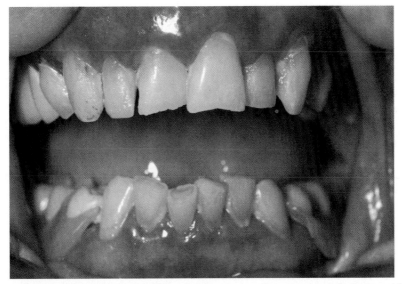

Figure 12-4 Oral lichen planus: erosive *Erythematous, edematous, eroded gingiva with retraction exposing a portion of the teeth. Brushing is very painful, resulting in accumulation of dental plaque, which also adds to chronic periodontal inflammation.*

GRANULOMA ANNULARE

Granuloma annulare (GA) is a self-limited asymptomatic chronic dermatosis of the dermis that exhibits papules in an annular arrangement, commonly arising on the dorsa of the hands and feet, elbows, and knees.

Epidemiology and Etiology

Age Children and young adults

Sex Female : male ratio 2:1

Etiology Unknown. The lesions are sometimes indistinguishable from necrobiosis lipoidica. Generalized GA may be associated with diabetes mellitus.

History

Duration of Lesions Months to years

Skin Symptoms Usually asymptomatic. Cosmetic disfigurement.

Physical Examination

Skin Lesions

TYPE
Firm, smooth, shiny dermal papules and plaques 1.0 to 5.0 cm (Figure 12-5). Keratotic papules and nodules are seen in perforating granuloma annulare.
Nodules, subcutaneous

COLOR Skin-colored, erythematous, violaceous

SHAPE Dome-shaped, annular

ARRANGEMENT Complete circle (annular) or half-circle (arciform)

DISTRIBUTION Isolated lesion, multiple lesions in certain regions, or generalized (older patients)

SITES OF PREDILECTION *Dermal Papules* Dorsa of hands, fingers, feet, extensor aspects of arms and legs, trunk
Subcutaneous Nodules Palms, legs, buttocks, scalp

Differential Diagnosis

Papular Lesions Necrobiosis lipoidica, papular sarcoid, lichen planus, lymphocytic infiltrate of Jessner

Subcutaneous Nodules Rheumatoid nodules

Annular Lesions Dermatophytosis

Laboratory and Special Examinations

KOH Preparation Rule out epidermal dermatophytosis.

Dermatopathology Foci of chronic inflammatory and histiocytic infiltrations in superficial and middermis with incomplete and reversible necrobiosis of connective tissue surrounded by a wall of palisading histiocytes and multinucleated giant cells

Pathogenesis

An inflammatory reaction occurs around blood vessels, altering collagen and elastic tissues.

Course

The disease disappears in 75 % of patients in 2 years, but recurrences are common (40 %).

Management

Patients should be reassured that GA is a local skin disorder and not a marker for internal disease and that spontaneous remission is the rule.

Topical Therapy

TOPICAL CORTICOSTEROIDS Applied under plastic occlusion or hydrocolloid

INTRALESIONAL TRIAMCINOLONE 3.0 mg/ml into lesions is very effective.

CRYOSPRAY Superficial lesions respond to liquid nitrogen, but atrophy may occur.

PUVA Photochemotherapy Effective in generalized GA

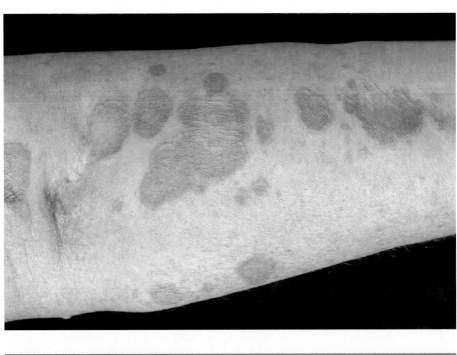

A

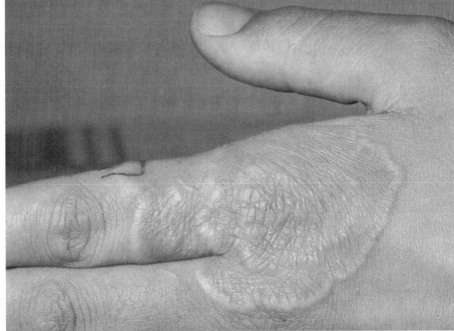

B

Figure 12-5 Granuloma annulare A. *Numerous large, tan-pink, dermal plaques with peripheral extension and central clearing (creating annular-shaped lesions) on forearm. B. Confluent, pearly white, firm papules forming two rings, 1.0 cm and 5.0 cm in diameter. There is no scaling.*

MORPHEA

Morphea is a localized cutaneous sclerosis characterized by early violaceous, later ivory-colored, plaques, which may be solitary, linear, generalized, and rarely, accompanied by atrophy of underlying structures.
Synonyms: Localized scleroderma, circumscribed scleroderma.

Epidemiology and Etiology

Age 75 % have their onset between the ages of 20 and 50; in linear morphea the onset is earlier. Pansclerotic morphea usually starts before age 14.

Sex Women are affected about 3 times as often as men.

Etiology Unknown. However, there is some evidence that at least some patients (predominantly in Europe) with classic morphea have sclerosis due to *Borrelia burgdorferi* infection.

History

Skin Symptoms Usually absent. No history of Raynaud's phenomenon.

Physical Examination

Skin, Hair, and Nail Lesions

CLASSIFICATION BY PATTERN OF INVOLVEMENT

Circumscribed or localized: plaques or bands
Linear: extremity
Frontoparietal (en coup de sabre): linear morphea occurring on the head with or without hemiatrophy of face
Generalized plaques
Pansclerotic: involvement (trunk, extremities, face, and scalp, with sparing of fingertips and toes) of dermis, fat, fascia, muscle, bone. Pansclerotic morphea is usually generalized.

TYPE *Plaques*—initially indurated, but poorly defined areas; 2.0 to 15.0 cm in diameter (Figures 12-6 and 12-7). In time, surface becomes smooth and shiny; hair follicles and sweat duct orifices disappear. *Purpura,*

telangiectasia, and very rarely, *bullae* may be seen later in course. Deep involvement of tissue may be associated with atrophy of muscle and bone, with resultant growth disturbance in children and flexion contracture; pseudoainhum-like lesion may occur circumferentially on limb with subsequent distal edema. Scalp involvement results in scarring alopecia.

COLOR Initially, purplish or mauve; after months to years, may be hyperpigmented. Ivory with lilac-colored edge. In lesions of rapid onset, may be erythematous. With generalized morphea, may have hyperpigmentation in involved areas.

SHAPE Round or oval

PALPATION Indurated, hard. May be hypesthetic. Rarely, lesions become atrophic and hyperpigmented without going through a sclerotic stage (atrophoderma of Pasini and Pierini) (Figure 12-7).

ARRANGEMENT Usually multiple, bilateral, asymmetric. May be linear on extremity or scalp.

HAIR AND NAILS Scarring alopecia with scalp involvement of plaque, generalized, or frontoparietal morphea. Nail dystrophy in linear lesions of extremity or in pansclerotic morphea.

DISTRIBUTION ***Circumscribed*** Trunk, limbs, face, genitalia; less commonly, axillae, perineum, areolae
Linear Usually on extremity
Frontoparietal Scalp and face
Generalized Initially on trunk (upper, breasts, abdomen), thighs

MUCOUS MEMBRANES With linear morphea of head, may have associated hemiatrophy of tongue.

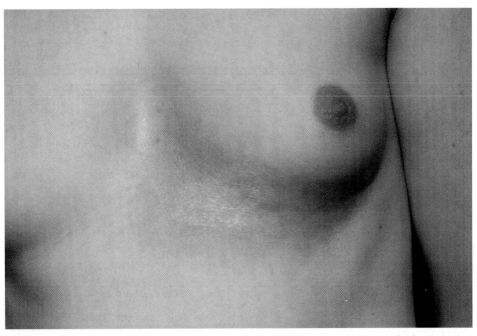

Figure 12-6 Morphea *Indurated, poorly defined plaque under the left breast. The lesion is multicolored with a central yellow "carnauba wax"-colored area surrounded by a lilac border.*

General Examination Involvement around joints may lead to flexion contractures, especially of hands and feet. Deeper involvement of tissue is associated with atrophy and fibrosis of muscle. Extensive involvement may result in restricted respiration. With linear morphea of the head, may have associated atrophy of ocular structures and atrophy of bone.

Differential Diagnosis

Sclerotic Plaque Sclerotic plaque associated with *B. burgdorferi* infection, acrodermatitis chronica atrophicans, progressive systemic sclerosis, lichen sclerosus et atrophicus, eosinophilic fasciitis, eosinophilia-myalgia syndrome associated with L-tryptophan ingestion, scleredema

Laboratory and Special Examinations

Serology Appropriate serologic testing to rule out *B. burgdorferi* infection

Dermatopathology

EPIDERMIS Normal to atrophic with loss of rete ridges

DERMIS Initially edematous with swelling and degeneration of collagen fibers; later these become homogeneous and eosinophilic. Slight infiltrate, perivascular or diffuse; lymphocytes, plasma cells, macrophages. Later, dermis thickened with few fibroblasts and dense collagen; inflammatory infiltrate at dermal-subcutis junction; dermal appendages disappear progressively. Pansclerotic lesions show fibrosis and disappearance of subcutaneous tissue, fibrosis broadening, as well as sclerosis of fascia. Silver stains should be performed to rule out *B. burgdorferi* infection.

Diagnosis

Clinical diagnosis, at times confirmed by skin biopsy

Course

May be slowly progressive, but spontaneous remissions occur.

Management

There is no effective treatment for morphea, i.e., symptomatic interventions when indicated.

Morphea-Like Lesions Associated with Lyme Borreliosis In patients with early involvement, there may be a reversal of sclerosis with high-dose parenteral penicillin or ceftriaxone treatment given in several courses over a time span of several months (see Etiology). Concomitant systemic corticosteroids reduce sclerosis.

Phototherapy using UVA-1 (340–400 nm) The mechanism of action of UVA-1 is thought to be by the induction of interstitial collagenase (matrix metalloproteinase 1, MMP1). Collagenase initiates degradation of types I and III collagen and plays a key role in the remodeling of dermal collagen. UVA-1 phototherapy, however, can induce a variety of cytokines and soluble factors, resulting in immunomodulation. [Gruss C et al. Induction of interstitial collagenase (MMP-1) by UVA-1 phototherapy in morphea fibroblasts. Lancet 1997; 350:1295–1296.]

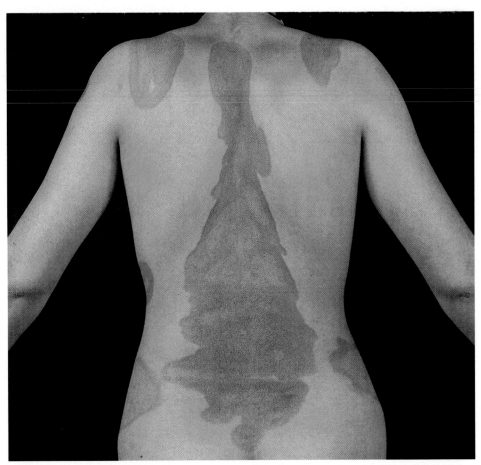

Figure 12-7 Generalized morphea *Multiple, sharply demarcated, indurated, brown trunkal plaques. In the Pasini-Pierini type of morphea, lesions have typical color and atrophy but lack induration.*

LICHEN SCLEROSUS ET ATROPHICUS

Lichen sclerosus et atrophicus (LSA) is a chronic atrophic mucocutaneous disorder, characterized by white, angular, well-defined, indurated papules and plaques and, at times, follicular keratotic plugs.

Epidemiology and Etiology

Age A disease of adults, but occurs in children 1 to 13 years of age. Mean age of onset: 50 years in females, 43 in males.

Sex Female: male ratio 10:1

Etiology Unknown

History

Duration of Lesions May be present for years prior to detection. May first be noted by gynecologist or internist doing pelvic examination.

Symptoms

NONGENITAL Usually asymptomatic

GENITAL Often asymptomatic, even with striking clinical changes. In females, vulvar lesions may be sensitive, especially while walking; pruritus; painful especially if erosions are present; dysuria; dyspareunia. In males, acquired phimosis, recurrent balanitis; in boys, may be discovered on pathologic examination of prepuce removed during circumcision.

Physical Examination

Skin Lesions

TYPE *Macules and papules:* whitish, sharply demarcated, individual lesions may become confluent, forming *plaques* (Figures 12-8 and 12-9). Surface of lesions may be elevated or in the same plane as normal skin; older lesions may be depressed. Puncta in the center. Dilated pilosebaceous or sweat duct orifices filled with keratin plugs (these are known as *dells*); if plugging is marked, surface appears verrucous. *Bullae* and *erosions*;

may heal with fusion of labia minora. *Purpura* is a characteristic feature; *telangiectasia.* On vulva, hyperkeratotic plaques may become macerated; vulva may become atrophic, shrunken, especially clitoris and labia minora, with vaginal introitus reduced in size. Fusion of labia minora and majora. In uncircumcised males, prepuce becomes sclerotic and cannot be retracted. This and involvement of the glans was called in the past *balanitis xerotica obliterans.* Uncommonly, *squamous cell carcinoma* may develop in genital LSA, predominantly in females.

COLOR Ivory or porcelain-white; semitransparent, resembling mother-of-pearl

ARRANGEMENT Keyhole or figure-of-eight in anogenital area of females

DISTRIBUTION *Nongenital* Trunk, especially upper back, periumbilical, neck, axillae; flexor surface of wrists; rarely palms and soles
   Genital Females: vulva and perianal regions as well as the perineum; inguinal line. Males: undersurface of prepuce and glans.

ORAL MUCOSA Bluish-white plaques on buccal or palatal mucosa; tongue. Superficial erosions. Hyperkeratotic, macerated lesions may have reticulate pattern resembling lichen planus.

Differential Diagnosis

Sclerotic/Atrophic Plaque Morphea (may coexist with LSA), lichen simplex chronicus, chronic cutaneous lupus erythematosus, leukoplakia, lichen planus, intraepithelial neoplasia (bowenoid papulosis), extramammary Paget's disease, intertrigo, candidiasis

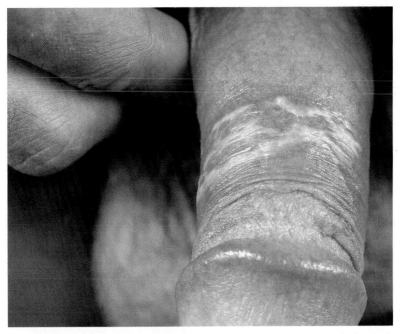

Figure 12-8 Lichen sclerosus et atrophicus: penis *Early involvement with shiny white plaques on the glans and prepuce; hemorrhage was also present within the lesion on the glans. Periurethral involvement can obstruct the flow of urine. Progressive involvement of the prepuce makes retraction over the glans impossible, i.e., phimosis.*

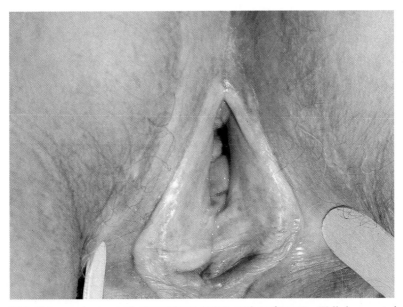

Figure 12-9 Lichen sclerosus et atrophicus: vulva and perineum *Well-demarcated, ivory/porcelain-white plaques involve the anogenital skin; the labia minora and clitoris have been virtually reabsorbed (referred to as agglutination). Hemorrhage and erosions are also commonly seen.*

Laboratory and Special Examinations

Dermatopathology *Epidermis:* early in course, variably thickened, hyperkeratotic, follicular plugging; later, epidermis atrophic. *Dermis:* band of homogenization of dermal collagen below epidermis; structureless, edematous; lymphocytic infiltrate, bandlike subepidermal in early lesions, later below the edematous, structureless, subepidermal zone. Dilated capillaries, hemorrhage.

Diagnosis

Clinical diagnosis at times confirmed by biopsy

Course and Prognosis

Waxes and wanes. In girls, may undergo spontaneous resolution. At times, coexisting lesions of morphea and vitiligo may be present. Patients should be followed every 12 months to check for occurrence of squamous cell carcinoma of the vulva. Extragenital lesions in adults are more likely to undergo remission.

Management

Symptomatic; no curative therapy.

Topical Corticosteroids Potent topical corticosteroid preparations have proved very effective for genital LSA. Signs of corticosteroid-induced atrophy should be monitored. Topical androgens admixed with corticosteroids

Systemic Therapy Antimalarials, e.g., hydroxychloroquine, 250 mg/day

Borrelia in Morphea and Lichen Sclerosus Various reports from Europe have documented an association between *Borrelia* species, morphea, and lichen sclerosus et atrophicus (LSA). Studies from the United States have not confirmed these findings. In the most recent European study, skin biopsy specimens (19 morphea and 34 LSA) were obtained from patients in the United States, Japan, and Germany. Genotype-specific sequences in the flagellin gene were determined for *Borrelia burgdorferi,* sensu stricto *Borrelia garinii,* and *Borrelia afzelii.* Five cases of morphea and two cases of LSA in Germany and Japan yielded positive results for *B. garinii* or *B. afzelii;* however, none of the American samples detected DNA for these spirochetes. (Fujiwara H et al. Arch Dermatol 1997;133:41–44.)

Circumcision In males, circumcision relieves symptoms of phimosis and in some cases can cause remission.

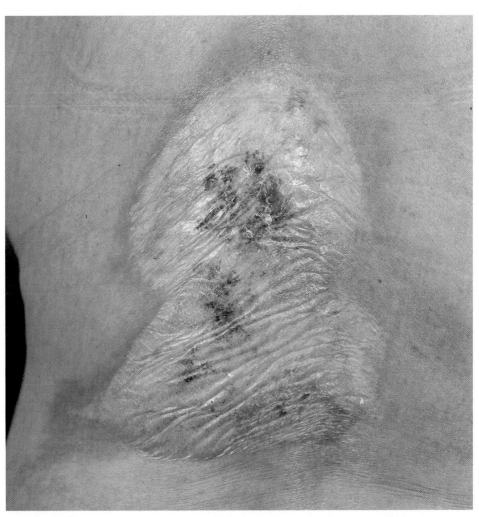

Figure 12-10 Lichen sclerosus et atrophicus: lower back *The entire involved skin has transformed into an ivory-white sclerotic plaque with central purpura.*

Section 13

ERYTHRODERMA

EXFOLIATIVE ERYTHRODERMA SYNDROME

The exfoliative erythroderma syndrome (EES) is a serious, at times life-threatening reaction pattern of the skin characterized by generalized and confluent redness and scaling involving practically the entire skin and associated with systemic "toxicity," generalized lymphadenopathy, and fever. Two stages, acute and chronic, merge one to the other. In the acute and subacute phases there is rapid onset of generalized vivid red erythema and fine branny scales; the patient feels hot and cold, shivers, and has fever. In the chronic EES, the skin thickens, there is a loss of scalp and body hair, the nails become thickened and separated from the nail bed (onycholysis), and there may be hyperpigmentation or patchy loss of pigment in patients whose normal skin color is brown or black. In about 50 % of the patients with EES there is a history of a preexisting dermatosis, and this is recognizable only in the acute or subacute stages. The most frequent preexisting skin disorders are (in order of frequency) eczematous dermatitis (atopic, allergic contact), psoriasis, lymphoma and leukemia, adverse cutaneous drug reaction, and pityriasis rubra pilaris. In 10 % to 20 % of patients it is not possible by the history or the histology to identify the cause. (See Sézary's Syndrome, page 550, for a special consideration of this form of EES.)

Epidemiology

Age >50 years; when in children, EES usually results from pityriasis rubra pilaris or atopic dermatitis.

Sex Males > females

History

Duration of Lesions Depending on the etiology, the acute phase may develop rapidly, as in a drug reaction, lymphoma, or eczema. At this early acute stage it is possible to identify the preexisting dermatosis (psoriasis, mycosis fungoides, lichen planus, etc.)

Skin Symptoms Pruritus

Constitutional Symptoms Fatigue, weakness, anorexia, weight loss, malaise, feeling cold

Physical Examination

Appearance of Patient Frightened, red, "toxic"

Skin

TYPE OF LESION   Skin is red, thickened, scaly. Dermatitis is confluent and diffuse, without recognizable borders (Figures 13-1 and 13-2), except for pityriasis rubra pilaris, where EES spares sharply defined areas of normal skin. Scaling may be fine and branny, and may be barely perceptible or large, up to 0.5 cm, and lamellar.

COLOR OF LESIONS   Bright red

PALMS AND SOLES   Usually involved, with massive hyperkeratosis and deep fissures in pityriasis rubra pilaris, Sézary's syndrome, and psoriasis

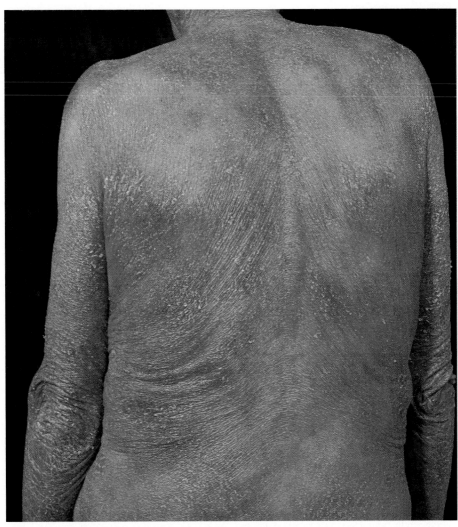

Figure 13-1 Erythroderma: cutaneous T-cell lymphoma *Universal erythema, thickening, and scaling. The degree of erythema and thickening is not uniform and the redness has a brownish-blue hue. Hair loss, involvement of palms/soles, and generalized lymphadenopathy were also present.*

Hair Thinning of hair, even alopecia, except for EES arising in eczema or psoriasis

Nails Onycholysis, shedding of nails

General Examination Lymph nodes generalized, rubbery, and usually small; enlarged in Sézary's syndrome

Differential Diagnosis

Eczematous dermatitis (atopic, contact), psoriasis, lymphoma and leukemia, adverse cutaneous drug reaction, pityriasis rubra pilaris, lichen planus, pemphigus foliaceus, lamellar ichthyosis, acute graft-versus-host disease

Laboratory and Special Examinations

Chemistry   Low serum albumin and increase in gamma globulins; electrolyte imbalance; acute-phase proteins increased

Bacterial Culture   *Skin:* Rule out secondary *Staphylococcus aureus* infection. *Blood:* rule out sepsis.

Dermatopathology   Depends on type of underlying disease. Parakeratosis, inter- and intracellular edema, acanthosis with elongation of the rete ridges, and exocytosis of cells. There is edema of the dermis and a chronic inflammatory infiltrate.

Imaging   CT scans or MRI should be used to find evidence of lymphoma.

Diagnosis

This is not easy, and the history of the preexisting dermatosis may be the only clue. Also, pathognomonic signs and symptoms of the preexisting dermatosis may help, e.g., dusky red color in psoriasis and yellowish-red in pityriasis rubra pilaris; typical nail changes of psoriasis; lichenification, erosions, and excoriations in atopic dermatitis and eczema; diffuse, relatively nonscaling palmar hyperkeratoses with fissures in CTCL and pityriasis rubra pilaris; sharply demarcated patches of noninvolved skin within the erythroderma in pityriasis rubra pilaris; massive hyperkeratotic scale of scalp usually without hair loss in psoriasis; and with hair loss in CTCL and pityriasis rubra pilaris; in the latter and in CTCL, ectropion may occur.

Pathogenesis

The metabolic response to exfoliative dermatitis may be profound. Large amounts of warm blood are present in the skin due to the dilatation of the capillaries, and there is considerable heat dissipation through insensible fluid loss and by convection. Also, there may be high output cardiac failure; the loss of scales through exfoliation can be considerable, up to 9.0 g/m^2 of body surface per day and this may contribute to the reduction in serum albumin and the edema of the lower extremities so often noted in these patients.

Significance

This is an important medical problem that should be dealt with using a modern inpatient dermatology facility and personnel.

Prognosis

Guarded, depends on underlying etiology. Despite the best attention to all details, patients may succumb to infections or, if they have cardiac problems, to cardiac failure ("high output" failure) or to the effects of the prolonged corticosteroid therapy that may be required.

Management

The patient should be hospitalized in a single room, at least for the beginning workup and during the development of a therapeutic program. The hospital room conditions (heat and cold) should be adjusted to the patient's needs; most often these patients need a warm room with many blankets.

Topical   Water baths with added bath oils, followed by application of bland emollients

Systemic

>   Oral corticosteroids for remission induction and for maintenance (except in psoriatic EES); systemic and topical therapy as required by underlying condition
>   Supportive (cardiac, fluid, electrolyte, protein replacement) therapy as required

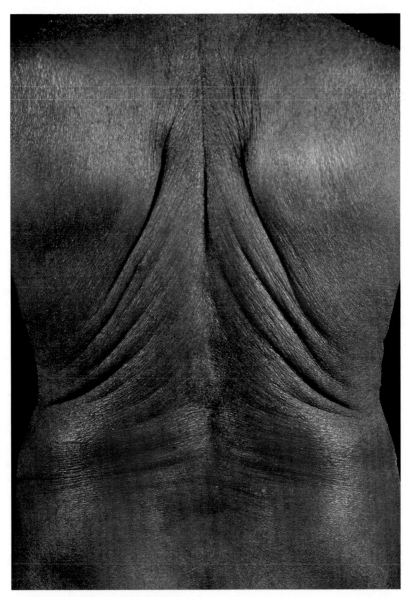

Figure 13-2 Erythroderma: drug-induced *Generalized erythroderma with thickening of skin and universal erythema following the injection of gold salts.*

Section 14

PIGMENTARY DISORDERS

While normal skin color is composed of a mixture of four biochromes, namely, (1) *reduced* (blue) and (2) *oxyhemoglobin* (red), (3) *carotenoids* (yellow) (exogenous from diet), and (4) *melanin* (brown), it is the total amount of melanin pigment that is the principal determinant of the skin color. Variations in the amount and distribution of melanin in the skin, furthermore, are the basis of the three racial colors: black, brown, and white. Basic skin color is genetically determined and is called *constitutive melanin pigmentation;* also, the normal melanin pigmentation can be increased deliberately by exposure to ultraviolet radiation, and this is called *inducible melanin pigmentation.* The degree of increase of melanin (*inducible* melanin pigmentation) determines the *skin phototype,* which is classified into four categories based solely on the ability to tan: skin phototype I cannot tan at all, and skin phototype IV develops deep tans. (For definitions of skin phototypes, see Section 11, Photosensitivity and Photo-Induced Disorders.)

Increase of melanin in the epidermis results in a disease state known as *hypermelanosis.* This occurs as a result of two types of changes: (1) An increase in the number of melanocytes in the epidermis that produces increased levels of melanin is called *melanocytotic hypermelanosis* (an example is *lentigo;* see page 236). (2) Another type of hypermelanosis in which there is no significant increase of melanocytes but an increase in the production of melanin is called *melanotic hypermelanosis* (an example is *melasma;* see page 300).

Alterations in hypermelanosis of both types (*melanocytotic* and *melanotic*) can result from three factors: *genetic; hormonal* (as in Addison's disease), when it is caused by an increase in circulating pituitary melanotropic hormones; and *ultraviolet radiation* (as in tanning, which is related to exposure to UVB, wavelengths 290 to 320 nm, and UVA, wavelengths 320 to 400 nm).

VITILIGO

Vitiligo is characterized clinically by development of totally white macules, microscopically by complete absence of melanocytes, and medically by an increased risk of certain diseases, particularly thyroid disease.

Epidemiology and Etiology

Age of Onset Vitiligo may begin at any age, but in 50 % of cases it begins between the ages of 10 and 30 years. A few cases of vitiligo have been reported to be present at birth; onset of vitiligo in old age also occurs but is unusual.

Sex Equal in both sexes. The predominance in women suggested by the literature likely reflects the greater willingness of women to express concern about cosmetic appearance.

Race Appears in all races. The apparently increased prevalence reported in some countries and among darker-skinned people results from a dramatic contrast between white vitiligo macules and dark skin and from marked social stigma in countries such as India, where the opportunities for advancement or marriage among affected individuals are even today very limited.

Incidence Common. Affects up to 1 % of the population.

Inheritance Vitiligo appears to be an inherited disease. Over 30 % of affected individuals have reported vitiligo in a parent, sibling, or child. Vitiligo in identical twins has been reported. As many as four genic loci may be responsible for vitiligo. The risk of vitiligo for children of affected individuals is unknown but may be less than 10 %. Individuals from families with an increased prevalence of thyroid disease, diabetes mellitus, and vitiligo appear to be at increased risk for development of vitiligo.

History

Characterizations of the onset of vitiligo suggest that there are both predisposing (genetic) and precipitating (environmental) factors. Many patients attribute onset of their vitiligo to physical trauma, illness, or emotional stress. Onset following the death of a relative or after severe physical injury is often mentioned. Even sunburn reaction may precipitate vitiligo.

Physical Examination

Skin Lesions

TYPE Macules; 5 mm to 5 cm or more in diameter (Figures 14-1 and 14-2)

COLOR Chalk white. Newly developed macules may be off-white in color; this represents a transitional phase. The disease progresses by gradual enlargement of the old macules or by development of new ones. Pigmentation around a hair follicle in a white macule may represent residual pigmentation or return of pigmentation (Figure 14-3). Confetti-sized hypomelanotic macules also may be observed. Inflammatory vitiligo has an elevated erythematous margin and may be pruritic; this appears to have no special significance.

SHAPE Convex margins (as if the pathologic process of depigmentation were flowing into normally pigmented skin). Round, oval, or elongated. Linear or artifactual macules represent the isomorphic or "Koebner" phenomenon.

DISTRIBUTION (SEE FIGURE VII) Depigmentation occurs in three general patterns. The *focal* type is characterized by one or several macules in a single site; this may be an early evolutionary stage of one of the other types in some cases. The *segmental* type is characterized by one or several macules in one band on one side of the body; this type is associated rarely with distant vitiligo macules

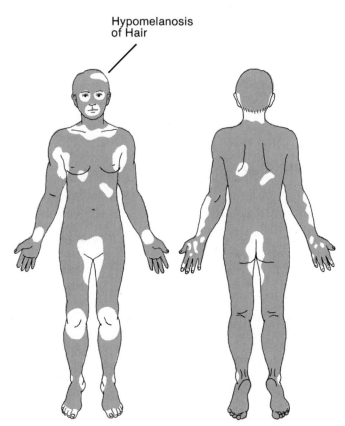

Hypomelanosis
of Hair

Figure VII Vitiligo

or with further evolution of the disease. The most common type is *generalized* vitiligo, characterized by widespread distribution of depigmented macules, often in a remarkably symmetric array. Typical macules occur around the eyes and mouth and on digits, elbows, and knees, as well as on the low back and in genital areas. The *"lip-tip" pattern* involves the skin around the mouth as well as on distal fingers and toes; lips, nipples, and genitalia (tip of the penis) may be involved. Extensive generalized vitiligo may leave only a few normally pigmented areas of skin; this is referred to as *vitiligo universalis* (Figure 14-4).

Associated Cutaneous Findings   White hair and prematurely gray hair, alopecia areata, and halo nevi. There is no increased risk for malignancy in the white skin. Skin cancers (all types) appear to be rare. In older patients, photoaging

may occur in vitiligo macules with long exposures to sunlight.

General Examination   Vitiligo is not uncommonly associated with thyroid disease (up to 30 % of all vitiligo cases, and especially in women), diabetes mellitus (probably less than 5 %), pernicious anemia (uncommon, but increased risk), Addison's disease (uncommon), and multiple endocrinopathy syndrome (rare). Ophthalmologic examination may reveal evidence of healed chorioretinitis or iritis (probably less than 10 % of all cases). Vision is unaffected. Hearing is normal.

Differential Diagnosis

Lupus erythematosus (atypical, asymmetrical pattern, serologic studies for ANA)

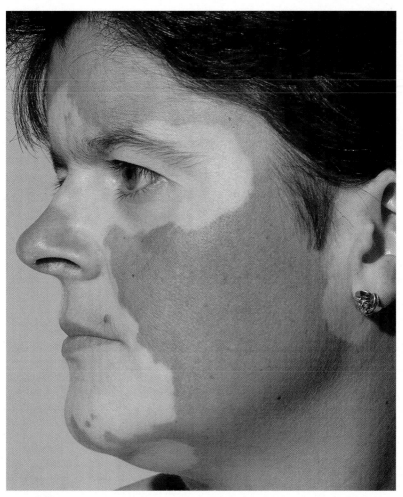

Figure 14-1 Vitiligo *Extensive depigmentation of the central face. Involved vitiliginous skin has convex borders, extending into the normal pigmented skin.*

Pityriasis alba (slight scaling, fuzzy margins, off-white color)

Piebaldism (congenital, white forelock, stable, dorsal pigmented stripe on back, distinctive pattern with large hyperpigmented macules in the center of the hypomelanotic areas)

Pityriasis versicolor alba (fine scales with greenish yellow fluorescence under Wood's lamp, positive KOH)

Chemical leukoderma (history of exposure to certain phenolic germicides, confetti macules). This is a difficult differential diagnosis.

Leprosy (endemic areas, off-white color, anesthetic macules)

Nevus depigmentosus (stable, congenital, off-white macules, Blaschko's line pattern)

Nevus anemicus (does not enhance with Wood's lamp; does not show erythema after rubbing)

Tuberous sclerosis [stable, congenital off-white macules (polygonal, ash-leaf shape), occasional segmental macules, and confetti macules]

Leukoderma associated with melanoma may be true vitiligo (may repigment spontaneously, melanocytes usually present)

Postinflammatory leukoderma (off-white macules, usually a history of psoriasis or eczema in the same macular area), not so sharply defined

Laboratory and Special Examinations

Diagnosis usually can be established on clinical grounds alone; however, in certain difficult cases, a skin biopsy may be required (see Dermatopathology, below). Chemical leukoderma (a vitiligo-like process caused by certain known chemicals) can only be diagnosed on clinical grounds and history.

Wood's Lamp Examination Wood's lamp examination is required to evaluate macules, particularly in lighter skin types, and to identify macules in sun-protected areas in all but the darkest skin types.

Dermatopathology Established vitiligo macules show normal skin except for an absence of melanocytes. There may be melanocytes at the margins (normal numbers of melanocytes that appear relatively inactive or reduced numbers that are very activated) and a mild lymphocytic response. These changes are not diagnostic for vitiligo, however—only consistent with it.

Electron Microscopy Electron microscopy has demonstrated other changes in skin affected by vitiligo; these include changes in keratinocytes: spongiosis, exocytosis, basilar vacuopathy,• and necrosis. Extracellular granules and lymphocytes have been seen in the epidermis.

Laboratory Studies T_4, TSH (radioimmunoassay), fasting blood glucose, complete blood count with indices (pernicious anemia), ACTH stimulation test (Addison's disease) if suspected

Diagnosis

Normally, diagnosis of vitiligo can be made readily on clinical examination of a patient with progressive, acquired chalk-white, sharply defined macules in typical sites.

Pathogenesis

Three principal theories have been presented about the mechanism of destruction of melanocytes in vitiligo. The *autoimmune theory* holds that selected melanocytes are destroyed by certain lymphocytes that have somehow been activated internally. The *neurogenic hypothesis* is based on an interaction of the melanocytes and the nerve cells. The *self-destruct hypothesis* suggests that melanocytes are destroyed by toxic substances formed as part of normal melanin biosynthesis. While the immediate mechanism for the evolving white macules involves progressive destruction of selected melanocytes by cytotoxic T cells, other genetically determined cytobiologic changes and cytokines must be involved. Because of differences in the extent and course of segmental and generalized vitiligo, the pathogenesis of these two types must be somewhat different.

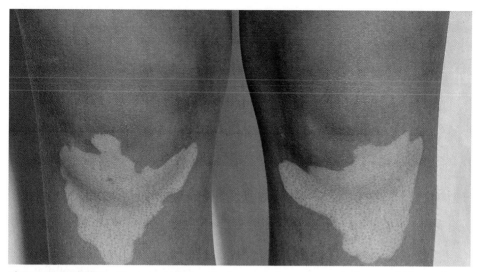

Figure 14-2 Vitiligo *Depigmented, sharply demarcated macules on the knees, which may have arose following minor trauma (Koebner phenomenon). Apart from the loss of pigment, vitiliginous skin appears normal.*

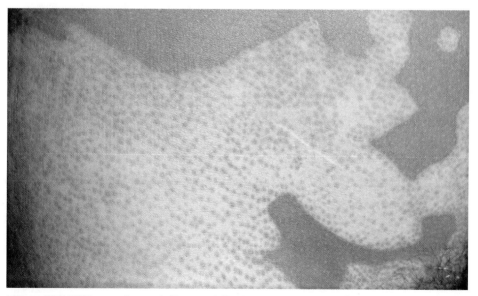

Figure 14-3 Vitiligo repigmentation *A follicular pattern of repigmentation extensively occurring in a large vitiliginous macule. Melanocytes persist in the hair follicle epithelium and serve to repopulate involved skin, spontaneously or with photochemotherapy.*

Course and Prognosis

Vitiligo is a chronic disease. The course is highly variable, but rapid onset followed by a period of stability or slow progression is most characteristic. Up to 30 % of patients may report some spontaneous repigmentation in a few areas—particularly areas that are exposed to the sun. Rarely is this satisfactory to the patient. Rapidly progressive or "galloping" vitiligo may quickly lead to extensive depigmentation.

Segmental vitiligo is a special subset that usually develops precipitously in one unilateral region, usually does not extend beyond that initial one-sided region, and once present is very stable.

The treatment of vitiligo-associated disease (i.e., thyroid disease) appears to have no impact on the course of vitiligo.

Management

The five general options for the management of vitiligo are sunscreens, coverup, repigmentation, minigrafting, and depigmentation.

Sunscreens The dual objectives of sunscreens are protection of involved skin from acute sunburn reaction and limitation of tanning of normally pigmented skin. Sunscreens with a sun protection factor of more than 30 are reasonable choices to prevent sunburn for most patients. However, since their ability to limit the tanning reaction is inversely proportional to skin phototype, opaque sunscreens should be more effective in limiting the tanning reaction in fairer-skinned individuals. While all skin phototypes have a need for sun protection, sunscreens alone are often perfectly adequate management for those vitiligo patients with skin phototypes I, II, and sometimes III (those who burn and then tan to some degree).

Cosmetic Coverup The objective of coverup with dyes or makeup is to hide the white macules so that the vitiligo is not apparent. Vitadye (ICN) and Dy-o-Derm (Owen Laboratories) each come in one color, are easy to apply, and

do not rub off but gradually wash or wear off. So-called self-tanning agents, which contain dihydroxyacetone, are available in a number of formulations; many contain sunscreens that will be effective for much less time than the dye is present. Estée Lauder preparations have been found particularly useful by patients. Covermark (Lydia O'Leary) and Dermablend (Flori Roberts) are cosmetics available to match most skin hues; they do not wash off but do rub off. Other preparations may be found at cosmetic counters.

Repigmentation The objective of repigmentation is the permanent return of normal melanin pigmentation. This may be achieved for local macules with topical steroids or topical psoralens and UVA (long-wave ultraviolet light) and for widespread macules with oral psoralens and UVA.

TOPICAL CORTICOSTEROIDS Initial treatment with topical Class I corticosteroid ointments is practical, simple, and safe. If there is no response in 2 months, it is unlikely to be effective. Physician monitoring every 2 months for signs of early steroid atrophy is required.

TOPICAL PHOTOCHEMOTHERAPY Much more complicated is the use of topical 8-methoxypsoralen (8-MOP), because this substance is so highly phototoxic and because the phototoxicity lasts for 3 days or more. This procedure should be undertaken for small macules only and by experienced physicians and well-informed patients. As with oral psoralens, it may require 15 or more treatments to initiate response and 100 or more to finish.

SYSTEMIC PHOTOCHEMOTHERAPY For more widespread vitiligo, oral PUVA is more practical and carries less risk of severe phototoxicity than topical phototherapy. Oral phototherapy may be done with sunlight and trimethylpsoralen (TMP) and 5-methoxy psoralen (5-MOP) (not available in the United States) or with artificial UVA (doctor's office or other approved unit) and TMP, 5-MOP, or 8-MOP (Figure 14-5). Ophthalmologic examination and an ANA blood test are required before starting therapy.

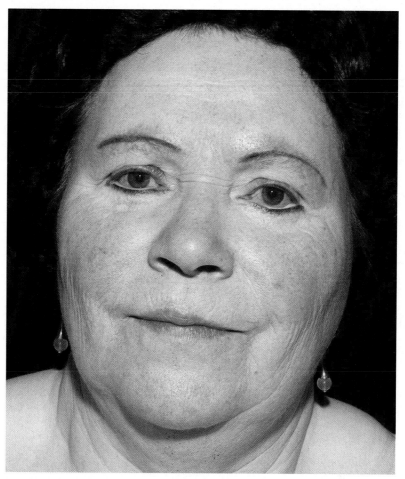

Figure 14-4 Universal vitiligo *Vitiliginous macules have coalesced to involve all skin sites with complete depigmentation of skin and hair in a female. The patient is wearing a black wig, and has darkened the brows with eyebrow pencil and eyelid margins with eye liner.*

Outdoor therapy may be initiated with 0.6 mg/kg TMP (or 1.2 mg/kg 5-MOP) followed 2 hours later by 5 minutes of New England sunlight (less in the southern regions). Treatments should be twice weekly, though not on 2 consecutive days, and sunlight exposure should increase by 3 to 5 minutes per treatment until a sign of response or of phototoxicity occurs. In some patients, mild phototoxicity is required for response, and in a few it causes koebnerization. Individualization of treatment is required.

Indoor PUVA is as effective in regimentation as is PUVA with sunlight; it can be controlled more rigorously but has the significant disadvantage of additional cost. Either 0.2 to 0.4 mg/kg 8-MOP (well absorbed, efficient, potentially very phototoxic, with significant risk of nausea) 1 hour before UVA exposure or 0.6 to 0.8 mg/kg TMP (variably absorbed, not very phototoxic, with very little risk of nausea) (or 1.2 mg/kg 5-MOP; less phototoxic than 8-MOP and no nausea) 2 hours before UVA exposure may be used. Initial UVA exposure should be 1.0 J/cm^2 and increments (twice weekly, not on 2 consecutive days) of 0.5 (8-MOP) to 1.0 J/cm^2 per treatment until evidence of response or of phototoxicity appears. The latter is the guide to sustaining or increasing the UVA dose until reasonable repigmentation has been established or until progress has stalled.

PUVA is up to 85 % effective in over 70 % of patients with vitiligo of the head, neck, upper arms and legs, and trunk. Distal hands and feet are poorly responsive and when present alone are not usually worth treating. Genital areas should be shielded and not treated.

Macules that have *totally* repigmented usually stay that way in the absence of injury or sunburn (85 % likelihood up to 10 years); macules less than fully repigmented will slowly reverse once treatments have been discontinued. Maintenance treatments are not required.

Risks of treatment with PUVA include nausea, gastrointestinal upset, sunburn reaction, hyperpigmentation of the normal skin, and dryness acutely. Chronic effects include photoaging, PUVA lentigines, keratoses (including leukokeratoses), skin cancers (we have seen 1 in over 30 years of collective experience with over 2000 patients), and cataracts (we have not observed any).

Standard PUVA precautions should apply; we advise against oral PUVA in children under age 10. Treatment is most likely to be successful in highly motivated patients who clearly have reasonable objectives and understand the risks and benefits. While PUVA is not a cure, most patients who are responding well to treatment do not at the same time develop new vitiligo macules.

Minigrafting Minigrafting may be a useful technique for refractory segmental vitiligo macules. PUVA may be required following the procedure to unify the color between the graft sites. The demonstrated occurrence of koebnerization in donor sites in generalized vitiligo restricts this procedure to those who have limited cutaneous areas at risk for vitiligo (that is, segmental vitiligo in which there is no koebnerization of normal skin). "Pebbling" of the grafted site may occur.

Depigmentation The objective of depigmentation is unification of skin color in patients with extensive vitiligo or in those who have failed PUVA, who cannot use PUVA, or who reject the PUVA option. Bleaching with monobenzylether of hydroquinone 20 % cream (monobenzone 20 %) *of normally pigmented skin* is a permanent, irreversible process. Since application of monobenzone 20 % may be associated with satellite depigmentation, this treatment cannot be used selectively to bleach certain areas of normal pigmentation, since there is a real likelihood that new and distant white macules will develop over the months of use. Bleaching with monobenzone 20 % normally requires application twice daily and takes 2 to 3 months to initiate response and up to 9 to 12 months or more to complete. Erythema, dryness, and itching are possible side effects. Contact dermatitis is observed uncommonly. The success rate is over 90 %. Periodically, following sun exposure, an occasional patient will observe focal repigmentation that requires a month or so of local use of monobenzone 20 % to reverse; use of a sunscreen containing titanium dioxide or zinc oxide should reduce this risk.

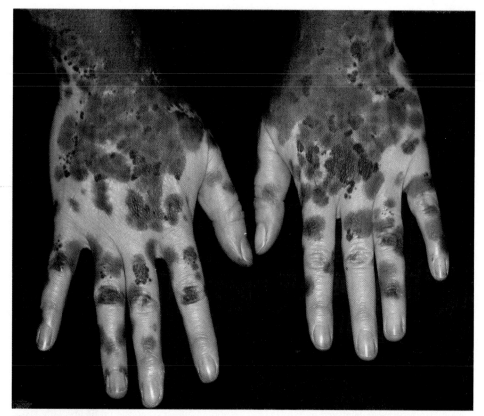

Figure 14-5 Vitiligo, repigmentation *The patient is being treated with photochemotherapy (PUVA). Repigmentation has been uniform except on the hands, sites which are often resistant to the treatment; islands of repigmentation have created spotted macules in a background of depigmentation, resulting in significant cosmetic disfigurement.*

The end-stage color of depigmentation with monobenzone 20 % is chalk white, as in vitiligo macules. Most patients are quite satisfied with the uniformity and the finality of the results. An occasional patient may wish to take 30 to 60 mg beta-carotene to impart an off-white color to the skin; other than the color change, the only side effect of beta-carotene is the uncommon risk of diarrhea.

All those who have bleached are at risk for sunburn from acute solar irradiation. Avoidance of midday sun exposure and use of a sunscreen with a high sun protection factor are urged.

No long-term untoward effects have been reported from the use of monobenzylether of hydroquinone 20 % cream. *But note that the differentiation achieved is permanent.*

ALBINISM

Albinism is a heritable disorder that affects skin, hair follicles, and eyes (iris and choroid). It principally involves the synthesis of melanin but also includes some alterations of the pathways of the CNS. Albinism can affect the eyes, *ocular albinism* (X-linked recessive or autosomal recessive), or the eyes and skin, *oculocutaneous albinism* (OCA). In OCA, the disorder is autosomal recessive, with dilution of normal amounts of skin, hair, and melanin pigment; nystagmus and iris translucency are always present, and there is a reduction of visual acuity, sometimes severe enough to cause severe impairment of vision.

Epidemiology

Incidence   The incidence of OCA is 1:16,000 to 20,000

Age   Present at birth

Race   There is no special predilection in any one skin color. Hermansky-Pudlak syndrome (OCA and a platelet disorder) is seen in Hispanics from Puerto Rico, in persons of Dutch origin, and in East Indians from Madras.

Classification of Albinism   Two groups: (1) Type I tyrosinase-negative OCA, type II tyrosinase-positive OCA, with defects in the tyrosinase-melanin pathway catalyzed by tyrosinase. Molecular studies have defined several types of OCA resulting in mutations of the tyrosinase gene, which are the basis of yellow, minimal-pigment, and temperature-sensitive OCA. (2) Changes that affect the membrane of the pigment organelle, the melanosome, and other organelles, *Chédiak-Higashi syndrome* (CHS), in which there are prominent hematologic abnormalities (giant granules in the platelets and thrombocytopenia) and repeated bacterial infections resulting from depressed degranulation response and bactericidal functions. Also, *Hermansky-Pudlak syndrome* (HPS), characterized by a mild to severe bleeding diathesis because of defective platelets; there is a lack of storage of granules or dense bodies, and platelets fail to undergo secondary aggregation when stimulated.

History

Duration   Present at birth. Patients with albinism early in life need to avoid the sun because of repeated sunburns, especially as toddlers.

Systems Review   *HPS:* epistaxis, gingival bleeding, excessive bleeding after childbirth or tooth extraction, fibrotic restrictive lung disease

Family History   There may be no family history of albinism in the autosomal recessive or X-linked recessive types.

Social History   Albinos live an essentially normal life, except for problems with vision and, in lower latitudes, the development of skin cancers and dermatoheliosis. There is a national volunteer group of albinos in the United States called the National Organization for Albinism and Hypomelanosis (NOAH)—Noah, builder of the ark in the Old Testament, was thought to be an albino). The volunteer group assists albinos in various ways, especially in dealing with vision problems: obtaining driver's license, etc. Many albinos appear to be musicians and to be high achievers (Rev. W. A. Spooner, head of New College, Oxford, was an albino and famous for his "spoonerisms," e.g., "well-oiled bicycle" transposed as "well-boiled icicle").

Physical Examination

Appearance of Patient   "Poring" (eyes half closed, squinting) when in sunlight

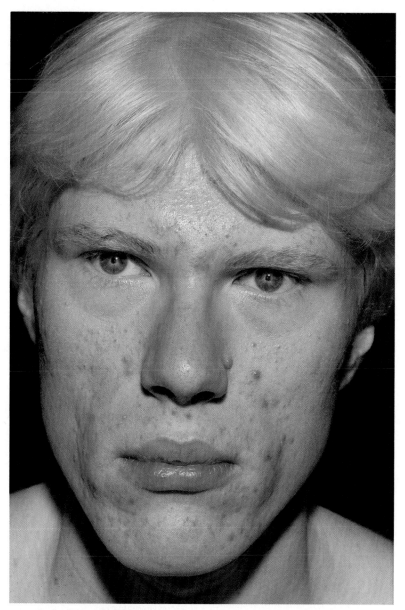

Figure 14-6 Oculocutaneous albinism   *White skin and white eyelashes; scalp hair and eyebrows have been darkened with dye. The irises appear translucent. Heme pigment gives the face a pinkish hue; mild papulopustular acne is present. Carotene colors the central face a yellow-orange hue. The slight divergent strabism is due to nystagmus.*

Skin "Snow" white, fair, cream, light tan (Figure 14-6)

Hair White (ty-neg), yellow, cream, or light brown (ty-pos), red, platinum

Eyes The eye changes are the essential physical finding that defines the syndrome of albinism; the skin color and hair color can vary from snow white to brown, but it is the eye findings that permit the diagnosis. Nystagmus, a feature virtually always present, results from hypoplasia of the fovea with reduction of visual acuity and alteration in the formation of the optic nerves; this misrouting of the optic paths is also associated with an alternating strabismus and diminished stereoacuity. The diagnostic features in the eye that identify albinism are therefore nystagmus, iris translucency (Figure 14-7), reduction of visual acuity, decreased retinal pigment, foveal hypoplasia, and strabismus.

Laboratory and Special Examinations

Dermatopathology

LIGHT MICROSCOPY Melanocytes are present in the skin and hair bulb in all types of albinism. The dopa reaction of the skin and hair is markedly reduced or absent in melanocytes of the skin and hair, depending on the type of albinism (ty-neg or ty-pos).

ELECTRON MICROSCOPY Melanosomes are present in melanocytes in all types of albinism, but depending on the type of albinism, there is a reduction of the melanization of melanosomes, with many being completely unmelanized (stage I) in ty-neg albinism. Melanosomes in the albino melanocytes are transferred in a normal manner to the keratinocytes.

Hematology Morphologic, chemical, and functional defects of platelets in HPS type of albinism

Tyrosinase Hair Bulb Test (Ty-Neg and Ty-Pos) Hair bulbs are incubated in tyrosine solutions for 12 to 24 hours and develop new pigment formation from normal and ty-pos patients, but no new pigment formation is present in ty-neg albinism. [For details of methods, see King RA et al: Albinism, in C Scriver et al (eds): *The Metabolic and Molecular Bases of Inherited Disease*, 7th ed, New York, McGraw-Hill, 1995, chap 147.]

Diagnosis

White persons with very fair skin (skin phototype I), blond hair, and blue eyes may mimic albinos, but they do not have iris translucency or nystagmus. Some persons with albinism who have constitutive black or brown skin color may have a dilution of their skin color from black to a light brown and have the capacity to tan; also, they may have brown irides but will still have iris translucency. Therefore, iris translucency and the presence of other eye findings in the fundus are the pathognomonic signs of albinism.

Etiology and Pathogenesis

The defect in melanin synthesis has been shown to result from absence of the activity of the enzyme tyrosinase. Tyrosinase is a copper-containing enzyme that catalyzes the oxidation of tyrosine to dopa and the subsequent dehydrogenation of dopa to dopa-quinone. Recent cloning of complementary DNAs (cDNAs) encoding tyrosinase has made it possible to directly characterize the mutations in the tyrosinase gene responsible for deficient tyrosinase activity in several types of albinism. In type IA, two different missense mutations, one from each parent, result in amino acid substitutions within one of the two copper-binding sites.

Significance

Albinism is an important disease to recognize early in life in order to start prophylactic measures to prevent dermatoheliosis and skin cancer.

Course and Prognosis

Albinos with ty-pos OCA form melanin pig-

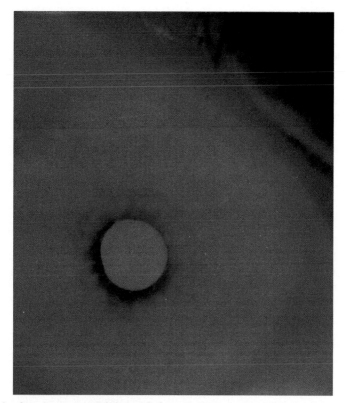

Figure 14-7 Oculocutaneous albinism: iris translucency *In a darkened room, illumination of the eye with a light placed beside the iris shows it to be transparent and devoid of any melanin pigmentation.*

ment in the hair, skin, and eyes during early life, the hair becoming cream, yellow, or light brown and the eye color changing from light gray to blue, hazel, or even brown.

Albinos living in central Africa who are unprotected from the sun develop squamous cell carcinomas early in life, and this significantly shortens their life span; few survive to the age of 40 years because of metastasizing squamous cell carcinoma. Dermatoheliosis and basal cell carcinomas are frequent in albinos living in temperate climates. Melanomas are curiously very rare in albinos living in Africa; they are usually amelanotic. Melanocytic nevi occur in albinism and also may be amelanotic.

Management

Skin A lifetime program beginning in in-

fancy, including

Daily application of topical, potent, broad-spectrum SPF > 30 sunblocks, including lip sunblocks

Avoidance of sun exposure in the high solar intensity season during the hours of 1000 to 1500

Yearly examination by a dermatologist to detect skin changes: skin cancers and dermatoheliosis

Use of topical tretinoin for dermatoheliosis and for its possible prophylactic effect against sun-induced epithelial skin cancers

Systemic Beta-carotene (30 to 60 mg t.i.d.) imparts a more normal color to the skin and may have some protective effect on the development of skin cancers, although this has been proved only in mice.

MELASMA

Melasma (Greek: "a black spot") is an acquired light- or dark-brown hyperpigmentation that occurs in the exposed areas, most often on the face, and results from exposure to sunlight; may be associated with pregnancy, with ingestion of contraceptive hormones, or possibly with certain medications such as diphenylhydantoin or be idiopathic.
Synonyms: Chloasma (Greek: "a green spot"), mask of pregnancy.

Epidemiology

Incidence Common, especially among persons with constitutive brown skin color and who are taking contraceptive regimens and who live in sunny areas. During the early clinical trials of estrogen–synthetic progesterone combinations, which were done in the Caribbean in brown-skinned Hispanic women, melasma occurred in 20 % of the patients. Melasma has recently been appearing in menopausal women as a result of regimens for prevention of osteoporosis using a combination of estrogens *and* progesterone (medroxyprogesterone, or Provera); melasma did not appear in those women who were given estrogen replacement treatment but without progesterone. Melasma is still occurring in women given the contraceptive agents that are combinations of estrogen-type compounds and progestational agents.

Age Young adults

Race Melasma is more apparent or more frequent in persons with brown or black constitutive skin color (people from Asia, the Middle East, India, South America).

Sex Females >> males; about 10 % of patients with melasma are men.

Geography More apparent or more frequent in sunny areas of the world, especially in the Caribbean and in countries bordering on the Mediterranean

Precipitating Factors Sun exposure plus pregnancy or oral contraceptives, diphenylhydantoin; cosmetics probably do not play a role.

History

Duration of Lesions The pigmentation usually evolves quite rapidly over weeks, particularly following exposure to sunlight.

Relationship of Melasma to Other Factors Season (more apparent in summer months in northern latitudes), medications (following or during ingestion of oral contraceptives), menses (during premenstrual period, a darkening of preexisting melasma may sometimes occur), pregnancy

Physical Examination

Skin Lesions

TYPE   Completely macular hyperpigmentation, the hue and intensity depending largely on the skin phototype of the patient (Figure 14-8)

COLOR   Light or dark brown or even black. Color is usually uniform but may be splotchy.

ARRANGEMENT   Most often symmetric

SHAPE AND BORDER OF INDIVIDUAL LESIONS   The pattern follows the areas of exposure, and the lesions have serrated, irregular, and geographic borders.

DISTRIBUTION   Two-thirds on central part of the face: cheeks, forehead, nose, upper lip, and chin; a smaller percentage involve the malar or mandibular areas of the face and occasionally the dorsa of the forearms.

WOOD'S LAMP EXAMINATION   A marked accentuation of the hyperpigmented macules. *This contrast is not accentuated in patients with a normal brown or black skin.* This has been mistakenly interpreted as a "dermal" melasma.

Differential Diagnosis

Postinflammatory hypermelanotic macules

Laboratory and Special Examinations

Dermatopathology Increase in production and transfer of melanosomes to the keratinocytes in the epidermis

Illumination Allow for dark adaptation

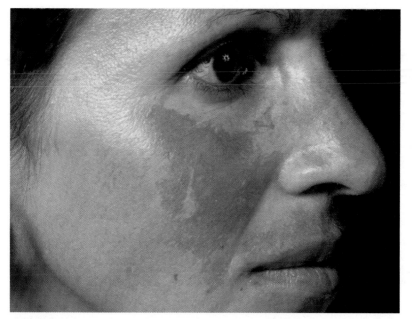

Figure 14-8 Melasma   *Well-demarcated, hyperpigmented macules are seen on the cheek, nose, and forehead.*

Diagnosis

Clinical findings

Pathogenesis

Unknown. *Estrogen preparations alone, however, given to postmenopausal women do not cause melasma, despite sun exposure.* However, pregnancy causes melasma, and combinations of estrogen and progestational agents, as used for contraception, are the most frequent cause of melasma.

Significance

While this is a strictly cosmetic problem, it is very disturbing to both males and females, especially persons with brown skin color and good tanning capacity (skin phototype V). For a discussion of how to determine skin phototype (SPT I to VI), see page 229.

Course and Prognosis

Melasma may disappear spontaneously over a period of months following delivery or after cessation of contraceptive hormones. Melasma may or may not return with each subsequent pregnancy.

Management

Topical   A commercially available (in the United States) 3 % hydroquinone solution is used in combination with topical tretinoin and is reasonably effective and at present the therapy of choice. *Under no circumstances should monobenzylether of hydroquinone or the other ethers of hydroquinone (monomethyl- or monoethyl-) be used in the treatment of melasma because these drugs can lead to a permanent loss of melanocytes with the development of a disfiguring spotty leukoderma.*

Prevention   It is essential that the patient use, every morning, an *opaque* sunblock containing titanium dioxide and/or zinc oxide; the action spectrum of pigment darkening extends into the visible range, and even the potent (with high SPF) transparent sunscreens are completely ineffective in blocking visible radiation.

BECKER'S NEVUS

Becker's nevus is a common acquired benign pigmentary hamartoma that occurs as a unilateral blotchy brown hyperpigmentation, usually on the shoulders of teenage boys. Hair is typically not present at the time of onset of the hyperpigmentation but usually appears within a year. Since there are no nevomelanocytes present, the lesion is not regarded as a melanocytic nevus.

Epidemiology and Etiology

Incidence 0.52 % in males aged 17 to 26 years

Age Onset appears before age 10 (50 %), ages 10 to 15 (25 %), and after age 15 (25 %)

Sex Male/female ratio 5:1

Heredity Familial cases have been reported.

History

Onset of Skin Lesions Pigmentation develops first at puberty; terminal hair appears often within a year.

Physical Examination

Skin Lesions (Figure 14-9)

TYPE Singular plaque, 125 cm^2 (mean), often with a barely detectable verrucous surface

COLOR Light tan or brown, not uniform as a café-au-lait macule

PALPATION Barely palpable, detectable elevation by oblique lighting

SHAPE Large lesion, usually with jagged, sharp ("coast of Maine") borders; long axes follow lines of cleavage.

DISTRIBUTION Shoulder and submammary area (32 %), lower back (23 %), upper back (19 %), arms (3 %), legs (3 %)

Hair Increased hair growth (56 %) localized to pigmented areas

Miscellaneous Physical Findings Rarely, hypoplasia of underlying structures, e.g., shortening of the arm or reduced breast development in areas under lesion

Differential Diagnosis

Large Brown Macule/Plaque *Giant congenital melanocytic nevus,* which is present at birth and distinctly elevated. *Albright's disease,* which is congenital, no hair is present, and pigmentation is uniform rather than splotchy.

Laboratory and Special Examinations

Dermatopathology

LIGHT MICROSCOPY *Site* Epidermis
  Process Acanthosis, regular with some hyperkeratosis and occasional horn cysts. No nevomelanocytes are present. Melanocytes are not increased. Basal layer keratinocytes are packed with melanin.

ELECTRON MICROSCOPY Increased number of melanosome complexes in the keratinocytes of the basal cell layer

Illumination Oblique lighting: place a flashlight at the side of the lesion to detect subtle elevation.

Significance

This lesion is confused with congenital nevomelanocytic nevus; biopsy may be necessary.

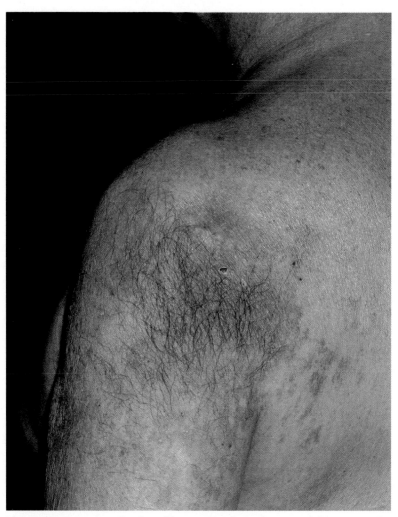

Figure 14-9 Becker's nevus *Patches of hyperpigmentation become confluent centrally on the shoulder associated with hypertrichosis; the lesion is hamartoma (i.e., nevus) of the epidermis and hair follicles.*

Course and Prognosis

Pigmentation extends for a year or two and then remains stable, only rarely fading. The lesion often (but not always) develops dark, coarse hairs, but this always follows the onset of the pigmentation.

Management

Melanoma does not develop in these lesions. The lesion is a cosmetic disfigurement but rarely, if ever, presents a problem for the patient.

GENITAL LENTIGINOSES

Genital lentiginoses are acquired multiple or single light brown, brown, dark brown, or black, oval or round, often fairly large (15 mm) macules that appear on the anogenital areas of women and men. These lesions have an adult onset and persist for years without change in size. The pathology does not show significant melanocytic hyperplasia, and nevus cells are not present; the pigmentation is the result of increased melanin in the basal cell layer.

Synonyms: Penile lentigo, vulvar melanosis.

Epidemiology

Incidence Uncommon

Age Adults

Sex Men and women

History

Onset In adults

Symptoms None

Systems Review Negative

Family History Not reported

Physical Examination

Skin Lesions

TYPE 5 to 15 mm macules (Figures 14-10 and 14-11)

COLOR Tan, brown, intense blue-black; usually variegated

SHAPE Oval or round

ARRANGEMENT In clusters

DISTRIBUTION Vulva (labia minora) (Figure 14-11), perianal areas, penis shaft and glans (Figure 14-10)

Differential Diagnosis

Melanoma *in situ,* PUVA lentigo, fixed drug reaction, lentiginosis as part of the LAMB syndrome (lentigo, atrial myxoma, myxoid neurofibromas, and blue nevi), HPV-induced SCC *in situ*

Laboratory Examinations

Dermatopathology

LIGHT MICROSCOPY *Site* Epidermis, papillary dermis
   Process Increased melanin pigment in basal layer without significant increase in melanocytes

Diagnosis

Multiple or single brown macular lesions localized to the penis or vulva without neoplasia of melanocytes

Etiology and Pathogenesis

Unknown

Significance

In women, these lesions are almost always a source of concern for the patient; they may indicate vulvar melanoma. Penile lentiginosis—especially a single lesion—also suggests the possibility of melanoma; epiluminescence microscopy rules out *in situ* melanoma, but, since experience is still limited, a biopsy should nevertheless be performed to establish that there are no nevus or melanoma cells present. These patients should be examined every 3 years.

Management

No treatment indicated

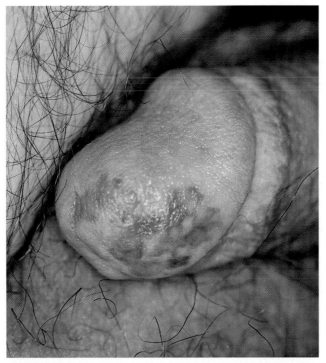

Figure 14-10 Genital lentiginosis: penis *Highly variegated tan-brown macules on the glans present for many years. In situ melanoma must be ruled out by lesional biopsy.*

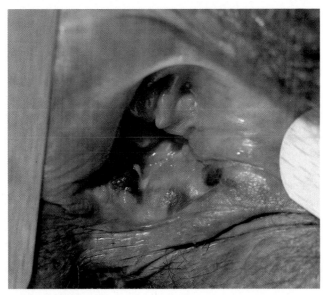

Figure 14-11 Genital lentiginosis: vulva *Multiple, sharply demarcated, variegated, dark-brown macules on the vulva for many years. In situ melanoma must be ruled out by lesional biopsy.*

PIGMENTED PURPURIC DERMATOSES

Pigmented purpuric dermatoses are distinguished by their clinical characteristics, having identical dermatopathologic findings, and include

- *Schamberg's disease,* also known as *progressive pigmented purpuric dermatosis* and *progressive pigmentary purpura*
- *Majocchi's disease,* also known as *purpura annularis telangiectodes*
- *Gougerot-Blum disease,* also known as *pigmented purpuric lichenoid dermatitis* and *purpura pigmentosa chronica*
- *Lichen aureus,* also known as *lichen purpuricus*

Clinically, each entity shows recent pinpoint cayenne pepper–colored hemorrhages associated with older hemorrhages and hemosiderin deposition and capillaritis histologically. Pigmented purpuric dermatoses are significant only if they are a cosmetic concern to the patient; they are often mistaken as manifestations of vasculitis or thrombocytopenia.
Synonym: Capillaritis of unknown cause.

Epidemiology and Etiology

Age 30 to 60 years; uncommon in children

Sex More common in males

Etiology Unknown. Primary process believed to be cell-mediated immune injury with subsequent vascular damage and erythrocyte extravasation. Other etiologic factors: pressure, trauma, eczematous dermatitis, drugs (acetaminophen, ampicillin, especially carbromal, diuretics, meprobamate, nonsteroidal anti-inflammatory drugs, zomepirac sodium)

History

Onset and Duration Insidious, slow to evolve—except drug-induced variant, which may develop rapidly and be more generalized in distribution. Persists for months to years. Most drug-induced purpuras resolve more quickly after discontinuation of the drug.

Symptoms

Usually asymptomatic, but may be mildly pruritic

Physical Examination

Schamberg's Disease

TYPE OF LESIONS Pinhead-sized macules (fresh hemorrhages) become confluent, coalescing into patches (Figure 14-13).

COLOR OF LESIONS Reddish brown, "cayenne pepper." New lesions are red, representing pinpoint hemorrhages. Older lesions are tan to brown, representing degradation of extravasated erythrocytes with the formation of hemosiderin.

ARRANGEMENT OF LESIONS Discrete clusters of macules and patches that can become confluent

DISTRIBUTION OF LESIONS Lower extremities (especially pretibial and on ankles) but may extend proximally to lower trunk. Usually bilateral but may be unilateral. Uncommonly, generalized.

Majocchi's Disease Essentially an annular form of Schamberg's disease. An arciform variant also has been described (Figure 14-12).

Gougerot-Blum Disease Lichenoid papules, plaques, macules in association with lesions of Schamberg's disease

Lichen Aureus Solitary or few patches or

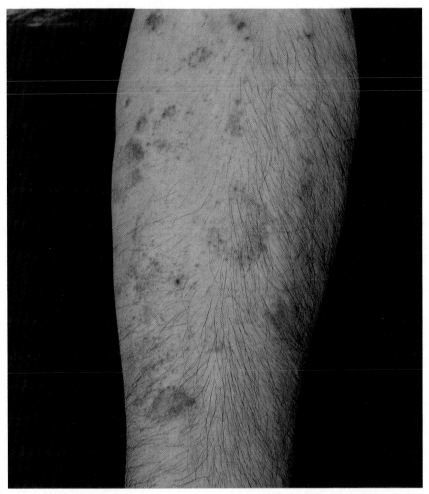

Figure 14-12 Pigmented purpuric dermatoses, Majocchi's disease *Petechiae of various ages with red-to-tan color are arranged in semiannular and annular configurations. Although the eruption appears to be acute, lesions had been present for many months.*

plaques, rust-colored, purple, or golden, arising on the extremities or trunk

Differential Diagnosis

Nonpalpable Purpura Chronic venous insufficiency with clotting abnormalities, corticosteroid usage, cutaneous T-cell lymphoma, dysproteinemias, nummular eczema, old fixed drug eruption, parapsoriasis, poikiloderma vasculare atrophicans, primary amyloidosis, scurvy, senile purpura, stasis dermatitis, thrombocytopenia, trauma

Palpable Purpura Atheroembolism, collagen vascular disease, cryoglobulinemias, infections, leukocytoclastic vasculitis

Laboratory Examinations

Dermatopathology Epidermal involvement varies, but dermal pathology (capillaritis) is common to all. Epidermis is normal in lichen aureus and drug-induced eruptions; in some cases there is vacuolar degradation of basal layer, spongiosis, and/or lymphocytic exocytosis. Dermal features present in all variants: extravasation of erythrocytes, hemosiderin pigment-laden macrophages (more extensive in lichen aureus), mild perivascular and interstitial lymphohistiocytic infiltrate in reticular dermis (more dense and bandlike lichenoid infiltrate observed in lichen aureus and Gougerot-Blum disease).

Immunohistochemistry Immunofluorescence is variable and nonspecific. Most common pattern: deposits in superficial dermal vessels of fibrinogen, IgM, and/or C3; keratinocytes express HLA-DR; CD4 cells are the predominant lymphocytes in the dermis and bear HECA-452–recognized antigen; B cells are absent or rare, suggesting that the role of humoral immunity is minimal.

Diagnosis

Usually made on clinical findings

Course

Chronic (months to years), slow to evolve and resolve; spontaneous resolution has been observed. Almost all cases due to drugs clear within months after discontinuation of the offending agent.

Management

Symptomatic. Long-standing lesions may be cosmetically disfiguring, and patients may choose to treat these lesions. Topical low- and middle-potency corticosteroid preparations inhibit new purpuric lesions. In lesions of long standing, hemosiderin deposits resolve very slowly (months to years). Systemic tetracycline *or* minocycline (50 mg b.i.d.); PUVA is effective but is indicated only in severe forms.

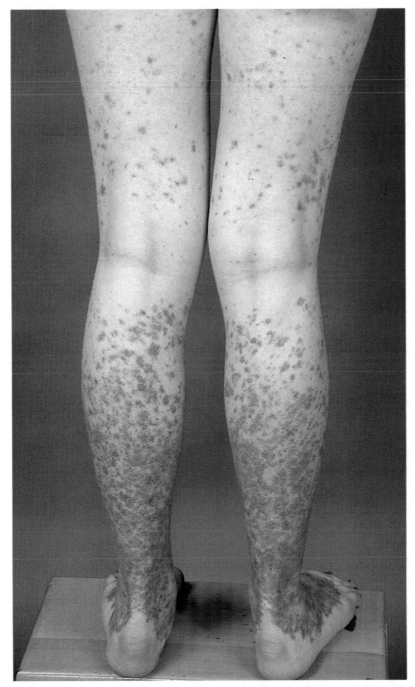

Figure 14-13 Pigmented purpuric dermatoses, Schamberg's disease *Multiple, discrete, nonpalpable, nonblanching purpuric lesions of many years' duration on the legs. Acute microhemorrhages resolve with deposition of hemosiderin, creating a disfiguring dark-brown stain.*

SKIN SIGNS OF IMMUNE, AUTOIMMUNE, AND RHEUMATIC DISEASES

SYSTEMIC AMYLOIDOSIS

Amyloidosis is an extracellular deposition in various tissues of amyloid fibril proteins and of a protein called *amyloid P component* (AP); the identical component of AP is present in the serum and is called *SAP.* These amyloid deposits can affect normal body function, and *acquired systemic amyloidosis (amyloidosis AL),* known previously as *primary amyloidosis,* occurs in patients with B-cell or plasma cell dyscrasias in whom fragments of monoclonal immunoglobulin light chains form amyloid fibrils. Amyloidosis AL also is associated with multiple myeloma. *AA,* or *secondary, amyloidosis* occurs in patients following chronic inflammatory disease, in whom the fibril protein is derived from the circulating acute-phase lipoprotein known as *serum amyloid A.* Clinical features include a combination of macroglossia and cardiac, renal, hepatic, and GI involvement, as well as carpal tunnel syndrome. Skin lesions occur in 30 % of patients with amyloidosis AL (primary), and since they occur early in the disease, they are an important clue to the diagnosis. There are few or no characteristic skin lesions in AA (secondary) amyloidosis.

Three not uncommon varieties of localized amyloidosis that are unrelated to the systemic amyloidoses are *lichenoid amyloidosis* (discrete, very pruritic, brownish-red papules on the legs), *nodular amyloidosis* (single or multiple, smooth, nodular lesions with or without purpura on limbs, face, or trunk), and *macular amyloidosis* (pruritic, gray-brown, reticulated macular lesions occurring principally on the upper back; the lesions often have a distinctive "ripple" pattern). As stated, these three localized forms of amyloidosis are confined to the skin and unrelated to systemic disease; however, the skin lesions of nodular amyloidosis are identical to those that also occur in amyloidosis AL (primary) described below.

Epidemiology

Age Sixth decade

Sex Equal incidence

Precipitating Factors Multiple myeloma in many but not all patients with amyloidosis AL

Systemic Involvement Chronic constitutional symptoms: fatigue, weakness, anorexia,

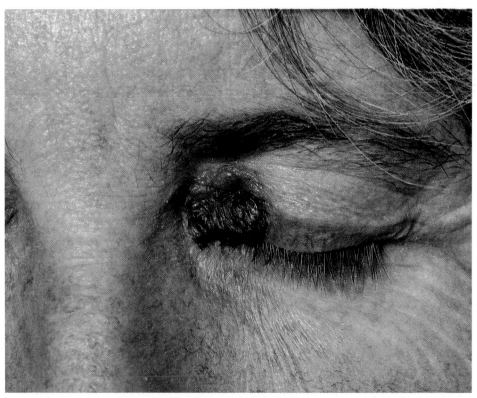

Figure 15-1 Primary systemic amyloidosis: "pinch purpura" *The topmost papule is yellowish and nonhemorrhagic; the lower portion is hemorrhagic. So-called "pinch purpura" of the upper eyelid can appear as hemorrhagic papules following pinching or rubbing the eyelid.*

weight loss, malaise. Dyspnea, paresthesia related to carpal tunnel syndrome.

Physical Examination

Skin Lesions

TYPES

  Purpura following trauma, "pinch" purpura (Figure 15-1), occurs on the face and especially around the eyes.
  Papules: smooth, waxy, with or without purpura, sometimes involving large surface areas
  Nodules

DISTRIBUTION Purpuric lesions around the eyes, central face, body folds, axillae, umbilicus, anogenital area

Mucous Membranes Macroglossia: diffusely enlarged and firm, "woody" (Figure 15-2). This also occurs in AA.

General Examination Kidney—nephrosis; nervous system—peripheral neuropathy, carpal tunnel syndrome; CVS—partial heart block, congestive heart failure; hepatic—hepatomegaly

Differential Diagnosis

Purpura Thrombocytopenic purpura, actinic (Bateman's) purpura, scurvy

Macroglossia Hypothyroidism

Laboratory and Special Examinations

Hematology Thrombocytosis > 500,000/μl may be present.

Urinalysis Proteinuria

Chemistry Increased serum creatinine; hypercalcemia

Immunoglobulin Studies Increased IgG. Monoclonal protein in two-thirds of patients with primary or myeloma-associated amyloidoses

Dermatopathology

Accumulation of faintly eosinophilic masses of amyloid near the epidermis, in sweat glands, around and within blood vessel walls

Use thioflavin and examine the sections for an apple-green birefringence using a simple polarization microscope.

Diagnosis

The combination of purpuric skin lesions, waxy papules, macroglossia, carpal tunnel syndrome, and cardiac symptoms and signs. A tissue diagnosis can be made from the skin biopsy. Scintigraphy after injection of ^{123}I SAP is now available for estimating the extent of the involvement and can serve as a guide for treatment.

Pathogenesis

The various manifestations of the disease result from the impairment of normal function of the various organs because of the extracellular accumulation of large amounts of amyloid.

Course and Prognosis

Poor, especially if there is renal involvement. Amyloidosis AL with multiple myeloma has an especially poor prognosis, with 18- to 24-month survival.

Management

Cytotoxic drugs can modify the course of amyloidosis AL associated with multiple myeloma.

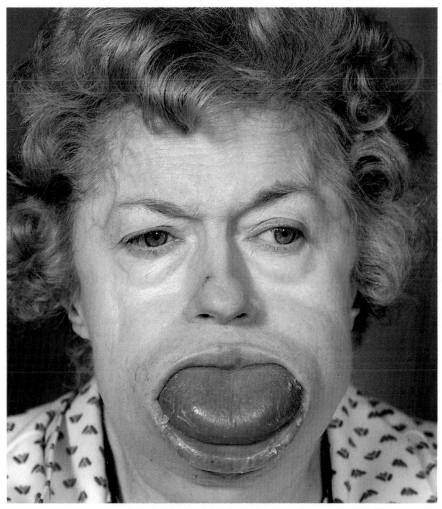

Figure 15-2 Primary systemic amyloidosis: macroglossia *Massive infiltration of the tongue with amyloid substance has caused immense enlargement; the tongue cannot be retracted completely into the mouth because of its size. (Courtesy of Evan Calkins, M.D.)*

URTICARIA AND ANGIOEDEMA

Urticaria and angioedema are composed of transient wheals (edematous papules and plaques, usually pruritic) and larger edematous areas that involve the dermis and subcutaneous tissue (angioedema). Urticaria and/or angioedema may be acute recurrent or chronic recurrent. There are some syndromes with angioedema in which urticarial wheals are rarely present (e.g., hereditary angioedema).

Incidence

15 % to 23 % of the population may have had this condition during their lifetime. Chronic urticaria is likely to be present at some time in about 25 % of patients with urticaria.

Etiology

Angioedema and urticaria can be classified as IgE-mediated, complement-mediated, related to physical stimuli (cold, sunlight, pressure), or idiosyncratic. The syndrome known as *angioedema-urticaria-eosinophilia syndrome* is related to action of the eosinophil major basic protein.

Special Types

IMMUNOLOGIC *IgE-Mediated* Often with atopic background. Antigens: food (milk, eggs, wheat, shellfish, nuts), therapeutic agents, drugs (penicillin!) (see Drug-Induced Urticaria, page 580), parasites

Complement-Mediated By way of immune complexes activating complement and releasing anaphylatoxins that induce mast cell degranulation. Serum sickness, administration of whole blood, immunoglobulins.

PHYSICAL URTICARIA *Dermographism* Although 4.2 % of the normal population have it, symptomatic dermographism is a nuisance. Fades in 30 minutes (Figure 15-3).

Cold Urticaria Usually in children or young adults; "ice cube" test establishes diagnosis.

Solar Urticaria Action spectrum 290 to 500 nm, histamine is one of the mediators.

Cholinergic Urticaria Exercise to the point of sweating provokes typical (small, papular) lesions and establishes diagnosis (Figure 15-4).

Vibratory (Pressure) Angioedema History of swelling induced by pressure (buttock swelling when seated, hand swelling after hammering, foot swelling after walking). No laboratory abnormalities; no fever. Antihistamines are ineffective, but corticosteroids are sometimes helpful. Biopsy reveals a prominent mononuclear infiltrate in the deep dermis. Urticaria may occur in addition to angioedema. Vibratory angioedema may be familial (autosomal dominant) or sporadic. It is believed to result from histamine release from mast cells caused by "vibrating" stimulus—rubbing a towel across the back will produce lesions, but direct pressure (without movements) will not cause a response.

URTICARIA DUE TO MAST CELL-RELEASING AGENTS Urticaria/angioedema and even anaphylaxis-like syndromes may occur with radiocontrast media and as a consequence of intolerance to salicylates, azo dyes, and benzoates (see Drug-Induced Uticaria, page 580).

URTICARIA ASSOCIATED WITH VASCULAR/CONNECTIVE TISSUE AUTOIMMUNE DISEASE Urticarial vasculitis is a form of cutaneous vasculitis associated with urticarial skin lesions that persist longer than 12 to 24 hours, can be associated with purpura, and can show residual pigmentation due to hemosiderin after involution. There is only slow change of size and configuration. Often associated with

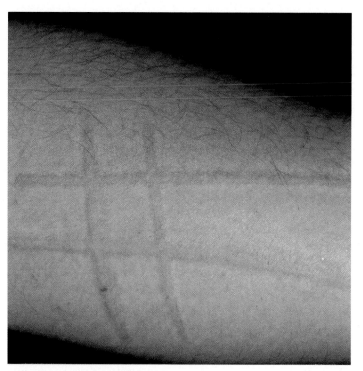

Figure 15-3 Urticaria: dermatographism *Urticaria as it appeared 5 minutes after stroking the skin with a wooden stick. The patient had experienced generalized pruritus for several months with no spontaneously occurring urticaria.*

hypocomplementemia and renal disease. Urticarial lesions also may be associated with SLE and Sjögren's syndrome, which usually, but not always, represent urticarial vasculitis (see page 384).

HEREDITARY ANGIOEDEMA A serious autosomal dominant (positive family history) disorder; involves angioedema of the face (Figure 15-5A and 5B) and extremities, episodes of laryngeal edema, and acute abdominal pain caused by angioedema of the bowel wall. Urticaria does not usually occur, but there may be an erythema marginatum-like eruption. Laboratory abnormalities involve the complement system: decreased levels of C1 esterease inhibitor (85 %) or dysfunctional inhibitor (15 %), low C4 value in the presence of normal C1 and C3 levels. Angioedema results from bradykinin formation, since C1 esterease inhibitor is also the major inhibitor of the Hageman factor and kallikrein, the two enzymes required for kinin formation.

ANGIOEDEMA-URTICARIA-EOSINOPHILIA SYNDROME Severe angioedema with pruritic urticaria involving the face, neck, extremities, and trunk that lasts for 7 to 10 days. There is fever and marked increase in normal weight (increased by 10 % to 18 %) owing to fluid retention. No other organs are involved. Laboratory abnormalities include striking leukocytosis (20,000 to 70,000/μl) and eosinophilia (60 % to 80 % eosinophils) which are related to the severity of attack. There is no family history. Prognosis good.

General Types

ACUTE URTICARIA (<30 DAYS) Usually large wheals, often IgE-dependent with atopic background, related to alimentary agents, parasites, and penicillin. Also, complement-mediated in serum sickness-like reactions (whole blood, immunoglobulins, penicillin). Often accompanied by angioedema.

CHRONIC URTICARIA (>30 DAYS) Rarely IgE-dependent; etiology unknown in 80 % to 90 % and therefore considered idiopathic; emotional stress often seems to be an exacerbating factor. Intolerance to salicylates, benzoates. Chronic urticaria affects predominantly adults and is approximately twice as common in women as in men. Up to 40 % of patients with chronic urticaria of more than 6 months' duration still have urticaria 10 years later.

History

Duration of Lesions Hours

Skin Symptoms Pruritus, pain on walking (in foot involvement), flushing, burning, and wheezing (in cholinergic urticaria)

Constitutional Symptoms Fever in serum sickness and in the angioedema-urticaria-eosinophilia syndrome; in angioedema, hoarseness, stridor, dyspnea

Systems Review Arthralgia (serum sickness, necrotizing vasculitis, hepatitis)

Physical Examination

Skin Lesions

TYPES

Transient papular wheals—many small (1.0 to 2.0 mm are typical in cholinergic urticaria), pruritic (Figure 15-4)
Wheals—small (1.0 cm) to large (8.0 cm), edematous plaques (Figure 15-6)
Angioedema—skin-colored enlargement of portion of face (eyelids, lips, tongue) (Figure 15-5A and 5B) or extremity

COLOR Pink with larger lesions having a white central area surrounded by an erythematous halo

SHAPE Oval, arciform, annular, polycyclic, serpiginous, and bizarre patterns

ARRANGEMENT Annular, arciform, linear (Figure 15-3)

DURATION Transient, hours

DISTRIBUTION Localized, regional, or generalized (see Figure 22-2)

SITES OF PREDILECTION Sites of pressure, exposed areas (solar urticaria), trunk, hands and feet, lips, tongue, ears

Differential Diagnosis

Urticarial Wheals Insect bites, adverse drug reactions, urticarial contact dermatitis, urticarial vasculitis

Laboratory and Special Examinations

For general medical workup, to rule out systemic disease in chronic urticaria (SLE, necrotizing vasculitis, lymphoma)

Dermatopathology Site: dermis. Edema of the dermis or subcutaneous tissue, dilatation of venules but no evidence of vascular damage, nuclear dust, or red cell extravasation. Mast cell degranulation. The predominant perivascular inflammatory cell types are lymphocytes of the T-helper phenotype that are HLA-DR positive. In spontaneous wheals there is a moderate expression of E-selectin and ICAM I on vascular endothelial cells and of VCAM I on perivascular cells.

Serology Search for hepatitis-associated antigen, assessment of the complement system, assessment of specific IgE antibodies by RAST.

Hematology The erythrocyte sedimentation rate (ESR) is often elevated in persistent urticaria (necrotizing vasculitis), and there may be hypocomplementemia; transient eosinophilia in urticaria from reactions to foods, parasites, and drugs; high levels of eosinophilia in the angioedema-urticaria-eosinophilia syndrome.

Complement Studies Screening for functional inhibitor

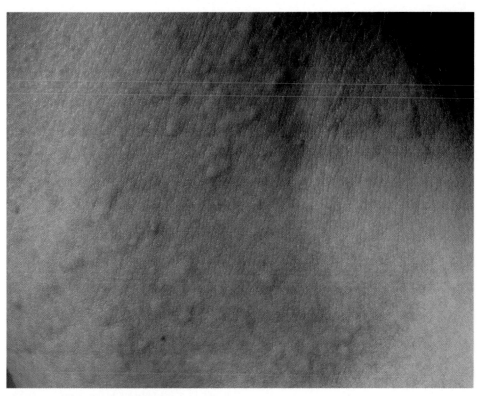

Figure 15-4 Cholinergic urticaria *Small urticarial papules on red skin (axon reflex erythema) occurring on the neck within 30 minutes of vigorous exercise.*

Ultrasonography For early diagnosis of bowel involvement; if abdominal pain is present, this may indicate edema of the bowel.

Parasitology Stool specimen for presence of parasites

Diagnosis

A practical approach to the diagnosis of chronic urticaria is shown in Table 15-A. A careful history of medications including aspirin and nonsteroidal anti-inflammatory drugs should be obtained. If physical urticaria is suspected, this should be assessed by appropriate challenge testing. *Cholinergic urticaria* can best be diagnosed by exercise to sweating and intracutaneous injection of acetylcholine or mecholyl, which will produce micropapular whealing. *Solar urticaria* is verified by testing with UVB, UVA, and visible light. *Cold urticaria* is verified by a wheal response to the application to the skin of an ice cube or a test tube containing ice water. If urticarial wheals do not disappear in 24 hours or less, urticarial vasculitis should be suspected and a biopsy done. The *angioedema-urticaria-eosinophilia syndrome* has high fever, high leukocytosis (mostly eosinophils), a striking increase in body weight due to retention of water, and a cyclic pattern that may occur and recur over a period of years. *Hereditary angioedema* has a positive family history and is characterized by angioedema of the face and extremities as the result of trauma or abdominal pain and shows decreased levels of C4 and of C1 esterease inhibitor or a dysfunctional inhibitor.

Pathophysiology

Lesions in acute IgE-mediated urticaria result from antigen-induced release of biologically active materials from mast cells or basophilic leukocytes sensitized with specific IgE antibodies (type I anaphylactic hypersensitivity). Mediators released increase venular permeability and modulate the release of biologically active materials from other cell types.

In complement-mediated urticaria, complement is activated by immune complexes; this results in the release of anaphylatoxins, which, in turn, induce mast cell degranulation.

In chronic urticaria, histamine derived from mast cells in the skin is considered the major mediator. Other mediators, including eicosanoids and neuropeptides, also may play a part in producing the lesions, but direct measurement of these mediators has not been reported. Intolerance to salicylates and food preservatives and additives, such as benzoic acid and sodium benzoate, as well as several azo dyes, including tartrazine and sunset yellow, is presumably mediated by abnormalities of the arachidonic acid pathway.

A wheal producing noncytokine mediator of a molecular weight of more than 1 million has been identified as IgG. It releases histamine from both basophils in normal blood and mast cells in skin (Hide M et al, *N Engl J Med* 1993; 328:1599). This is an autoantibody that interacts with IgE cross-linked subunits of adjacent high-affinity IgE receptors. Such functional anti-IgE autoantibodies or anti-FCϵ REα autoantibodies have been identified in 48 % of serum samples from patients with chronic urticaria, and a positive correlation between histamine-releasing activity and disease activity has been demonstrated. Clinically, patients with these autoantibodies are indistinguishable from those without them. These autoantibodies may explain why plasmapheresis, intravenous immunoglobulin, or cyclosporine induces remission of disease activity in these patients. The concept that some chronic urticaria is a manifestation of autoimmune mast cell disease is also supported by the association of chronic urticaria with autoimmune thyroid disease (14 %).

In hereditary angioedema, decreased or dysfunctional esterase inhibitor leads to increased kinin formation. The angioedema-urticaria-eosinophilia syndrome may result from the eosinophilia that is markedly elevated in the skin. In this syndrome, the eosinophilia increases and decreases with the angioedema and urticaria; there are morphologic changes in the eosinophils, including destruction and release of their contents in the dermis; major basic protein is distributed following release from the eosinophil into the collagen bundles, and mast cells in the dermis show degranulation.

Course and Prognosis

Half the patients with urticaria alone are free of lesions in 1 year, but 20 % have lesions for more than 20 years. Prognosis is good in most syndromes except hereditary angioedema, which may be fatal if untreated.

Management

Prevention   Try to prevent attacks by elimination of etiologic chemicals or drugs: aspirin and food additives, especially in chronic recurrent urticaria—rarely successful.

Antihistamines   H$_1$ blockers, e.g., hydroxyzine, terfenadine; and if they fail, H$_1$ and H$_2$ blockers (cimetidine) and/or mast cell stabilizing agents (ketotifen). Doxepin, a tricyclic antidepressant with marked H$_1$ antihistaminic activity, is valuable when severe urticaria is associated with anxiety and depression.

Prednisone   Indicated   for   angioedema-urticaria-eosinophilia syndrome.

Danazol   Long-term therapy for hereditary angioedema; whole fresh plasma or C1 esterase inhibitor in the acute attack

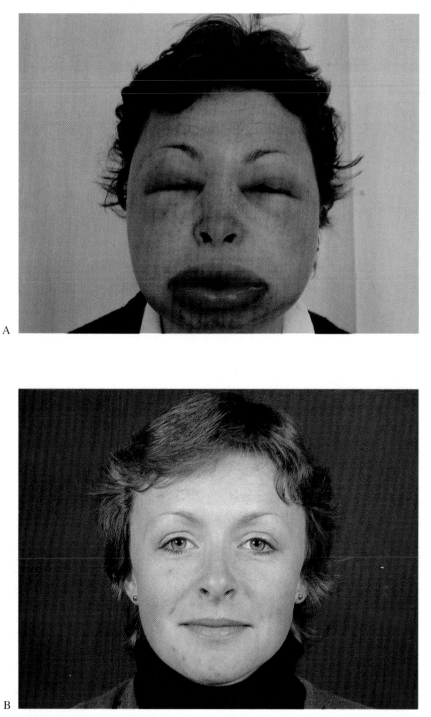

A

B

Figure 15-5 Hereditary angioedema A. *Severe edema of the face during episode.* B. *This grotesque looking involvement is to be contrasted to the same patient's normal facies.*

TABLE 15-A FEATURES OF COMMON TYPES OF CHRONIC URTICARIA

Type of Urticaria	Age Range of Patients (yrs)	Principal Clinical Features	Associated Angioedema	Diagnostic Test
Chronic idiopathic	20–50	Profuse or sparse generalized, pink or pale edematous papules or wheals, often annular with itching	Yes	—
Symptomatic dermographism	20–50	Itchy, linear wheals with a surrounding bright-red flare at sites of scratching or rubbing	No	Light stroking of skin causes an immediate wheal with itching
Other physical urticarias:				
Cold	10-40	Itchy pale or red swelling at sites of contact with cold surfaces or fluids	Yes	Ten-minute application of an ice pack causes a wheal within 5 minutes of the removal of ice
Pressure[1]	20–50	Large painful or itchy red swelling at sites of pressure (soles, palms, or waist)	No	Application of pressure perpendicular to skin produces persistent red swelling after a latent period of 1 to 4 hours
Solar	20–50	Itchy pale or red swelling at site of exposure to UV or visible light	Yes	Irradiation by a 2.5-kW solar simulator (290–690 nm) for 30 to 120 seconds causes wheals in 30 minutes
Cholinergic	10–50	Itchy, small (<5 mm) monomorphic pale or pink wheals on trunk, neck, and limbs	Yes	Exercise or a hot shower elicits an eruption, acute stressful situation

[1] A 1993 study indicates that pressure-induced and spontaneous wheals appear concurrently in 37 % of patients with chronic idiopathic urticaria.

SOURCE: Greaves MW. Chronic urticaria: A review. *N Engl J Med* 1995; 332:1767.

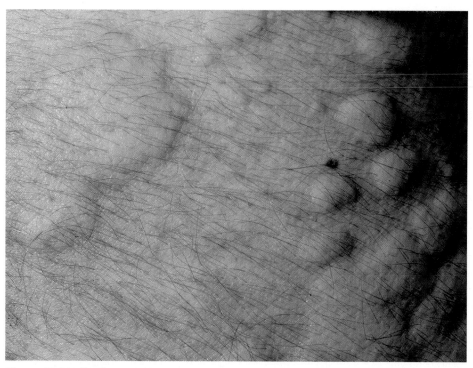

Figure 15-6 Urticaria   *Wheals with white-to-light-pink color centrally and peripheral erythema in a close-up view.*

BEHÇET'S SYNDROME

Behçet's syndrome (BS) is a perplexing multisystem inflammation which, in the most recent definition of diagnostic criteria, has one basic major feature—recurrent *oral* aphthous ulcers (AU)—and two of the following features: recurrent genital AU, eye lesions (posterior uveitis), skin lesions (erythema nodosum or cutaneous pustular vasculitis). Other manifestations include synovitis, neurologic disorders, and thrombophlebitis.
Synonym: Behçet's disease.

Epidemiology

Prevalence Highest in Japan (1:10,000), Southeast Asia, the Middle East, southern Europe. Rare in northern Europe, United States.

Age Third and fourth decades

Sex Males > females

History

Duration of Lesions AU: weeks to months

Skin Symptoms Oral AU and/or genital AU associated with moderate to severe pain; odynophagia; present in 100 % of cases. Other skin lesions present in 80 % of cases.

Systems Review Highly variable, dependent on organ system involved

Physical Examination

Skin and Mucous Membranes

TYPES OF LESIONS *AU* Punched out ulcers (3.0 to >10 mm) with rolled or overhanging borders and necrotic base; red rim; occur in crops (2 to 10) on mucous membranes
Erythema Nodosum-Like Lesions Painful nodules on the arms and legs (40 %)

Other Cutaneous pustular vasculitis, inflammatory plaques resembling those seen in Sweet's syndrome (acute febrile neutrophilic dermatosis), pyoderma gangrenosum-like lesions, palpable purpuric lesions of necrotizing venulitis

DISTRIBUTION OF LESIONS Mouth (see Figure 7-4), vulva (Figure 15-7), penis, and scrotum

Systemic Findings

EYE Posterior uveitis (retinal vasculitis), anterior uveitis, vitreitis hypopyon, secondary cataracts, glaucoma, neovascular lesions

MUSCULOSKELETAL Nonerosive, asymmetric oligoarthritis

NEUROLOGIC Onset delayed, occurring in one-quarter of patients. Meningoencephalitis, benign intracranial hypertension, cranial nerve palsies, brain stem lesions, pyramidal/extrapyramidal lesions, psychosis

VASCULAR Aneurysms, arterial occlusions, venous occlusions, varices; hemoptysis. Coronary vasculitis: myocarditis, coronary arteritis, endocarditis, valvular disease.

GI TRACT Aphthous ulcers throughout

Differential Diagnosis

Mouth Ulcers Viral infection (HSV), VZV, hand-foot-and-mouth disease, herpangina, chancre, histoplasmosis, SCC

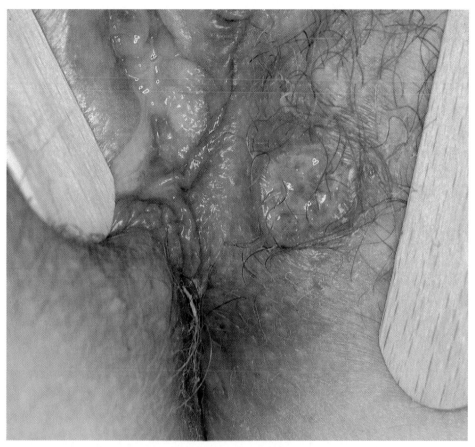

Figure 15-7 Behçet's syndrome: genital ulcers *Multiple large aphthous type ulcers on the labial and perineal epithelium.*

Laboratory and Special Examinations

Dermatopathology Earliest mucocutaneous lesions: neutrophilic vascular reaction with endothelial swelling, extravasation of erythrocytes, leukocytoclasia. Later: fully developed leukocytoclastic vasculitis in addition to features of earlier lesions and, in some cases, fibrinoid necrosis of blood vessel walls.

Pathergy Test Positive pathergy test read by physician at 24 or 48 hours, performed with oblique insertion of a 20-gauge or smaller needle under sterile conditions. Leads to inflammatory pustule.

Other Examinations Nonspecific, varying with specific organ system involved

Diagnosis

Proposed criteria for Behçet's syndrome include the presence of oral AU plus two of the following: recurrent genital AU, eye lesions, skin lesions, or positive pathergy test.

Criteria	Description
Skin	Erythema nodosum-like lesions observed by physician or papulopustular lesions consistent with BS observed by physician
Pathergy	See above
Oral	Minor aphthae, major aphthae, or herpetiform ulcers observed by physician or reported reliably by patient; recurrent at least three times in one 12-month period
Genital	Recurrent genital aphthae or scarring, especially scrotal in males, observed by physician or reliably reported by patient
Eye	Anterior uveitis, posterior uveitis, cells in vitreous on slit-lamp examination or retinal vasculitis observed by qualified physician

Etiology and Pathogenesis

Etiology unknown. In the eastern Mediterranean and East Asia, HLA-B5 and HLA-B51 association; in the United States and Europe, no consistent HLA association. The lesions could be the result of an accumulation of neutrophils in the sites of immune complex–mediated vasculitis.

Course and Prognosis

Highly variable course, with recurrences and remissions; the mouth lesions are always present; remissions may last for weeks, months, or years. With CNS involvement, there is a higher mortality. In the eastern Mediterranean and East Asia, severe course, one of leading causes of blindness.

Management

Aphthous Ulcers Potent topical corticosteroids. Intralesional triamcinolone 3 to 10 mg/ml injected into ulcer base. Thalidomide: 100 mg PO b.i.d. Colchicine: 0.6 mg PO 2 to 3 times a day. Dapsone.

Systemic Complications Prednisone with or without azathioprine, cyclophosphamide, azathioprine alone, chlorambucil, cyclosporine

DERMATITIS HERPETIFORMIS

Dermatitis herpetiformis (DH) is a chronic, recurrent, intensely pruritic eruption on extensor surfaces occurring often in *symmetric* groups and comprising three types of lesions: tiny vesicles, papules, and urticarial wheals.

Epidemiology

Age of Onset   20 to 60 years, but most common at 30 to 40 years; may occur in children

Sex   Male : female ratio 2 : 1

History

Duration of Lesions   Days, weeks

Skin Symptoms   Pruritus, intense, episodic; burning or stinging of the skin; rarely, pruritus may not occur. Local symptoms often precede the appearance of skin lesions by 8 to 12 hours.

Exacerbating Factors   Ingestion of iodides and overload of gluten. Provocation with iodides administered orally has been used diagnostically in the past. The availability of immunopathologic techniques and the detection of IgA deposits in the skin have made such provocation tests obsolete.

Systems Review   Laboratory evidence of small-bowel malabsorption is detected in 10 % to 20 %. Gluten-sensitive enteropathy occurs in nearly all patients and is demonstrated by small-bowel biopsy. There are usually no systemic symptoms.

Physical Examination

Skin Lesions   (Figure 15-8)

TYPES   Erythematous papule. Tiny firm-topped vesicle, sometimes hemorrhagic; occasionally bullae. Urticaria-like wheal. Scratching results in excoriations, crusts. Postinflammatory hyper- and hypopigmentation at sites of healed lesions.

COLOR   Red

ARRANGEMENT   In groups (hence the name *herpetiformis*)

DISTRIBUTION   Strikingly symmetric.

SITES OF PREDILECTION   Extensor areas—elbows, knees. Buttocks, scapular, sacral area. Scalp, face, and hairline.

Differential Diagnosis

Allergic contact dermatitis, atopic dermatitis, scabies, neurotic excoriations, papular urticaria, bullous pemphigoid, herpes gestationis

Laboratory and Special Examinations

Immunogenetics   Association with HLA-B8 and HLA-DR3

Dermatopathology   Biopsy is best from early erythematous papule. (1) Microabscesses (polymorphonuclear cells and eosinophils) at the tips of the dermal papillae. Fibrin accumulation and necrosis occur also. (2) Dermal infiltration (severe) of neutrophils and eosinophils. (3) Subepidermal vesicle.

Immunofluorescence (of Normal-Appearing Skin, Usually the Buttocks)   IgA deposits: (1) *Granular* in tips of papillae—this correlates well with small-bowel disease. Granular IgA is found in the large majority of patients. In addition, complement is also deposited. (2) *Linear,* bandlike along the dermal-epidermal junction (other bullous diseases have, in addition, IgG in bandlike pattern at the basement membrane zone). This pattern is not associated with small-bowel disease. Patients with linear IgA constitute only a minority of patients.

Circulating Autoantibodies Circulating basement membrane zone antibodies are generally not detectable in the sera of dermatitis herpetiformis patients. Antireticulin antibodies of the IgA and IgG types can be present, and antimicrosomal antibodies and antinuclear antibodies have all been detected. Immune complexes have been detected in 20 % to 40 % of patients. IgA antibodies binding to the intermyofibril substance of smooth muscles (antiendomysial antibodies) are present in the majority of patients and seem to correlate with the severity of the intestinal disease.

Malabsorption Studies Steatorrhea (20 % to 30 %) and abnormal D-xylose absorption (10 % to 73 %)

Hematology Anemia secondary to iron or folate deficiency. Obtain G-6-PD level before starting treatment with sulfones; follow blood counts carefully during first few months of therapy with weekly CBC for 1 month and then every 6 to 8 weeks.

Imaging Small bowel: in the proximal areas of the small intestine there is blunting and flattening of the villi (80 % to 90 %), as in celiac disease. Lesions are focal and best seen by endoscopy. Verification by small-bowel biopsy.

Diagnosis

Often difficult. Biopsy of early lesions is usually pathognomonic, but immunofluorescence detecting IgA deposits in normal-appearing or perilesional skin is the best confirming evidence.

Pathophysiology

The relationship of the gluten-sensitive enteropathy to the skin lesions has been controversial. It is now known that circulating immune complexes are always found in patients with dermatitis herpetiformis. It is not known whether IgA binds to antigens in the bowel and complexes then circulate to bind in the skin or whether IgA has specificity for skin proteins. In skin, IgA is associated with microfibrils. IgA and complement mediate a cascade of events (possibly through the alternative complement pathway) leading to tissue injury by chemotaxis of neutrophils and release of enzymes. The absence of gluten sensitivity and gluten-sensitive enteropathy in patients with linear IgA deposits who also have normal prevalence of HLA-B8 and HLA-DR3 suggests that these patients have a different disease (linear IgA disease).

Course

Prolonged, for years, with a third of the patients eventually having a spontaneous remission

Management

Systemic Therapy

DAPSONE   100 to 200 mg daily with gradual reduction to 25 to 50 mg

SULFAPYRIDINE   1.0 to 1.5 g daily, with plenty of fluids, if dapsone contraindicated or not tolerated

Diet A gluten-free diet may completely suppress the disease or allow reduction of the dosage of dapsone or sulfapyridine, but response is slow.

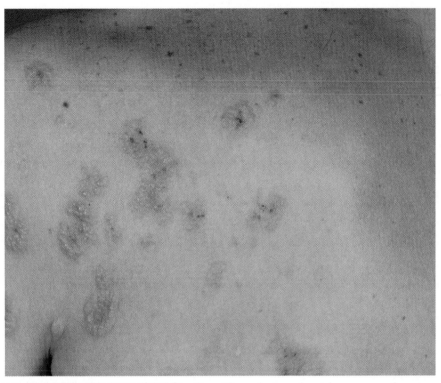

Figure 15-8 Dermatitis herpetiformis *Herpetiform clusters of vesicles on an erythematous, edematous base with crusts and postinflammatory pigmentation on the upper back and shoulder.*

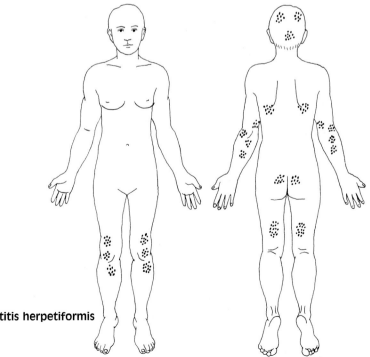

Figure VIII Dermatitis herpetiformis

DERMATOMYOSITIS

Dermatomyositis (DM) is a systemic disease characterized by violaceous (heliotrope) inflammatory changes of the eyelids and periorbital area; erythema of the face, neck, and upper trunk; and flat-topped violaceous papules over the knuckles, associated with a polymyositis, interstitial pneumonitis, myocardial involvement, vasculitis.

Epidemiology and Etiology

Age Juvenile. Adult >40 years

Etiology Unknown. Cases >55 years often associated with malignancy. Associated malignant tumors: breast, lung, ovary, stomach, colon, uterus.

Clinical Spectrum Ranges from DM with only cutaneous inflammation to polymyositis with only muscle inflammation

History

History ±Photosensitivity, muscle weakness

Systems Review Difficulty in rising from supine position, climbing stairs, raising arms over head, turning in bed. Dysphagia.

Physical Examination

Skin Lesions

TYPES Periorbital heliotrope (reddish purple) flush usually associated with some degree of edema (Figure 15-9). Papular dermatitis with varying degrees of erythema (Figure 15-10) and scaling; may evolve to erosions and ulcers that heal with stellate, bizarre scarring. Flat-topped, violaceous papules (Gottron's papule/sign) (Figure 15-11) with varying degrees of atrophy. Periungual erythema, telangiectasia, thrombosis of capillary loops, infarctions. Calcification in subcutaneous/fascial tissues common later in course of juvenile DM; may evolve to calcinosis universalis.

COLOR Facial lesions have a heliotrope hue.

PALPATION ± Muscle atrophy, ± muscle tenderness

DISTRIBUTION Pressure points—elbows, knuckles. Dermatitis—forehead, scalp, malar area, neck, upper chest (Figure 15-9). Gottron's papules—dorsa of knuckles (sparing interarticular areas, Figure 15-11) and nape of neck (Figure 15-10). With or without sparing of dermatitis under chin and adjacent neck, i.e., photoprotection; accentuation in the V area of neck; subcutaneous calcifications about elbows, trochanteric region.

Nails Periungual telangiectasia (see Figure 18-9)

General Examination Progressive muscle weakness affecting proximal/limb girdle muscles. Difficulty or inability to rise from sitting or supine position without using arms. Occasional involvement of facial/bulbar, pharyngeal, and esophageal muscles. Deep tendon reflexes—within normal limits.

Differential Diagnosis

Lupus erythematosus, mixed connective tissue disease, steroid myopathy, trichinosis, toxoplasmosis

Laboratory and Special Examinations

Chemistry During acute active phase: elevation of creatine phosphokinase (65 %) most specific for muscle disease; also, aldolase (40 %), glutamic oxaloacetic transaminase, lactate dehydrogenase.

Urine Elevated 24-hour creatine excretion (>200 mg per 24 hours)

Electromyography Increased irritability on insertion of electrodes, spontaneous fibrilla-

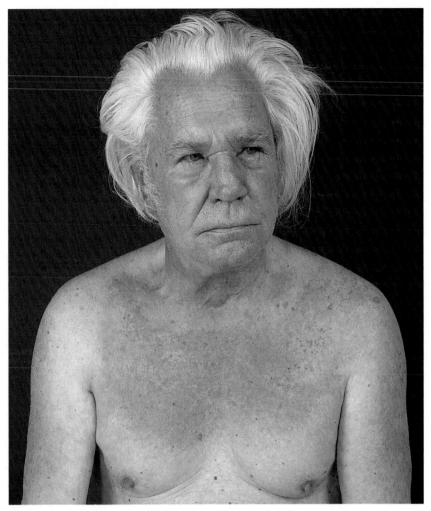

Figure 15-9 Dermatomyositis   *Violaceous erythema on the upper chest, neck, and face; periorbital heliotrope (violet color) with edema.*

tions, pseudomyotonic discharges, positive sharp waves: excludes neuromyopathy. With evidence of denervation, suspect coexisting tumor.

ECG Evidence of myocarditis; atrial, ventricular irritability, atrioventricular block

X-Ray of Chest ± Interstitial fibrosis

Pathology

SKIN Flattening of epidermis, hydropic degeneration of basal cell layer, edema of upper dermis, scattered inflammatory infiltrate, PAS-positive fibrinoid deposits at dermal-epidermal junction and around upper dermal capillaries, accumulation of acid mucopolysaccharides in dermis

MUSCLE Biopsy shoulder/pelvic girdle; one that is weak or tender, i.e., deltoid, supraspinatus, gluteus, quadriceps. Histology—segmental necrosis within muscle fibers with loss of cross-striations; waxy/coagulative type of eosinophilic staining; with or without regenerating fibers; inflammatory cells, histiocytes, macrophages, lymphocytes, plasma cells. Histology of adult DM, polymyositis, and myositis in patients with other connective tissue diseases is indistinguishable. Vasculitis may be seen in juvenile DM.

Diagnosis

Proximal muscle weakness with two of three laboratory criteria, i.e., elevated serum "muscle enzyme" levels, characteristic electromyographic changes, diagnostic muscle biopsy

Pathophysiology

Acute and chronic inflammation of striated muscle accompanied by segmental necrosis of myofibers resulting in progressive muscle weakness

Course and Prognosis

Dermatitis and polymyositis usually are detected at the same time; however, skin or muscle involvement can occur alone initially, followed at some time by the other. However, patients with dermatomyositis have a higher risk of developing cancer than do patients with polymyositis. Prognosis is good except in patients with malignancy and those with pulmonary involvement. Current recommendation is that patients over 50 years of age be investigated for associated malignancy: carcinoma of the breast, ovary, bronchopulmonary, GI tract. Most cancers occur within 2 years of diagnosis. Successful treatment of the neoplasm often followed by improvement/resolution of DM. Otherwise, course unpredictable. Two-thirds respond to steroid therapy. Subcutaneous calcification is a complication, especially in children.

Management

Prednisone 0.5 to 1.0 mg/kg of body weight per day increasing to 1.5 mg/kg if lower dose ineffective. Taper when "muscle enzyme" levels approach normal. Best if combined with azathioprine, 2 to 3 mg/kg per day.

Note: Onset of steroid myopathy may occur after 4 to 6 weeks of therapy.

Alternative Methotrexate, cyclophosphamide. High-dose IV immunoglobulin bolus therapy at monthly intervals saves corticosteroid doses to achieve or maintain remissions

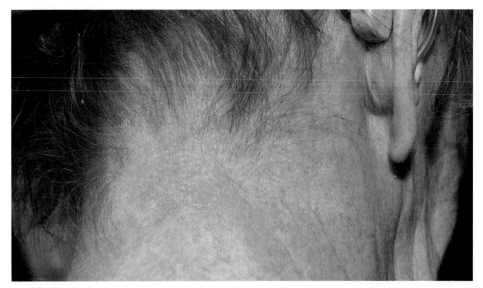

Figure 15-10 Dermatomyositis *Confluent, small, violaceous lichen planus-like papules of violaceous color involving the entire scalp and contiguous neck, pathognomonic signs for dermatomyositis. Scalp involvement may preceed and be the only manifestation for months.*

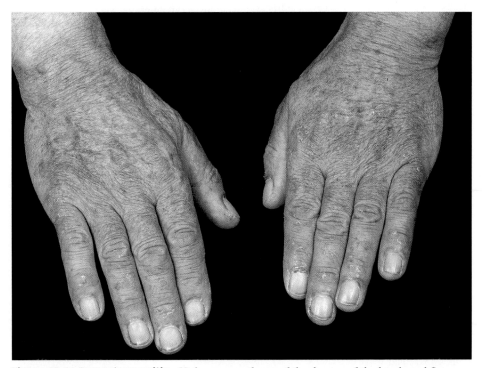

Figure 15-11 Dermatomyositis *Violaceous erythema of the dorsum of the hands and fingers, especially over the metacarpophalangeal and interphalangeal joints; the light-protected areas of the forearms are not involved. Violaceous papules over knuckle prominences, i.e., Gottron's papules. Periungual erythema and telangiectasis.*

ERYTHEMA MULTIFORME SYNDROME

This reaction pattern of blood vessels in the dermis with secondary epidermal changes is exhibited clinically as characteristic erythematous iris-shaped papules and vesicolobullous lesions typically involving the extremities (especially the palms and soles) and the mucous membranes.

Epidemiology and Etiology

Age 50 % under 20 years

Sex More frequent in males than in females

Etiologies

DRUGS Sulfonamides, phenytoin, barbiturates, phenylbutazone, penicillin, allopurinol

INFECTION Especially following herpes simplex, *Mycoplasma*

IDIOPATHIC >50 %

History

Duration of Lesions Several days. May have history of prior episode of erythema multiforme (EM).

Skin Symptoms May be pruritic or painful

Mucous Membrane Symptoms Mouth lesions are painful, tender.

Constitutional Symptoms Fever, weakness, malaise

Physical Examination

Skin Lesions Lesions may develop over 10 days or more (Figure 15-12).

TYPE

Macule (48 hours)→papule, 1.0 to 2.0 cm; lesions may appear for 2 weeks (Figure 15-14).
Vesicles and bullae (in the center of the papule) (Figure 15-13)

COLOR Dull red

SHAPE Iris or target lesions are typical (Figures 15-13 and 15-14)

ARRANGEMENT Localized to hands or generalized

DISTRIBUTION Bilateral and often symmetric

SITES OF PREDILECTION Dorsa of hands, palms, and soles; forearms; feet; face (Figures 15-12 and 15-13); elbows and knees; penis (50 %) and vulva (see Figure IX)

Mucous Membranes Erosions with fibrin membranes: lips, oropharynx, nasal, conjunctival, vulvar, anal

Other Organs Pulmonary, eyes with corneal ulcers, anterior uveitis

Differential Diagnosis

Acute Erythematous Plaques Drug eruption, psoriasis, secondary syphilis, urticaria

Acute Oral Erosions Primary herpes, pemphigus, acute lupus erythematosus

Course

Mild Forms (EM Minor) Little or no mucous membrane involvement, no bullae or systemic symptoms. Eruption usually confined to extensor aspects of extremities, classic target lesions (Figure 15-14). Recurrent EM minor is usually associated with an outbreak of herpes simplex preceding it by several days. Chronic suppressive acyclovir therapy prevents recurrence of herpes as well as EM.

Severe Forms (EM Major) Most often occurs as a drug reaction, always with mucous membrane involvement, severe, extensive, tendency to become confluent and bullous, positive Nikolsky sign in erythematous lesions, systemic symptoms, fever, prostration (Figure 15-12). Cheilitis and stomatitis interfere with eating; vulvitis and balanitis, with micturition.

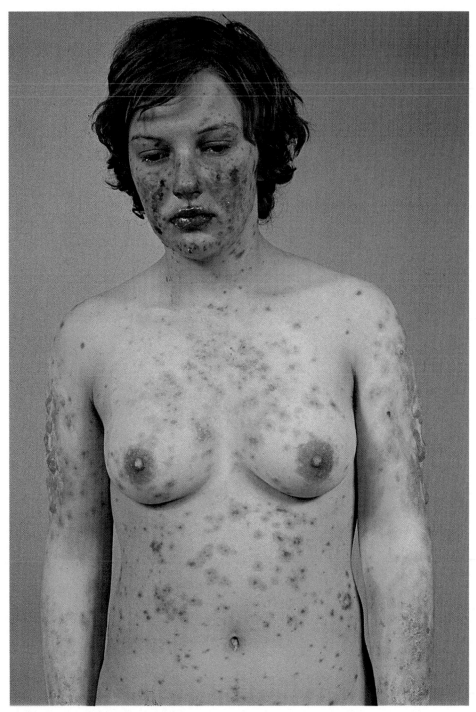

Figure 15-12 Erythema multiforme *Erythematous iris and target papules, plaques, bullae, and erosions on the trunk, arms, neck, and face. Mucosal involvement is manifested by erosive lip lesions.*

Conjunctivitis can lead to keratitis and ulceration; lesions also in pharynx, larynx, and trachea.

Maximal Variant Life-threatening. In addition to the preceding, necrotizing tracheobronchitis, meningitis, renal tubular necrosis (Stevens-Johnson syndrome, see Section 22).

Dermatopathology

Site Epidermis and dermis

Process Inflammation characterized by perivascular mononuclear infiltrate, edema of the upper dermis; if bulla formation, there is eosinophilic necrosis of keratinocytes with subepidermal bulla formation. In severe cases, complete necrosis of epidermis as in toxic epidermal necrolysis.

Differential Diagnosis

The target lesion and the symmetry are quite typical, and the diagnosis is not difficult. In the absence of skin lesions, the mucous membrane lesions may present a difficult differential diagnosis: bullous diseases, fixed drug eruption, and primary herpetic gingivostomatitis. Urticaria.

Management

Prevention Control of herpes simplex using oral acyclovir may prevent development of recurrent erythema multiforme.

Corticosteroids In severely ill patients, systemic corticosteroids are usually given (prednisone 50 to 80 mg daily in divided doses, quickly tapered), but their effectiveness has not been established by controlled studies.

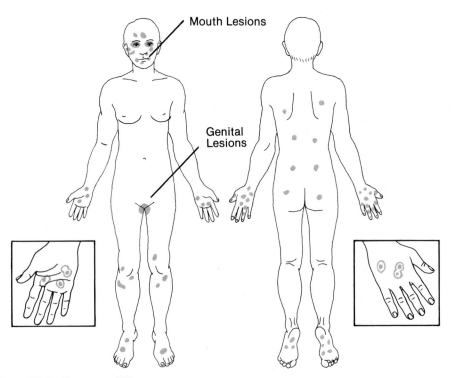

Mouth Lesions

Genital Lesions

Figure IX Erythema multiforme

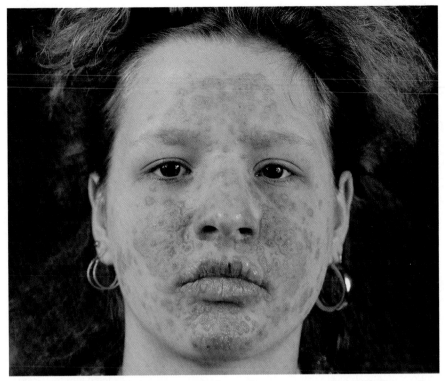

Figure 15-13 Erythema multiforme *Multiple, confluent target papules and bullae on the central facies. Bullae are seen on the lips and were also present on the buccal mucosa.*

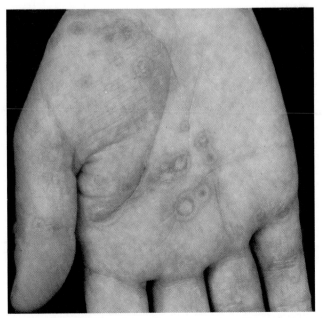

Figure 15-14 Erythema multiforme *Iris and target patterns within papules and bullae on the palm.*

ERYTHEMA NODOSUM SYNDROME

Erythema nodosum is an important acute inflammatory/immunologic reaction pattern of the panniculus characterized by the appearance of painful, tender nodules on the lower legs and caused by multiple and diverse etiologies.

Epidemiology and Etiology

Age   15 to 30 years, but age distribution related to etiology

Sex   Three times more common in females than in males

Etiologic Associations

INFECTIOUS AGENTS   Rarely primary tuberculosis (children), coccidioidomycosis, histoplasmosis, beta-hemolytic streptococcus, *Yersinia* organisms, lymphogranuloma venereum, leprosy (erythema nodosum leprosum)

DRUGS   Sulfonamides, oral contraceptives

MISCELLANEOUS   Sarcoidosis (quite often), ulcerative colitis, Behçet's syndrome, idiopathic ±40 %

History

Duration of Lesions   Days

Skin Symptoms   Painful, tender lesions

Constitutional Symptoms   Fever, malaise

Systems Review   Arthralgia (50 %) most frequently of ankle joints, other symptoms depending on etiology

Physical Examination

Skin Lesions

TYPE   Nodules (3.0 to 20.0 cm) not sharply marginated (Figure 15-15), deep-seated. Nodules are located in the subcutaneous fat and are appreciated as such only upon palpation. The term erythema nodosum best describes the skin lesions: they look like erythema but *feel* like nodules.

COLOR   Bright to deep red, later violaceous and even later, brownish, yellow-green, like resolving hematomas (Figure 15-15).

PALPATION   Indurated, tender

SHAPE   Oval, round, arciform

ARRANGEMENT   Scattered discrete lesions (2 to 50)

DISTRIBUTION   Bilateral but not symmetric

SITES OF PREDILECTION   Lower legs (most frequently) (Figure 15-15), knees, arms, rarely face and neck

Laboratory and Special Examinations

Bacterial Culture   Culture throat for GABHS (group A beta-hemolytic streptococcus), stool for *Yersinia*.

Imaging   Radiologic examination of the chest is important to rule out sarcoidosis.

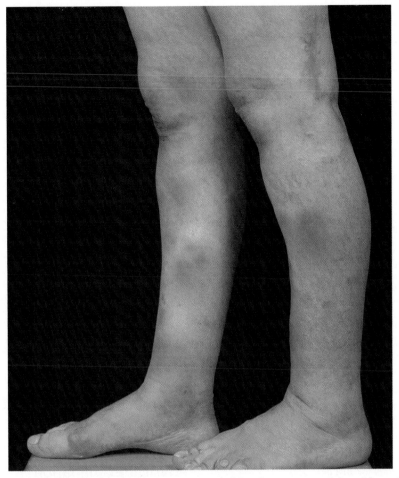

Figure 15-15 Erythema nodosum *Large, very painful, subcutaneous nodules with overlying erythema on the legs with ankle edema. Color ranges from bright red (new lesions) to tan to yellow-green (resolving lesions).*

Dermatopathology

Acute (polymorphonuclear) and chronic (granulomatous) inflammation in the panniculus and around blood vessels in the septum and adjacent fat

Course

Spontaneous resolution occurs in 6 weeks, but the course depends on the etiology.

Management

Symptomatic Bed rest or compressive bandages (lower legs).

Anti-inflammatory Treatment Salicylates, NSAIDs.

Prednisone Response to systemic corticosteroids is rapid but their use is indicated only when the etiology is known (and infectious agents are excluded).

GRAFT-VERSUS-HOST DISEASE

Graft-versus-host disease (GVHD) is an immune disorder caused by the response of histoincompatible, immunocompetent donor cells against the tissues of an immunoincompetent host (graft-versus-host reaction, GVHR), characterized by acute cutaneous changes ranging from maculopapular eruption to toxic epidermal necrolysis, diarrhea, and liver dysfunction, as well as chronic changes comprising lichenoid eruptions and sclerodermatous changes.

Epidemiology and Etiology

Types of Bone Marrow Transplants (BMT)

ALLOGENEIC BMT   Donor and recipient are of different genetic origins (usually family members).

AUTOLOGOUS BMT   Individuals are reinfused with their own marrow cells.

SYNGENEIC BMT   Donor and recipient are genetically identical (identical twins).

MATCHED UNRELATED BMT   Donor and recipient genetically unrelated but histocompatible antigens have been matched.

Incidence of GVHD   Allogeneic BMT: 60 % to 80 % of successful engraftments. Autologous BMT: mild cutaneous GVHD occurs in 8 %. Low incidence following blood transfusion in immunosuppressed patient, maternal-fetal transfer in immunodeficiency disease.

Indications for BMT

GENETICALLY DETERMINED HEMATOLOGIC DIS-EASES   Thalassemia major, sickle cell disease, congenital aplastic anemia, storage diseases due to enzyme deficiencies

SEVERE APLASTIC ANEMIA

LEUKEMIA   Acute and chronic myeloid and lymphoid

OTHER MALIGNANT DISEASES   Lymphomas, Hodgkin's disease, multiple myeloma, myelodysplastic syndromes, breast cancer, ovarian cancer, testicular cancer, small cell lung cancer

History

Onset of GVHD

ACUTE   During first 3 months after BMT (usually between 14 and 21 days)

CHRONIC   >100 days after BMT. Either evolving from acute GVHD or arising *de novo*. Acute GVHD is not always followed by chronic GVHD. Clinical classification thus distinguishes between quiescent onset, progressive onset, and *de novo* chronic cutaneous GVHD.

History   Mild pruritus, localized/generalized; pain on pressure, palms/soles

Systems Review   Nausea/vomiting, right upper quadrant pain/tenderness; cramping abdominal pain, watery diarrhea. Jaundice; dark yellow urine.

Physical Examination

Skin Lesions

ACUTE GVHD
Clinical Grading

1. Erythematous maculopapular eruption involving <25 % of body surface
2. Erythematous maculopapular eruption involving 25 % to 50 % of body surface
3. Erythroderma
4. Bulla formation

Types   Initially, subtle, discrete macules and/or papules (Figure 15-16); mild edema/violaceous hue, periungual and pinna. If controlled/resolved, erythema diminishes with subsequent desquamation and postinflammatory hyperpigmen-

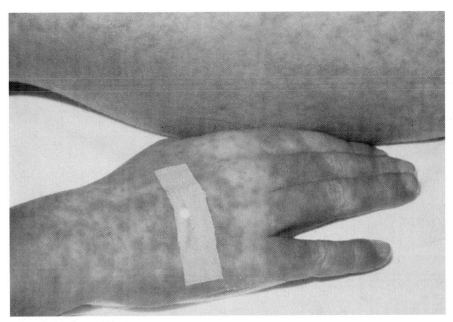

Figure 15-16 Acute graft-versus-host disease *Discrete and confluent, erythematous, blanchable macules and papules involving the hands and the trunk. Note the relative sparing over the wrist and metacarpophalangeal and proximal interphalangeal joints. These relatively mild cutaneous lesions were not associated with intestinal or hepatic involvement.*

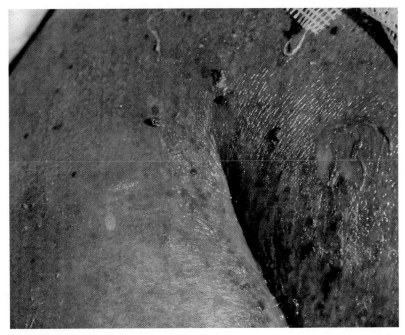

Figure 15-17 Acute graft-versus-host disease *Confluent epidermal necrosis and sloughing, resembling toxic epidermal necrolysis, on the upper trunk near the axilla after allogeneic BMT.*

tation. If progresses, macules/papules become confluent and then generalized, i.e., erythrodermic. Subepidermal bullae, especially over pressure/trauma sites, palms/soles. If bullae widespread with rupture/erosion, toxic epidermal necrolysis–like (TEN-like) form of acute cutaneous GVHR (Figure 15-17).

Color: Erythematous
Palpation: Pain upon pressure
Distribution: Earliest findings—upper trunk, hands/feet, especially palms/soles

CHRONIC GVHD
Types

Skin: Flat-topped (lichen planus-like) papules (Figure 15-18). Confluent areas of dermal sclerosis (Figure 15-19) with overlying scale resembling scleroderma. With more severe disease, severe sclerodermoid changes with necrosis and ulceration on acral and pressure sites. Hair loss; anhidrosis, vitiligo-like hypopigmentation.
Mucosa: Lichen planus-like lesions in buccal mucosa; erosive stomatitis, oral and ocular sicca-like syndrome; esophagitis/esophageal strictures. Keratoconjunctivitis.

Color: Violaceous (lichenoid type)
Palpation: Sclerotic
Distribution: Distal extremities. Sclerosis—trunk, buttocks, hips, thighs

General Findings

ACUTE GVHD   Fever, jaundice, diarrhea, serositis, pulmonary insufficiency

CHRONIC GVHD   Chronic liver disease, general wasting

Differential Diagnosis

Acute GVHD   Exanthematous drug reaction, viral exanthem, TEN, erythroderma

Chronic GVHD   Lichen planus, lichenoid drug reaction, scleroderma, poikiloderma

Laboratory and Special Examinations

Chemistry   Elevated SGOT, bilirubin, alkaline phosphatase

Dermatopathology

ACUTE GVHD   Basal vacuolization several days before clinically detectable lesions — focal vacuolization of basal cell layer, *apoptosis of individual keratinocytes;* mild perivenular mononuclear cell infiltrate—increasing vacuolization/cellular necrosis; apposition of lymphocytes to necrotic keratinocytes (satellitosis); vacuoles coalesce forming subepidermal clefts; endothelial cell swelling — subepidermal blister formation. Immunocytochemistry: HLA-DR expression of keratinocytes precedes morphologic changes and thus represents important, early diagnostic sign.

CHRONIC GVHD   Hyperkeratosis, mild hypergranulosis, mild irregular acanthosis, moderate basal vacuolization; mild perivascular mononuclear cell infiltrate; melanin incontinence — hyperkeratosis, epidermal atrophy or acanthosis, rare individual cell necrosis, mild perivascular mononuclear cell infiltrate, melanin incontinence; loss of hair follicles, entrapment of sweat glands; dense dermal sclerosis.

Diagnosis

Clinical findings confirmed by skin biopsy

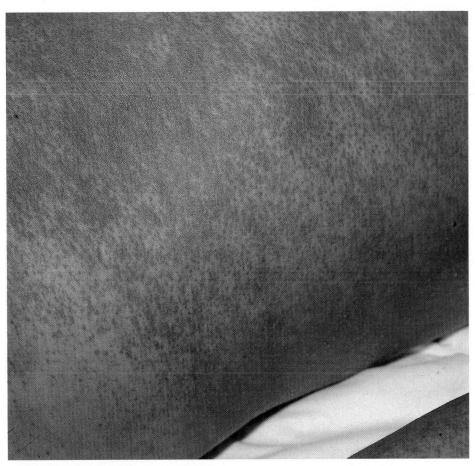

Figure 15-18 Chronic graft-versus-host disease *Violaceous (lichen planus-like or lichenoid), perifollicular macules and papules becoming confluent on the trunk, occurring 3 months after allogeneic BMT.*

Pathophysiology

GVHR associated with inflammatory reaction mounted by the donor cells against specific host organs—skin, liver, or GI tract. Severity of GVHD related to histocompatibility match between donor and recipient and preparatory regimen used. With successful engraftment, there is replacement of host marrow by immunocompetent donor cells capable of reacting against the "foreign" tissue antigens of the host.

Course and Prognosis

Acute GVHD Mild to moderate GVHD responds well to treatment. Prognosis of TEN-like GVHR grave. Severe GVHD susceptible to infections—bacterial, fungal, viral (CMV, HSV, VZV). Acute GVHD is primary or associated cause of death in 15 % to 70 % of BMT patients.

Chronic GVHD Sclerodermoid with tight skin/joint contracture may result in impaired mobility, ulcerations. Permanent hair loss; xerostomia, xerophthalmia → corneal ulcers → blindness. Malabsorption. Chronic GVHD occurs in 25 % of recipients of marrow from an HLA-identical sibling who survive beyond 100 days. Mild chronic cutaneous GVHD may resolve spontaneously. Chronic GVHD may be associated with recurrent and occasionally fatal bacterial infections.

Management

Topical Corticosteroids Potent corticosteroid ointment gives symptomatic relief and adequate control in cases of mild to moderate cutaneous GVHD.

Prednisone 80 to 100 mg/day for mild to moderate cutaneous GVHD

Cyclosporine Added to prednisone for severe cutaneous disease, ±GI or liver GVHD

PUVA Systemic PUVA is very effective for subacute and chronic GVHD. Extracorporeal photopheresis is being evaluated. Once cutaneous as well as GI and liver manifestations of GVHD have been controlled, cyclosporine and prednisone can be tapered and eventually discontinued.

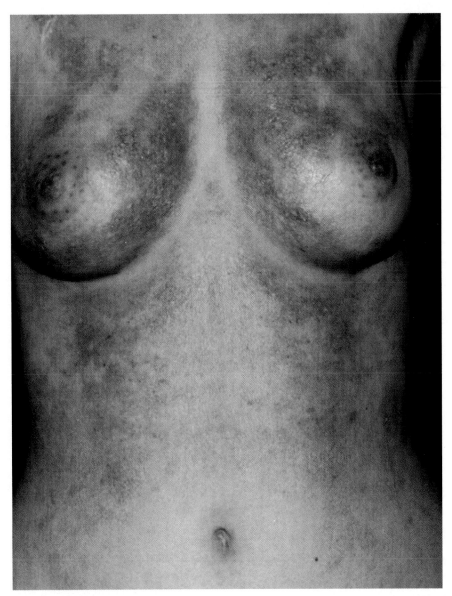

Figure 15-19 Chronic graft-versus-host disease *A lichenoid GVHR has partially resolved leading to pronounced macular gray-brown follicular hyperpigmentation, confluent on the breasts, upper chest, and anterior abdomen. Sclerosis of the tissue now supervenes, the skin feels bound down on palpation, similar to progressive systemic sclerosis (scleroderma).*

LIVEDO RETICULARIS

Livedo reticularis (LR) is a mottled bluish (livid) discoloration of the skin that occurs in a netlike pattern. It is not a diagnosis in itself but a reaction pattern.
Synonyms: Livedo racemosa, livedo annularis.

Epidemiology and Etiology

Classification

Idiopathic livedo reticularis (ILR): permanent bluish mottling for which no underlying disease is found

Secondary or symptomatic livedo reticularis (SLR): associated with underlying disorder such as *intravascular obstruction* [viscosity changes, stasis (paralysis, cardiac failure), organic (atheroemboli, thrombocythemia, cryoglobulinemia, cold agglutininemia, air)]; *vessel wall disease* [arteriosclerosis, hyperparathyroidism, vasculitis syndromes (polyarteritis nodosa, cutaneous polyarteritis nodosa, rheumatoid vasculitis), lupus erythematosus, anticardiolipin antibody syndrome, dermatomyositis, lymphoma, syphilis, tuberculosis, pancreatitis]; *drugs* (amantadine, quinine, quinidine)

Sneddon's syndrome: extensive livedo reticularis, hypertension, cerebrovascular accidents, and transient ischemic attacks

Age *ILR:* 20s to 50s

Sex *ILR:* more common in females

Etiology *ILR:* unknown. *SLR:* that of associated disorder.

Season Worse during winter months

History

Appearance or worsening with cold exposure. ± Numbness, tingling associated.

Physical Examination

Skin Lesions

TYPE Netlike, blotchy, arborizing, lightning-like or mottled pattern of cyanosis. Skin within webs of net (Figure 15-20) is normal to pallid. ILR: May be associated with livedoid vasculitis, and ulceration about the ankles and forefeet may occur in winter or spring/summer months.

COLOR Reddish blue

PALPATION Skin feels cool.

DISTRIBUTION Symmetric, arms/legs, buttocks; less commonly, body; ulceration on lower legs. Patchy, asymmetric on extremities

General Examination *ILR:* noncontributory. *SLR:* symptoms of underlying disease, thromboembolitic disease. *Sneddon's syndrome:* neurologic lesions (palsy, aphasia).

Differential Diagnosis

Mottled Pigmentation Cutis marmorata (transient physiologic mottling of skin that resolves on warming), livedoid vasculitis (segmental hyalinizing vasculitis causing atrophie blanche), erythema ab igne

Laboratory and Special Examinations

Laboratory *SLR:* varies with associated disorders

Dermatopathology ILR with livedoid vasculitis: arteriolar intimal proliferation with dilated numerous capillaries, thickening of walls of venules, hyalinization of walls of small arterial vessels, lymphocytic perivascular infiltration. In Sneddon's syndrome: vascular changes

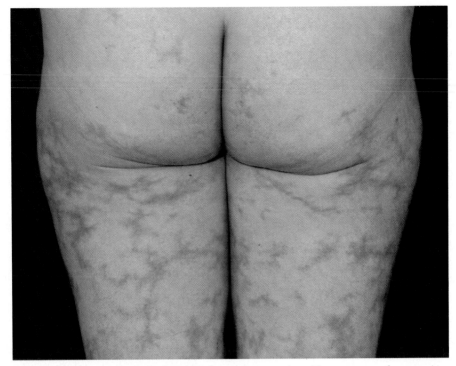

Figure 15-20 Livedo reticularis: Sneddon's syndrome *A netlike pattern on the posterior thighs and buttocks defined by violaceous, erythematous macules in a patient with labile hypertension and cerebrovascular ischemic attacks. The skin within the erythematous areas is normally pale.*

as in endarteritis obliterans. In SLR vascular pathology of underlying disease.

Diagnosis

Clinical diagnosis confirmed by laboratory data supporting diagnosis of associated disorder

Pathophysiology

LR pattern due to vasospasm of perpendicular arterioles, perforating dermis from below. Cyanotic periphery of each web of net caused by deoxygenated blood in surrounding horizontally arranged venous plexuses. When factors such as cold cause increased viscosity/low flow rates in superficial venous plexus, further deoxygenation occurs and cyanotic reticular pattern becomes more pronounced. Elevation of

limb decreases intensity of color due to increased venous drainage. LR may result from arteriolar disease causing obstruction to inflow and blood hyperviscosity or from obstruction to outflow of blood in venules.

Course and Prognosis

ILR occurs on exposure to cold but in time may become permanent. Course/prognosis of SLR depends on that of associated disorder.

Management

ILR: Keep from chilling extremity. Pentoxifylline 400 mg PO t.i.d. and low-dose aspirin may be helpful.

SLR: Treat associated disorder.

LUPUS ERYTHEMATOSUS

SYSTEMIC LUPUS ERYTHEMATOSUS

This serious multisystem disease involves connective tissue and blood vessels; the clinical manifestations include fever (90 %), skin lesions (85 %), arthritis, and renal, cardiac, and pulmonary disease. Systemic lupus erythematosus (SLE) may uncommonly develop in patients with chronic cutaneous lupus erythematosus (CCLE), but lesions of CCLE are common in SLE.

Epidemiology and Etiology

Age 30 (females), 40 (males)

Sex Male : female ratio 1 : 8

Race More common in blacks

Other Features Family history (<5 %); SLE syndrome can be induced by drugs (hydralazine, certain anticonvulsants, and procainamide), although rash is an uncommon feature of drug-induced SLE. Sunlight may cause an exacerbation of SLE (36 %).

History

Duration of Lesions Weeks (acute), months

Skin Symptoms Pruritus (especially papular lesions)

Constitutional Symptoms Fatigue (100 %), fever (100 %), weight loss, and malaise

Systems Review Arthralgia or arthritis, abdominal pain

Physical Examination

Skin Lesions

TYPES

Erythematous, confluent, macular butterfly eruption (face) (Figure 15-21) with fine scaling; erosions and crusts
Erythematous, discrete, papular or urticarial lesions (face, dorsa of hands, and arms) (Figure 15-22)
Bullae, often hemorrhagic (acute flares)
Papules and discoid plaques as in CCLE (face and arms)

"Palpable" purpura (vasculitis)
Urticarial lesions with purpura ("urticarial vasculitis")

COLOR Bright red (Figure 15-21)

SHAPE Round or oval

ARRANGEMENT Diffuse involvement of the face in light-exposed areas. Scattered discrete lesions (Figure 15-22) (face, forearms, and dorsa of hands).

DISTRIBUTION Localized or generalized

SITES OF PREDILECTION Face (80 %); scalp (discoid lesions); presternal, shoulders; dorsa of the forearms, hands, fingers, fingertips (vasculitis); palms; periungual telangiectases and palmar erythema are also seen.

Hair Discoid lesions associated with patchy alopecia. Diffuse alopecia

Mucous Membranes Ulcers arising in purpuric necrotic lesions on palate (80 %), buccal mucosa, or gums

Extracutaneous Multisystem Involvement Arthralgia or arthritis (15 %), renal disease (50 %), pericarditis (20 %), pneumonitis (20 %), gastrointestinal (due to arteritis and sterile peritonitis), hepatomegaly (30 %), myopathy (30 %), splenomegaly (20 %), lymphadenopathy (50 %), peripheral neuropathy (14 %), CNS disease (10 %), seizures or organic brain disease (14 %)

Laboratory and Special Examinations

Pathology

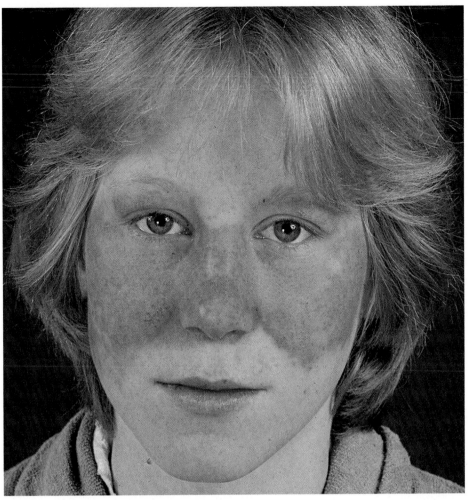

Figure 15-21 Acute systemic lupus erythematosus *Bright red, slightly edematous, sharply demarcated plaques in a "butterfly pattern" on the face.*

SKIN Atrophy of epidermis, liquefaction degeneration of the dermal-epidermal junction, edema of the dermis, dermal inflammatory infiltrate (lymphocytes), and fibrinoid degeneration of the connective tissue and walls of the blood vessels

IMMUNOFLUORESCENCE OF SKIN The lupus band test (direct immunofluorescence demonstrating IgG, IgM, C1q) shows granular or globular deposits of immune reactants in a bandlike pattern along the dermal-epidermal junction. This is positive in lesional skin in 90 % and in the clinically normal skin (sun-exposed, 70 % to 80 %; non-sun-exposed, 50 %); in the latter case indicative of renal disease and hypocomplementemia.

OTHER ORGANS The fundamental lesion is fibrinoid degeneration of connective tissue and walls of the blood vessels, which is associated with an inflammatory infiltrate of plasma cells and lymphocytes.

Serology ANA positive (>95 %); peripheral pattern of nuclear fluorescence and anti-double-stranded DNA antibodies are specific for SLE; low levels of complement (especially with renal involvement). Anticardiolipin autoantibodies (lupus anticoagulant) are present in a specific subset (anticardiolipin syndrome); SS-A(Ro) autoantibodies in the subset of subacute cutaneous lupus erythematosus (SCLE) in which there is extensive skin involvement and photosensitivity. SS-B(La) antibodies also co-exist in 50 % of the cases.

Hematology Anemia [normocytic, normochromic, or rarely, hemolytic Coombs-positive, leukopenia (<4000/μl)], thrombocytopenia, elevated ESR (a good guide to activity of the disease)

Pathophysiology

The tissue injury in the epidermis results from the deposition of immune complexes at the dermal-epidermal junction. Immune complexes selectively generate the assembly of the membrane-attack complex, which mediates membrane injury. CD3+ lymphocytes of the cytotoxic suppressor type.

Prognosis

Five-year survival is 93 %.

Management

General Measures Rest, avoidance of sun exposure

Indications for Prednisone (60 mg daily in divided doses): (1) CNS involvement, (2) renal involvement, (3) severely ill patients without CNS involvement, (4) hemolytic crisis

Concomitant Immunosuppressive Drugs Azathioprine or cyclophosphamide, depending on organ involvement and activity of disease

Antimalarials Hydroxychloroquine is useful for treatment of the skin lesions in subacute and chronic SLE but do not reduce the need for prednisone. See precautions in the use of hydroxychloroquine on page 354.

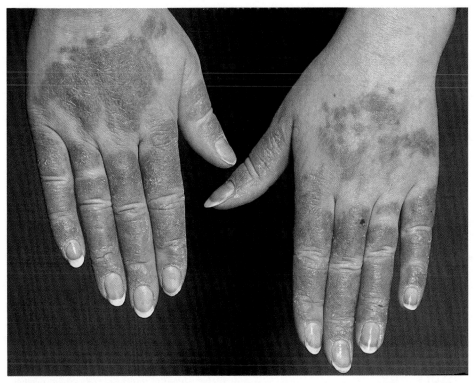

Figure 15-22 Acute systemic lupus erythematosus *Red-to-violaceous, well-demarcated papules and plaques on the dorsa of the fingers and hands, characteristically sparing the skin overlying the joints, an important differential diagnostic sign when considering dermatomyositis, which characteristically involves these sites.*

CUTANEOUS LUPUS ERYTHEMATOSUS

Subacute Cutaneous Lupus Erythematosus

Skin lesions of subacute cutaneous lupus erythematosus (SCLE) are annular or psoriasiform. There is no follicular plugging, no scarring, and little atrophy, as is frequently noted in CCLE. Patients with SCLE may have a few of the criteria of SLE as defined by the American Rheumatism Association, including photosensitivity, arthralgias, serositis, renal disease, and serologic abnormalities, and practically all have anti-Ro (SS-A) and anti-La (SS-B) antibodies. The serious criteria of SLE are uncommon: severe vasculitis, severe CNS disease, or progressive renal disease. The clinical skin lesions are the distinctive feature of SCLE.
Synonyms: Subacute LE, subacute disseminated LE.

Epidemiology

Incidence   About 10 % of the LE population

Age   Young and middle-aged

Race   Uncommon in blacks or Hispanics

Sex   Females > males

Precipitating Factors   Sunlight exposure

History

Duration   Rather sudden onset with diffuse, annular, or psoriasiform plaques eruption appearing on the upper trunk, arms, dorsa of the hands

Constitutional Symptoms   Chronic: mild fatigue, malaise

Systems Review   Some arthralgia, fever of unknown origin

Physical Examination

Skin Lesions

TYPES   Psoriasiform. Papulosquamous, with slight delicate scaling (Figure 15-23), and/or annular. Telangiectasia. No scarring or follicular plugging; sharply marginated but not as indurated as in CCLE. Hypopigmentation and mild atrophy.

SHAPE   Oval, annular, arciform, iris-shaped (erythema multiforme–like)

ARRANGEMENT   Scattered disseminated (Figure 15-23)

DISTRIBUTION   In light-exposed areas (Figure 15-23): shoulders, extensor surface of the arms, dorsal surface of the hands, upper back, V-neck area of the upper chest.

Hair   Diffuse nonscarring alopecia

Nails   Periungual telangiectasia

Differential Diagnosis

Scaly Red Plaques   Dermatomyositis, secondary syphilis, psoriasis, seborrheic dermatitis, tinea corporis

Laboratory Examinations

Dermatopathology

Liquefaction degeneration of the basal layer and edema of the upper dermis that can sometimes lead to vesicle formation. Colloid bodies in the epidermis. Only 40 % have immune deposits in dermal-epidermal junction.

UV Testing   Most patients have a lower than normal UVB MED. Typical SCLE lesions may develop in UVB test sites.

SEROLOGY   Low titers of ANA. Antibodies to Ro/SS-A antigen present in more than 80 %, as well as high levels of circulating immune complexes.

Diagnosis

The extensive involvement is far more than is ever seen in CCLE, and the distinctive eruption

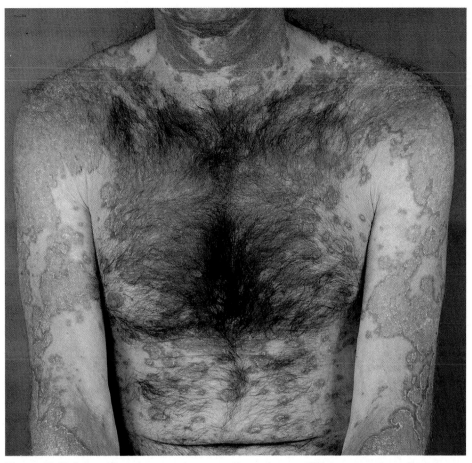

Figure 15-23 Subacute cutaneous lupus erythematosus *Widely scattered, erythematous-to-violaceous scaling, well-demarcated plaques on the trunk, neck, and arms, mimicking the clinical appearance of psoriasis vulgaris.*

is a marker for SCLE. The skin lesions could, however, be confused with atypical psoriasis or dermatomyositis.

Course and Prognosis

A better prognosis than for SLE. Some patients may have renal (and CNS) involvement and thus have a guarded prognosis. The skin lesions can disappear completely, but occasionally, a vitiligo-like leukoderma remains for some months. Women with Ro/SS-A–positive SCLE may give birth to babies with neonatal lupus and congenital heart block.

Diagnosis

Clinical findings confirmed by histology

Management

Topical Anti-inflammatory corticosteroids are somewhat helpful.

Systemic This is usually required. Thalidomide (100 to 300 mg/day) is very effective for skin lesions but not for systemic involvement. Hydroxychloroquine 400 mg/day; if this does not control the skin lesions, quinacrine hydrochloride, 100 mg/day, can be added. The bizarre yellow skin color caused by quinacrine can be somewhat modified by beta-carotene, 60 mg t.i.d.

Chronic Cutaneous Lupus Erythematosus

This chronic, indolent skin disease is characterized by sharply marginated, scaly, atrophic, red ("discoid") plaques, usually occurring on habitually exposed areas.

Epidemiology

Age   20 to 45 years

Sex   Females > males

Race   Possibly more severe in blacks

Classification

Discoid lupus erythematosus (localized and generalized)

Lupus erythematosus panniculitis (lupus profundus)

History

Duration of Lesions   Months to years

Skin Symptoms   Usually none, sometimes slightly pruritic or smarting

Systems Review   Negative

Physical Examination

Skin Lesions

TYPES   *Early*   Papules and plaques, sharply marginated, with adherent scaling (Figure 15-24) Scales are difficult to remove and show spines on undersurface (magnifying lens) resembling carpet tacks.
   Late   Atrophy and depression of lesions, with slightly raised border (Figure 15-25). Erythema contains fine telangiectases. Follicular plugging (closely set and often in clusters), dilated follicles, and scarring. Chronic untreated cutaneous lupus erythematosus results in marked scarring, with depressed and contracted lesions on the face, creating a wolflike, or lupus, facies.

COLOR   Active lesions bright red. "Burned out" lesions may be pink or white (hypome-lanosis) macules and scars. Lesions may show hyperpigmentation, especially in persons with brown or black skin.

SHAPE   Round, oval, annular, polycyclic with irregular borders

DISTRIBUTION   Scattered discrete lesions

SITES OF PREDILECTION   Face and scalp; otherwise: dorsa of forearms, hands, fingers, toes, and less frequently, the trunk

Hair   Scarring alopecia associated with lesions in the scalp skin

Mucous Membranes   Less than 5 % of patients have lip involvement (hyperkeratosis, hypermelanotic scarring, erythema) and atrophic erythematous or whitish areas with or without ulceration on the buccal mucosa, tongue, and palate.

Differential Diagnosis

The lesions of chronic cutaneous lupus erythematosus (CCLE) may closely mimic *actinic keratosis*. *Plaque psoriasis* and scaling discoid lupus erythematosus without atrophy and scarring may be difficult to distinguish, especially on the dorsa of the hands; histopathology permits distinction. *Polymorphous light eruption* (PMLE) may pose a problem. PMLE disappears in the winter in northern latitudes, does not develop atrophy or follicular plugging, and does not occur in unexposed areas—mouth, hairy scalp. *Lichen planus* can be confusing, but the biopsy is distinctive. *Lupus vulgaris* and *tinea facialis*.

Laboratory and Special Examinations

Dermatopathology   Hyperkeratosis, atrophy of the epidermis, follicular plugging, liquefac-

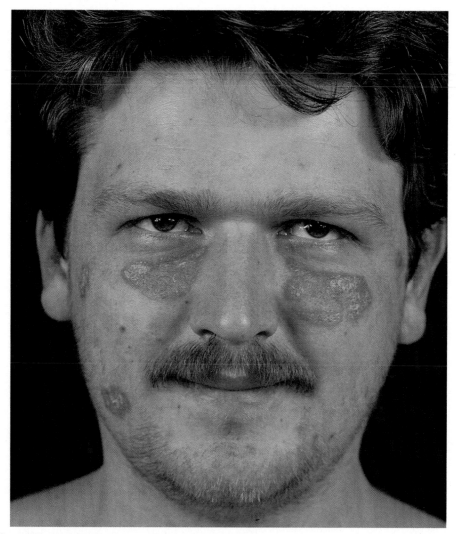

Figure 15-24 Chronic cutaneous lupus erythematosus *Well-demarcated, erythematous, hyperkeratotic plaques with atrophy, follicular plugging, and adherent scale on both cheeks.*

tion degeneration of the basal cell layer. In the dermis there is edema, dilatation of small blood vessels, and perifollicular and periappendageal inflammatory infiltrate (lymphocytes and histiocytes). Strong PAS reaction of the subepidermal, thickened basement zone.

Immunofluorescence Positive in active lesions at least 6 weeks old. Granular deposits of IgG (>IgM) at the dermal-epidermal junction. This is known as the *lupus band test* (LBT) and is positive in 90 % of active lesions not recently treated with topical corticosteroids but *negative in burnt-out (scarred) lesions and in the normal skin,* both sun-exposed and nonexposed. SLE, in contrast, has a positive LBT in lesional as well as both normal sun-exposed (70 % to 80 %) and nonexposed (50 %) skin.

SEROLOGY Low incidence of ANA in a titer more than 1:16

HEMATOLOGY Occasionally leukopenia (<4500/μl)

Diagnosis

Clinical findings confirmed by histology

Course and Prognosis

Only 1 % to 5 % may develop SLE; with localized lesions, complete remission occurs in 50 %; with generalized lesions, remissions are less frequent (<10 %). *Note:* CCLE lesions may be the presenting cutaneous sign of SLE.

Management

Prevention Topical sunscreens (SPF 30) routinely

Local Corticosteroids Topical fluorinated corticosteroids (with caution)

Intralesional triamcinolone acetonide, 3 to 5 mg/ml, for small lesions

Antimalarial Hydroxychloroquine ≤ 6.5 mg/kg of body weight per day. If hydroxychloroquine is ineffective, add quinacrine 100 mg t.i.d. (Quinacrine is an excellent agent and can be obtained from Panorama Pharmacy, Fax No. 818-787 7256.)

Retinoid Hyperkeratotic CCLE lesions respond well to systemic etretinate (1 mg/kg of body weight).

PRETREATMENT AND POSTTREATMENT SCREENING WHEN USING ANTIMALARIALS

Liver function tests
Slit-lamp and funduscopic examination
Assessment of visual acuity
Visual field testing by both static and kinetic techniques with a 3-mm red test object
Have patients test themselves with the Amsler grid every 4 weeks
Pretreatment eye examinations and ophthalmologic monitoring are important because retinopathy has been reported.
Follow-up (every 6 months)
Review subjective visual complaints, slit-lamp and funduscopic test results, and visual acuity.
Repeat visual testing if patient complains of difficulty in reading ("missing" words and letters) and demonstrates reproducible bilateral "fading" of Amsler grid squares.

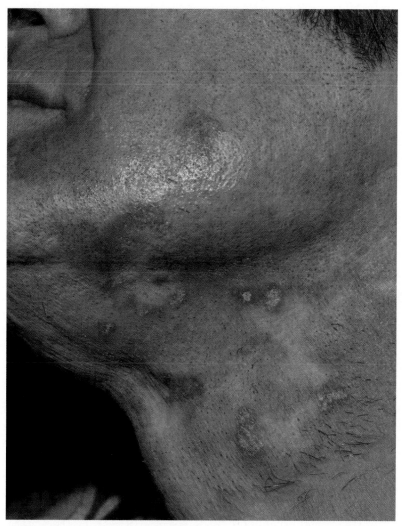

Figure 15-25 Chronic cutaneous lupus erythematosus *Round-to-oval, slightly indurated, red-to-violaceous, sharply demarcated plaques on the cheek and neck. Other characteristic features present are hyperkeratosis, central atrophy with loss of hair follicles, depressed scarring, and postinflammatory hypopigmentation.*

Chronic Lupus Panniculitis

This is a form of chronic cutaneous lupus erythematosus in which there are firm, circumscribed nodules on the face, scalp, breast, upper arms, thighs, and buttocks. Most patients also have typical lesions of discoid lupus erythematosus. Usually a form of cutaneous lupus but may occur in systemic lupus erythematosus.

Synonym: Lupus erythematosus profundus.

History

Duration of Lesions   May precede or follow the onset of discoid lesions by several years.

Skin Symptoms   Pain, slight tenderness

Systems Review   In one series, 35 % of the patients had SLE mild.

Physical Examination

Skin Lesions   '

TYPES

Deep-seated nodules or platelike infiltrations with or without grossly visible epidermal changes; these evolve into deep depressions. In a completely darkened room, place a flashlight at the side of the lesion to detect subtle surface changes (elevation or depression) (Figure 15-26).
Ulcers may develop in the plaques or nodules.

PALPATION   Plaques or nodules are better felt than seen; the overlying skin may be normal or exhibit typical lesions of chronic discoid lupus erythematosus.

SHAPE   Platelike lesions or round nodules, linear plaques

ARRANGEMENT   Scattered discrete lesions

DISTRIBUTION   Scalp, face, upper arms, trunk (especially the breasts), thighs, and buttocks

Differential Diagnosis

Morphea, erythema nodosum, sarcoid, miscellaneous types of panniculitis

Laboratory and Special Examinations

Dermatopathology   Subcutaneous layer
Necrobiosis with fibrinoid deposits, dense lymphocytic infiltrates; later, hyalinization of the fat lobules; there may be considerable mucinous deposits and also rarely vasculitis. In patients with SLE there are typical hematologic and serologic abnormalities.

Management

Systemic   Same as for chronic cutaneous lupus erythematosus, discoid type

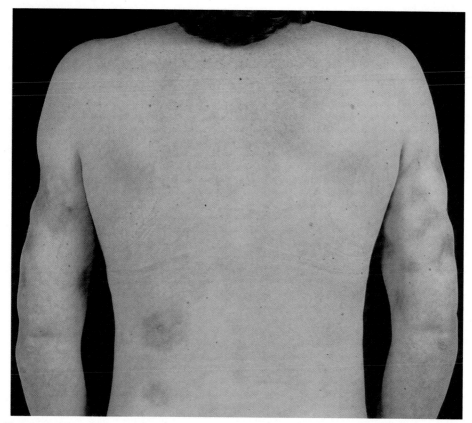

Figure 15-26 Lupus panniculitis *Chronic panniculitis with large areas of atrophy of the subcutaneous tissue, resulting in large sunken areas of overlying skin, representing resolving lesions. Where erythema is still visible, palpation reveals firm subcutaneous nodules and plaques.*

SCLERODERMA

Scleroderma is a multisystem disorder characterized by inflammatory, vascular, and sclerotic changes of the skin and a variety of internal organs, especially the lungs, heart, and GI tract.

Synonyms: Progressive systemic sclerosis, systemic sclerosis, systemic scleroderma.

Epidemiology and Etiology

Age Onset 30 to 50 years

Sex Female : males 4 : 1

Etiology Unknown

Classification

Systemic scleroderma can be divided into two subsets: *limited systemic scleroderma* (lSSc) and *diffuse systemic scleroderma* (dSSc). lSSc comprises 60 % of scleroderma patients; patients are usually female, older than those with dSSc, and have a long history of Raynaud's phenomenon with skin involvement limited to hands, feet, face, and forearms (acrosclerosis). lSSc includes the CREST syndrome, and systemic involvement may not appear for years; patients usually die of other causes. There is a high incidence of anticentromere antibodies. dSSc patients have a relatively rapid onset and diffuse involvement, not only of hands and feet but also of the trunk, synovitis, tendosynovitis, and early onset of internal involvement. Anticentromere antibodies are uncommon, but Scl-70 (antitopoisomerase I) antibodies are present in 30 %.

Clinical Variant CREST syndrome, i.e., *C*alcinosis cutis + *R*aynaud's phenomenon + *E*sophageal dysfunction + *S*clerodactyly + *T*elangiectasia

History

Skin Symptoms Raynaud's phenomenon with digital pain, coldness, rubor with pain and tingling

Systems Review Pain/stiffness of fingers, knees. Migratory polyarthritis. Heartburn, dysphagia, especially with solid foods. Constipation, diarrhea, abdominal bloating, malabsorption, weight loss. Exertional dyspnea, dry cough.

Physical Examination

Skin, Hair, and Nail Findings

TYPES OF LESIONS *Hands/Feet   Early:* Raynaud's phenomenon with triphasic color changes, i.e., pallor, cyanosis, rubor (Figure 15-27). Nonpitting edema of hands/feet. Painful ulcerations at fingertips (Figure 15-28), knuckles; heal with pitted scars. *Late:* sclerodactyly with tapering fingers, waxy, shiny atrophic skin, which is tightly bound down; flexion contractures; bony resorption results in loss of distal phalanges (Figure 15-27).

Face   Early: periorbital edema. *Late:* edema and fibrosis result in loss of normal facial lines, masklike (Figure 15-29), thinning of lips, microstomia, radial perioral furrowing, small sharp nose.

Ulceration Secondary to vascular occlusion, acrally (Figure 15-28)

Cutaneous Calcification Occurs over bony prominences or any sclerodermatous site; may ulcerate and extrude white paste.

CREST Syndrome Matlike telangiectasia (Figure 15-30), especially on face, neck, upper trunk, hands; also, lips, oral mucous membranes, GI tract

COLOR Hyperpigmentation, generalized. In areas of sclerosis, postinflammatory hyper- and hypopigmentation

PALPATION *Early:* skin feels indurated, stiff. *Late:* tense, smooth, hardened, bound down.

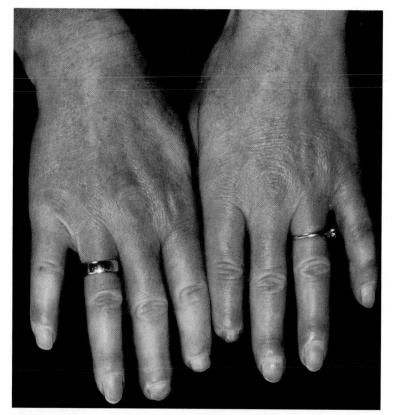

Figure 15-27 Scleroderma: Raynaud's phenomenon and acrosclerosis *Hands and fingers are edematous (nonpitting) with both erythema and vasoconstriction; skin is shiny, bound down; hair is absent due to sclerosis. Distal fingers are taped and the phalanges on some fingers shortened (index fingers), which is associated with bony resorption, with nail dystrophy*

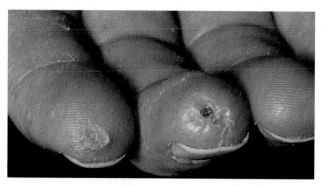

Figure 15-28 Scleroderma: acrosclerosis *Typical "rat bite" necroses and ulcerations of fingertips.*

Leathery crepitation over joints, especially knees.

DISTRIBUTION OF LESIONS *Early:* fingers, hands. *Late:* upper extremities, trunk, face, lower extremities

HAIR AND NAILS Thinning/complete loss of hair on distal extremities. Loss of sweat glands with anhidrosis. Periungual telangiectasia with giant sausage-shaped capillary loops. Nails grow clawlike over shortened distal phalanges (Figure 15-27).

MUCOUS MEMBRANES Sclerosis of sublingual ligament; uncommonly, painful induration of gums, tongue

General Examination

ESOPHAGUS Dysphagia, diminished peristalsis, reflux esophagitis

GASTROINTESTINAL SYSTEM Small intestine involvement may produce constipation, diarrhea, bloating, and malabsorption.

LUNG Pulmonary fibrosis and alveolitis. Reduction of pulmonary function due to restricted movement of chest wall

HEART Cardiac conduction defects, heart failure, pericarditis

KIDNEY Renal involvement occurs in 45 %. Slowly progressive uremia, malignant hypertension.

MUSCULOSKELETAL SYSTEM Carpal tunnel syndrome. Muscle weakness.

Differential Diagnosis

Diffuse Sclerosis Mixed connective tissue disease, eosinophilic fasciitis, scleromyxedema, lupus erythematosus, dermatomyositis, morphea, chronic graft-versus-host disease, lichen sclerosus et atrophicus, polyvinyl chloride exposure, adverse drug reaction (pentazocine, bleomycin)

Scleroderma-Like Conditions A scleroderma-like condition, as is seen in systemic sclerosis, occurs in persons exposed to *polyvinyl chloride*. *Bleomycin* also produces pulmonary fibrosis, Raynaud's phenomenon, and cutaneous changes indistinguishable from dSSc-like sclerosis of skin, myalgia, pulmonitis, myocarditis, neuropathy, and encephalopathy are related to the ingestion of certain lots of L-tryptophan (arthralgia-myalgia syndrome); the *toxic oil syndrome* that occurred in an epidemic in Spain in 1981 affecting 25,000 people was due to the consumption of denatured rape seed oil. After an acute phase, with rash, fever, pulmonitis, and myalgia, it progresses to a condition with neuromuscular abnormalities and scleroderma-like skin lesions.

Laboratory and Special Examinations

Dermatopathology *Early:* mild cellular infiltrate around dermal blood vessels, eccrine coils, subcutaneous tissue. *Late:* epidermis shows disappearance of rete ridges, increased eosinophilia, broadening and homogenization of collagen bundles, obliteration and decrease of interbundle spaces, thickening of dermis with replacement of upper or total subcutaneous fat by hyalinized collagen. Paucity of blood vessels, thickening/hyalinization of vessel walls, narrowing of lumen; dermal appendages atrophied; sweat glands are situated in upper dermis; calcium in sclerotic, homogeneous collagen of subcutaneous tissue.

Autoantibodies Patients with dSSc have circulating autoantibodies by ANA testing. Autoantibodies react with centromere proteins or DNA topoisomerase I; fewer patients have antinucleolar antibodies. Anticentromeric autoantibodies occur in 21 % of dSSc and 71 % of CREST, DNA topoisomerase I (Scl-70) antibodies in 33 % of dSSc and 18 % of CREST.

Cardiac Studies

Pulmonary Studies Diffusion studies: reduced O_2 transport

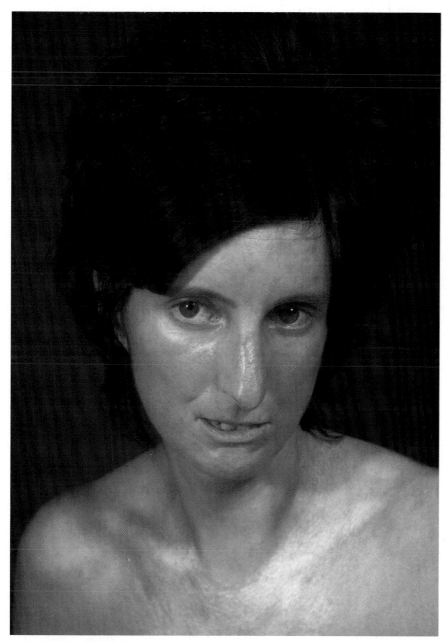

Figure 15-29 Scleroderma *Masklike facies with stretched, shiny skin and loss of normal facial lines giving a younger appearance than actual age; the hair and eyebrows are dyed black. Thinning of the lips and perioral sclerosis result in small mouth, which is asymmetric, creating a snarling appearance. Sclerosis and multiple telangiectases are also present on the shoulders and chest.*

Diagnosis

Clinical findings confirmed by dermatopathology.

Pathophysiology

Pathogenesis unknown. Primary event might be endothelial cell injury in blood vessels, the cause of which is unknown. Early in course, target organ edema occurs, followed by fibrosis; cutaneous capillaries are reduced in number; remainder dilate and proliferate, becoming visible telangiectasia. Fibrosis due to overproduction of collagen by fibroblasts.

Course and Prognosis

Course characterized by slow, relentless progression of skin and/or visceral sclerosis; how-ever, the 10-year survival is more than 50 %. Renal disease is the leading cause of death; also, cardiac and pulmonary involvement. Spontaneous remissions do occur. CREST syndrome progresses more slowly and has a more favorable prognosis; some cases do develop visceral involvement.

Management

Symptomatic. Systemic corticosteroids may be of benefit for limited periods early in the disease. All other systemic treatments (EDTA, aminocaproic acid, D-penicillamine, *para*-aminobenzoate, colchicine, immunosuppressive drugs) have not been shown to be of lasting benefit. Presently, interferon-gamma is being tested clinically, and so is photopheresis.

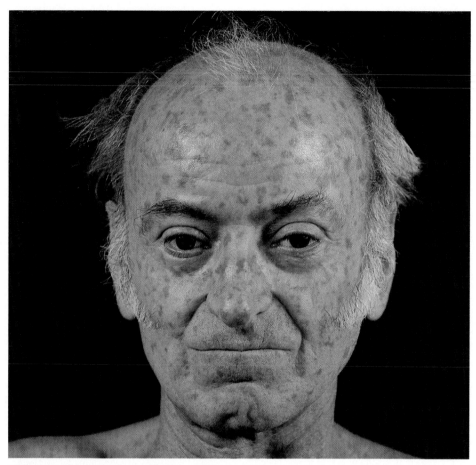

Figure 15-30 Scleroderma: CREST syndrome *Numerous macular or matlike telangiectases without other findings of scleroderma on the face. Complete features include* **c***alcinosis cutis,* **R***aynaud's phenomenon,* **e***sophageal dysmotility,* **s***clerosis, and* **t***elangiectasias.*

RAYNAUD'S DISEASE/RAYNAUD'S PHENOMENON

Raynaud's phenomenon (RP) is digital ischemia that occurs on exposure to cold and/or due to emotional stress. RP may be associated with other diseases, but when no etiology is found, the term *Raynaud's disease* (RD) is used. RD is the most common cause of RP, and this précis will largely summarize RD. The various causes of RP include *rheumatic disorders* [systemic scleroderma (85 %), SLE (35 %), dermatomyositis (30 %), Sjögren's syndrome, rheumatoid arthritis, polyarteritis nodosa], *diseases with abnormal blood proteins* (cryoproteins, cold agglutinins, macroglobulins), *drugs* (beta-adrenergic blockers, nicotine), *arterial diseases* (arteriosclerosis obliterans, thromboangiitis obliterans), and *carpal tunnel syndrome.*

Epidemiology

Incidence   As high as 20 % in young women

Age   Young adults or at menopause

Sex   Female >> male

Occupation   RP may occur in persons using vibratory tools (chain saw users), meat cutters, typists, and pianists.

Precipitating Factors   Cold, mental stress, certain occupations (see above), smoking

History

Relationship of Skin Changes to Other Factors   Season (worse in winter in temperate climates), cold (meat cutters), previous treatment (drugs), occupation (using vibratory tools). Skin symptoms: numbness, pain.

Systems Review   Careful review is important to detect diseases in which RP is associated: arthralgia, fatigue, dysphagia, muscle weakness, etc.

Physical Examination

Skin

TYPES OF SKIN CHANGES   *The Episodic Attack* There is sharply demarcated blanching or cyanosis of the fingers or toes, extending from the tip to varying levels of the finger or toe. The finger distal to the line of ischemia is white or blue and cold (Figure 15-31); the proximal skin is pink and warm. When the digits are rewarmed, the blanching may be replaced by cyanosis because of slow blood flow; at the end of the attack, the normal color or a red color reflects the reactive hyperemic phase. To recapitulate, the sequence of color changes is often white → blue → red. Rarely, the tip of the nose, earlobes, or the tongue may be involved. Blanching may occur in one or two digits or all the digits; often the thumb is spared. The feet are involved only 40 %

Repeated or Persistent Vascular Vasospasm Patients with RP often have a persistent vasospasm rather than episodic attacks. Skin changes include trophic changes with development of taut, atrophic skin and shortening of the terminal phalanges—this is called *sclerodactyly* (see Scleroderma, page 358).

Acrogangrene is rare in RD (<1 %). In RP associated with scleroderma, painful ulcers and fissures develop (Figure 15-32); sequestration of the terminal phalanges or the development of gangrene may lead to autoamputation of the fingertips.

Nails   Pterygium, clubbing

Differential Diagnosis

See Table 15-B

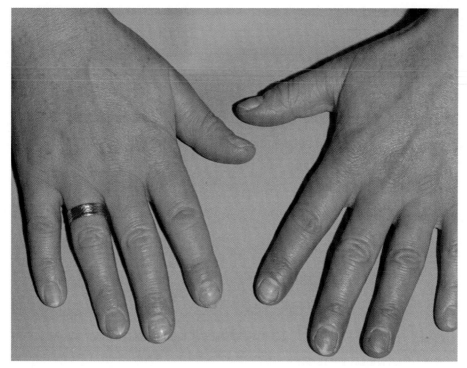

Figure 15-31 Raynaud's disease *The left hand exhibits a cyanosis compared to the right hand; it is seen especially well in the nail beds. Unilateral episodes such as this may occur after contact with a cold object.*

Laboratory Examinations

SEROLOGY   ANA and other tests to rule out scleroderma, lupus erythematosus, immunoproteins

Diagnosis

The vascular changes in RP are characteristic, and when no other disease is discovered (see above), the diagnosis is RD.

Pathogenesis

The vasomotor tone is regulated by the sympathetic nervous system. The centers for vasomotor tone are located in the brain, in the spinal cord, and in the peripheral nerves. Vasodilatation occurs only on withdrawal of the sympathetic activity. It is conjectured that there may be a "local fault" in which blood vessels are abnormally sensitive to cold.

Course and Prognosis

RP may disappear spontaneously; it progresses in about 1 of 3 patients.

Management

Prevention   Education regarding the use of loose-fitting clothing, avoiding cold and pressure on the fingers. Giving up smoking is necessary.

Systemic Therapy   Drug therapy such as reserpine and nifedipine should be used only in patients who have severe RD.

TABLE 15-B
Causes of Raynaud's Phenomenon

Connective tissue disease	Methysergide
Scleroderma	Bleomycin and vinblastine
Systemic lupus erythematosus	Clonidine
Dermatomyositis and polymyositis	Bromocriptine
Mixed connective tissue disease	Cyclosporine
Rheumatoid arthritis	Trauma
Polyarteritis and vasculitis	Vibratory tools
Sjogren syndrome	Hypothenar hammer syndrome
Obstructive arterial disease	Pianists, typists
Arteriosclerosis obliterans	Meat cutters
Thromboangiitis obliterans	Hematologic causes
Arterial embolism	Cryoproteins
Thoracic outlet syndrome	Cold agglutinins
Neurogenic disorders	Macroglobulins
Carpal tunnel syndrome	Polycythemia
Reflex sympathetic dystrophy	Miscellaneous
Hemiplegia	Hypothyroidism
Poliomyelitis	Vinyl chloride disease
Multiple sclerosis	Neoplasms
Syringomyelia	Vasculitis and hepatitis B
Drugs	antigenemia
Beta-adrenergic blockers	Arteriovenous fistula
Ergot preparations	Intraarterial injections

SOURCE: TD Coffman: Cutaneous changes in peripheral vascular disease, in TB Fitzpatrick et al (eds): *Dermatology in General Medicine,* 4th edition. New York, McGraw-Hill, 1993; Chapter 167.

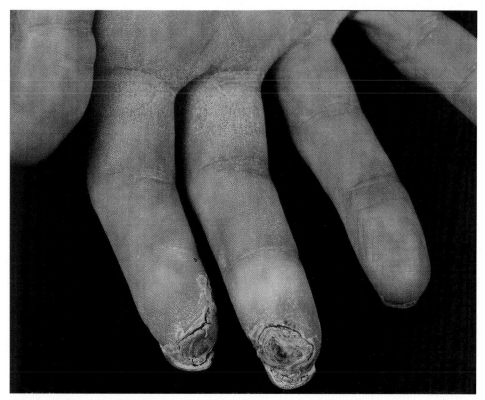

Figure 15-32 Raynaud's phenomenon: acrogangrene *Persistent vasospasm of medium-sized arterioles can sometimes lead to gangrene of the terminal digits as illustrated in this patient with scleroderma.*

VASCULITIS

HYPERSENSITIVITY VASCULITIS

Hypersensitivity vasculitis (HV) encompasses a heterogeneous group of vasculitides associated with hypersensitivity to antigens from infectious agents, drugs, or other exogenous or endogenous sources, characterized pathologically by involvement of small blood vessels (principally venules) and segmental inflammation and fibrinoid necrosis. Clinically, skin involvement is characteristic of HV, manifested by "palpable purpura" in the skin; systemic vascular involvement occurs, chiefly in the kidney, muscles, joints, GI tract, and peripheral nerves. Henoch-Schönlein purpura (HSP) is a type of HV associated with IgA.

Synonyms: Allergic cutaneous vasculitis, necrotizing vasculitis.

Epidemiology and Etiology

Age   All ages. HSP: usually 20 years.

Sex   Equal incidence in males and in females

Etiology   Idiopathic 50 %

Classification

Exogenous Stimuli Proved or Suspected

Henoch-Schönlein purpura: group A streptococci
Serum sickness/serum sickness–like reactions: sulfonamides, penicillin, serum
Other drug-induced vasculitides
Vasculitis associated with infectious diseases: hepatitis B virus, hepatitis C virus, group A hemolytic streptococcus, *Staphylococcus aureus, Mycobacterium leprae*

Endogenous Antigens Likely Involved   Vasculitis associated with

Neoplasms: lymphoproliferative disorders, carcinoma of kidney
Connective tissue diseases: SLE, rheumatoid arthritis, Sjögren's syndrome
Other underlying diseases: cryoglobulinemia, paraproteinemia, hypergammaglobulinemic purpura
Congenital deficiencies of the complement system

History

History of Drug Ingestion   A new drug taken during the few weeks prior to the onset of HV is a likely etiologic agent.

Duration of Lesions   Acute (days, as in drug-induced or idiopathic), subacute (weeks, especially urticarial types), chronic (recurrent over years)

Symptoms   Pruritus, burning pain, or no symptoms

Constitutional Symptoms   Fever, malaise

Systems Review   Symptoms of peripheral neuritis, abdominal pain (bowel ischemia), arthralgia, myalgia, kidney involvement (microhematuria), CNS involvement

Physical Findings

Skin Lesions

TYPES   (Figures 15-33 and 15-34) Palpable purpura. Petechiae due to coagulation defects or thrombocytopenia are macular and, therefore, not palpable. In HV, there is an inflammatory infiltrate, the petechiae are therefore palpable and actually papular, hence the term palpable purpura, which is pathognomonic. Urticarial wheals (persist more than 24 hours) (urticarial vasculitis). In case of massive inflammation, palpable purpura (papules) converts to hemorrhagic blisters (Figure 15-34) and necrosis → ulcers.

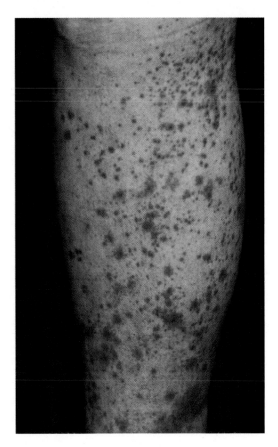

Figure 15-33 Hypersensitivity vasculitis *Multiple sites of cutaneous vasculitis present clinically as "palpable purpura" on the lower extremity. Crusted sites represent cutaneous infarction associated with necrotizing vasculitis.*

COLOR Red initially. Purpuric lesions do not blanch (using a glass slide).

SHAPE Round, oval, annular, arciform

ARRANGEMENT Scattered, discrete lesions or dense and confluent

DISTRIBUTION Usually regional localization: lower third of legs, ankles, buttocks, arms. Stasis factor aggravates or precipitates lesions.

General Examination Should include search for underlying disease and organ involvement (kidney)

Differential Diagnosis

Palpable Purpura Thrombocytopenic purpura, rash such as exanthematous drug eruption in setting of thrombocytopenia, disseminated intravascular coagulation (DIC) with purpura fulminans, septic vasculitis (rickettsial spotted fevers), septic emboli (infective endocarditis), bacteremia [disseminated gonococcal infection, meningococcemia (acute/chronic)], other non-infectious vasculitides

Laboratory and Special Examinations

Hematology Rule out thrombocytopenic purpura.

ESR Elevated

Serology Serum complement is reduced or normal in some patients, depending on associated disorders.

Urinalysis RBC casts, albuminuria

Dermatopathology Deposition of eosinophilic material (fibrinoid) in the walls of postcapillary venules in the upper dermis and perivenular and intramural inflammatory infiltrate consisting predominantly of neutrophils. Extravasated RBC and fragmented neutrophils (nuclear "dust"). Frank necrosis of vessel walls. Intramural C3 and immunoglobulin deposition is seen with immunofluorescent techniques. In Henoch-Schönlein syndrome, the immunoglobulins are predominantly IgA.

Diagnosis

The American College of Rheumatology 1990 criteria for diagnosis of HV are as follows; a diagnosis of HV is made if at least three of these criteria are present (Table 15-C).

Pathophysiology

The most frequently postulated mechanism for the production of necrotizing vasculitis is the deposition in tissues of circulating immune complexes. Initial alterations in venular permeability, which may facilitate the deposition of complexes at such sites, may be due to the release of vasoactive amines from platelets, basophils, and/or mast cells. Immune complexes may activate the complement system or may interact directly with Fc receptors on cell membranes. When the complement system is activated, the generation of anaphylatoxins C3a and C5a could degranulate mast cells. Also, C5a can

TABLE 15-C

Criteria	Definition
1. Age at disease onset >16 years	Development of symptoms after age 16
2. Medication at disease onset	Medication was taken at the onset of symptoms that may have been a precipitating factor
3. Palpable purpura	Slightly elevated purpuric rash over one or more areas of the skin; does not blanch with pressure and is not related to thrombocytopenia
4. Maculopapular rash	Flat and raised lesions of various sizes over one or more areas of the skin
5. Biopsy including arteriole and venule	Histologic changes showing granulocytes in a perivascular or extravascular location

Henoch-Schönlein purpura is a specific subtype of HV; the diagnosis is made if two of these four criteria are present:

Criteria	Definition
1. Palpable purpura	Slightly raised "palpable" hemorrhagic skin lesions, not related to thrombocytopenia
2. Age ≤ 20 at disease onset	Patient 20 years or younger at onset of first symptoms
3. Bowel angina	Diffuse abdominal pain, worse after meals, or the diagnosis of bowel ischemia, usually including bloody diarrhea
4. Wall granulocytes on biopsy	Histologic changes showing granulocytes in the walls of arterioles or venules

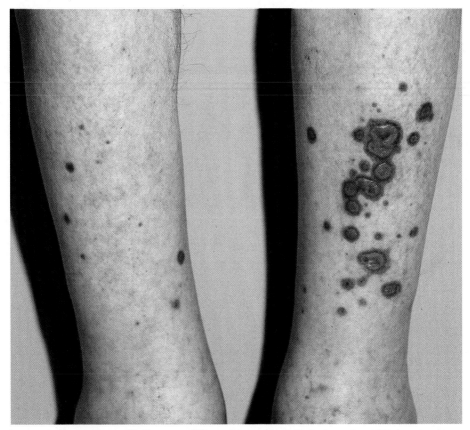

Figure 15-34 Hypersensitivity vasculitis: cutaneous *A limited number of lesions on the shins with palpable purpura and hemorrhagic bullae. Bilateral ankle edema is also present and may be associated with vasculitis.*

attract neutrophils that could release lysosomal enzymes during phagocytosis of complexes and subsequently damage vascular tissue.

Course and Prognosis

Depends on underlying disease. In the idiopathic variant, multiple episodes can occur over the course of years. Usually self-limited, but irreversible damage to kidneys can occur.

Management

Antibiotics   Antibiotics for patients in whom vasculitis follows bacterial infection

Prednisone   For patients with moderate to severe disease

Cytotoxic Immunosuppressives   Cyclophosphamide, azathioprine have been used, usually in combination with prednisone.

POLYARTERITIS NODOSA

Polyarteritis nodosa (PAN) is a multisystem, necrotizing vasculitis of small and medium-sized muscular arteries characterized by its involvement of the renal and visceral arteries. There is a form of PAN that is restricted to skin (*cutaneous* PAN).
Synonyms: Periarteritis nodosa, panarteritis nodosa.

Epidemiology and Etiology

Age   Mean age 45 years

Sex   Male : female ratio 2.5 : 1

Etiology   Unknown

Clinical Variants   *Cutaneous PAN* is a rare variant with symptomatic vasculitis limited to skin and at times peripheral nerves.

History

Systems Review   *Chronic disease syndrome.* GI involvement: nausea, vomiting, abdominal pain, hemorrhage, perforation, infarction. CVS: congestive heart failure, pericarditis, conduction system defects, myocardial infarction. Paresthesias, numbness. *Cutaneous PAN:* pain in nodules, ulcers, involved extremities; aching during flares, physical activity. Myalgia. Neuralgia, numbness, mild paresthesia.

Physical Examination

Skin Lesions   Occur in 15 % of cases

TYPES   Subcutaneous nodules that follow the course of involved arteries; may ulcerate (Figure 15-35). Palpable purpura. Violaceous macule, confluent with livedo reticularis pattern. *Cutaneous PAN:* inflammatory nodules (0.5 to 2.0 cm). Livedo reticularis (Figure 15-36); "starburst" livedo follows at site of cluster of nodular lesions (Figure 15-35). Ulcers may follow ischemia of nodules. Duration—days to months. Resolves with residual violaceous or postinflammatory hyperpigmentation.

COLOR   Nodules bright red to light pink; blue

PALPATION   Nodules often more palpable than visible. Tender.

DISTRIBUTION   Lower extremities, usually bilateral. Lower legs > thighs. Other: arms > trunk > head/neck > buttocks.

General Examination   Elevated blood pressure

NEUROLOGIC EXAMINATION   CNS: cerebrovascular accident. Peripheral nerves: mixed motor/sensory involvement with mononeuritis multiplex pattern.

EYE   Hypertensive changes, ocular vasculitis, retinal artery aneurysm, optic disc edema/atrophy

Differential Diagnosis

Other vasculitides

Laboratory and Special Examinations

Dermatopathology   *Best yield: biopsy of nodular skin lesion (deep wedge biopsy).* Polymorphonuclear neutrophils infiltrate all layers of muscular vessel wall and perivascular areas. Later, infiltrates, mononuclear cells. Fibrinoid necrosis of vessel wall with compromise of lumen, thrombosis, infarction of tissues supplied by involved vessel, with or without hemorrhage. Skin pathology is identical in systemic and cutaneous PAN.

CBC   Commonly neutrophilic leukocytosis; rarely eosinophilia; anemia of chronic disease. ± Elevated ESR

Serology   Antineutrophil cytoplasmic autoantibodies (ANCA) in serum. Hepatitis B surface antigenemia in 30 % of cases.

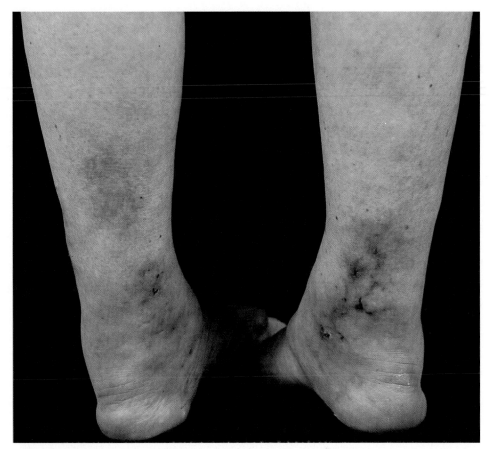

Figure 15-35 Polyarteritis nodosa *Multiple, confluent, dermal and subcutaneous nodules with ulceration (note starburst pattern of lesions) occurring on the medial aspect of the lower legs; lesions represent cutaneous infarctions. Scar on the left posterior calf represents a previous site of cutaneous polyarteritis nodosa.*

Chemistry Elevated creatinine, BUN

Arteriography Aneurysms in small and medium-sized muscular arteries of kidney/hepatic/visceral vasculature

Diagnosis

ARA 1990 criteria for the classification* of polyarteritis nodosa (traditional format): Table 15-D

TABLE 15-D

Criteria	Definition
1. Weight loss ≥4 kg	Loss of 4 kg or more of body weight since illness began, not due to dieting or other factors
2. Livedo reticularis	Mottled reticular pattern over the skin of portions of the extremities or torso
3. Testicular pain or tenderness	Pain or tenderness of the testicles, not due to infection, trauma, or other causes
4. Myalgias, weakness, or leg tenderness	Diffuse myalgias (excluding shoulder and hip girdle) or weakness of muscles or tenderness of leg muscles
5. Mononeuropathy or polyneuropathy	Development of mononeuropathy, multiple mononeuropathies, or polyneuropathy
6. Diastolic bp >90 mmHg	Development of hypertension with the diastolic bp higher than 90 mmHg
7. Elevated BUN or creatinine	Elevation of BUN >40.0 mg/dl or creatinine >1.5 mg/dl, not due to dehydration or obstruction
8. Hepatitis B virus	Presence of hepatitis B surface antigen or antibody in serum
9. Arteriographic abnormality	Arteriogram showing aneurysms or occlusions of the visceral arteries, not due to arteriosclerosis, fibromuscular dysplasia, or other noninflammatory causes
10. Biopsy of small or medium-sized artery containing polymorphonuclear neutrophils	Histologic changes showing the presence of granulocytes or granulocytes and mononuclear leukocytes in the artery wall

Pathophysiology

Necrotizing inflammation of small and medium-sized muscular arteries; may spread circumferentially to involve adjacent veins. Lesions segmental, tend to involve bifurcations of arteries. About 30 % of cases associated with hepatitis B antigenemia, i.e., immune complex formation.

Course and Prognosis

Untreated, very high morbidity and mortality characterized by fulminant deterioration or by relentless progression associated with intermittent acute exacerbations. Mortality from renal failure, bowel infarction and perforation, cardiovascular complications, intractable hypertension. Lesions may heal with scarring and further occlusion or aneurysmal dilatations. Effective treatment improves morbidity and mortality. *Cutaneous PAN:* chronic relapsing benign course.

*For classification purposes, a patient shall be said to have polyarteritis nodosa if at least 3 of these 10 criteria are present. The presence of any 3 or more criteria yields a sensitivity of 82.2 % and a specificity of 86.6 %.

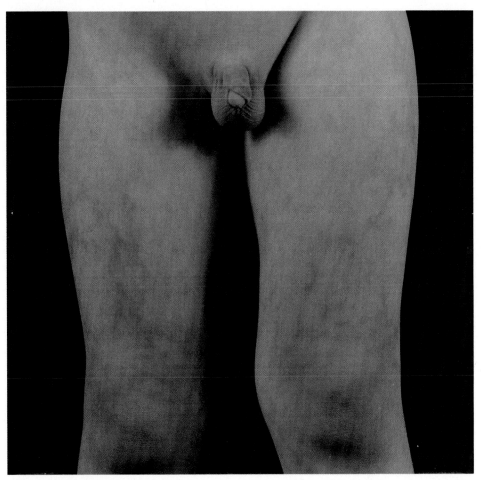

Figure 15-36 Polyarteritis nodosa *A netlike or livedo pattern of violaceous erythema on the anterior thighs of a boy.*

Management

Systemic PAN

COMBINED THERAPY   Prednisone, 1 mg/kg of body weight per day, and cyclophosphamide, 2 mg/kg per day

CUTANEOUS PAN   Nonsteroidal anti-inflammatory agent, prednisone

WEGENER'S GRANULOMATOSIS

Wegener's granulomatosis (WG) is a systemic vasculitis, defined by a clinical triad of manifestations that includes involvement of the upper airways, lungs, and kidneys and by a pathologic triad consisting of necrotizing granulomas in the upper respiratory tract and lungs, vasculitis involving both arteries and veins, and glomerulitis.

Epidemiology and Etiology

Age Mean age 40 years, but occurs at any age

Sex Male : female ratio 1.3:1

Race Rare in blacks

Etiology Unknown

Clinical Variants Variants limited to kidneys; i.e., glomerulitis occurs in 15 % of cases. Limited to respiratory tract.

History

Systems Review Chronic disease syndrome. Fever. Paranasal sinus pain, purulent or bloody nasal discharge. Cough, hemoptysis, dyspnea, chest discomfort.

Physical Examination

Skin Lesions Overall in 45 % of patients, but in only 13 % of patients at initial presentation

TYPES Ulcers most typical; resemble pyoderma gangrenosum. Papules, vesicles, palpable purpura (Figures 15-37 and 15-38) as in hypersensitivity (necrotizing) vasculitis, subcutaneous nodules, plaques, noduloulcerative lesions as in PAN.

DISTRIBUTION Most common on lower extremities. Also, face, trunk, upper limbs.

MUCOUS MEMBRANES Oral ulcerations (Figure 15-39). Often first symptom.

General Examination

EAR-NOSE-THROAT ±Nasal mucosal ulceration, crusting, blood clots; nasal septal perforation; saddle-nose deformity. Eustachian tube occlusion with serous otitis media; ±pain. External auditory canal: pain, erythema, swelling. Marked gingival hyperplasia.

EYE 65 %. Mild conjunctivitis, episcleritis, scleritis, granulomatous sclerouveitis, ciliary vessel vasculitis, retroorbital mass lesion with proptosis

NERVOUS SYSTEM Cranial neuritis, mononeuritis multiplex, cerebral vasculitis

RENAL DISEASE 85 %. Signs of renal failure in advanced WG.

Differential Diagnosis

Cutaneous Necrosis + Respiratory Tract Disease Other vasculitides, Goodpasture's syndrome, tumors of the upper airway/lung, infectious/noninfectious granulomatous diseases (especially blastomycosis), midline granuloma

Angiocentric Lymphoma Allergic granulomatosis

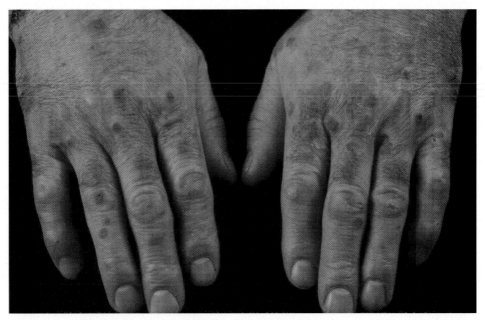

Figure 15-37 Wegener's granulomatosis *A limited number of erythematous, purpuric, non-blanchable papules and nodules on the dorsa of fingers and hands; a few lesions have central areas of infarction.*

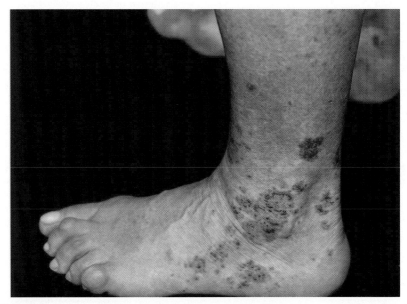

Figure 15-38 Wegener's granulomatosis *Confluent areas of cutaneous vasculitis presenting as palpable purpura are seen on the lower leg and the foot; the dark-violet, small papules represent infarcts with areas of vasculitis.*

Laboratory and Special Examinations

Hematology Mild anemia. Leukocytosis. ±Thrombocytosis.

ESR Markedly elevated

Chemistry Impaired renal function

Urinalysis Proteinuria, hematuria, RBC casts

Serology

> Antineutrophil cytoplasmic autoantibodies (ANCA) are seromarkers for WG. Two ANCA patterns occur in ethanol-fixed neutrophils: cytoplasmic pattern (c-ANCA) and perinuclear pattern (p-ANCA). A 29-kDa protease is the major antigen for c-ANCA; myeloperoxidase, that for p-ANCA. c-ANCA has been associated predominantly with WG; p-ANCA with microscopic polyarteritis, other vasculitides, idiopathic necrotizing and crescentic glomerulonephritis. Titers correlate with disease activity.
>
> Hypergammaglobulinemia, particularly IgA class

Pathology All involved tissues: necrotizing vasculitis of small arteries/veins with intra- or extravascular granuloma formation. Kidneys: focal/segmental glomerulonephritis.

Imaging *Paranasal sinuses:* opacification, with or without sclerosis. *Chest:* pulmonary infiltrates, nodules, consolidation, cavitation; upper lobes.

Diagnosis

Disease triad of necrotizing granulomatous vasculitis of upper and lower respiratory tract associated with glomerulonephritis.

ARA 1990 criteria for the classification* of Wegener's granulomatosis (traditional format): see Table 15-E

Pathophysiology

Immunopathogenesis unclear. Possibly an aberrant hypersensitivity response to an exogenous or endogenous antigen that enters through or resides in upper airways. Clinical symptomatology caused by necrotizing vasculitis of small arteries and veins. Pulmonary involvement: multiple, bilateral, nodular infiltrates. Similar infiltrates in paranasal sinuses, nasopharynx.

Course and Prognosis

Untreated, usually fatal because of rapidly progressive renal failure. With combination cyclophosphamide plus prednisone therapy, long-term remission is achieved in 90 % of cases.

Management

Treatment of Choice Cyclophosphamide plus prednisone

CYCLOPHOSPHAMIDE 2 mg/kg of body weight per day. Dose should be adjusted to keep leukocyte count >5000/μl (neutrophil count >1500/μl) to avoid infections associated with neutropenia. Therapy should be continued for 1 year after complete remission, then tapered and discontinued. *Alternative drug:* azathioprine given in similar doses if cyclophosphamide is not tolerated.

PREDNISONE 1 mg/kg of body weight per day is given for 1 month and then changed to alternate-day dosing, tapering, and discontinuing the drug after 6 months of therapy.

*For purposes of classification, a patient shall be said to have Wegener's granulomatosis if at least two of these four criteria are present. The presence of any two or more criteria yields a sensitivity of 88.2 % and a specificity of 92.0 %.

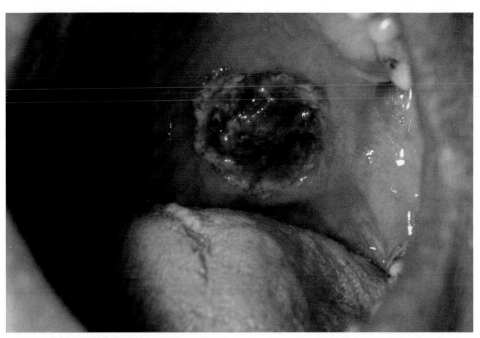

Figure 15-39 Wegener's granulomatosis *A large ulcer on the palate covered by a dense, adherent, necrotic mass; similar lesions occur in the sinuses and tracheobronchial tree.*

TABLE 15-E

Criteria	Definition
1. Nasal or oral inflammation	Development of painful or painless oral ulcers or purulent or bloody nasal discharge
2. Abnormal chest radiograph	Chest radiograph showing the presence of nodules, fixed infiltrates, or cavities
3. Urinary sediment	Microhematuria (>5 red blood cells per high-power field) or red cell casts in urine sediment
4. Granulomatous inflammation on biopsy	Histologic changes showing granulomatous inflammation within the wall of an artery or in the perivascular or extravascular area (artery or arteriole)

GIANT CELL ARTERITIS

Giant cell arteritis is a systemic granulomatous vasculitis of medium- and large-sized arteries, most notably the temporal artery and other branches of the carotid artery, characterized by headaches, fatigue, fever, anemia, and high ESR, in elderly patients.
Synonyms: Temporal arteritis, cranial arteritis.

Epidemiology and Etiology

Age Elderly, usually >55 years

Sex Females > males

Etiology Unknown. Probably via cell-mediated immunity.

Clinical Variants Temporal arteritis is a characteristic regional expression of giant cell arteritis affecting the temporal and other cranial arteries, which may or may not be accompanied by clinical symptoms of systemic involvement. Association with polymyalgia rheumatica

History

Systems Review Fatigue. Fever. Chronic disease syndrome. Headache usually bilateral. Scalp pain. Claudication of jaw/tongue while talking/chewing. Eye involvement: transient impairment of vision, ischemic optic neuritis, retrobulbar neuritis, persistent blindness. Systemic vasculitis: claudication of extremities, stroke, myocardial infarction, aortic aneurysms/dissections, visceral organ infarction. Polymyalgia rheumatica syndrome: stiffness, aching, pain in the muscles of the neck, shoulders, lower back, hips, thighs.

Physical Examination

Skin Lesions

TYPES Superficial temporal arteries are swollen, prominent, tortuous, ±nodular thickenings (Figure 15-40). ±Erythema of overlying skin. Scalp gangrene, i.e., skin infarction with sharp, irregular borders; ulceration with exposure of bone (Figure 15-41). Scars at sites of old ulcerations. Postinflammatory hyperpigmentation over involved artery.

PALPATION Tender. Initially, involved artery pulsates; later, occluded with loss of pulsation.

DISTRIBUTION Skin supplied by superficial temporal/occipital arteries in the temporal/parietal scalp

General Examination Findings in other organ systems related to tissue ischemia/infarction

Differential Diagnosis

Other vasculitides

Laboratory and Special Examinations

CBC Normochromic/slightly hypochromic anemia

ESR Marked elevation

Temporal Artery Biopsy Biopsy tender nodule of involved artery with or without overlying affected skin after Doppler flow examination. Lesions focal; section serially. Panarteritis with inflammatory mononuclear cell infiltrates within the vessel wall with frequent giant cell granuloma formation. Intimal proliferation with vascular occlusion, fragmentation of internal elastic lamina, extensive necrosis of intima and media.

Diagnosis

ARA 1990 criteria for the classification* of giant cell (temporal) arteritis (traditional format): Table 15-F

*For purposes of classification, a patient shall be said to have giant cell arteries (temporal) arteritis if at least three of these five criteria are present. The presence of any three or more criteria yields a sensitivity of 93.5 % and a specificity of 91.2 %.

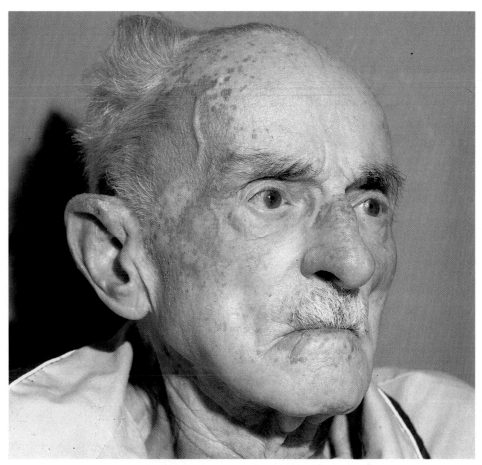

Figure 15-40 Giant cell arteritis *The superficial temporal artery is prominent, and on palpation is tender and pulseless in an elderly male. An incidental finding is extensive vitiligo with islands of repigmentation.*

TABLE 15-F

Criteria	Definition
1. Age at disease onset $\geq$ 50 years	Development of symptoms or findings beginning at age 50 or older
2. New headache	New onset or new type of localized pain in the head
3. Temporal artery abnormality	Temporal artery tenderness to palpation or decreased pulsation, unrelated to arteriosclerosis of cervical arteries
4. Elevated ESR	Erythrocyte sedimentation rate $\geq$ 50 mm/h by the Westergren method
5. Abnormal artery biopsy	Biopsy specimen with artery showing vasculitis characterized by a predominance of mononuclear cell infiltration or granulomatous inflammation, usually with multinucleated giant cells

Pathophysiology

Systemic vasculitis of multiple medium- and large-sized arteries. Symptoms secondary to ischemia.

Course and Prognosis

Untreated can result in blindness secondary to ischemic optic neuritis. Excellent response to adequate therapy. Remission following several years.

Management

Prednisone Initially 40 to 60 mg/day; taper when symptoms abate; continue 7.5 to 10 mg/day for 1 to 2 years.

Methotrexate Initial observations indicate that low-dose (0.15 to 0.30 mg/kg) methotrexate, once a week, may have a considerable corticosteroid-sparing effect in giant cell arteritis.

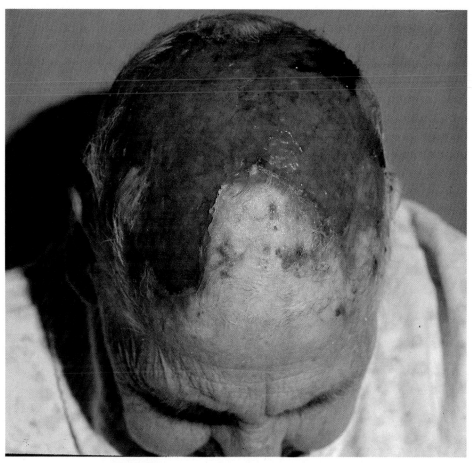

Figure 15-41 Giant cell arteritis *Extensive bilateral infarction and ulceration of the scalp of an elderly female secondary to vascular occlusion of temporal arteries.*

URTICARIAL VASCULITIS

Urticarial vasculitis is a multisystem disease characterized by cutaneous lesions resembling urticaria, except that they persist more than 24 hours, generally up to 3 to 4 days. There are also fever, arthralgia, elevated sedimentation rate, and histologic findings of a leukocytoclastic vasculitis. The syndrome is often accompanied by varying degrees of extracutaneous involvement.
Synonym: Urticaria perstans.

Epidemiology and Etiology

Age   Majority 30 to 50 years

Sex   Female : male ratio 3 : 1

Etiology   In patients with serum sickness, in collagen vascular diseases, with certain infections (e.g., hepatitis B), and idiopathic

Incidence   <5 % of patients with urticaria

History

Systems Review   *Lesions may be associated with itching, burning, stinging sensation, pain, tenderness.* Fever (10 % to 15 %). Arthralgias with or without arthritis in one or more joints (ankles, knees, elbows, wrists, small joints of fingers). Nausea, abdominal pain. Cough, dyspnea, chest pain, hemoptysis. Pseudotumor cerebri. Cold sensitivity. Renal involvement: diffuse glomerulonephritis. May be cutaneous manifestations of SLE.

Physical Examination

Skin Lesions

TYPES   Urticaria-like (i.e., edematous) lesions: raised, occasionally indurated, erythematous, circumscribed wheals (Figure 15-42); macular erythema; angioedema. Eruption occurs in transient crops, *usually lasting more than 24 hours and up to 3 to 4 days,* changing shape slowly, may or may not resolve with purpura; hyperpigmentation.

COLOR   Erythematous. Resolving lesions, yellowish-green stain.

PALPATION   Indurated. Blanch when pressed, but purpura remains.

General Examination   Extracutaneous manifestations: joints (70 %), GI tract (20 % to 30 %), CNS (>10 %), ocular system (>10 %), kidneys (10 % to 20 %), lymphadenopathy (5 %)

Differential Diagnosis

Urticaria-Like Lesion of Several Days Duration   Urticaria, serum sickness, other vasculitides, SLE, urticaria in acute hepatitis B infection

Laboratory and Special Examination

Dermatopathology   Biopsy several early lesions, which may show inflammation of dermal venules primarily with neutrophils without necrotic vasculitis. Later features may show frank leukocytoclastic vasculitis: perivascular infiltrate consisting primarily of neutrophils; leukocytoclasia; fibrinoid deposition in/around vessel walls; endothelial cell swelling; slight to moderate extravasation of RBC. In some patients there is no histologic evidence of leukocytoclastic vasculitis, and these lesions are most often related to circulating immune complex (Gell and Coombs type III) immunologic reactions that occur 1 to 2 weeks after exposure to antigens such as heterologous serum or certain infectious agents or drugs. In contrast, common urticaria exhibits dermal edema; sparse perivascular lymphohistiocytic infiltrate with or without eosinophils.

Urinalysis   10 % of patients—microhematuria, proteinuria

ESR   Elevated

Serologic Findings   Hypocomplementemia (70 %); circulating immune complexes

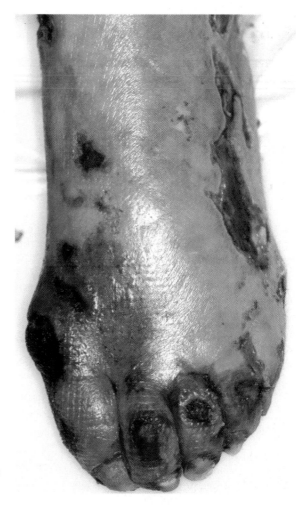

Figure 15-45 Cryoglobulinemia, mixed *Associated Raynaud's phenomenon and arterial occlusion have resulted in extensive necroses, hemorrhage, and ulcerations on the skin of the foot.*

REITER'S SYNDROME

Reiter's syndrome (RS) is defined by an episode of peripheral arthritis of more than 1 month's duration occurring in association with urethritis and/or cervicitis, which is frequently accompanied by keratoderma blennorrhagicum, circinate balanitis, conjunctivitis, and stomatitis, that is to say, the classic triad of arthritis, urethritis, and conjunctivitis.

Epidemiology and Etiology

Age 22 years (median) in postvenereal type

Sex 90 % of patients are males (postvenereal type).

Race Most common in Caucasians from northern Europe; rare in Asians and African blacks

Genetic Diathesis HLA-B27 occurs in up to 75 % of Caucasians with RS but in only 8 % of normal whites. B27-negative patients have a milder course, with significantly less sacroiliitis, uveitis, and carditis.

Associated Disorders Incidence of RS may be increased in HIV-infected individuals.

Etiology Unknown

History

Onset of Symptoms 1 to 4 weeks following infection: enterocolitis (shigellosis or other enteric pathogen infection); nongonococcal urethritis (*Chlamydia* or *Ureaplasma urealyticum*). Urethritis and/or conjunctivitis usually first to appear, followed by arthritis.

History Malaise, fever. Dysuria, urethral discharge. Eyes: red, slightly sensitive. Arthritis: tendon/fascia inflammation results in pain over ischial tuberosities, iliac crest, long bones, rib; heel pain at site of attachment of plantar aponeurosis and/or Achilles tendon; back pain; joint pains.

Physical Examination

Skin Lesions Lesions resemble those of psoriasis, especially on palms/soles, glans penis, mouth.

TYPES *Keratoderma blennorrhagicum* (KDB): early papules, vesicles, or macules that enlarge; centers of lesions become pustular and/or hyperkeratotic, crusted (Figure 15-46), i.e., resembling mollusk shells or ostraceous. Erosive patches resembling pustular psoriasis may occur, especially on shaft of penis, scrotum. *Circinate balanitis* (Figure 15-47): shallow erosions with serpiginous borders if uncircumcised; crusted and/or hyperkeratotic plaques if circumcised, i.e., psoriasiform.

COLOR Eroded lesions erythematous. Hyperkeratotic lesions yellow-tan

ARRANGEMENT Random; lesions may be scanty or numerous to the point of confluence.

DISTRIBUTION KDB: soles and palms. Scaling plaques: scalp, elbows, knees, buttocks.

Nails Small subungual pustules; extensive involvement may result in onycholysis and extensive subungual hyperkeratosis with erythema surrounding the nail.

Mucous Membranes *Urethra* Sterile serous or mucopurulent discharge
   Mouth Erosive lesions on tongue or hard palate resembling migratory glossitis
   Eyes Conjunctivitis (Figure 15-48), mild, evanescent, bilateral; anterior uveitis

Systemic Findings Arthritis: oligoarticular, involving up to six joints, asymmetric; most commonly knees, ankles, small joints of feet, diffuse swelling of fingers and toes

Differential Diagnosis

Arthritis Plus Skin Lesions Psoriasis vulgaris with psoriatic arthritis, disseminating

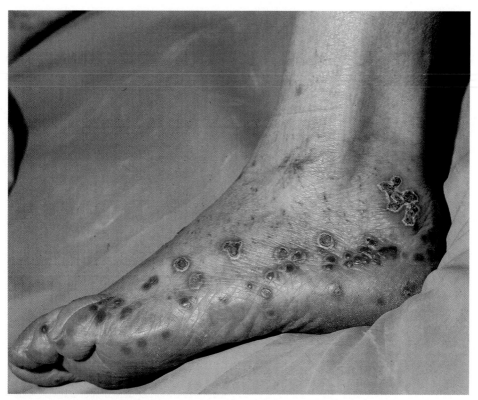

Figure 15-46 Reiter's syndrome: keratoderma blennorrhagicum *Red-to-brown papules, vesicles, and pustules with central erosion and characteristic crusting and peripheral scaling on the dorsilateral and plantar foot.*

gonococcal infection, SLE, ankylosing spondylitis, rheumatoid arthritis, gout, Behçet's disease

Laboratory and Special Examinations

Hematology   Nonspecific findings: anemia, leukocytosis, thrombocytosis, elevated ESR

Culture   Urethral culture negative for gonococcus

Serology   ANA, rheumatoid factor negative. Rule out HIV infection.

Dermatopathology   *Epidermis:* acutely, spongiosis, vesiculation; later, psoriasiform epidermal hyperplasia, spongiform pustules, parakeratosis. *Dermis:* perivascular neutrophilic infiltrate in superficial dermis; edema.

Diagnosis

Clinical findings; ruling out other spondylo- and reactive arthropathies.

Pathophysiology

RS appears linked to two factors: *genetic factors,* i.e., HLA-B27 in up to 75 % of Caucasians (8 % incidence in normal whites); *enteric pathogens* such as *Salmonella enteritidis, S. typhimurium, S. heidelberg; Yersinia enterocolitica, Y. pseudotuberculosis; Campylobacter fe-*

tus, Shigella flexneri. Two patterns are observed: the *epidemic form,* which follows venereal exposure, the most common type in the United States and the United Kingdom, and the *postdysenteric form,* the most common type of RS seen in continental Europe and North Africa.

Course and Prognosis

Only 30 % of RS patients develop complete triad of arthritis, urethritis, conjunctivitis; 40 % have only one manifestation, i.e., incomplete RS. Majority have self-limited course, with resolution in 3 to 12 months. RS may relapse over many years in 30 %. Chronic deforming arthritis in 10 % to 20 %.

Management

Prior Infection   Role of antibiotic therapy unproven in altering course of postvenereal RS

Cutaneous Manifestations   Similar to management of psoriasis (see Section 4). Balanitis: low-potency corticosteroids. Palmar/plantar: potent corticosteroid preparations, which are more effective under plastic occlusion. Extensive or refractory disease: phototherapy and PUVA.

Prevent Articular Inflammatory/Joint Deformity   Rest, nonsteroidal anti-inflammatory agents. Occasionally, phenylbutazone, methotrexate, or etretinate is indicated. In HIV-infected, zidovudine may improve RS.

Methotrexate, Etretinate   Effective in treatment of arthritis and cutaneous manifestations

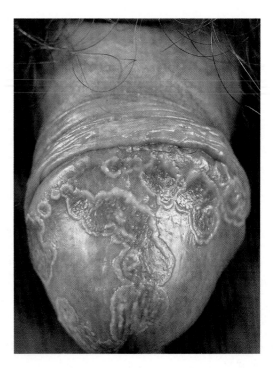

Figure 15-47 Reiter's syndrome: balanitis circinata *Moist, well-demarcated erosions with a slightly raised micropustular circinate border on the glans penis.*

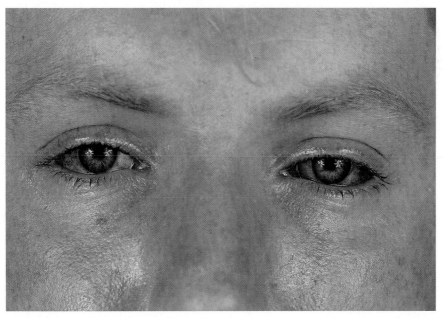

Figure 15-48 Reiter's syndrome: conjunctivitis *Bilateral conjunctivitis associated with anterior uveitis.*

PYODERMA GANGRENOSUM

Pyoderma gangrenosum (PG) is a rapidly evolving, idiopathic, chronic, and severely debilitating skin disease occurring most commonly in association with a systemic disease, especially chronic ulcerative colitis, and characterized by the presence of irregular, boggy, blue-red ulcers with undermined borders surrounding purulent necrotic bases.

Etiology

Unknown

History

Acute onset with painful hemorrhagic pustule or painful nodule either *de novo* or following minimal trauma.

Physical Examination

Skin Lesions

TYPES   *Primary lesion:* deep-seated nodule or superficial hemorrhagic pustule (Figure 15-49). Breakdown of this lesion occurs with ulcer formation (Figure 15-50). *Ulcer borders:* irregular and raised, undermined, boggy, with perforations that drain pus. *Ulcer base:* purulent, hemorrhagic exudate; partially covered by necrotic eschar; with or without granulation tissue. Pustules may be seen at the advancing border and in the ulcer base. Healing of ulcers results in thin, atrophic, $\pm$ cribriform scar. Pathergy, i.e., slight trauma initiating new PG lesion, noted at sites of minor trauma, biopsy sites, needle sticks.

COLOR   *Ulcer border:* dusky red or purple. Halo of erythema spreads centrifugally at the advancing edge of ulcer.

PALPATION   Primary nodule and ulcer are painful.

SHAPE   Ulcer margin may be irregular or serpiginous.

ARRANGEMENT   Usually solitary. May form in clusters that coalesce.

DISTRIBUTION   Most common sites: lower extremities >buttocks >abdomen >face

Mucous Membranes   Rarely, aphthous stomatitis–like lesions; massive ulceration of oral mucosa and conjunctivae

General Examination   Patient may appear ill.

Associated Systemic Diseases   Up to 50 % occur without associated disease. Remainder of cases associated with large- and small-bowel disease (Crohn's disease, ulcerative colitis), diverticulosis (diverticulitis), arthritis, paraproteinemia and myeloma, leukemia, active chronic hepatitis, Behçet's syndrome.

Differential Diagnosis

Large Cutaneous Ulcer(s)   Progressive synergistic gangrene, ecthyma gangrenosum, atypical mycobacterial infection, clostridial infection, deep mycoses, amebiasis, bromoderma, pemphigus vegetans, stasis ulcers, Wegener's granulomatosis

Laboratory and Special Examinations

CBC, ESR   Variably elevated

Dermatopathology   Not diagnostic. Neutrophilic inflammation with abscess formation and necrosis

Diagnosis

Clinical findings plus course of illness

Course and Prognosis

Untreated, course may last months to years. Ulceration may extend rapidly within a few days

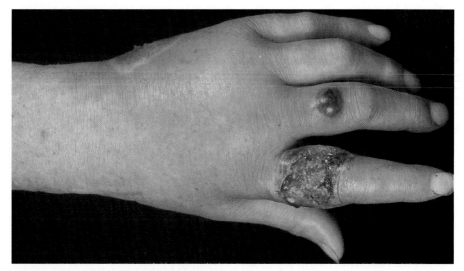

Figure 15-49 Pyoderma gangrenosum: early *Three large hemorrhagic bullae on the dorsum of the hand and fingers. The bulla on the index finger has ruptured, resulting in a large erosion with an irregular, raised, pustular border and a purulent hemorrhagic exudate.*

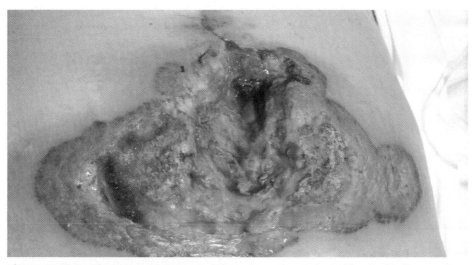

Figure 15-50 Pyoderma gangrenosum: later *A very large ulcer with raised bullous, undermined, boggy border covered with a purulent hemorrhagic exudate; the lesion arose at a recent operative site and extends deeply into the subcutaneous fat.*

or slowly. Healing may occur centrally with peripheral extension. New ulcers may appear as older lesions resolve.

Management

With Associated Underlying Disease Treat underlying disease.

For PG High doses of oral corticosteroids or IV corticosteroid pulse therapy (1 to 2 g prednisolone per day) may be required. ±Intralesional triamcinolone. Sulfasalazine, sulfones, and cyclosporine have been shown to be effective in uncontrolled studies.

SWEET'S SYNDROME

Sweet's syndrome (SS) is an uncommon, recurrent skin disease characterized by painful plaque-forming inflammatory papules and associated with fever, arthralgia, and peripheral leukocytosis. *Synonym:* Acute febrile neutrophilic dermatosis.

Epidemiology and Etiology

Age   Majority 30 to 60 years

Sex   Women > men

Etiology   Unknown, possibly hypersensitivity reaction. In some cases associated with *Yersinia* infection

Associated Disorders   Febrile upper respiratory tract infection. Hematologic malignancy

History

Prodrome   Febrile upper respiratory tract infection, GI symptoms (diarrhea), tonsillitis, influenza-like illness, 1 to 3 weeks prior to skin lesions

Systems Review   Lesions tender/painful. Fever, headache, arthralgia, general malaise.

Physical Examination

Skin Lesions

TYPES   Papules or nodules that coalesce to form irregular, sharply bordered inflammatory plaques (Figure 15-51). Intense edema gives appearance of vesiculation (Figure 15-52). ±Tiny pustules. If associated with leukemia, bullous lesions may occur, and lesions may mimic pyoderma gangrenosum.

COLOR   Red, bluish red

PALPATION   *Lesions are tender.*

SHAPE   As lesions evolve, central clearing may lead to annular or arcuate patterns.

ARRANGEMENT   May present as single lesion or multiple lesions, asymmetrically distributed.

DISTRIBUTION   Most commonly, face, neck (Figure 15-51), upper extremities (Figure 15-52); also, lower extremities, where lesions may be deep in the panniculus and thus mimic panniculitis or erythema nodosum. Truncal lesions uncommon. Widespread and generalized forms occur.

Mucous Membranes   ±Conjunctivitis, episcleritis

General Examination   Patient may appear ill.

Differential Diagnosis

Very Edematous Acute Nodules/Plaques
Erythema multiforme, erythema nodosum, prevesicular herpes simplex infection, preulcerative pyoderma gangrenosum, bowel-bypass syndrome, urticaria, serum sickness, other vasculitides, SLE panniculitis

Laboratory and Special Examinations

CBC   Leukocytosis with neutrophilia

ESR   Elevated

Dermatopathology   Epidermis usually normal but may show subcorneal pustulation. Massive edema of papillary body, dense leukocytic infiltrate with starburst pattern of lower dermis. Infiltrate: diffuse or perivascular, consisting of neutrophils with occasional eosinophils/lymphoid cells. Leukocytoclasia leading to nuclear dust, but other signs of vasculitis absent. ± Neutrophilic infiltrates in subcutaneous tissue.

Diagnosis

Clinical impression plus skin biopsy confirmation

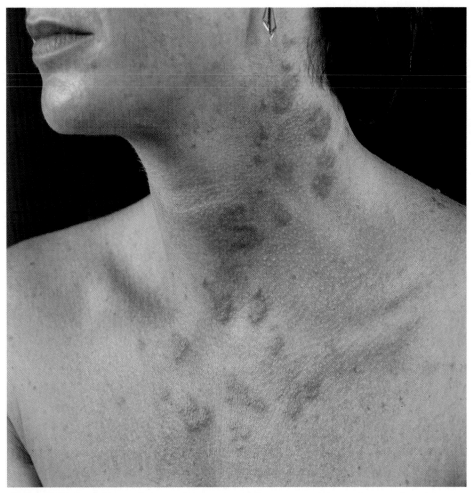

Figure 15-51 Sweet's syndrome *Edematous, erythematous papules coalesce to form irregular, inflammatory, mammillated (covered with nipple-like protuberances) plaques on the neck and upper chest.*

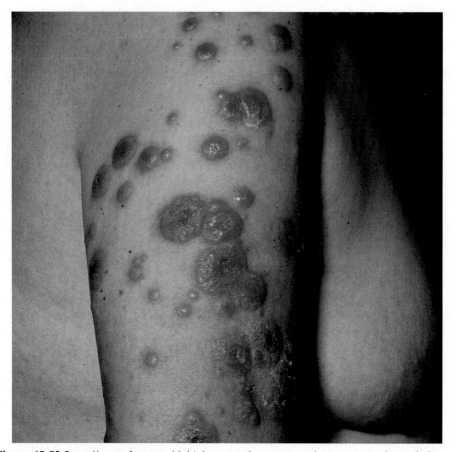

Figure 15-52 Sweet's syndrome *Multiple, very edematous, erythematous papules and plaques on the upper arm with areas of epidermal necrosis, erosion, exudation, and crusting. The lesions appear to be bullous but are firm on palpation, i.e., pseudovesiculation.*

Course and Prognosis

Untreated, lesions enlarge over a period of days or weeks and eventually resolve without scarring after weeks or months. Treated with oral prednisone, lesions resolve within a few days. Recurrences occur in 50 % of patients, often in previously involved sites. Some cases follow *Yersinia* infection or are associated with acute myeloid leukemia, transient myeloid proliferation, various malignant tumors, ulcerative colitis, benign monoclonal gammopathy.

Management

Rule out sepsis.

Prednisone   30 to 60 mg daily, tapering in 2 to 3 weeks; some but not all cases respond to dapsone, 100 mg/day, or to potassium iodide.

Antibiotic Therapy Clears eruption in *Yersinia*-associated cases; in all other cases antibiotics are ineffective.

PEMPHIGUS VULGARIS

Pemphigus vulgaris (PV) is a serious, acute or chronic, bullous, autoimmune disease of skin and mucous membranes that is often fatal unless treated with immunosuppressive agents.

Epidemiology and Etiology

Age   40 to 60 years

Sex   Equal incidence in males and in females

Etiology   Autoimmune disorder

History

Duration of Lesions   PV starts usually in oral mucosa, and months may elapse before skin lesions occur; these may be localized for 6 to 12 months, following which generalized bullae occur. Less frequently there may be a generalized, acute eruption of bullae from the beginning.

Skin Symptoms   No pruritus; painful and tender mouth lesions may prevent adequate food intake. Skin lesions: burning, pain

Constitutional Symptoms   Weakness, malaise, weight loss (if prolonged mouth involvement)

Systems Review   Epistaxis, hoarseness, dysphagia

Physical Examination

Skin Lesions

TYPES   Vesicles and bullae (Figure 15-53), flaccid (flabby), easily ruptured, and weeping, arising on normal skin. Extensive erosions that bleed easily, crusts particularly on scalp.

COLOR   Skin-colored

SHAPE   Round or oval

ARRANGEMENT   Randomly scattered, discrete lesions (Figure 15-54)

DISTRIBUTION   Localized (e.g., to mouth) or generalized with a random pattern (Figure 15-54)

NIKOLSKY'S SIGN   Dislodging of epidermis by lateral finger pressure in the vicinity of lesions, which leads to an erosion. Pressure on bulla leads to lateral extension of blister.

SITES OF PREDILECTION   Scalp, face, chest, axillae, groin, umbilicus

Mucous Membranes   Bullae rarely seen, erosions of mouth (Figure 15-55) and nose, pharynx and larynx, vagina

Laboratory and Special Examinations

Dermatopathology   Light microscopy (select early small bulla or, if not present, margin of larger bulla or erosion): (1) loss of intercellular cohesion in lower part of epidermis, leading to (2) acantholysis (separation of keratinocytes) and to (3) bulla that is split just *above* the basal cell layer and contains separated, rounded-up (acantholytic) keratinocytes.

Immunofluorescence (IF)   Direct IF staining reveals IgG and often C3 deposited in lesional and paralesional skin in *the intercellular substance of the epidermis.*

Serum   Autoantibodies (IgG) detected by indirect immunofluorescence. Titer usually correlates with activity of disease process. Autoantibodies are directed against a 130-kDa glycoprotein designated Desmoglein III, a member of the cadherin superfamily.

Diagnosis

Can be a difficult, subtle problem if only mouth lesions are present. Biopsy of the skin and mucous membrane, direct immunofluorescence, and demonstration of circulating autoantibodies confirm a high index of suspicion.

Pathophysiology

A loss of the normal cell-to-cell adhesion in the epidermis occurs as a result of circulating antibodies of the IgG class; these antibodies bind to cell surface glycoproteins (pemphigus antigens) of the epidermis and induce acantholysis, probably by the activation of serine proteases.

Course

The disease inexorably progresses to death unless treated aggressively with immunosuppressive agents. The mortality has been markedly reduced since treatment has become available.

Variants

Pemphigus Vegetans (PVeg) Usually confined to intertriginous regions, perioral area, neck, and scalp. Granulomatous vegetating purulent plaques that extend centrifugally. Suprabasal acantholysis with intraepidermal abscesses containing mostly eosinophils. Pseudoepitheliomatous hyperplasia of the epidermis, exuberant granulation tissue with abscess formation. IgG autoantibodies as in PV. PV may evolve into PVeg and vice versa.

Pemphigus Foliaceus (PF) Most commonly on face, scalp, upper chest, and abdomen but may involve entire skin, presenting as exfoliative erythroderma. Superficial form of pemphigus with acantholysis in the granular layer of the epidermis. Bullae hardly ever present; lesions consist of erythematous patches and erosions covered with crusts. PF is also mediated by circulating autoantibodies to an intercellular (cell surface) antigen, Desmoglein I, in the desmosomes of keratinocytes but PV (130 kDa) and PF (160 kDa) antigens differ. This explains the different sites of acantholysis and thus the different clinical appearances of the two conditions.

Brazilian Pemphigus (Fogo Selvagem) A distinctive form of pemphigus foliaceus endemic to south central Brazil. Clinically, histologically, and immunopathologically the disease is identical to PF. Patients improve when moved to urban areas but relapse after returning to endemic regions. It is speculated that the disease is somehow related to an arthropod-borne infectious agent. More than 1000 new cases per year are estimated to occur in the endemic regions.

Pemphigus Erythematosus (PE) *Synonym:* Senear-Usher syndrome. A localized variety of PF largely confined to seborrheic sites. Erythematous, crusted, and erosive lesions in the "butterfly" area of the face, forehead, presternal, and interscapular regions. Despite clinical, histopathologic, and immunopathologic similarity to PF, PE may be unique, since patients have immunoglobulin and complement deposits at the dermal-epidermal junction in addition to intercellular pemphigus antibody in the epidermis and antinuclear antibodies, as is the case in lupus erythematosus. In addition, PE may be associated with thymoma and myasthenia gravis.

Drug-Induced Pemphigus A PV- and PF/PE-like syndrome can be induced by D-penicillamine and less frequently by captopril and other drugs. In most, but not all, instances the eruption resolves after termination of therapy with the offending drug.

Management

Corticosteroids 2.0 to 3.0 mg/kg of body weight of prednisone until cessation of new blister formation and disappearance of Nikolsky's sign. Then rapid reduction to about half the initial dose until patient is almost clear, followed by slow tapering of dose to minimal effective maintenance dose.

Concomitant Immunosuppressive Therapy Immunosuppressive agents are given concomitantly for their corticosteroid-saving effect:

Azathioprine, 2.0 to 3.0 mg/kg of body weight until complete clearing; tapering

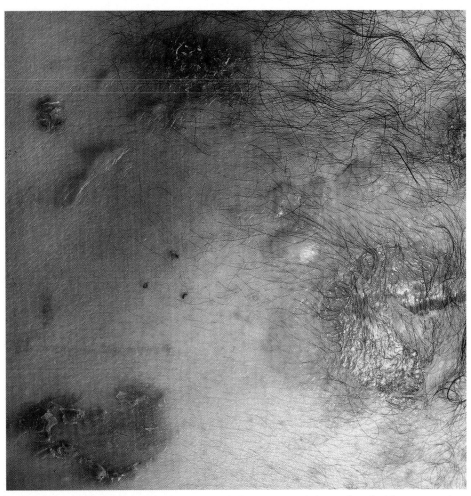

Figure 15-53 Pemphigus vulgaris *Flaccid bullae on normal skin with and without an erythematous base. The largest bullae has ruptured and collapsed; mild trauma to the site will result in denudation of the epidermis in the bulla roof and a large erosion. In contrast with the bullae of bullous pemphigoid which are tense and intact, those of pemphigus vulgaris arise within the epidermis, are more fragile and flaccid, and may be few in number compared with the number of eroded sites.*

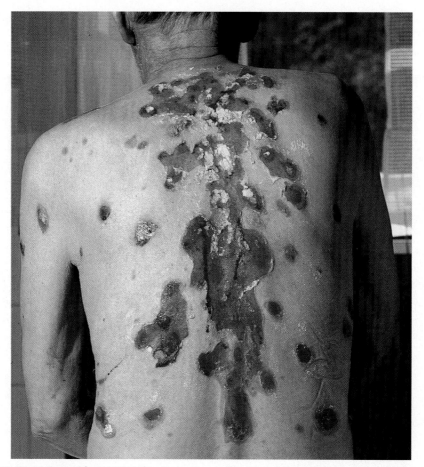

Figure 15-54 Pemphigus vulgaris *Extensive confluent erosions and crusts with a few large, intact, flaccid bullae on the back; eroded sites tend to bleed with minimal trauma and are quite painful.*

of dose to 1.0 mg/kg. Azathioprine alone is continued even after cessation of corticosteroid treatment and may have to be continued for many months. Clinical freedom from disease and a negative pemphigus antibody titer for at least 3 months permit cessation of therapy.

Methotrexate, either PO or IM at doses of 25 to 35 mg per week. Dose adjustments are made as with azathioprine.

Cyclophosphamide, 100 to 200 mg daily, with reduction to maintenance doses of 50 to 100 mg/day. Alternatively, cyclophosphamide "bolus" therapy with 1000 mg IV once a week or every 2 weeks in the initial phases, followed by 50 to 100 mg/day PO as maintenance.

Plasmapheresis, in conjunction with corticosteroids and immunosuppressives in poorly controlled patients, in the initial phases of treatment to reduce antibody titers.

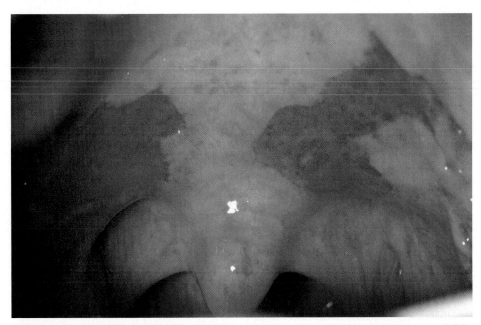

Figure 15-55 Pemphigus vulgaris *Extensive erosions on the soft palate that are very painful.*

Gold therapy, for milder cases. After an initial test dose of 10 mg IM, 25 to 50 mg of gold sodium thiomalate is given IM at weekly intervals to a maximum cumulative dose of 1 g.

Other measures: cleansing baths, wet dressings, topical and intralesional corticosteroids, antibiotics to combat bacterial infections. Correction of fluid and electrolyte imbalance.

Monitoring Clinical, for improvement of skin lesions and development of drug-related side effects. Laboratory monitoring of pemphigus antibody titers and for hematologic and metabolic indicators of corticosteroid- and/or immunosuppressive-induced adverse effects

BULLOUS PEMPHIGOID

Bullous pemphigoid is an autoimmune disorder presenting as a chronic bullous eruption mostly in patients over 60 years of age.
Synonym: parapemphigus.

Epidemiology

Age 60 to 80 years or childhood

Sex Equal incidence in males and in females

History

Duration of Lesions Often starts with a prodromal eruption (urticarial lesions) and evolves in weeks to months to bullae that may appear suddenly as a generalized eruption

Skin Symptoms Initially, usually none except mouth lesions; occasionally, moderate pruritus and tenderness of eroded lesions

Constitutional Symptoms None, except in widespread, severe disease

Physical Examination

Skin Lesions

TYPES Erosions. Erythematous, urticarial-type lesions, not unlike the lesions in erythema multiforme (Figure 15-56), may precede bullae formation by months. Bullae, large, tense, firm-topped (Figure 15-57); may arise in normal or erythematous skin.

SHAPE Bullae are oval or round.

ARRANGEMENT Arciform, annular, or serpiginous lesions are scattered and discrete.

DISTRIBUTION Generalized or localized and randomly distributed

SITES OF PREDILECTION Axillae; medial aspects of thighs, groins, abdomen; flexor aspects of forearms; lower legs (often first manifestation)

Mucous Membranes Mouth, anus, vagina; less common and less severe and painful than in pemphigus, the bullae less easily ruptured.

Differential Diagnosis

Histopathology and immunology permit a differentiation from pemphigus, erythema multiforme, or dermatitis herpetiformis.

Diagnosis

Clinical, confirmed by histopathology and immunopathology

Laboratory and Special Examinations

Dermatopathology

LIGHT MICROSCOPY Neutrophils in "Indian-file" alignment at dermal-epidermal junction; neutrophils, eosinophils, and lymphocytes in papillary dermis; subepidermal bullae, with regeneration of the floor of the bulla

ELECTRON MICROSCOPY Junctional cleavage, i.e., split occurs in lamina lucida of basement membrane.

IMMUNOPATHOLOGY IgG deposits along the basement membrane zone. Also, C3, which may occur in the absence of IgG.

SERUM Circulating anti-basement membrane IgG antibodies detected by indirect immunofluorescence in 70 % of patients. Titers do not correlate with course of disease. Autoantibodies in bullous pemphigoid recognize two types of antigens. BP-Ag1 is a 230-kDa glycoprotein (gene on short arm of

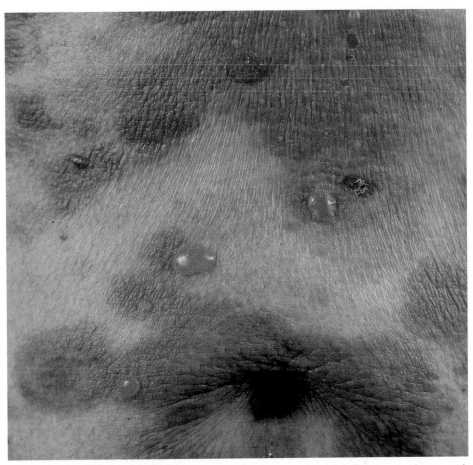

Figure 15-56 Bullous pemphigoid *Large, erythematous, urticarial, inflammatory plaques with only occasional vesiculation and some crusting. These nonbullous lesions may occur months to years before bulla formation.*

chromosome 6) that has high homology with desmoplakin I/II and is part of hemidesmosomes. BP-Ag2 is a transmembranous 180-kDa polypeptide encoded by a gene on the long arm of chromosome 10.

Hematology   Eosinophilia

Pathogenesis

Interaction of autoantibody with bullous pemphigoid antigen on the surface of basal keratinocytes (extending into the lamina lucida of basement membrane) is followed by complement activation and attraction of neutrophils and eosinophils. Bullous lesion results from interaction of multiple bioactive molecules released by mast cells and eosinophils.

Management

Systemic prednisone with starting doses of 50 to 100 mg to clear, either alone or combined with azathioprine 150 mg daily for remission induction and 50 to 100 mg for maintenance; in milder cases, sulfones (dapsone), 100 to 150 mg/day. In very mild cases and for local recurrences, topical corticosteroid therapy may have a beneficial effect. Tetracycline ± nicotinamide has been reported to be effective in some cases.

For patients under 50 years, systemic prednisone alone in divided doses of 50 to 100 mg is highly effective to initially control this autoimmune disease. Patients usually achieve remission in a few weeks, and the dose is gradually tapered. For patients older than 50 to 60 years, systemic prednisone in divided doses of 50 to 100 mg is started until remission occurs. Azathioprine is started simultaneously and continued after the clinical remission has been achieved. Patients will often go into a permanent remission and not require any therapy; the local recurrences can be controlled with topical corticosteroids or intralesional corticosteroids (triamcinolone suspensions).

Systemic prednisone alone can be a problem in older patients because of compression fractures, which may be disabling. Azathioprine, 150 mg daily, avoids this complication, but it takes about 4 to 6 weeks to become effective and this may not be possible if the disease is severe, generalized, and rapidly progressive. We have used methotrexate in older patients as the beginning and sole medication in the event that systemic prednisone is a problem for whatever reason: age, psychotic symptoms. After clearing has been accomplished with methotrexate, the patients are then shifted to tetracycline and nicotinic acid, which, however, is not always effective.

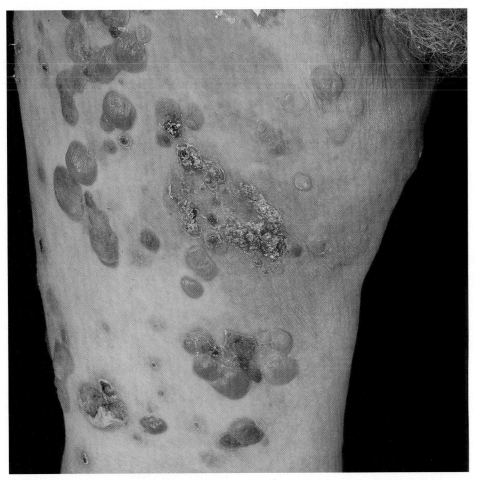

Figure 15-57 Bullous pemphigoid *Multiple tense bullae with a serous and partially hemorrhagic content on the thigh of an elderly woman. Some lesions have ruptured and the eroded sites are crusted. Postinflammatory hyperpigmentation is present at sites of prior erythematous urticarial-type lesions and bullae.*

SARCOIDOSIS

Sarcoidosis is a chronic granulomatous inflammation affecting diverse organs, but it presents primarily as skin lesions, eye lesions, bilateral hilar lymphadenopathy, and pulmonary infiltration.

Epidemiology and Etiology

Age   Under 40 years (range 12 to 70 years)

Sex   Equal incidence in males and in females

Race   All races. In the United States and South Africa, much more frequent in blacks. Frequent in Scandinavia.

Other Factors   The disease occurs worldwide, and there is no clue as to the etiology. The disease can occur in families.

History

Onset of Lesions   Days (presenting as acute erythema nodosum) or months (presenting as papules or plaques on skin or pulmonary infiltrate discovered on routine chest radiography)

Skin Symptoms   Asymptomatic

Constitutional Symptoms   Fever, fatigue, weight loss, arrhythmia

Systems Review   Enlarged parotids, cardiac dyspnea, neuropathy, kidney stones, uveitis, arthralgia (with erythema nodosum)

Physical Examination

Skin Lesions

TYPE AND COLOR

Brownish purple infiltrated plaques (Figure 15-58)

Lupus pernio—violaceous, soft, doughy infiltration of the nose (Figure 15-59), cheek, and earlobes

Multiple maculopapular lesions, 0.5 to 1.0 cm, yellowish brown

"Scar sarcoidosis"—translucent purple-red nodules occurring in an old scar (Figure 15-60)

Note: Upon blanching with glass slide, all cutaneous lesions of sarcoidosis reveal "apple jelly" yellowish brown color.

SHAPE   Annular, polycyclic, serpiginous

ARRANGEMENT   Scattered discrete lesions (maculopapular and nodular types) and diffuse infiltration (lupus pernio)

DISTRIBUTION *Plaques* Extremities, buttocks, trunk
Papular Face, extremities
Lupus Pernio Nose, cheeks, and earlobes
"Scar Sarcoidosis" Anywhere
Scalp May have scarring alopecia

Associations   In acute, bilateral hilar sarcoidosis, particularly in young women, the first clinical manifestation of sarcoidosis may be erythema nodosum (see page 336) and arthritis (Löfgren's syndrome). The Heerford syndrome describes patients with fever, parotid enlargement, uveitis, and facial nerve palsy.

Laboratory and Special Examinations

Dermatopathology   Large islands of epithelioid cells with a few giant cells, and lymphocytes (so-called naked tubercles). Asteroid bodies in large histiocytes; occasionally fibrinoid necrosis.

Skin Tests   Intracutaneous tests for recall antigens usually but not always negative. The Kveim-Silzbach test (antigen prepared from sarcoid spleen injected intracutaneously) is of historical interest only.

Imaging   Systemic involvement is verified radiologically by gallium scan and transbronchial, liver, or lymph node biopsy. In 90 % of patients: hilar lymphadenopathy, pulmonary infiltrate

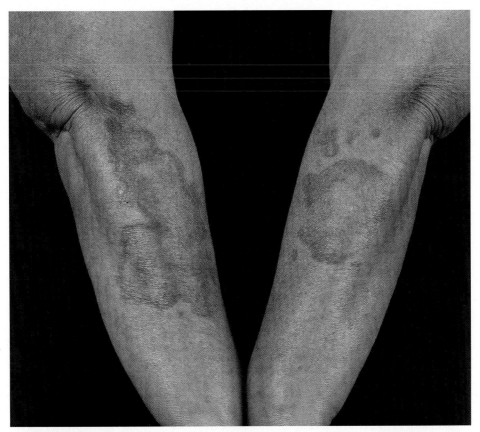

Figure 15-58 Sarcoidosis: granulomatous lesions *Multiple, circinate, confluent, firm, brownish-red, infiltrated plaques that show a tendency to resolve in the center. The lesions are diascopy positive, i.e., an "apple-jelly" tan-pink color remains in lesions after compression with glass.*

Blood Chemistry

Increase in serum angiotensin-converting enzyme (ACE)
Hypergammaglobulinemia
Hypercalcemia

Diagnosis

Tissue biopsy of skin or lymph nodes is the best criterion for diagnosis of sarcoidosis.

Management

Systemic Sarcoidosis Systemic corticosteroids for active ocular disease, active pulmonary disease, cardiac arrhythmia, CNS involvement, or hypercalcemia

Cutaneous Sarcoidosis

CORTICOSTEROIDS *Local* Intralesional triamcinolone 3 mg/ml effective for small lesions

Systemic For widespread or disfiguring involvement, prednisone

HYDROXYCHLOROQUINE 100 mg b.i.d. for widespread or disfiguring lesions refractory to intralesional triamcinolone. Not always effective.

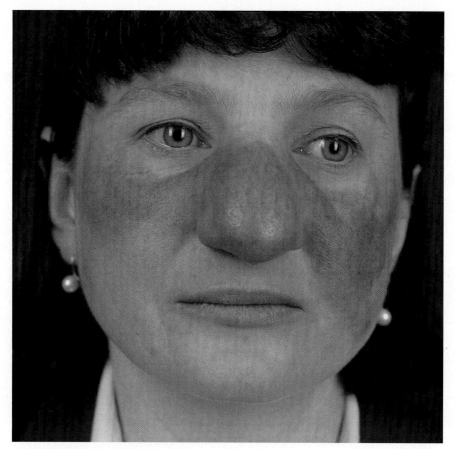

Figure 15-59 Sarcoidosis: lupus pernio *Extensive infiltration of the nose and cheeks by gran-ulomatous inflammation. (Pernio or chilblains is a congestion and swelling of the skin following cold exposure; lupus pernio arises on the nose and resembles cold-induced changes.)*

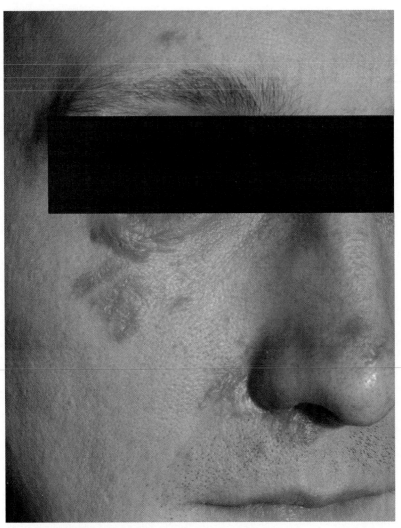

Figure 15-60 Sarcoidosis: granulomatous lesions arising in a scar *Yellowish-brown papules and plaques on the face in old atrophic posttraumatic scars. Upon diascopy these lesions exhibit an "apple-jelly"-like color.*

DISEASES IN PREGNANCY

PRURITIC URTICARIAL PAPULES AND PLAQUES OF PREGNANCY

Pruritic urticarial papules and plaques of pregnancy (PUPPP) is a distinct pruritic eruption of pregnancy that usually begins in the third trimester, most often in primigravidae. There is no increased risk of fetal morbidity or mortality.

Synonyms: Polymorphic eruption of pregnancy, toxemic rash of pregnancy, late-onset prurigo of pregnancy.

Epidemiology and Etiology

Age Average age 27 years

Etiology Unknown. The development of striae has been theorized to be a trigger for PUPPP. A relationship with maternal and fetal weight gain has been proposed but challenged.

Incidence Estimated to be 1:120 to 240 pregnancies

Risk Factors 76 % of patients are primigravidae. Some cases have been associated with polyhydramnions.

History

Signs and Symptoms Symptoms of pruritus develop on the abdomen, often in the striae distensae. The pruritus is severe enough to disrupt sleep.

Onset Average time of onset is 36 weeks of gestation, usually 1 to 2 weeks prior to delivery. Symptoms can start in the postpartum period.

Duration The skin lesions evolve over 1 to 2 weeks and taper off over 7 to 10 days.

Physical Examination

Skin Lesions

TYPES 1- to 3-mm erythematous papules (Figure 15-61), quickly coalescing into urticarial plaques (Figure 15-62) with polycyclic shape and arrangement; 2-mm vesicles oc-

cur in the plaques in 40 % of the cases. Target lesions are observed in 19 %. Bullae are absent. Although pruritus is the chief symptom, excoriations are infrequent.

COLOR Erythematous with hypopigmented halos around the periphery of lesions

DISTRIBUTION 50 % of the women affected have papules and plaques in the striae distensae (Figure 15-61); the abdomen, the buttocks, thighs (Figure 15-62), upper inner arms, and lower back also may be affected. The face, breasts, palms, and soles are rarely involved. The periumbilical area is usually spared.

Mucous Membranes No lesions

Differential Diagnosis

Pruritic Abdominal Rash in Late Pregnancy Herpes gestationis, adverse cutaneous drug reaction, allergic contact dermatitis, metabolic pruritus, atopic dermatitis

Laboratory Studies

Laboratory Findings Moderately elevated leukocyte count and sedimentation rate consistent with third-trimester pregnancy. Normal human chorionic gonadotropin, estrogen, and progesterone. No circulating complement-binding herpes gestationis (HG) factor.

Histology Superficial or middermal, loosely arranged perivascular lymphohistiocytic infiltrate with rare eosinophils. Some specimens

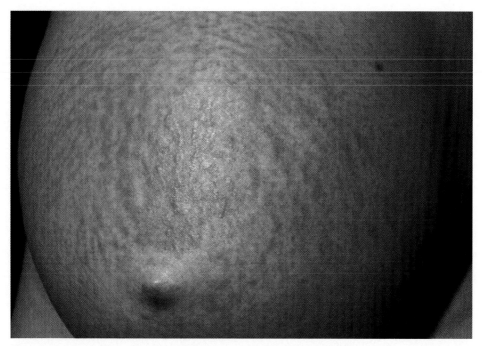

Figure 15-61 Pruritic urticarial papules and plaques of pregnancy *Small papules distributed and confluent within striae distensae on the abdomen in pregnant woman (35 weeks of gestation).*

may show dermal edema, with focal parakeratosis, spongiosis, microvesiculation, or exocytosis. Overall the histologic findings are nondiagnostic.

Direct Immunofluorescence No consistent findings of immunoreactants in lesional or perilesional skin. One case detected intercellular IgG epidermal immunoglobulins.

Pathophysiology There is little evidence to suggest that PUPPP is an autoimmune disease. This reaction may represent a maternal response to paternal antigens expressed in the fetal placenta. No HLA subtypes appear to be predisposed when patients are compared with North American controls. The pathophysiology of PUPPP is not understood.

Diagnosis

Clinical; immunofluorescence studies may be needed to differentiate PUPPP from herpes gestationis (HG), especially if there is evidence of papulovesicular lesions. HG may be associated with increased fetal morbidity and mortality. It often starts in the periumbilical areas, and involvement of the striae is not prominent. HG will always have C3 deposition at the basement membrane zone and is associated with HLA-B8, -DR3.

Course and Prognosis

The majority of women studied do not have a recurrence in the postpartum period or with subsequent pregnancies or the use of oral contraceptives. A recurrence is usually much milder than the original episode. The symptoms usually resolve within 10 days of delivery.

In one large series, there were no premature or postmature infants or spontaneous abortions; one stillborn (one of a set of twins) was reported. No consistent congenital abnormalities have been observed.

Management

Topical High-potency topical steroids may relieve the pruritus within 24 to 72 hours. Application of topical steroids often can be tapered off after 1 week of therapy. Baths and emollients may be helpful as supportive measures.

Systemic Oral prednisone in doses of 10 to 40 mg/day has been used for severe cases; often the symptoms are relieved in 24 hours. Oral antihistamines are generally ineffective.

Delivery The symptoms can be so severe and exhausting for the pregnant woman that early delivery may be a consideration; often the patient is better within several days.

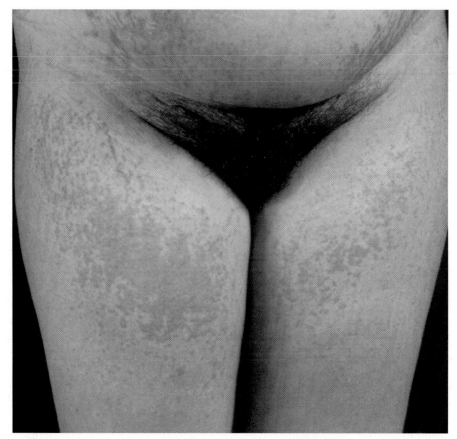

Figure 15-62 Pruritic urticarial papules and plaques of pregnancy *Papular urticaria-like lesions characteristically localized within striae distensae are also present on the upper thighs.*

HERPES GESTATIONIS

Herpes gestationis (HG) is a pruritic polymorphic inflammatory dermatosis of pregnancy and the postpartum period. It is an autoimmune process with circulating complement-fixing IgG antibodies in the serum and is unrelated to any known viral infection. It creates severe discomfort for the affected, but it is debated whether fetal prognosis is impaired.

Epidemiology

Incidence   Estimated to be 1:10,000 deliveries

Age and Sex   Pregnant women

Race   All races

Onset   Usually between the fourth and seventh months of pregnancy but has been reported also during the first trimester and in the postpartum period. Postpartum exacerbations are common. HG may or may not recur in subsequent pregnancies and is exacerbated by the use of estrogen- or progesterone-containing medications (e.g., contraceptives).

History

Skin Symptoms   Extremely pruritic eruption that causes great anxiety, particularly in primigravidae

Family History   Noncontributory

Systems Review   Negative

Physical Examination

Skin Lesions

TYPES   Papulovesicular eruption. Lesions vary from erythematous, edematous papules to urticarial lesions and large, tense bullae (Figure 15-63), erosions, and crusts. Grouping of lesions is pronounced, hence the name *herpes gestationis*. Milder cases present with only a few erythematous papules or isolated edematous urticarial plaques.

DISTRIBUTION   Mainly on the abdomen and lateral sides of the trunk but also involves other areas, including palms, soles, chest, back, and face.

Mucous Membranes   Spared

Hair and Nails   Spared

Differential Diagnosis

Pruritic Eruption in Pregnancy   Pruritic urticarial papules and plaques of pregnancy that occur usually late in pregnancy are also severely pruritic, are not vesicular, and have no immunoreactants at the epidermal-dermal junction. Other papular eruptions in pregnancy: erythema multiforme, dermatitis herpetiformis, bullous pemphigoid, adverse cutaneous drug reaction, atopic dermatitis.

Laboratory and Special Examinations

Dermatopathology   Variable. Lymphohistiocytic infiltrates with eosinophils and occasional neutrophils around superficial and deep dermal-vascular plexus. Edema of the dermal papillae and epidermis with vesicular lesions showing subepidermal blister formation in a bulbous teardrop shape, liquefaction, degeneration of basal cells of variable degree, and characteristic foci of basal cell necrosis over the tips of the dermal papillae, spongiosis.

Immunopathology   Heavy homogeneous linear deposition of C3 along basement membrane zone in peribullous and urticarial lesions and perilesional normal-appearing skin. Concomitant deposition of IgG in 30 % to 40 % of patients that is IgG1. Occasional IgA and IgM and rarely properdin, properdin factor B, or C1q and C4. Immunofluorescence findings persist for months and up to a year after lesions have resolved.

A serum complement-fixing factor, termed *HG factor*, is an avidly complement-fixing IgG antibody, presumably IgG1 (which often escapes detection by routine indirect immunofluorescence because of low concentration) in all patients. This factor binds to amniotic epithelial basement membrane.

Immunogenetic Studies   Marked increase in HLA-B8, HLA-DR3, and HLA-DR4

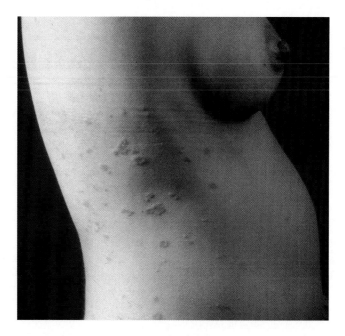

Figure 15-63 Herpes gestationis *Urticarial pruritic papules and plaques in a pregnant woman (28 weeks gestation).*

Diagnosis

Clinical setting confirmed by histology

Fetal Involvement

One study reveals significant fetal death and premature deliveries in a larger series of HG patients, whereas other studies suggested that there is no increase in fetal mortality. Children born of affected mothers usually have no skin lesions, but in some reports, babies have been described with urticarial, vesicular, and bullous lesions that resolve spontaneously. C3 deposition has been noted in clinically normal as well as affected infant skin, and HG factor has been detected in the sera of some infants born of affected mothers.

Pathogenesis

Etiology unknown. The C3 deposition at the basement membrane and HG factor suggest an immunologic mechanism similar to that in bullous pemphigoid. It is postulated that IgG antibodies arise in response to antigenic stimulus peculiar to pregnancy, perhaps in the amnion. These antibodies have specificity for a 180-kDa antigen, presumably a hemidesmosomal peptide. An-

tibodies deposited on the basement membrane zone activate the complement cascade, which in turn generates an inflammatory response.

Relationship between HG and bullous pemphigoid is unresolved. This is suggested by the morphologic similarity of lesions, similar immunopathology, and the fact that the HG antigen is very closely related to, if not identical with, the 180-kDa bullous pemphigoid antigen.

Hormonal factors undoubtedly play an important role. Onset in pregnancy or thereafter, postpartum flares, and exacerbations with hormone-producing tumors or contraceptives.

Management

Systemic corticosteroids given orally in doses equivalent to 20 to 40 mg or prednisone. Exacerbation during remission may require higher doses. Prednisone is gradually tapered during the postpartum period. A few patients do not require systemic prednisone and can be controlled with antihistamines and topical steroids.

Infants born to affected mothers who have received high doses of prednisone should be examined carefully by a neonatologist for adrenal insufficiency. Cutaneous lesions in infants are transient and do not require therapy.

Section 16

GENETIC, METABOLIC, ENDOCRINE, AND NUTRITIONAL DISEASES

DIABETES MELLITUS

Classification of Diabetes Mellitus (DM)

Primary
Insulin-dependent DM (IDDM, type 1)
Non-insulin-dependent DM (NIDDM, type 2): nonobese NIDDM, obese NIDDM, maturity-onset DM of the young (MODY)

Secondary
Pancreatic disease, hormonal abnormalities, drug-/chemical-induced, insulin receptor abnormalities, genetic syndromes

Classification of the Cutaneous Complications or Skin Diseases Associated with Diabetes Mellitus

NECROBIOSIS LIPOIDICA (See page 422.)

SCLEREDEMA
Synonym: Scleredema adultorum of Buschke. Onset correlates with duration of DM and with presence of microangiopathy. Skin findings: poorly demarcated scleroderma-like induration of the skin and subcutaneous tissue of the upper back, neck, proximal extremities. Rapid onset and progression.

CALCIPHYLAXIS (See page 426.)

GRANULOMA ANNULARE (See page 272.)
Disseminated, varied, associated with DM

CUTANEOUS PERFORATING DISORDERS (See Kyrle's Disease, page 110.)

ACANTHOSIS NIGRICANS AND LIPODYSTROPHY (See page 505.)
Associated with insulin resistance in DM. Insulin-like epidermal growth factors may cause epidermal hyperplasia.

ERUPTIVE XANTHOMAS (See page 470.)
Occur in setting of grossly uncontrolled DM and very high serum triglycerides.

DIABETIC BULLAE *(Bullosis diabeticorum)*
Large, intact bullae (Figure 16-1) arise on the dorsum of the hand, fingers, legs, and feet on a noninflamed bases. Histologically, bullae show intra- or subepidermal clefting without acantholysis.

PERIPHERAL VASCULAR DISEASE (See Section 17.)
Small-Vessel Vasculopathy (Microangiopathy) Involves arterioles, venules, and capillaries. Characterized by basement membrane thickening and endothelial cell proliferation. Presents clinically as acral erysipelas-like erythema, ± ulceration
Large-Vessel Vasculopathy Incidence greatly increased in DM. Ischemia is most often symptomatic on lower legs and feet with gangrene and ulceration. Predisposes to infections.

INFECTIONS (See Sections 24 and 25.)
Poorly controlled DM associated with increased incidence of primary (furuncles, carbuncles) and secondary *Staphylococcus aureus* infections (paronychia, wound/ulcer infection, cellulitis (*S. aureus,* group A streptococcus), erythrasma, dermatophytoses (tinea pedis,

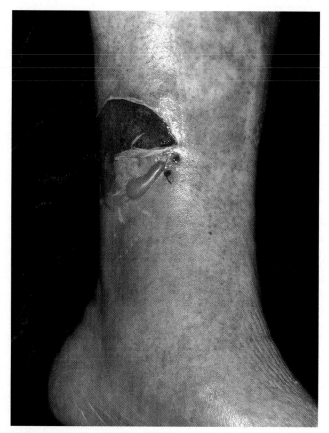

Figure 16-1 Diabetic bulla *Large bulla which has ruptured with formation of an extensive erosion on the leg of an elderly male diabetic; the skin is atrophic and hair is absent secondary to diabetes-associated peripheral vascular disease.*

onychomycosis), candidiasis (mucosal and cutaneous), mucormycosis with necrotizing nasopharyngeal infections.

PERIPHERAL NEUROPATHY
Combined motor and sensory. Motor neuropathy: weakness and muscle wasting distally. Sensory neuropathy predisposes to neurotrophic ulcers over bony prominences of feet, usually on the soles. Autonomic neuropathy: causes localized anhidrosis.

ADVERSE CUTANEOUS DRUG REACTION
(See Section 22.)
 Insulin   Local reactions: lipodystrophy with decreased adipose tissue at sites of sub-

cutaneous injection; Arthus-like reaction with urticarial lesion at site of injection
Systemic Insulin Allergy   Urticaria, serum sickness-like reactions
Oral Hypoglycemic Agent   Exanthematous eruptions, urticaria, erythema multiforme, photosensitivity

DIABETIC DERMOPATHY
Circumscribed, atrophic, slightly depressed, brownish lesions on the anterior lower legs. The pathogenic significance of diabetic angiopathy remains to be established but is often accompanied with microangiopathy.

NECROBIOSIS LIPOIDICA

Necrobiosis lipoidica (NL) is a cutaneous disorder often, but not always, associated with diabetes mellitus. The lesions are distinctive, sharply circumscribed, multicolored (red, yellow, brown) plaques occurring on the anterior and lateral surfaces of the lower legs.

Synonym: Necrobiosis lipoidica diabeticorum.

Epidemiology and Etiology

Incidence <1.0 % of diabetics

Age Young adults, early middle age, but not uncommon in juvenile diabetics

Sex Female : male ratio is 3 : 1 in both diabetic and nondiabetic forms.

Etiology Unknown

Precipitating Factors A history of preceding trauma to the site can be a factor in the initial development of the lesions, and for this reason, NL is often present on the shins and over the bony areas of the feet.

History

Onset of Lesions In the majority of individuals, NL occurs in the setting of long-standing juvenile-onset diabetes.

Duration of Lesions Slowly evolving and enlarging over months, persisting for years

Skin Symptoms Cosmetic disfigurement. Pain in lesions that d]evelop ulcers

Relationship to DM One-third of patients have clinical DM; one-third have abnormal glucose tolerance only; one-third have normal glucose tolerance.

Physical Examination

Skin Lesions

TYPES

Early lesions: well-demarcated waxy plaques of variable size (Figure 16-2). Epidermis shiny and atrophic with telangiectatic dermal vessels visible.

Older lesions: larger lesions formed by centrifugal enlargement or merging of early lesions. Ulceration commonly occurs within plaques (Figure 16-3). Healed ulcers result in depressed scars. Many well-marked telangiectases are seen throughout the center of the lesion where the atrophy is most prominent.

Treated/burned-out lesions: yellow color resolves, plaques flatten. Old burned-out lesions appear as tan-brown areas with telangiectasia.

COLOR Yellow-orange is the diagnostic and dominant color of early NL. Older lesions have tan-brown hues.

SHAPE Serpiginous, irregular with merging of smaller lesions

ARRANGEMENT At times symmetric

DISTRIBUTION >80 % occur on the shin; less commonly, on feet, arms, trunk, or face and scalp; rarely may be generalized

Differential Diagnosis

Cutaneous Yellow-Brown Plaques Sarcoidosis, granuloma annulare (not infrequently coexists with NL), xanthoma

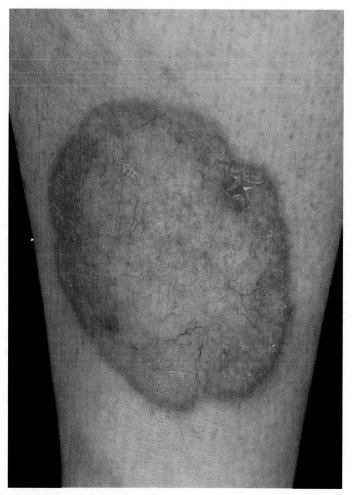

Figure 16-2 Necrobiosis lipoidica, diabeticorum: early *A large plaque with an active yellow-orange to tan-pink, well-demarcated, raised, firm border on the calf of a diabetic female. The central part of the lesion has resolved with atrophic changes of epidermal thinning and telangiectasias against yellow background.*

Laboratory and Special Examinations

Dermatopathology Sclerotic collagen and obliteration of the bundle pattern, necrobiosis of connective tissue, and concomitant granulomatous infiltration in lower dermis. Fat-containing foam cells are often present, imparting the yellow color to the clinical lesion. Dermal blood vessels show "microangiopathy" with endothelial thickening and focal deposits of PAS-positive material.

Immunofluorescence Presence of immunoglobulins and complement (C3). Immune complexes may occur in the walls of the small blood vessels.

Chemistry Abnormal glucose tolerance test

Diagnosis

The lesions are so distinctive that biopsy confirmation is not necessary; may be required to rule out granuloma annulare.

Pathogenesis

The granulomatous inflammatory reaction is believed to be due to alterations in the collagen.

The arteriolar changes in the areas of necrobiosis of the collagen have been thought by some to be precipitated by aggregation of platelets. The severity of NL is not related to the severity of the diabetes mellitus. Furthermore, control of the diabetes has no effect on the course of NL.

Course and Prognosis

The lesions are indolent and can enlarge to involve large areas of the skin surface unless treated. The lesions are unsightly, and patients are usually upset about the cosmetic appearance. Ulcerated areas within NL are painful but usually can be healed over time.

Management

Corticosteroids

TOPICAL Potent corticosteroid under occlusion is helpful in some cases; however, ulcerations may rarely occur when NL is occluded.

INTRALESIONAL Intralesional triamcinolone 5 mg/ml into active yellow lesions usually arrests extension of plaques of NL.

Ulceration The majority of ulcerations within NL lesions heal with local wound care; if not, excision of entire lesion with grafting may be required.

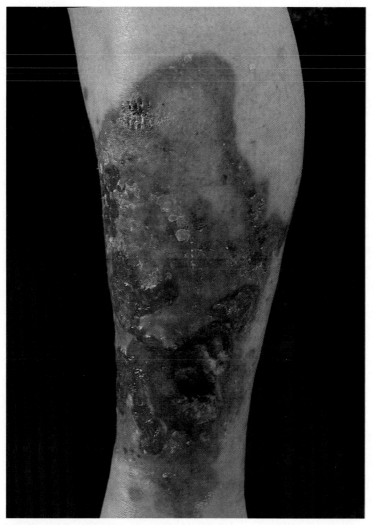

Figure 16-3 Necrobiosis lipoidica, late with ulceration *A very extensive plaque of necrobiosis lipoidica on the lower leg of a diabetic female. The lower portion has undergone necrosis with extensive, deep ulceration.*

CALCIPHYLAXIS

Calciphylaxis is characterized by progressive cutaneous necrosis associated with small and medium-sized vessel calcification occurring in the setting of end-stage renal disease and hyperparathyroidism. Cutaneous involvement presents as initial painful geographic areas of ischemia that progress to gangrene and ulceration of the subcutaneous fat, dermis, and epidermis; secondary infection and sepsis are common.

Synonym: Widespread systemic calcification.

Epidemiology and Etiology

Sex Equal

Age Middle to old age

Risk Factors End-stage renal disease, diabetes mellitus, advanced HIV disease

History

History Even early infarctive lesions are exquisitely tender.

Systems Review End-stage renal disease. The majority of patients are diabetic. Onset often closely follows initiation of hemo- or peritoneal dialysis.

Physical Examination

Skin Findings

TYPES OF LESIONS Initially preinfarctive ischemic plaques occur, appearing as mottling or having a livedo reticularis pattern (Figure 16-4*A*). Bullae may form over ischemic tissue. Epidermis/dermis eventually becomes necrotic, resulting in slough of tissue, which forms an ulcer when debrided (Figure 16-4*B*). Ulcers and surrounding ischemic skin frequently become secondarily infected, which can remain localized or invade, causing cellulitis and bacteremia.

COLOR OF LESIONS *Early:* dusky erythema to violaceous. *Later:* Central infarcted sites are black. Lesions gradually enlarge over weeks to months.

PALPATION OF LESIONS Even early lesions are extremely tender, unless advanced sensory neuropathy coexists. Large areas of induration can be defined on palpation. Margins of pregangrene and gangrene are poorly defined.

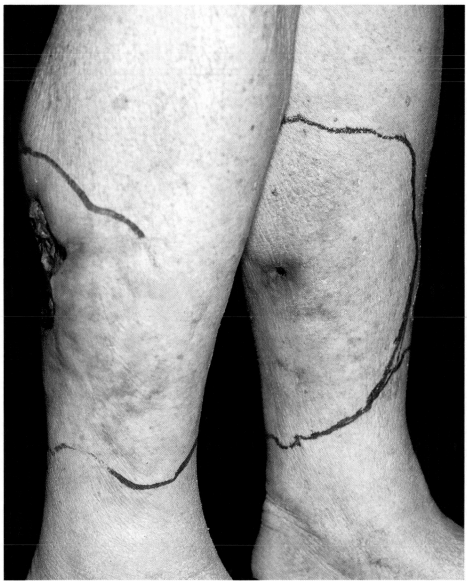

A

Figure 16-4 Calciphylaxis A. *A very large ulceration of the right calf and a small necrotic lesion of the left, surrounded by a mottled violaceous zone of ischemia, in a diabetic female with renal failure. The areas outlined in blue demarcated subcutaneous induration corresponding to sites of early calciphylaxis.*

DISTRIBUTION OF LESIONS   Distal extremities, most commonly on the lateral and posterior calves. Abdomen, buttocks. Fingers. Glans penis.

Differential Diagnosis

Painful Ischemic Plaque(s)   Panniculitis, vasculitides, necrobiosis lipoidica with ulceration, dystrophic calcinosis cutis, metastatic calcification (calcium deposited in dermis and not the subcutaneous fat), scleroderma, atheroembolization, atherosclerosis obliterans, disseminated intravascular coagulation (purpura fulminans), pyoderma gangrenosum, warfarin necrosis, heparin necrosis, phaeohyphomycosis, *Vibrio vulnificus* cellulitis, other necrotizing cellulitides

Laboratory and Special Examinations

Chemistry   Azotemia. Calcium $\times$ phosphate ion product usually elevated.

Parathormone (PTH)   Levels usually elevated.

Cultures   Rule out secondary infection.

Dermatopathology   Incisional biopsy is recommended. Calcification of the media of small and medium-sized blood vessels is noted within the dermis and subcutaneous tissue. Intraluminal fibrin thrombi are present. Ischemic results in intralobular or septal fat necrosis, accompanied by a sparse lymphohistiocytic infiltrate.

Imaging   Radiographs of affected extremities show calcium deposition outlining small and large vessels. Microcalcification of calciphylaxis is difficult to visualize.

Diagnosis

Made on history of renal failure, clinical findings, elevated PTH level, elevated calcium $\times$ phosphate ion product, and histologic features.

Pathophysiology

The pathogenesis is poorly understood. In animal models, calciphylaxis is described as a condition of induced systemic hypersensitivity in which tissues respond to appropriate challenging agents with calcium deposition. In humans, calciphylaxis is associated with chronic renal failure, secondary hyperparathyroidism, and an elevated calcium phosphate end product. Implicated "challenging agents" include corticosteroids, albumin infusions, intramuscular tobramycin, iron dextran complex, calcium heparinate, immunosuppressive agents, and vitamin D.

Course and Prognosis

The course in the majority of patients tends to be slowly progressive despite all therapeutic interventions. Pain is a constant feature, associated with ischemia and secondary infection. In advanced disease, gangrene of fingers, toes, and penis may result in autoamputation. Local infection and sepsis are common complications. Overall, the prognosis is poor, and the mortality rate is very high.

Management

Calciphylaxis is best managed by early diagnosis, treatment of renal failure, partial parathyroidectomy when indicated, aggressive debridement of necrotic tissue, and avoidance of precipitating factors such as systemic corticosteroids.

Medical

CALCIUM $\times$ ION PHOSPHATE LEVELS   Reduce calcium phosphate ion product by administration of oral phosphate binders and/or by decreasing the calcium level in dialysate.

ANTIMICROBIAL AGENTS   Identify secondary infection and treat with appropriate agents.

RENAL FAILURE   Treat with dialysis.

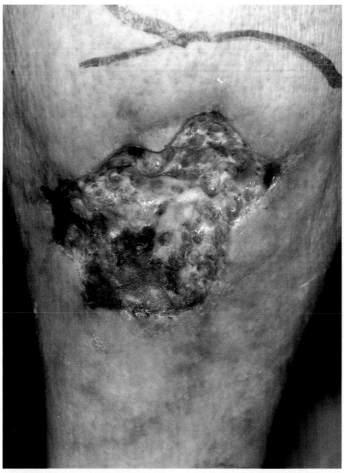

B

Figure 16-4 Calciphylaxis B. Close-up. *The ulcer is sharply demarcated with eschar in a portion and extending into the subcutaneous fat; the lesion was extremely painful and secondarily infected with* Xanthomonas maltophilia. *The reticulated or mottled surrounding skin is ischemic and may become necrotic.*

Surgical

DEBRIDEMENT All necrotic tissue should be debrided and the resultant defect covered with split-thickness grafts.

SUBTOTAL PARATHYROIDECTOMY May be helpful in some patients with secondary hyperparathyroidism. Best performed soon after onset of calciphylaxis

AMPUTATION Indicated for extensive areas of gangrene, uncontrollable infection, and uncontrollable pain

RENAL TRANSPLANTATION Has been helpful in some patients

HEREDITARY HEMORRHAGIC TELANGIECTASIA

Hereditary hemorrhagic telangiectasia (HHT) is an autosomal dominant condition affecting blood vessels, especially in the mucous membranes of the mouth and the gastrointestinal (GI) tract. The disease is frequently heralded by recurrent epistaxis that appears often in childhood. The diagnostic lesions are small, pulsating, macular and papular, usually punctate, and vascular telangiectases. *Synonym:* Osler-Weber-Rendu syndrome.

Epidemiology

Inheritance   Autosomal dominant, gene locus 9q33–34

Age of Onset   Cutaneous telangiectases begin to appear after puberty but peak in the third or fourth decade.

Incidence   1 to 2 : 100,000

History

Age at Presentation   Childhood to early adulthood

Duration of Lesions   Telangiectases persist throughout life unless treated.

Symptoms   Recurrent epistaxis often in childhood in 50 %. GI bleeding (12 % to 50 %). Hemoptysis from pulmonary arteriovenous (A-V) malformations

Family History   Similar symptoms in family members

Physical Examination

Skin Lesions

TYPES   Macular or papular telangiectases (Figure 16-5) up to 3.0 mm in diameter that usually pulsate; often can be blanched.

COLOR   Red

SHAPE   Punctate (most frequent), stellate, or linear

ARRANGEMENT   Symmetric and scattered, nonpatterned

DISTRIBUTION   *Skin*   Face, palms/soles, fingers/toes, nail beds
   Mucous Membranes   Nasopharynx, vermilion border of lips, tip and dorsum of tongue, conjunctivae, throughout the GI tract, genitourinary (GU) tract

Systemic Findings   Pulmonary. A-V fistulas

Differential Diagnosis

CREST syndrome, generalized essential telangiectasia, Fabry's disease, ataxia telangiectasia

Laboratory and Special Examinations

Hematology   Anemia from chronic blood loss

Stool Guaiac Screen   Check for occult bleeding.

Dermatopathology   Capillaries and venules, irregularly dilated and lined by flattened endothelial cells in papillary dermis

Imaging   Chest x-ray or CT or MRI of chest to discover pulmonary A-V fistula

Endoscopy   Tracheobronchial tree or GI tract for symptomatic bleeding

Diagnosis

Triad of (1) typical telangiectases on skin (fingers and palms) *and* mucous membranes (lips and tongue), (2) repeated GI hemorrhages, and (3) family history

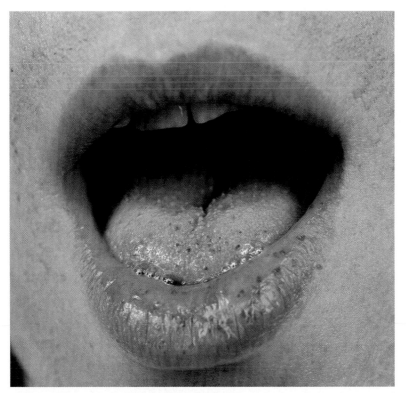

Figure 16-5 Hereditary hemorrhagic telangiectasia *Multiple 1–2-mm, discrete, red macular and papular telangiectases on the lower lip and tongue.*

Pathogenesis

Mutation in a transforming growth factor beta (TGF-β)–binding protein (endoglin) that is present on endothelial cells. The mutation results in a breakdown of the junction between the endothelial cells because of a lack of perivascular support (pericytes, smooth muscle, and elastic fibers). The abnormal telangiectatic capillaries rupture easily, and this is the basis for the repeated nasal and GI hemorrhages.

Course

More than 80 % of patients experience recurrent epistaxis. GI bleeding associated with significant risk of morbidity and mortality. Highest morbidity from pulmonary A-V fistulas.

Management

Destruction of Abnormal Vessels Electrosurgery or laser surgery with pulse dye laser can be used to destroy cutaneous and mucosal telangiectases.

Epistaxis Packing, cautery, septal dermoplasty for recurrent epistaxis

GI Hemorrhage If accessible, treat bleeding lesions with Nd:YAG laser.

Pulmonary A-V Fistulas Resection, embolization

Estrogen Has been used to treat recalcitrant bleeding.

CUSHING'S SYNDROME AND HYPERCORTICISM

Cushing's syndrome (CS) is characterized by truncal obesity, moon face, acne, abdominal striae, hypertension, decreased carbohydrate tolerance, protein catabolism, psychiatric disturbances, and amenorrhea and hirsutism in females, associated with excess adrenocorticosteroid of endogenous or exogenous source. Cushing's disease refers to CS associated with a pituitary adrenocorticotropic hormone (ACTH)–producing adenoma. CS medicamentosum refers to CS caused by exogenous administration of glucocorticosteroids.

Synonym: Pituitary basophilism.

Etiology

Endogenous

Adrenal hyperplasia
Secondary to pituitary ACTH overproduction
Pituitary-hypothalamic dysfunction
Pituitary ACTH-producing micro- or macroadenomas
Secondary to nonendocrine tumors secreting ACTH or corticotropin (ACTH)-releasing hormone (CRH), producing: small cell (oat cell) type of bronchogenic carcinoma, carcinoma of thymus, pancreatic carcinoma, bronchial adenoma, medullary carcinoma of thyroid
Adrenal nodular hyperplasia
Adrenal neoplasia
Adenoma
Carcinoma

Exogenous (Iatrogenic)

Prolonged use of glucocorticoids
Systemic
Topical with systemic absorption
Prolonged use of ACTH

History

Onset Usually gradual. May be sudden, associated with oat cell carcinoma of lung.

Skin Symptoms Weight gain (94 %), especially truncal, face, neck obesity. Easy bruising (65 %). New pink-purple striae (67 %). Hair: thinning of scalp hair in females; hirsutism (80 %). Acne: recent onset, flaring of existing acne. Menses: amenorrhea (77 %). Polyuria, polydipsia (19 %).

General Symptoms Fatigue and muscle weakness (87 %), and often, personality changes (66 %)

Physical Examination

Typical Habitus A plethoric obese person with a "classic" habitus that results from the redistribution of fat: moon facies (Figure 16-6), "buffalo" hump, truncal obesity, and thin arms (97 %)

Skin Findings

Cutaneous atrophy: purple striae, mostly on the abdomen, similar to striae produced by topical application of corticosteroids; thin skin (epidermal and dermal atrophy); ecchymoses usually at sites of trauma; telangiectasia (plethoric facies)
Deposition of subcutaneous fat: face, neck, trunk due to fat in mesenteric bed (central obesity), intrascapular area ("buffalo" hump)
Hair: hirsutism; facial hypertrichosis with pigmented hairs and often increased lanugo hairs on the face and arms; androgenetic alopecia in females
Steroid acne (differs from acne vulgaris): monomorphous lesions with few or no comedones
Pigmentation: addisonian pigmentation when CS is associated with increased ACTH production (intra- or extracranial)
Associated findings: pityriasis versicolor and dermatophytoses common

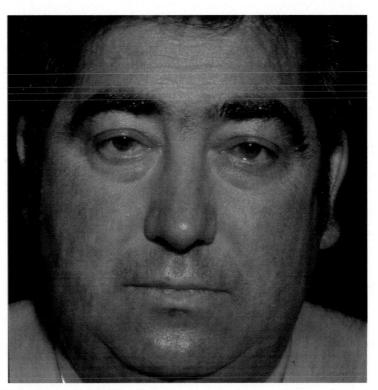

Figure 16-6 Cushing's syndrome *Plethoric moon facies with erythema and telangiectases of cheek and forehead; the face, neck, and supraclavicular areas show increased deposition of fat.*

General Examination Hypertension ≥150/90 (82 %). Hypertrophy of the clitoris (19 %). Edema (62 %). Psychiatric changes: emotional lability, depression, confusion, psychosis. Muscle weakness due to myopathy

Differential Diagnosis

Pseudo-CS Obesity, chronic alcoholism, depression

Laboratory Examinations

Chemistry Blood glucose: about 20 % have diabetes mellitus. Hypokalemia

Hormone Studies Corticosteroids: elevated urinary free cortisol in 24-hour urine. Abnormal dexamethasone suppression test with failure to suppress endogenous cortisol secretion when dexamethasone is administered. Elevated ACTH.

Imaging CT scan of the abdomen and the pituitary. Osteoporosis

Diagnosis

Clinical features confirmed by demonstration of increased cortisol production and failure to suppress endogenous cortisol production normally when dexamethasone is administered

Pathophysiology

Clinical findings caused by glucocorticoids. Many of the cutaneous findings secondary to weakening of collagen fibers in dermis

Course and Prognosis

Variable, depending on the etiology

Management

Depends on detection and correction of underlying cause

GRAVES' DISEASE AND HYPERTHYROIDISM

Graves' disease (GD) is a disorder with three major manifestations: hyperthyroidism with diffuse goiter, ophthalmopathy, and dermopathy. The manifestations often do not occur together, may not occur at all, and run courses that are independent of each other.
Synonyms: Parry's disease, Basedow's disease.

Epidemiology and Etiology

Incidence   Relatively common. Dermopathy occurs in about 5 % of patients with GD.

Age   Third and fourth decades

Race   Haplotypes: Caucasians—HLA-B8 and -DRw3; Japanese—HLA-Bw36; Chinese—HLA-Bw46

Sex   Female > males

Etiology   Unknown. Considered to be autoimmune

Associated Disorders   Primary thyroprivic hypothyroidism, Hashimoto's disease, pernicious anemia, vitiligo

History

Onset of Dermopathy   In half of cases it occurs during the active stage of GD and in the other half after treatment of the GD.

General Symptoms   Nervousness, emotional lability, insomnia, tremors, especially in younger patients. Weight loss despite an increased appetite. Older patients more often have cardiac manifestations: dyspnea, palpitations, and angina pectoris.

Symptoms Relating to the Skin   Pruritus, hyperhidrosis, heat intolerance

Family History   There is an association with other autoimmune diseases: pernicious anemia, Hashimoto's thyroiditis.

Physical Examination

Appearance of Patient   The patient appears anxious, is irritable and tremulous. There is often a persistent facial flush, palmar erythema, increased sweating on the palms and soles.

Skin Findings   Warm, moist (hyperhidrosis), soft, smooth

TYPES OF LESIONS   Dermopathy of GD (pretibial myxedema): early lesions bilateral, asymmetric firm nodules and plaques. Late lesions: confluence of early lesions, which may, in extreme cases, result in grotesque involvement of entire lower legs and dorsa of feet (Figure 16-7); surface smooth with orange peel-like appearance, later becomes verrucous.

COLOR OF LESIONS   Pink or skin-colored or purple

PALPATION OF LESIONS   Firm, plus nonpitting brawny edema in the normal skin

DISTRIBUTION OF LESIONS   Dermopathy usually begins in pretibial region; may extensively involve lower legs; dorsa of feet, rarely as preradial myxedema

Hair   Scalp hair is fine and soft, with an altered texture. Diffuse alopecia is not uncommon. Hypertrichosis in area of pretibial myxedema.

Nails   A special type of onycholysis (Plummer's nail) (see Section 18) in which free edge of the nail becomes undulated and curves upward. Clubbing of the nails, which may be associated with diaphyseal proliferation of the periosteum in the acral (Figure 16-7) and long bones; this is known as *thyroid acropachy.*

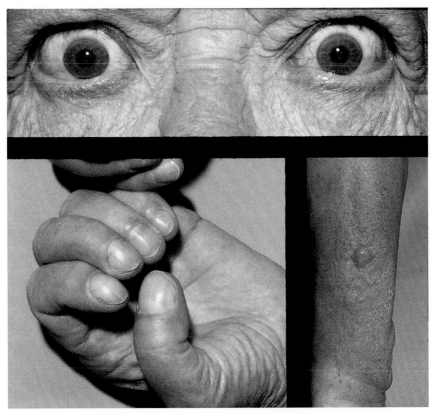

Figure 16-7 Graves' disease *A composite image illustrates: proptosis, lid retraction; thyroid acropachy (osteoarthropathy) with clubbing; and the pink- and skin-colored papules, plaques, and nodules of pretibial myxedema.*

Thyroid Examination GD: diffuse toxic goiter, asymmetric, lobular. Asymmetric and lobular thyroid enlargement, often with the presence of a bruit

Eyes Ophthalmopathy of GD has two components, spastic and mechanical. Spastic findings: stare, lid lag, lid retraction (Figure 16-7). Mechanical components: proptosis, ophthalmoplegia, congestive oculopathy (chemosis, conjunctivitis, periorbital swelling, and potential complications of corneal ulceration, optic neuritis, optic atrophy). Exophthalmic ophthalmoplegia: ocular muscle weakness with inward gaze, convergence, strabismus, diplopia

Cardiovascular Findings Atrial arrhythmias, systolic murmurs

Mental Status Anxiety, depression

Differential Diagnosis

Dermopathy Edema, stasis dermatitis, elephantiasis nostras verrucosa, deep fungal infection

Thyrotoxicosis Anxiety, metastatic carcinoma, cirrhosis, hyperparathyroidism, sprue, myasthenia gravis, muscular dystrophy, pheochromocytoma

Laboratory and Special Examinations

Chemistry

THYROID FUNCTION TESTS

Increased radioactive iodine uptake, increased serum T_4, increased T_3, RT3U, and FT421
Antithyroid antibodies

Dermatopathology Pretibial myxedema shows "edematous" separation of collagen bundles and stellate fibroblasts with accumulation of hyaluronic acid and chondroitin sulfate in the lesions and in normal skin.

Pathogenesis

This is not settled, but autoimmune processes appear to play an important role. In some patients, Hashimoto's thyroiditis develops in Graves' disease; in some, Graves' disease follows Hashimoto's thyroiditis. Thus Graves' disease, Hashimoto's thyroiditis, and primary myxedema are considered closely related autoimmune entities. There is a disturbance of the homeostasis of thyroid secretion by the presence of an abnormal thyroid stimulator. Long-acting thyroid stimulators (LATS) are thyroid-stimulating immunoglobulins (TSI) of the IgG class elaborated by lymphocytes. TSI are antibodies against the TSH receptor (TRAb), thus mediating thyroid stimulation. The pathogeneses of pretibial myxedema and exophthalmus are not clear, but factors in patients' sera stimulate the deposition of mucopolysaccharides by dermal fibroblasts.

Management

Thyrotoxicosis Antithyroid agents block thyroid hormone synthesis. Ablation of thyroid tissue, surgically or by radioactive iodine

Ophthalmopathy Symptomatic treatment in mild cases. Severe cases: prednisone 100 to 120 mg/day initially tapering to 5 mg/day. Orbital radiation. Orbital decompression.

Dermopathy Topical corticosteroid preparations under plastic occlusion for several months are usually effective. Low-dose corticosteroids (prednisone) 5 mg/day

HYPOTHYROIDISM AND MYXEDEMA

Myxedema results from insufficient production of thyroid hormones and can be caused by multiple disturbances, characterized by accumulation of water binding mucopolysaccharides in the dermis, resulting in thickening of facial features and doughy induration of the skin. *Cretinism* denotes hypothyroidism dating from birth, resulting from developmental abnormalities.

Epidemiology

Age   40 to 60 years

Sex   Female : male ratio 10 : 1

Incidence   1 : 5000 neonates

Classification of Etiology

THYROID (95 % of cases)   ***Thyroprivic***   Congenital development defect, primary idiopathic, postablative (radioiodine, surgery), postradiation

Goitrous   Heritable biosynthetic defects, maternally transmitted (iodides, antithyroid agents), iodine deficiency, drug-induced (aminosalicylic acid, iodides, phenylbutazone, iodoantipyrine, lithium), chronic thyroiditis (Hashimoto's disease)

SUPRATHYROID (TROPHOPRIVIC) (5 % of cases)   *Pituitary*   Panhypopituitarism, isolated TSH deficiency

Hypothalamic   Congenital defects, infection (encephalitis), neoplasm, infiltrative (sarcoidosis)

History

Systems Review

CRETINISM   Usually becomes manifest within first few months of life. Physiologic jaundice, hoarse cry, constipation, somnolence, feeding problems

MYXEDEMA   Early symptoms are slow in developing and are nonspecific and often overlooked: fatigue, lethargy, cold intolerance, constipation, stiffness and cramping of muscles, carpal tunnel syndrome, menorrhagia. Later: intellectual and motor activity slow, appetite declines, weight increases. Dry skin; dry hair, hair loss. The voice may become deeper.

Physical Examination

Appearance of Patient

CRETINISM   Short stature, coarse features with protruding tongue, broad flat nose, widely set eyes, sparse hair, dry skin, protuberant abdomen with umbilical hernia, impaired mental development, retarded bone age, epiphyseal dysgenesis, delayed dentition

MYXEDEMA   Dull, expressionless facies (Figure 16-8), with puffiness of the eyelids; the puffiness may be unilateral. The nose is broadened, and the lips are thick. There is a slowing down of bodily activity.

Skin Lesions

TYPES   Skin appears swollen, waxy, rough, dry, coarse (xeroderma or ichthyosiform), increased skin creases (Figure 16-8). Palmoplantar keratoderma

COLOR   Pale: due to increased concentration of water and mucopolysaccharides and vasoconstriction. Yellow-orange: palms and soles, associated with carotenemia

PALPATION   The skin is dry due to decreased sebum and sweat secretion. Cool. Doughy induration; boggy, nonpitting edema in acral parts

DISTRIBUTION   Generalized

Associated Condition

VITILIGO   May occur associated with subclinical hypothyroidism, especially in women >50 years of age.

Hair   Dry, coarse, and brittle. Alopecia: thinning of hair due to slow growth in the scalp, beard, and sexual areas; increase in the number of telogen hairs. Eyebrows: alopecia of the lateral one-third

Nails Brittle, grow slowly

Mucous Membranes The tongue is large, smooth, red, and clumsy

General Examination

CRETINISM Short stature, coarse features with protruding tongue, broad flat nose, widely set eyes, protuberant abdomen with umbilical hernia, impaired mental development, delayed dentition

MYXEDEMA Thyroid is not usually palpable unless a goiter is present. Heart rate: decreased. "Hung-up" reflex: relaxation phase of deep tendon reflexes (ankle) is prolonged, a brisk contraction with a slow relaxation time

Differential Diagnosis

Cretinism Down's syndrome

Myxedema Nephrotic syndrome, depression, Parkinson's disease, Alzheimer's disease

Laboratory and Special Examinations

Chemistry

THYROID FUNCTION TESTS It is recommended that all infants be screened with T_4 or TSH.

THYROID-STIMULATING HORMONE (TSH) Elevated in thyroprivic hypothyroidism. Low or undetectable in pituitary hypothyroidism. Pituitary hypothyroidism usually accompanied by hyposecretion of other pituitary hormones. T_3, T_4 decreased

SERUM CHOLESTEROL Elevated

Dermatopathology Papillary dermis, around hair follicles and blood vessels. Chondroitin sulfate and hyaluronic acid accumulate with separation of the collagen bundles.

Imaging

CRETINISM Retarded bone age, epiphyseal dysgenesis

MYXEDEMA Enlarged heart due to dilatation and pericardial effusion. Megacolon, intestinal obstruction

Diagnosis

Clinical findings confirmed by TSH levels

Pathogenesis

Accumulation of acid mucopolysaccharides associated with changes in skin, vocal cords, and oropharynx. Pale color of skin is due to increased mucopolysaccharides (hyaluronic acid and chondroitin sulfate) in the skin, which change the refraction of incident light. Carotenemia results from a reduction in the conversion of beta-carotene to vitamin A.

Course and Prognosis

Untreated, long-standing hypothyroidism can progress to a hypothermic, stuporous state, i.e., myxedema coma, that may be fatal.

Management

Neonates, infants, juveniles: full thyroid replacement should be given immediately to minimize chance for abnormal intellectual development and growth. Adults/elderly: metabolic state should be restored gradually to minimize stress on cardiac and coronary reserve

Hypothyroidism (Adult)
Average daily oral maintenance dose:

Levothyroxine 125 μg **or**
Thyroid extract 120 to 180 mg

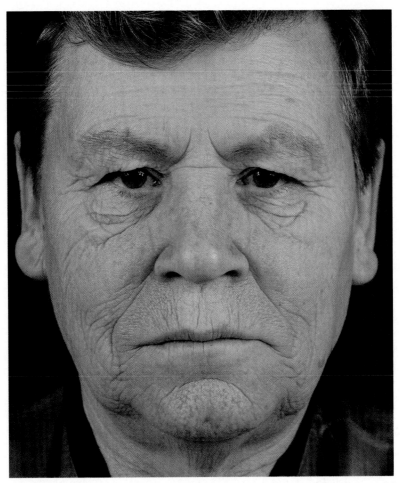

Figure 16-8 Myxedema *Dry, pale skin; thinning of the lateral eyebrows; puffiness of the face and eyelids; increased number of skin creases; dull, expressionless, beardless facies.*

SCURVY

Scurvy is an acute or chronic disease of infancy and of middle and old age caused by dietary deficiency of ascorbic acid (vitamin C). The disorder is characterized principally by anemia, hemorrhagic manifestations in the skin (ecchymoses and perifollicular hemorrhage) and in the musculoskeletal system (hemorrhage into periosteum and muscles), and changes in the gums (loosening of teeth, bleeding gums).
Synonym: Vitamin C deficiency.

Epidemiology and Etiology

Age   6 to 12 months; middle to old age

Etiology

INFANCY/CHILDHOOD   Diet consisting of only processed milk with no added citrus fruit or vegetables. Result of maternal neglect.

ADULTHOOD   Edentulous single persons who live alone, cook for themselves, and do not eat salads and uncooked vegetables. Affected individuals often have other dietary deficiencies as well.

Precipitating Factors   Pregnancy, lactation, and thyrotoxicosis increase requirements of ascorbic acid; alcoholism

History

Dietary Intake   Lack of intake of food containing vitamin C

Onset   With no vitamin C intake, symptoms of scurvy occur after 1 to 3 months.

Symptoms   Those associated with medical problems. Lassitude, weakness, arthralgia, and myalgia

Physical Examination

Appearance of Patient   Lethargic and weak

Skin Lesions

TYPES

Hemorrhage: petechiae, ecchymoses of arms and legs (Figure 16-9)
Hyperkeratosis: follicular, hyperkeratotic papules with hemorrhage, especially on the backs of lower legs

COLOR   Red-brown of recent ecchymoses. Yellow-green of resolving hemorrhage

ARRANGEMENT   Follicular keratoses. Perifollicular hemorrhages

DISTRIBUTION   Hemorrhages on arms and legs, especially inner thighs

Hair   Hair becomes fragmented and buried in perifollicular hyperkeratotic papules. Perifollicular hemorrhage

Nails   Splinter hemorrhages

Mouth   Gingiva: swollen, purple, spongy, and bleeds easily; findings occur in more advanced scurvy. Loosening and loss of teeth

Infancy/Childhood

MUSCULOSKELETAL   Hemorrhage into periosteum of long bones causes painful swellings and epiphyseal separation. Sternum may sink inward; scorbutic rosary (elevation at rib margins).

HEMORRHAGE   Ecchymoses. Gum lesions occur only if teeth have erupted. Retrobulbar, subarachnoid, intracerebral can cause death.

Differential Diagnosis

Hemorrhagic Leg Lesions   Thrombocytopenia, senile purpura, coagulopathy, anticoagulant drug therapy (warfarin, heparin), cryoglobulinemia

Gingival Hypertrophy   Poor dental hygiene, drug-induced gingival hyperplasia, leukemia, pregnancy

Laboratory and Special Examinations

Hematology   Normocytic, normochromatic anemia resulting from bleeding into tissues. Fo-

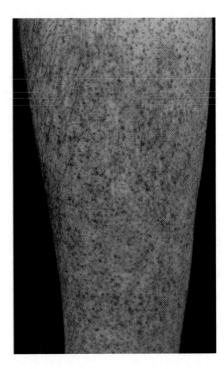

Figure 16-9 Scurvy *Perifollicular hemorrhage on the leg. The follicles are often plugged by keratin (follicular hyperkeratosis).*

late deficiency is also common, resulting in macrocytic anemia. Positive capillary fragility test

Chemistry Platelet ascorbic acid level usually <25 % of normal value

Imaging X-ray findings diagnostic

Diagnosis

Clinical findings confirmed by low ascorbic acid level

Pathophysiology

Humans are unable to synthesize ascorbic acid and require it as an essential dietary vitamin. Total-body pool of vitamin C varies from 1.5 to 3 g. First symptoms of depletion (i.e., petechial hemorrhages and ecchymoses) occur when pool size is <0.5 g. With further depletion of pool size to 0.1 to 0.5 g, gum hyperplasia, hyperkeratosis, follicular keratoses, corkscrew hairs, arthralgias, joint effusions. With severe depletion of pool to <0.1 g, dyspnea, edema, oliguria, neuropathy occur, at which point death may ensue rapidly.

The best-understood function of vitamin C is in synthesis of collagen. Deficiency leads to impairment of peptidyl hydroxylation of procollagen, reduction in collagen formation, and secretion with associated capillary fragility.

Course and Prognosis

Unless treated, scurvy is fatal. Upon treatment spontaneous bleeding ceases within 24 hours; muscle and bone pain fade quickly; bleeding from gums stops in 2 to 3 days.

Management

In suspected cases, blood should be obtained for ascorbic acid level and therapy begun immediately.

Ascorbic Acid 100 mg 3 to 5 times daily until 4 g is given, then 100 mg/day is curative in days to weeks.

Diet High vitamin C–rich diet should be given simultaneously.

ZINC DEFICIENCY AND ACRODERMATITIS ENTEROPATHICA

Acrodermatitis enteropathica (AE) is a genetic disorder of zinc absorption, presenting in infancy, characterized by a triad of acral dermatitis (face, hands, feet, anogenital area), alopecia, and diarrhea; nearly identical clinical findings occur in other individuals with acquired zinc deficiency (AZD) due either to dietary deficiency or failure of intestinal absorption.

Epidemiology and Etiology

Age *AE:* in infants bottle-fed with bovine milk, days to few weeks. In breast-fed infants, soon after weaning. *AZD:* older individuals

Etiology *AE:* autosomal recessive trait resulting in failure to absorb zinc. *AZD:* secondary to reduced dietary intake of zinc, malabsorption (regional enteritis, following intestinal bypass surgery for obesity), chronic alcoholism, increased urinary loss (nephrotic syndrome), hypoalbuminemic states, penicillamine therapy, high catabolic states (trauma, burns, surgery), hemolytic anemias, adolescents who eat dirt, prolonged parenteral nutrition without supplemental zinc

Predisposition *AZD:* pregnancy, growing child, or adolescent

History

AE usually starts when infant is weaned and placed on cow's milk. Sometimes in earlier *AZD* concomitant with dietary change or underlying illness.

Clinical Findings

Skin Findings

TYPES OF LESIONS   Patches and plaques of dry, scaly, eczematous skin. Evolve to vesiculob- ullous, pustular, erosive, and crusted lesions (Figure 16-10). Sharply marginated dermatitis; paronychia, fissures on fingertips (Figure 16-11). Annular lesions with collarette scaling. Lesions become secondarily infected with *Candida albicans, Staphylococcus aureus.* Impaired wound healing

COLOR OF LESIONS   Initially pink. Later, brightly erythematous

DISTRIBUTION OF LESIONS   Initially, face (particularly perioral) (Figure 16-12), scalp, anogenital area (Figure 16-10). Later, hands and feet, flexural regions, trunk.

Hair and Nails   Diffuse alopecia, graying of hair. Paronychia, nail ridging, loss of nails

Mucous Membranes   Oral: perlèche; red, glossy tongue; superficial aphthous-like erosions; oral candidiasis. Photophobia

General Examination   Irritable, depressed mood. Children with AE whine and cry constantly. Failure of growth

Differential Diagnosis

Atopic dermatitis, seborrheic dermatitis, mucocutaneous candidiasis, glucagonoma

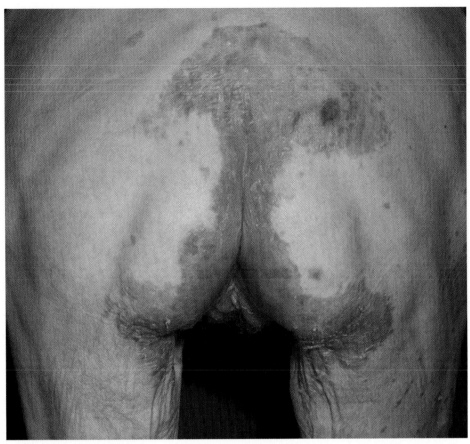

Figure 16-10 Zinc deficiency *Well-demarcated, psoriasiform and eczematous-like plaques overlying the sacrum, intergluteal cleft, buttocks, and hip.*

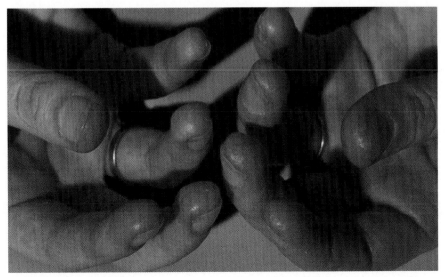

Figure 16-11 Zinc deficiency *Fingertips are red, shiny, fissured, and oozing; paronychia occur commonly.*

Laboratory and Special Examinations

CBC Anemia

Chemistry Low serum/plasma zinc levels

Urine Reduced urinary zinc excretion

Dermatopathology Psoriasiform dermatitis with large, pale keratinocytes in the upper epidermis; dyskeratotic cells; prominent parakeratosis. There may be intraepidermal clefts with acantholysis and blisters. Sparse superficial perivascular lymphohistiocytic infiltrate and tortuous capillaries in the papillary dermis

Diagnosis

Clinical diagnosis confirmed by zinc blood levels

Pathophysiology

In AE, patients do not absorb enough zinc from the diet. The specific ligand involved in basic transport mechanisms for zinc that might be abnormal in AE is not known. The defect appears to be somewhere in the early stages of zinc nutriture, where zinc is presented to the intestinal brush border. This defect can be overcome by increased zinc supply in the diet. It is also not known how zinc deficiency leads to skin and other lesions.

Course and Prognosis

Before it was known that AE is due to a deficient zinc uptake from the diet, it was usually fatal in infancy or early childhood. Patients failed to thrive and suffered from severe candidal and bacterial infections. Following zinc replacement: severely infected and erosive skin lesions heal within 1 to 2 weeks, diarrhea ceases, and irritability and depression of mood improve within 24 hours.

Management

Dietary or IV supplementation with zinc salts with 2 to 3 times the required daily amount restores normal zinc status in days to weeks.

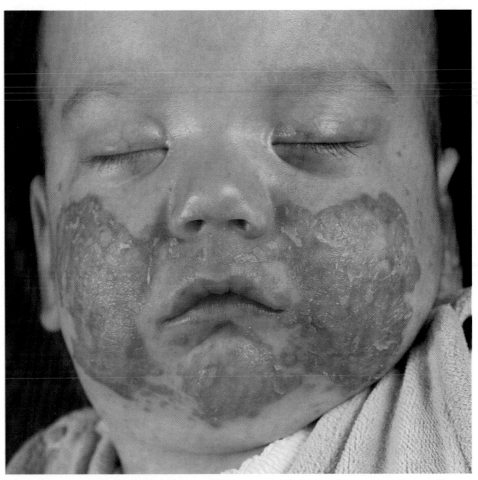

Figure 16-12 Acrodermatitis enteropathica *Sharply demarcated, symmetrical, partially erosive, scaly and crusted plaques on the face. Similar lesions are also found in the perigenital and perianal regions and on the fingertips. Zinc supplementation usually results in prompt clearing of these lesions within a matter of a few days.*

PANCREATIC PANNICULITIS

Pancreatic panniculitis is characterized clinically by painful erythematous nodules occurring at any site, frequently accompanied by arthritis and polyserositis, associated with either pancreatitis or pancreatic carcinoma, and histologically by a lobular panniculitis.

Epidemiology and Etiology

Age   Middle-aged to elderly

Sex   Males > females

Etiology   Associated with chronic pancreatitis or carcinoma of the pancreas

History

Alcoholism, abdominal pain, weight loss, recent-onset diabetes mellitus. Lesions are quite tender.

Physical Examination

Skin Findings

TYPES OF LESIONS   Nodules (Figure 16-13), and plaques. Following biopsy of lesion, liquefied fat drains from lesion.

COLOR OF LESIONS   Erythematous

PALPATION OF LESIONS   Lesions tender, warm. ±Fluctuant (Figure 16-13)

DISTRIBUTION OF LESIONS   Occur at any site; however, predilection for legs and buttocks

General Examination   Pleural effusion, ascites, arthritis (especially ankles)

Differential Diagnosis

Panniculitis   Erythema nodosum, subacute nodular migratory panniculitis (Villanova's disease), lupus erythematosus panniculitis, post-steroid panniculitis, relapsing febrile nonsuppurative nodular panniculitis (alpha-antitrypsin deficiency), Sweet's syndrome

Laboratory and Special Examinations

CBC   Eosinophilia

Chemistry   Hyperlipasemia, hyperamylasemia

Urine   Increased amylase, lipase

Dermatopathology   Lobular panniculitis with necrosis of lipocytes and varying degrees of calcification. Foci of granular basophilic degeneration of lipocytes occur in lobular area, leading to loss of nuclear staining and formation of ghostlike fat cells with thick walls and no nuclei. ±Calcification. Polymorphic lobular infiltrate surrounds foci of necrosis. Contiguous lobules may be spared.

Diagnosis

Clinical diagnosis confirmed by histologic examination of an adequate biopsy including subcutaneous tissue

Pathophysiology

Breakdown of subcutaneous fat caused by enzymes (amylase, trypsin, lipase) released to the circulation from the diseased pancreas

Course and Prognosis

Depends on pancreatic disease. Crops of painful lesions recur.

Management

Directed at treatment of underlying pancreatic disorder

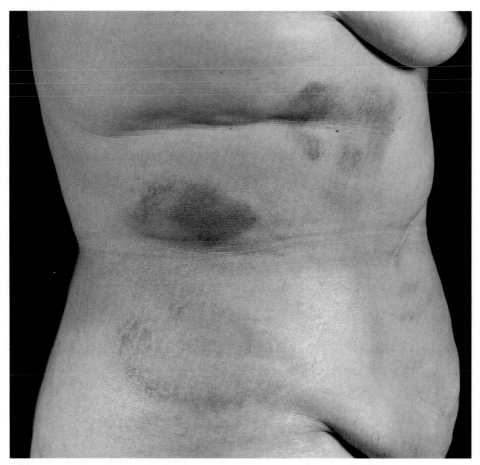

Figure 16-13 Pancreatic panniculitis *Three erythematous, tender, subcutaneous plaques on the trunk. Hemorrhage within the lesions produces various color changes associated with extravasated blood: red, violet, and yellow-green.*

PSEUDOXANTHOMA ELASTICUM

Pseudoxanthoma elasticum (PXE) is a serious hereditary disorder of connective tissue that involves the elastic tissue in the skin, blood vessels, and eyes. The principal skin manifestations are a distinctive *peau d'orange* surface pattern resulting from closely grouped clusters of yellow (chamois-colored) papules in a reticular pattern on the neck, axillae, and other body folds. The effects on the vascular system include gastrointestinal (GI) hemorrhage, hypertension occurring in young persons and resulting from involvement of renal arteries, and claudication. Ocular manifestations ("angioid" streaks and retinal hemorrhages) can lead to blindness.

Epidemiology

Incidence 1:40,000 to 1:160,000

Age of Onset 20 to 30 years

Inheritance Autosomal recessive (most common) and autosomal dominant

History

History Asymptomatic skin lesions, which may at first be overlooked, may develop in early childhood. Skin lesions are usually present by age 30 but may go undetected until old age.

Systems Review Symptoms relating to multisystem involvement. Decrease of visual acuity in a young person. Coronary artery disease: angina pectoris, myocardial infarction. Peripheral vascular disease: claudication, such as cardiac disease, hematemesis and melena, symptoms associated with hypertension. History of miscarriages

Physical Examination

Skin

TYPES OF LESIONS Papules. Coalesce to form larger plaques (Figure 16-14). Skin of involved sites becomes redundant, lax, soft.

COLOR OF LESIONS Yellow, chamois-colored

PALPATION The skin is soft and lax and hangs in folds.

ARRANGEMENT OF MULTIPLE LESIONS Reticulated or linear, furrows between individual plaques

DISTRIBUTION OF LESIONS *Skin* Sides of the neck, axillae, abdomen, groins, and thighs *Mucous Membranes* Yellow papules may be present on the soft palate, labial mucosa, rectum, and vagina.

General Examination Decrease of peripheral pulses

Eyes Angioid streaks (Figure 16-15), which are slate-gray, wider than blood vessels, and extend across the fundus, radiating from the optic disc (streaks represent rupture of Bruch's membrane secondary to elastic fiber defect). Macular degeneration. Retinal hemorrhages. Diminished visual acuity; blindness. Alteration of retinal pigmentation

Cardiovascular Decreased or absent peripheral pulses. Hypertension. Mitral valve prolapse

Differential Diagnosis

Lax Yellow Plaque(s) Cutis laxa, Ehlers-Danlos syndrome, xanthomatosis

Angioid Streaks Sickle cell anemia, Paget's disease of bone, hyperphosphatemia

Laboratory and Special Examinations

Dermatopathology Biopsy lesional skin, normal skin, or scar. Biopsy of scar can detect characteristic changes of PXE before typical skin changes are apparent. Swelling and irregular clumping of elastic fibers in reticular dermis can be seen with routine stains as a faintly basophilic staining of fibers; with von Kossa

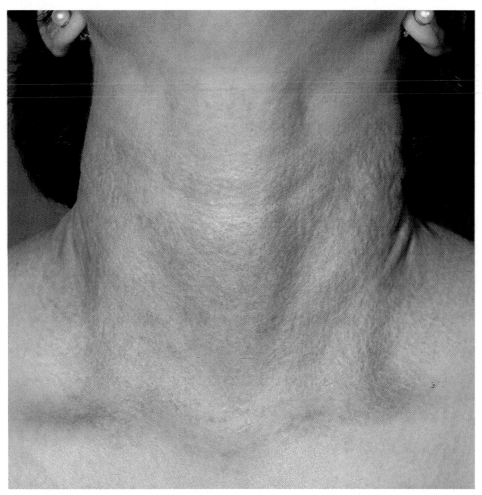

Figure 16-14 Pseudoxanthoma elasticum *Multiple, confluent, chamois-colored or yellow papules (pseudoxanthomatous) created a large, circumferential, pebbled plaque on the neck. Changes in the connective tissue in this condition lead to excessive folds on the lateral neck.*

stain, elastic fibers appear curled and "chopped up" with calcium deposition

Imaging   X-ray: extensive calcification of the peripheral arteries of the lower extremities. Arteriography of symptomatic vessels

Diagnosis

By the skin lesions, which are distinctive, but the diagnosis of PXE is confirmed by biopsy. Angioid streaks are also characteristic.

Etiology and Pathogenesis

Biochemical defect is not known. Abnormalities of both collagen and elastic tissues result in fragmented and calcified elastic fibers in skin, eyes, arteries.

Course and Prognosis

The course is inexorably progressive. Gastric artery hemorrhage occurs commonly, resulting in epistaxis and/or hematemesis. Peripheral vascular disease presents as premature cerebrovascular accidents, atherosclerosis obliterans, or bowel angina. Pregnancies are complicated by miscarriage, cardiovascular complications. Life span is often shortened due to myocardial infarction or massive GI hemorrhage.

Management

Genetic counseling. Evaluate family members for PXE. Obstetrician should be aware of PXE diagnosis and follow patient carefully. Regular reevaluation by primary care physician is mandatory. For symptomatic involvement by various systems, patient should be referred to dermatologist, ophthalmologist, gastroenterologist, cardiologist, neurologist. Surgery can correct some disfiguring cutaneous changes.

Eye   Laser surgery for retinal hemorrhages

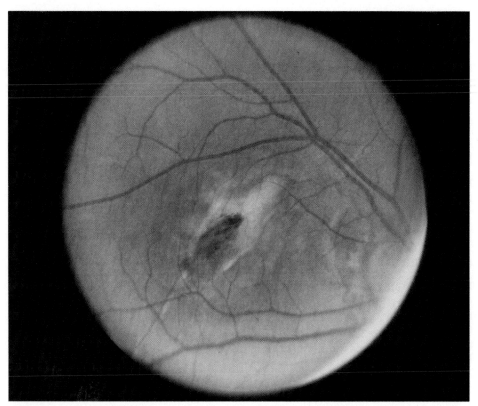

Figure 16-15 Pseudoxanthoma elasticum: angioid streak in retina *Yellowish streaks wider than blood vessels extend across the fundus in a distribution more or less radial from the optic disk.*

TUBEROUS SCLEROSIS

Tuberous sclerosis is an autosomal dominant disease arising from a genetically programmed hyperplasia of ectodermal and mesodermal cells and manifested by a variety of lesions in the skin, CNS (hamartoma), heart, kidney, and other organs. The principal early manifestations are the triad of seizures, mental retardation, and congenital white spots (macules). Facial angiofibromata are pathognomonic but do not appear until the third or fourth year.

Epidemiology

Incidence   In institutions, 1 : 100 to 1 : 300; in general population, 1 : 20,000 to 1 : 100,000

Age   Infancy

Sex   Equal incidence

Race   All races

Heredity   Autosomal dominant. The genes for tuberous sclerosis have been located in chromosomes 16p13 and 9q34.

History

Onset of Lesions

White macules are present at birth or appear in infancy (80 % occur by 1 year of age, 100 % appear by the age of 2 years).

Other skin lesions: angiofibromata (>20 % are present at 1 year of age, 50 % occur by age of 3 years)

Systems Review

Seizures (infantile spasms) 86 %; the earlier the onset of seizures, the worse the mental retardation

Mental retardation (49 %)

Physical Examination

Skin   96 % incidence of skin lesions

TYPES OF LESIONS

Hypomelanotic macules (present in >80 % of patients)—"off-white"; one or many, usually more than three

Papules/nodules on the face (adenoma sebaceum or angiofibromas) (Figure 16-16) (present in 70 %)—red and skin-colored

Plaques representing connective tissue nevi ("shagreen" patch) (present in 40 %)—skin-colored

Periungual papules or nodules—ungual fibromas (Koenen's tumors) present in 22 %, arise late in childhood and have the same pathology (angiofibroma) as the facial papules

SHAPE AND SIZE OF WHITE MACULES

Polygonal or "thumbprint," 0.5 to 2.0 cm

Lance ovate or "ash-leaf" spots (Figures 16-17 and16-18), 3.0 to 4.0 cm (range from 1.0 to 12.0 mm)

Tiny white spots or "confetti" (Figure 16-19), 1.0 to 2.0 mm

DISTRIBUTION OF LESIONS

White macules occur on the trunk (56 %), lower extremities (32 %), upper extremities (7 %), head and neck (5 %).

Angiofibromatous papules and nodules occur on the face and around the toe- and fingernails.

"Shagreen" patches occur on the back or buttocks.

Hair   Depigmented tufts of hair present at birth

Associated Systems   CNS (tumors producing seizures), eye (gray or yellow retinal plaques, 50 %), heart (benign rhabdomyomas), hamartomas of mixed-cell type (kidney, liver, thyroid, testes, and GI system)

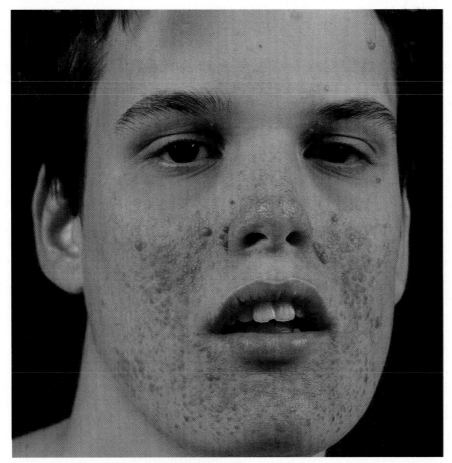

Figure 16-16 Tuberous sclerosis: angiofibromata *Confluent, small, angiomatous (erythematous, glistening) papules on the lower half of the face. These lesions are not present at birth but occur only later during infancy and childhood.*

Differential Diagnosis

White Spots Focal vitiligo, nevus anemicus, tinea versicolor, nevus depigmentosus, postinflammatory hypomelanosis

Angiofibromas Tricholemmoma, syringoma, skin-colored papules on the face, dermal nevi

Periungual Fibromas Verruca vulgaris

Laboratory Examinations

Dermatopathology

LIGHT MICROSCOPY *White Macules* Decreased number of melanocytes, decreased melanosome size, decreased melanin in melanocytes and keratinocytes
Angiofibromata Proliferation of fibroblasts, increased collagen, angioneogenesis, capillary dilatation, absence of elastic tissue
Brain "Tubers" are gliomas.

Imaging

Skull X-Ray Multiple calcific densities

CT Scan Ventricular deformity and tumor deposits along the striothalamic borders

Renal Ultrasound Reveals renal hamartoma

Electroencephalography Abnormal

Special Examinations

Illumination (allow for dark adaptation) Wood's lamp examination should always be used to detect white macules with a deceased melanin pigmentation. This examination is essential for light-skinned persons, since white spots will be detected (Figure 16-18).

The diagnosis may be difficult or impossible in an infant or child if one or two white macules are the only cutaneous finding. More than five is highly suggestive.

Even when typical white "ash-leaf" or "thumb-print" macules are present, it is necessary to confirm the diagnosis. Confetti spots (Figure 16-19) are virtually pathognomonic. A pediatric neurologist can then evaluate the patient with a study of the family members and by obtaining various types of imaging as well as electroencephalography. It should be noted that mental retardation and seizures may be absent.

Etiology and Pathogenesis

Genetic alterations of ectodermal and mesodermal cells with hyperplasia, with a disturbance in embryonic cellular differentiation

Significance

A serious autosomal disorder that causes major problems in behavior, because of mental retardation, and in therapy, to control the serious seizure problem present in many patients

Course and Prognosis

In severe cases, 30 % die before the fifth year of life, and 50 % to 75 % die before reaching adult age. Malignant gliomas are not uncommon. Genetic counseling is imperative.

Management

Prevention Counseling

Treatment Laser surgery for angiofibromas

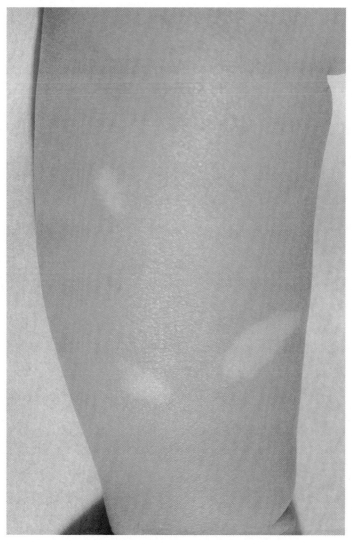

Figure 16-17 Tuberous sclerosis: ash-leaflet hypopigmented macules *Three well-demarcated, elongated (ash-leaflet shaped), hypomelanotic macules on the lower leg of child with tan skin.*

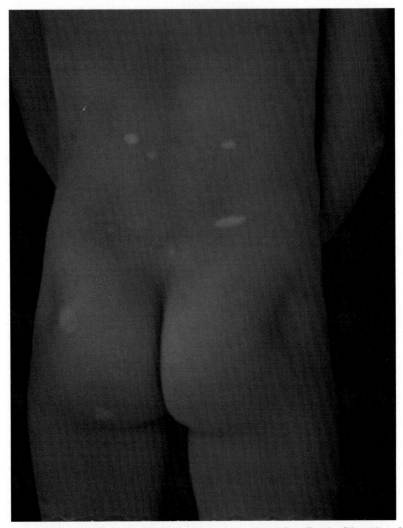

Figure 16-18 Tuberous sclerosis: hypopigmented macules visualized with a Wood's lamp *Hypopigmented macules are difficult to visualize in light-skinned individuals. In this case, the lesions were barely perceptible in this white child until the skin was examined with long-wave UVA light source: thumbprint- and ash-leaf-shaped macules are seen on the trunk and buttocks.*

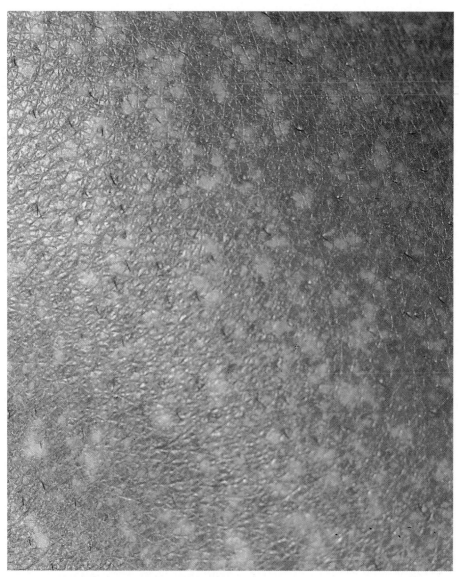

Figure 16-19 Tuberous sclerosis: "confetti" macules *Multiple, discrete, small, confetti-like, hypopigmented macules of variable size on the leg.*

NEUROFIBROMATOSIS

Neurofibromatosis (NF) is an autosomal dominant trait manifested by changes in the skin, nervous system, bones, and endocrine glands. These changes include a variety of congenital abnormalities, tumors, and hamartomas. Two major forms of NF are now recognized: (1) classic von Recklinghausen's NF, termed *NF1* and first described in 1882, and (2) central, or acoustic, NF, termed *NF2*. Both types have café-au-lait macules and neurofibromas, but only NF2 has *bilateral* acoustic neuromas (unilateral acoustic neuromas are a variable feature of NF1). An important diagnostic sign present only in NF1 is pigmented hamartomas of the iris (Lisch nodules).

Epidemiology

Incidence *NF1:* 1:4,000; *NF2:* 1:50,000

Race All races

Sex Males slightly more than females

Heredity Autosomal dominant; the gene for NF1 is on chromosome 17 and that for NF2 is on chromosome 22.

History

Onset of Lesions Café-au-lait (CAL) macules are not usually present at birth but appear during the first 3 years; neurofibromata appear during late adolescence.

Skin Symptoms Neurofibromata may be tender to firm; pressure causes pain.

Systems Review Clinical manifestations in various organs related to pathology: hypertensive headaches (pheochromocytomas), pathologic fractures (bone cysts), mental retardation, brain tumor (astrocytoma), short stature, precocious puberty (early menses, clitoral hypertrophy)

Physical Examination

Appearance of Patient Patients not uncommonly consult physician only because of the physical disfigurement.

Skin Lesions

TYPES

CAL macules: light- or dark-brown *uniform* melanin pigmentation. Lesions vary in size from multiple "freckle-like" tiny macules (Figure 16-20) <2.0 mm to very large >20-cm brown macules (Figure 16-21). The common size, however, is 2.0 to 5.0 cm. Tiny freckle-like lesions in the axillae are highly characteristic (Figure 16-20). A few CAL macules (three or less) may be present in 10 % to 20 % of the normal population.

Nodules: skin-colored, pink, or brown (Figure 16-21); pedunculated; soft or firm; "buttonhole sign"—invagination with the tip of the index finger is pathognomonic.

Plexiform neuromas: drooping, soft, doughy (Figure 16-22); may be massive, involving entire extremity, the head, or a portion of the trunk.

PALPATION Nodules are very soft and compressible.

DISTRIBUTION Randomly distributed (Figures 16-20 to 16-22) but may be localized to one region (segmental NF1). The segmental type may be heritable or a localized hamartoma; therefore, to do genetic counseling, it is necessary to rule out the heritable type by a complete study, including eye examination and family history.

Other Physical Findings

EYES Pigmented hamartomas of the iris (Lisch nodules) begin to appear at age 5 and are present in 20 % of children with NF before age 6; they can be found in 95 % of patients after age 6 in NF1, but Lisch nodules are not present in NF2. These are visible only with slit-lamp examination and appear as "glassy," transparent, dome-shaped, yellow-to-brown papules up to 2.0 mm. They do not correlate with the severity of the disease.

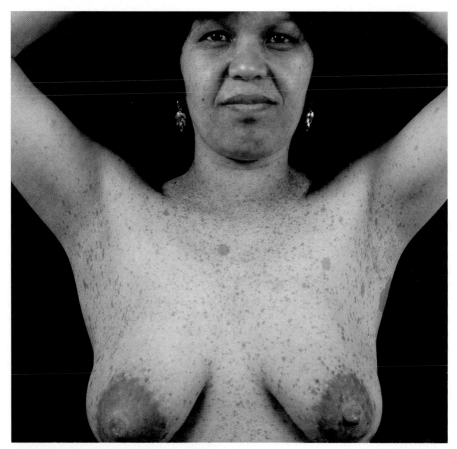

Figure 16-20 von Recklinghausen's disease (NF1) *Several larger (>1.0 cm) café-au-lait macules on the upper chest and multiple small macules in the axillae (axillary "freckling") in a brown-skinned female. Myriads of early, small, pink-tan neurofibromata on the chest, breasts, and neck.*

MUSCULOSKELETAL   Cervicothoracic kyphoscoliosis, segmental hypertrophy

ADRENAL   PHEOCHROMOCYTOMA   Elevated blood pressure and episodic flushing

PERIPHERAL NERVOUS SYSTEM   Elephantiasis neuromatosa (gross disfigurement from neurofibromatosis of the nerve trunks)

CENTRAL NERVOUS SYSTEM   Optic glioma, acoustic neuroma (rare in NF1 and unilateral, bilateral in NF2), astrocytoma, meningioma, neurofibroma

Differential Diagnosis

Brown CAL-Type Macules   Albright's syndrome (polyostotic fibroma, dysplasia, and precocious puberty), normal (present in 10 % to 20 % of population)

The CAL macules present in Albright's syndrome (polyostotic fibrous dysplasia) are impossible to differentiate clinically from the CAL macules in neurofibromatosis. Other criteria listed under Diagnosis are required to establish a diagnosis of neurofibromatosis.

Laboratory and Special Examinations

Dermatopathology   More than 10 *melanin macroglobules* per 5 high-power fields in "split" dopa preparations. The melanin macroglobules also can be seen in routine H&E sections. These do not occur in Albright's syndrome.

Wood's Lamp Examination   In white persons with pale skin, the CAL macules are more easily visualized with Wood's lamp examination.

Diagnosis

Two of the following criteria:

1. Multiple CAL macules, more than six lesions with a diameter of 1.5 cm in adults and more than five lesions with a diameter of 0.5 cm or more in children younger than 5 years
2. Multiple freckles in the axillary and inguinal regions
3. Based on clinical and histologic grounds, two or more neurofibromas of any type, or one plexiform neurofibroma
4. Sphenoid wing dysplasia or congenital bowing or thinning of long bone cortex, with or without pseudoarthrosis
5. Bilateral optic nerve gliomas
6. Two or more Lisch nodules on slit-lamp examination
7. First-degree relative (parent, sibling, or child) with NF1 by the preceding criteria

Etiology and Pathogenesis

Action of an abnormal gene on cellular elements derived from the neural crest: melanocytes, Schwann cells, endoneurial fibroblasts

Significance

It is important to establish the diagnosis in order to do genetic counseling and to follow patients for development of malignancy. Also, neurofibromatosis support groups help with social adjustment in severely affected persons.

Course and Prognosis

There is a variable involvement of the organs affected over time, from only a few pigmented macules to marked disfigurement with thousands of nodules, segmental hypertrophy, and plexiform neuromas. The mortality rate is higher than in the normal population, principally because of the development of neurofibrosarcoma during adult life. Other serious complications are relatively infrequent.

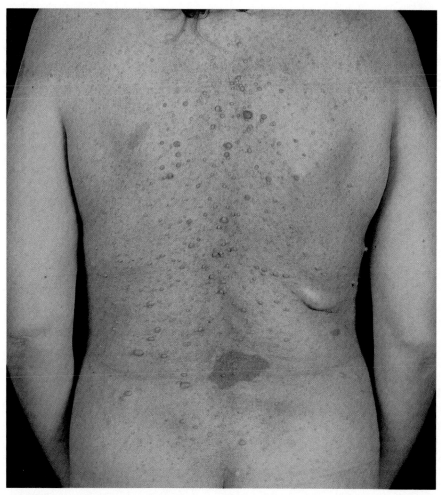

Figure 16-21 von Recklinghausen's disease (NF1) *Skin-colored and pink-tan, soft papules and nodules on the back are neurofibromata; the lesions first appeared during late childhood. Three large café-au-lait macules on the back and right arm. The large, soft, ill-defined, subcutaneous nodule on the right lower back and on the right posterior axillary line are plexiform neuroma.*

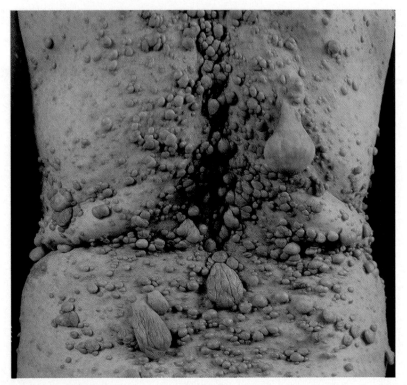

Figure 16-22 von Recklinghausen's disease (NF2) *Myriads of large, pink-violet neurofibromas and pedunculated neuromas on the back; the lesions cause severe, grostesque, cosmetic disfigurement for the individual.*

Management

An orthopedic physician should manage the two major bone problems: kyphoscoliosis and tibial bowing. The plastic surgeon can do reconstructive surgery on the facial asymmetry. The language disorders and learning disabilities should be evaluated by psychological assessment. Close follow-up annually should be mandatory to detect sarcomas that may arise within plexiform neuromas. Surgical removal of pheochromocytoma

XANTHOMAS

Cutaneous xanthomas are yellow-brown, pinkish, or orange macules (as in xanthoma striatum), papules (as in xanthoma papuloeruptivum), plaques (as in xanthelasma palpebrarum), nodules (xanthoma tuberosum), or infiltrations in tendons (xanthoma tendineum). Xanthomas are characterized histologically by accumulations of xanthoma cells—macrophages containing droplets of lipids. A xanthoma may be a symptom of a general metabolic disease, a generalized histiocytosis, or a local cell dysfunction. The following classification is based on this principle: (1) xanthomas due to hyperlipoproteinemia (hyperlipidemia) and (2) normolipoproteinemic xanthomas. Of the latter group, only the normolipoproteinemic xanthelasmata of the eyelids are common enough to be discussed in detail, but reference is made to diffuse normolipemic xanthoma as a sign of lymphoma. Although the hyperlipoproteinemic xanthomas are relatively rare, they are important for two reasons: (1) they may be the first symptom of a serious metabolic disease, and (2) they may be regarded as an experiment of nature that may enable us to study the pathogenesis of atherosclerotic disease.

The causes of hyperlipoproteinemia may be divided into primary, in most cases genetically determined, and secondary, those caused by severe hyperthyroidism, biliary cirrhosis, grossly deranged diabetes, and a number of still rarer conditions.

In 1972, Frederickson and Lees considerably furthered the study of hyperlipoproteinemias by dividing them into five phenotypes depending on the distribution of the lipoprotein classes. Lipids, which are insoluble in water, are transported in the blood and bound in various proportions to proteins, resulting in so-called lipoproteins (see Table 16-A).

From Table 16-A it can be calculated that a hypercholesterolemia may be caused by an excess of low-density lipoprotein (LDL) as well as by an excess of very low density lipoprotein (VLDL). However, in the first case, the triglycerides are normal; in the second case, cholesterol *and* triglycerides are elevated. It is important to recognize this because a hypercholesterolemia caused by LDL has more serious consequences than one caused by VLDL.

Apoproteins

The lipids, which are insoluble in water, are coated with proteins that have three functions: (1) causing water solubility, (2) fixing lipoproteins to cellular receptors, and (3) exercising enzymatic activity.

The sources of the lipids and apoproteins are the gut and the liver. Lipids and apoproteins interact in two cascades: one originates from the chylomicrons from the gut and the other from the VLDL synthesized in the liver. The principal apoprotein of the chylomicrons is apoprotein β48; of the VLDL, the apoproteins B100, E, and C11. During the transformation of VLDL via IDL (floating β, VLDL remnant) to LDL, apoproteins E and C11 are lost.

In the past decade it has been recognized that Fredrickson's phenotypes are symptoms of genetic metabolic diseases with distinct and different pathogeneses (Tables 16-B and 16-C).

TABLE 16-A COMMON ABNORMAL LIPOPROTEIN PATTERNS IN HYPERLIPOPROTEINEMIA

Type	Lipoprotein Abnormalities	Appearance of Plasma[1]	Usual Changes in Lipid Concentrations
I	Massive chylomicronemia, VLDL normal, LDL, HDL normal or decreased	Cream layer on top, clear below	C normal, TG↑↑
II^a	LDL increased, VLDL normal	Clear	C↑, TG normal
II^b	LDL increased, VLDL increased	May be slightly turbid	C↑, TG↑
III	Presence of β-VLDL	Usually turbid, often with faint cream layer	C↑, TG↑↑
IV	VLDL increased	Usually turbid, no cream layer	C normal, TG↑↑
V	Chylomicrons present, VLDL increased	Cream layer on top, turbid below	C↑, TG↑↑

NOTE: VLDL = very low density pre-β-lipoproteins; LDL = low-density (β) lipoproteins; HDL = high-density (alpha) lipoproteins; C = cholesterol; TG = triglycerides; β-VLDL = IDL = intermediate-density lipoproteins, floating β.
[1]After standing at 4°C for 18 hours or more.
SOURCE: Modified from Fredrickson DS: Plasma lipid abnormalities and cutaneous and subcutaneous xanthomas, in *Dermatology in General Medicine*, 2d ed, edited by TB Fitzpatrick et al. New York, McGraw-Hill, 1979, p 1120.

TABLE 16-B CLASSIFICATION OF GENETIC LIPOPROTEIN DISTURBANCES

1. Familial hypercholesterolemia (FH): type II^a
2. Familial dyslipoproteinemia (FD): type III
3. Familial combined hyperlipoproteinemia (FCL): types II$^{a\ or\ b,}$ or IV
4. Familial hypertriglyceridemia (FHT): type IV/V
5. Familial lipoproteinlipase deficiency (FLD) (very rare): type I

TABLE 16-C RELATION OF THE TYPE OF XANTHOMATOSIS TO THE VARIOUS PHENOTYPES OF LIPOPROTEIN DISTURBANCE AND THEIR NOSOLOGIC CAUSE

Xanthelasma palpebrarum	Normolipemic or FH, FD
Xanthoma tendineum	FH (type II$^{a)}$
Xanthoma tuberosum	FD, FHT, FH (if homozygous) (types III, IV, II^a)
Xanthoma papuloeruptivum	FD, FHT, FLD (types II, IV/V, I)
Xanthochromia and xanthoma striatum palmare	FD (type III)

XANTHELASMA

Xanthelasma palpebrarum *may* or *may not* be associated with hyperlipoproteinemia.
Synonyms: Xantheloma palpebrarum, eyelid xanthoma.

Epidemiology and Etiology

Age   Over 50 years; when in children or young adults, it is associated with FH or FD

Sex   Either

Incidence   Most common of all xanthomas

Significance   May be an isolated finding unrelated to hyperlipoproteinemia, but sometimes there is an elevation of LDL. When the LDL is markedly elevated, it is a sign of FH or FD.

History

Duration of Lesions   Months, with slow enlargement from tiny spot

Skin Symptoms   None

Physical Examination

Skin Lesions (Figure 16-23)

TYPE   Papules, plaques, soft

COLOR   Yellow-orange

SHAPE   Polygonal

DISTRIBUTION   Localized to eyelids

Laboratory Examination

Cholesterol estimation in plasma, if enhanced screening for type of hyperlipoproteinemia

Course and Prognosis

If due to hyperlipoproteinemia, complication with atherosclerotic cardiovascular disease may be expected.

In a larger percentage of the patients with xanthelasmata palpebralia, no metabolic disturbances are found. In others, xanthelasmata palpebralia are a sign of familial hyperlipoproteinemia FH or FD. When total lipids and total cholesterol content of the serum are within normal limits, no further lipid analysis is necessary.

Management

Excision, electrodesiccation, laser, and application of trichloroacetic acid are the treatments of choice; recurrences are uncommon.

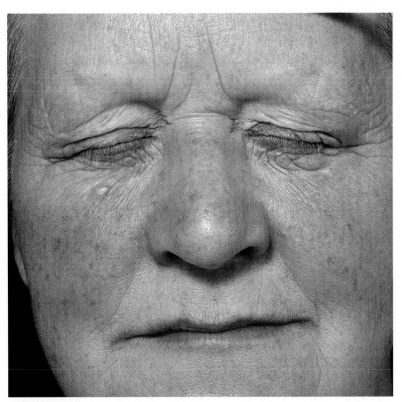

Figure 16-23 Xanthelasma *Multiple, longitudinal, creamy-orange, slightly elevated dermal papules on the eyelids of a normolipemic individual.*

XANTHOMA TENDINEUM

Xanthomata tendinea are yellow or skin-colored subcutaneous tumors that move with the extensor tendons (Figure 16-24). They are a symptom of familiar hypercholesterolemia (FH) that presents as a type II^a hyperlipoproteinemia. This condition is autosomal recessive, with a different phenotype in the heterozygote and homozygote. In the heterozygote, the xanthomata appear in adult life, as do the cardiovascular complications. In the homozygote, the xanthomata appear in early childhood, and the cardiovascular complications in early adolescence; the elevation of the LDL content of the plasma is extreme. These patients rarely attain ages above 20 years.

FH is caused by a defect in the LDL receptors on the cell membrane localized in coated pits. This defect is partial in the heterozygotes, total in the homozygotes. Due to this defect, the cholesterol-rich LDL is insufficiently cleared from the blood, which again results in an insufficient checking of the endocellular cholesterol synthesis. Recent investigations have shown that different deletions on the DNA cause different defects in the LDL receptors.

Management

A diet low in cholesterol and saturated fats is necessary but insufficient. This should be supplemented with a bile acid sequestrant, cholestyramine, and an HMG CoA reductase inhibitor (simvastine, pravastine). In this way, the production of LDL receptors is stimulated. This stimulation is impossible in homozygous patients, due to the total absence of LDL receptors. Here, heroic measures such as portacaval shunt or liver transplantation have to be considered.

XANTHOMA TUBEROSUM

This comprises yellowish nodules (Figure 16-25) located especially on the elbows and knees originating by confluence of concomitant eruptive xanthomata. They are to be found in patients with FD, FHT, and FLD. In homozygous patients with FH, the tuberous xanthomata are flatter and skin-colored. They are not accompanied by eruptive xanthomata.

Management

Treatment of the underlying condition

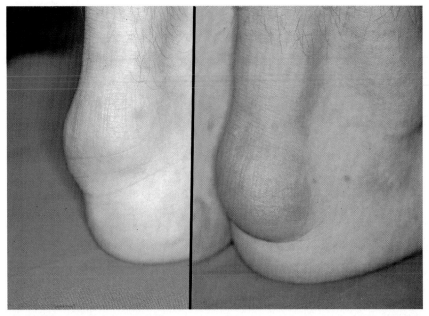

Figure 16-24 Tendinous xanthomas *Large subcutaneous tumors adherent to the Achilles tendons.*

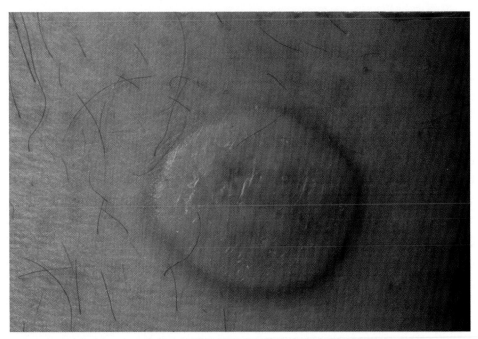

Figure 16-25 Tuberous xanthoma *Flat-topped, yellow, firm tumor with an erythematous margin.*

ERUPTIVE XANTHOMA

These discrete, inflammatory-type papules "erupt" suddenly and in showers, appearing typically on the buttocks.

Synonym: Xanthoma papuloeruptivum.

Etiology

A sign of FHT, FD, and the very rare FLD (exogenous hyperchylomicronemia) and diabetes out of control

History

Lesions appear suddenly.

Physical Examination

Skin Lesions

TYPES

Papules, discrete
Nodules represent confluent papules.

COLOR   Initially red, then yellow center with red halo

SHAPE   Dome-shaped

ARRANGEMENT

Scattered, discrete lesions in a localized region (e.g., elbows, buttocks) (Figure 16-26), may coalesce to form large plaques (Figure 16-27)
"Tight" clusters may become confluent to form "tuberoeruptive" xanthomata.

DISTRIBUTION

Papules: buttocks, elbows, knees, back, or anywhere
"Tuberoeruptive" lesions: elbows

Management

React very favorably on a low-caloric and low-fat diet

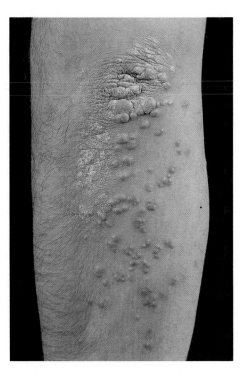

Figure 16-26 Papular eruptive xanthomas
Multiple, discrete, red-to-yellow papules be-coming confluent on the elbow of an individ-ual with uncontrolled diabetes mellitus; le-sions were present on both elbows and buttock.

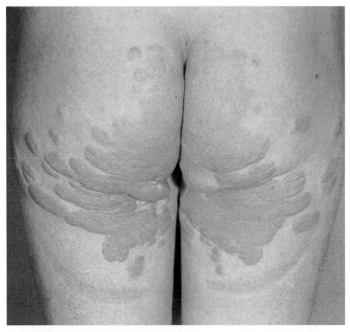

Figure 16-27 Papular eruptive xanthomas *Yellow-orange (due to fat in the dermis), sharply demarcated plaque xanthomata on the buttocks and thighs.*

XANTHOMA STRIATUM PALMARE

Xanthoma striatum palmare presents as yellow-orange, flat or elevated infiltrations of the volar creases of palms and fingers (Figure 16-28). This is highly characteristic for FD. FD is characterized by a type III phenotype of lipoprotein disturbance due to the presence of chylomicron and VLD remnants in the plasma (IDL, β-VLDL, with an enhanced ratio of cholesterol/triglycerides). These particles are present in the plasma due to defective binding in the liver. The deficient binding is caused by a hereditary abnormality in the E apoprotein, which is responsible for the binding of the VLDL remnants in the liver. Investigation on the molecular-genetic level has shown a variation in alleles causing different types of apoprotein E patterns.

Next to the highly characteristic xanthomata striata palmaria, FD also presents with tuberous xanthoma (Figure 16-25), eruptive xanthoma (Figure 16-26), and xanthelasma palpebrarum (Figure 16-23).

Patients with FD are prone to atherosclerotic cardiovascular disease, especially ischemia of the arteries of the legs and coronary vessels.

Management

Patients with FD react very favorably to a diet low in fats and carbohydrates. If necessary, this may be supplemented with clofibrate, an aryloxylid derivative, that inhibits VLDL synthesis in the liver.

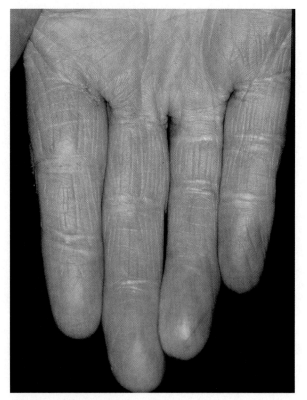

Figure 16-28 Xanthoma striatum palmare *The palmar creases are yellow, often a subtle lesion noticeable only upon close examination.*

NORMOLIPEMIC PLANE XANTHOMA

Xanthoma planum is a normolipemic xanthoma that consists of diffuse orange-yellow pigmentation of the skin. There is a recognizable border. These lesions can be idiopathic or secondary to leukemia, but the most common association is with multiple myeloma. The lesions may precede the onset of multiple myeloma by many years.

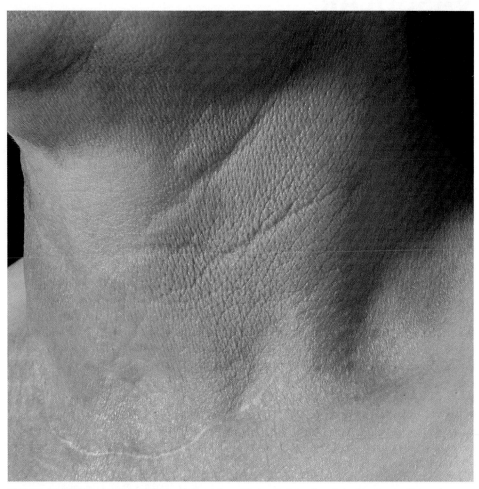

Figure 16-29 Plane xanthomas *Yellowish-reddish, slightly elevated plaques on the neck, noticeable mainly because of the accentuation of the skin texture in a normolipemic patient with lymphoma. Plane xanthomas occur most commonly on the upper trunk and neck and also occur in individuals with myeloma.*

CUTANEOUS MANIFESTATIONS OF VASCULAR INSUFFICIENCY

ATHEROSCLEROSIS, ATHEROEMBOLIZATION, AND ARTERIAL INSUFFICIENCY

Atherosclerosis obliterans (ASO), especially of the lower extremities, is associated with a spectrum of cutaneous findings, ranging from slowly progressive ischemic changes to the sudden appearance of ischemic lesions following atheroembolization. Atheroembolism is the phenomenon of dislodgement of atheromatous debris from an affected artery or aneurysm with centrifugal microembolization and resultant ischemic and infarctive cutaneous lesions.

Epidemiology and Etiology

Sex Males > females

Age Middle-aged to elderly

Incidence Atherosclerosis is the cause of 90 % of arterial disease in developed countries, affecting 5 % of men >50 years of age; 10 % (20 % of diabetics) of all men with atherosclerosis develop critical limb ischemia.

Risk Factors for Atherosclerosis Cigarette smoking, hyperlipidemia, low HDL cholesterol, high alpha-lipoprotein, hypertension, diabetes mellitus, hyperinsulinemia, abdominal obesity, family history of premature ischemic heart disease, personal history of cerebrovascular disease or occlusive peripheral vascular disease

Diabetes Mellitus and Lower Leg Ischemia Gangrene of lower extremities is estimated to be from 8 to 150 times more frequent in diabetics than in nondiabetics, most often occurring in those who smoke.

History

Symptoms

ATHEROSCLEROSIS OF LOWER EXTREMITY ARTERIES Early symptom is usually pain on exercise, i.e., intermittent claudication. With progressive arterial insufficiency, pain and/or paresthesias at rest occur in leg and/or foot, especially at night.

ATHEROEMBOLISM Often occurs following an intraarterial procedure. Acute pain and tenderness at site of embolization. "Blue toe," "purple toe" syndrome: peripheral ischemia, livedo reticularis of sudden onset.

Systems Review Individuals with arterial insufficiency of the lower extremities often have symptoms of ischemic heart disease (coronary artery disease or arteriosclerotic heart disease), atherosclerosis obliterans, diabetes mellitus. An episode of cutaneous atheroembolization may be accompanied by embolization to kidney, pancreas, muscle, etc.

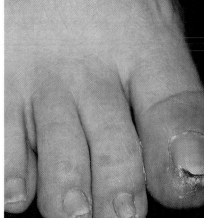

Figure 17-1 Atherosclerosis obliterans with ischemic skin changes *The great toe shows ischemic and preinfarctive changes of violaceous discoloration and early ulceration; the iliac artery was occluded. The changes were reversed following surgical correction of the vascular occlusion.*

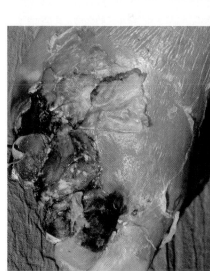

Figure 17-2 Atherosclerosis obliterans with infarction *Arterial occlusion has led to distal gangrene. The great toe is ischemic and the lateral toes infarcted with necrosis of the skin and deeper tissues.*

Physical Examination

Atherosclerosis/Arterial Insufficiency

SKIN LESIONS **Types** General findings associated with ischemia include pallor, cyanosis, loss of hair on affected limb. Earliest infarctive changes (Figure 17-1) include well-demarcated maplike areas of epidermal necrosis. Later, dry gangrene may occur over the infarcted skin through which underlying structures such as tendons can be seen. With shedding of slough, well-demarcated ulcers are seen (Figure 17-2). Microangiopathy in diabetics may present as acral erysipelas-like erythema.

Color Dusky to red; white

Palpation Pulse of large vessels usually diminished or absent. In diabetics with mainly microangiopathy, gangrene may occur in the setting of adequate pulses. Temperature of foot: cool to cold, room temperature. Pain: early infarctive lesions painful on palpation; eschemic ulcers are painful; in diabetics with neuropathy and ischemic ulcers, pain may be minimal or absent.

Distribution Arteriosclerosis of femoral, popliteal, dorsalis pedis, posterior tibial, which are most commonly associated with cutaneous, usually acral, ischemia, present as diminished or absent pulses. Ischemic ulcers may first appear between toes at sites of pressure and beginning on fissures on plantar heel. Dry gangrene of feet, especially of toes.

GENERAL EXAMINATION *Pulses* Buerger's sign: with significant reduction in arterial blood flow, limb elevation causes pallor (best noted on plantar foot); dependency causes delayed and exaggerated hyperemia. Auscultation over stenotic arteries reveals bruits.

Atheroembolization

SKIN LESIONS *Types* Livedo reticularis (Figures 17-3A and 3B). Ischemic changes with poor return of color after compression of skin. Necrosis and gangrene: indurated nodules and plaques, which may undergo necrosis (Figure 17-4A), become crusted, and ulcerate (Figure 17-4B). Cyanosis and gangrene.

Color Nodules/plaques/livedo: violaceous. Ulcers: erythematous halo.

Palpation Nodules/plaques and underlying muscles: tenderness

Distribution Livedo reticularis: lower abdomen/back, buttocks, legs, feet. Plaques/nodules: thighs, calves. Gangrene: digits.

GENERAL EXAMINATION *Pulses* Distal pulses may remain intact.

Differential Diagnosis

Intermittent Claudication Pseudoxanthoma elasticum, Buerger's disease (thromboangiitis obliterans), arthritis, gout

Painful Foot Gout, interdigital neuroma, onychomycosis with ingrowing great toenails, flat feet, calcanean bursitis, plantar fasciitis

Ischemic and Infarctive Lesions of Leg/Foot Vasculitis, ecchymosis, chilblains, Raynaud's phenomenon (vasospasm), disseminated intravascular coagulation (purpura fulminans), cryoglobulinemia, hyperviscosity syndrome (macroglobulinemia), septic embolization (infective endocarditis), nonseptic embolization (ventricular mural thrombus with myocardial infarction, atrial thrombus with atrial fibrillation), aneurysms (dissecting, thrombosed), drug-induced necrosis (warfarin, heparin), ergot poisoning, intraarterial injection, livedo reticularis syndromes, external compression (popliteal entrapment, cervical rib)

Laboratory and Special Examinations

Hematology Rule out anemia, polycythemia

Lipid Studies Hypercholesterolemia (>240 mg/dl), often associated with rise in low-density lipoprotein (LDL). Hypertriglyceridemia (250 mg/dl), often associated with rise in very low-density lipoproteins (VLDL) and remnants of their catabolism (mainly intermediate-density lipoprotein, IDL).

Dermatopathology of Atheroembolism Deep skin and muscle biopsy specimen shows arterioles occluded by multinucleated foreign-body giant cells and fibrosis surrounding biconvex, needle-shaped clefts corresponding to the cholesterol crystal microemboli.

Doppler Studies Noninvasive technique that measures velocity and volume of flow

Digital Plethysmography With exercise can unmask significant atherosclerotic involvement of lower extremity arteries.

X-Ray Calcification can be demonstrated intramurally; often the calcification represents medial sclerosis that may be present in the absence of significant atherosclerosis.

Arteriography Atherosclerosis is best visualized by angiography. With atheroemboliza-

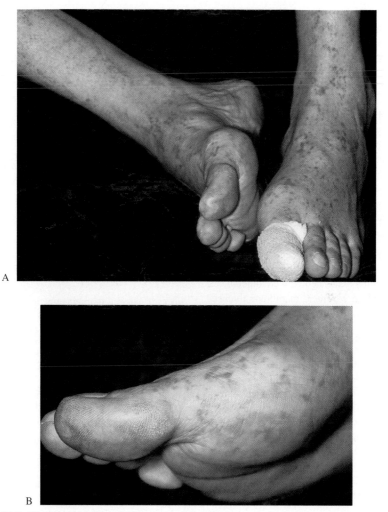

Figure 17-3 Atheroembolism following angiography A. *A mottled, violaceous, vascular pattern on the feet and ankles. The findings were noted following intravascular catheterization and angiography in an individual with ASO. The dressing on the great toe protects an ischemic ulcer.* B. *Close-up of the mottled, violaceous, vascular pattern on the foot.*

tion, ulceration of atheromatous plaques seen in abdominal aorta or more distally.

Diagnosis

Clinical suspicion confirmed by arteriography and deep skin biopsy (atheroembolism)

Pathophysiology

Atherosclerosis is the most common cause of arterial insufficiency and may be generalized or localize to the coronary arteries, aortic arch vessels to the head and neck, or those supplying the lower extremities, i.e., femoral, popliteal, anterior and posterior tibial arteries. Atheromatous narrowing of arteries supplying the upper extremities is much less common. Atheromatous deposits and thromboses occur commonly in the femoral artery in Hunter's canal and in the popliteal artery just above the knee joint. The posterior tibial is most often occluded where it rounds the internal malleolus, the anterior tibial where it is superficial and becomes the dorsalis pedis artery. Atheromatous material in the abdominal or iliac arteries also can diminish blood flow to the lower extremities as well as break off and embolize (atheroembolization) downstream to the lower extremities. Detection of atherosclerosis often delayed until an ischemic event occurs, related to critical decrease in blood flow.

In addition to large-vessel arterial obstruction, individuals with diabetes mellitus often have microvasculopathy associated with endothelial cell proliferation and basement membrane thickening of arterioles, venules, and capillaries.

Atheroembolism Multiple small deposits of fibrin, platelet, and cholesterol debris embolize from proximal atherosclerotic lesions or aneurysmal sites. Occurs spontaneously or after intravascular surgery or procedures such as arteriography, fibrinolysis, or anticoagulation. Emboli tend to lodge in small vessels of skin and muscle and usually do not occlude large vessels.

Course and Prognosis

Arterial insufficiency can be a slowly progressive disease or punctuated by episodes of complete occlusion or embolism. Approximately 5 % per year of individuals with intermittent claudication progress to pain at rest or gangrene. A much higher percentage die from other complications of atherosclerosis such as ischemic heart disease.

Poor tissue perfusion makes infection more likely, with interdigital tinea pedis, leg/foot ulcers, or small breaks and fissures in the skin. Chronic lymphedema, prior saphenous venous harvesting, and prior episodes of cellulitis increase the likelihood of cellulitis.

Atherosclerosis of coronary and carotid arteries usually determines survival of patient; involvement of lower extremity arteries often causes significant morbidity and is commonly associated with coronary artery involvement as well. Balloon angioplasty, endarterectomy, and bypass procedure have improved prognosis of patients with atherosclerosis. Amputation rates have been lowered from 80 % to less than 40 % by aggressive vascular surgery.

Atheroembolism May be a single episode if atheroembolization follows intraarterial procedure. May be recurrent if spontaneous and associated with significant tissue necrosis

Management

Prevention Goal of management is prevention of atherosclerosis rather than treatment of ischemic complications.

DIET First step in management of primary hyperlipidemia: Reduce intake of saturated fats and cholesterol as well as calories.

EXERCISE Useful adjunct to diet. Walking increases new collateral vessels in ischemic muscle.

HYPERTENSION Reduce elevated blood pressure.

CIGARETTE SMOKING Discontinue.

BLOOD Correct anemia or polycythemia.

POSITIONING OF ISCHEMIC FOOT As low as possible without edema

DRUG THERAPY Recommended for adults with LDL cholesterol >190 mg/dl or greater than 160 mg/dl in the presence of two or more risk factors after an adequate trial of at least 3 months of diet therapy alone. Initiation of drug therapy usually commits patients to lifelong treatment. Drugs act primarily by lowering LDL cholesterol and include bile acid-binding resins, nicotinic acid, and HMG-CoA reductase inhibitors.

Intermittent Claudication

MEDICAL MANAGEMENT Encourage walking to create new collateral vessels

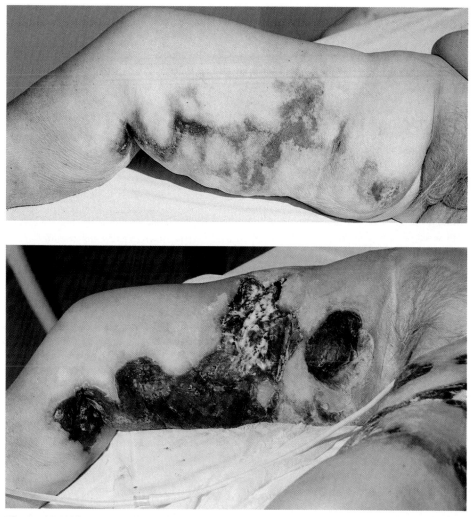

A

B

Figure 17-4 Atheroembolism with cutaneous infarction A. *Violaceous plaques and cutaneous infarctions with a linear arrangement on the medial thigh of an individual with atherosclerosis, heart failure, and diabetes. B. Within 48 hours the initial changes progressed to become far more extensive with large areas of infarction.*

SURGICAL MANAGEMENT Endarterectomy or bypass for aortic iliac occlusions and for extensive femoral popliteal disease.

Ischemia/Infarction of Foot/Leg

SURGICAL MANAGEMENT Distal bypass surgery of three crural arteries

Atheroembolization Response to surgical revascularization or thrombolytic therapy often poor

MEDICAL MANAGEMENT Heparin and warfarin. Analgesics.

SURGICAL MANAGEMENT Debridement of necrotic tissue locally or amputation if indicated. Remove or bypass atherosclerotic vessel or aneurysm. Amputation of leg/foot: indicated when medical and surgical management has failed.

CHRONIC VENOUS INSUFFICIENCY

Chronic venous insufficiency (CVI) results from failure of return of venous blood and increased capillary pressure; the resultant changes include edema, stasis dermatitis, hyperpigmentation, fibrosis of the skin and subcutaneous tissue (lipodermatosclerosis) of the leg, and ulceration.

Epidemiology and Etiology

Sex Varicose veins are three times more common in women than in men.

Age Varicose veins: peak incidence of onset 30 to 40 years

Etiology CVI is most commonly associated with varicose veins and the postphlebitic syndrome. Varicose veins are an inherited characteristic; pregnancy aggravates existing venous disease.

Aggravating Factors Varicose veins: pregnancy, increased blood volume, increased cardiac output, increased venocaval pressure, effect of progesterone on smooth muscle of vein wall

History

History Prior episode(s) of deep vein thrombosis. Risk factors for deep leg vein thrombosis include antepartum/postpartum state, minor leg injuries, pelvic lower abdominal operations, medical illnesses, prolonged recumbency.

CVI commonly associated with heaviness or aching of leg, which is aggravated by standing (dependency) and relieved by walking. Lipodermatosclerosis may limit movement of ankle and cause pain and limitation of movement. History of leg edema aggravated by dependency (end of the day, standing), summer season. Shoes feel tight in the evening. Night cramps. Atrophie blanche may occur at sites of trauma.

Physical Examination

Skin Lesions Arterial pulses in patients with CVI in that arterial as well as venous insufficiency exists in some.

TYPES

Varicose veins: Superficial leg veins are enlarged, tortuous, with incompetent valves; best evaluated with the patient standing (Figure 17-5). Brodie-Trendelenburg tourniquet test (used to demonstrate incompetence of long saphenous vein): release of midthigh tourniquet shows varicose veins fill from above downward.

Edema: dependent; improved or resolved in the morning after a night in the horizontal position

Pigmentation: stippled with recent and old hemorrhage

Eczematous (stasis) dermatitis: occurs in setting of CVI about the lower legs and ankles (Figure 17-6); must be distinguished from allergic contact dermatitis secondary to topically applied agents; if extensive, may be associated with a generalized eczematous dermatitis, i.e., "id" reaction or autosensitization.

Atrophie blanche: ivory-white plaques (Figure 17-7) on the ankle and/or foot; stippled pigmentation, hemosiderin-pigmented border

Ulceration: occurs in 30 % of cases; very painful "hyperalgesic microulcer" in area of atrophie blanche; larger superficial or deep ulcers (Figure 17-9)

Lipodermatosclerosis: inflammation, induration, pigmentation of lower third of leg creating "champagne bottle" or "piano leg" appearance with edema above and below the sclerotic region (Figure 17-8). A verrucous epidermal change can occur overlying the sclerosis, referred to as elephantiasis nostras verrucosa.

COLOR Extravasated blood: acutely red, fades to red-brown, and brown (hemosiderin). Melanin: postinflammatory hyperpigmentation, especially in individuals with darker skin types.

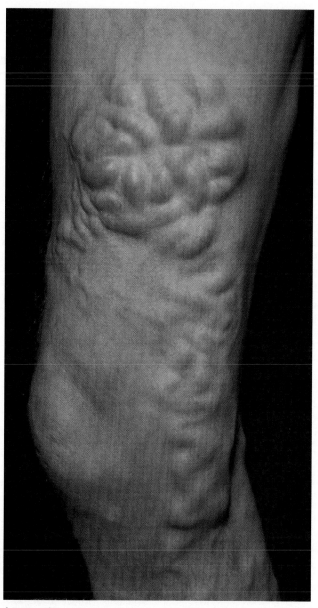

Figure 17-5 Varicose veins *Greatly dilated venous varicosities forming a cerebriform mass on the medial thigh and leg.*

Edema: dorsa of feet, ankles, legs. Pigmentation: over varices, at ankles, around the legs.

Differential Diagnosis

Varicose Veins Post-thrombotic syndrome, Klippel-Trenaunay-Weber syndrome, Parkes-Weber syndrome (congenital arteriovenous fistulas)

Deep Vein Phlebitis Superficial thrombophlebitis, muscle trauma, hematoma

Edema Right-sided heart failure, hypoalbuminemia, Kaposi's sarcoma, pretibial myxedema (Graves' disease), iliac vein compression

Pigmentation Progressive pigmentary purpura, minocycline pigmentation

Stasis Dermatitis Nummular eczema, atopic dermatitis, asteatotic eczema, allergic contact dermatitis, irritant dermatitis

Leg Ulcer (See Leg Ulcers, page 486.)

Laboratory and Special Examinations

Cultures Rule out secondary bacterial infection.

Doppler Studies Evaluate arterial flow in patients with poor peripheral pulses.

Varicography Contrast medium is injected into varicosities to detect incompetent veins, especially following recurrence after surgery.

Color-Coded Duplex Sonography Detects incompetent veins. Venous occlusion due to thrombus

Arteriography Rule out significant arterial insufficiency.

Imaging X-ray may (10 % of chronic cases) show subcutaneous calcification, i.e., postphlebitic subcutaneous calcinosis. Bony changes include periostitis underlying ulceration, osteoporosis as a result of disuse, osteomyelitis, fibrous ankylosis of ankle.

Tourniquet Test A tourniquet is applied to the leg that has been elevated to empty the veins; when the patient stands up and the tourniquet is released, there is an instant filling of a varicose vein due to absence of or ill-functioning valves.

Dermatopathology Early: small venules and lymphatic spaces appear dilated; edema of extracellular space with swelling and separation of collagen bundles. Subsequently: capillaries dilated, congested with tuft formation and tortuosity of venules; deposition of fibrin. Endothelial cell hypertrophy: may be associated with venous thrombosis; angioendotheliomatous proliferation mimicking Kaposi's sarcoma. In all stages, extravasation of RBCs that break down forming hemosiderin, which is taken up by macrophages. Lymphatic vessels become encased in a fibrotic stroma, i.e., dermatoliposclerosis. Calcification of fat and fibrous tissue may occur. Rule out Kaposi's sarcoma, calciphylaxis.

Diagnosis

Usually made on history, clinical findings, and Doppler sonography

Pathophysiology

The valves of the deep veins of the calf are damaged and incompetent at restricting backflow of blood. The communicating veins that connect deep and superficial calf veins are damaged, which also causes CVI. Fibrin is deposited in the extravascular space and undergoes organization, resulting in sclerosis and obliteration of lymphatics and microvasculature. Perivascular fibrosis results in diminished nutrition of the epidermis, which breaks down with ulcer formation.

Course and Prognosis

Acute deep vein thrombosis commonly results in lipodermatosclerosis one to two decades after the acute event; ulceration develops in a smaller percentage.

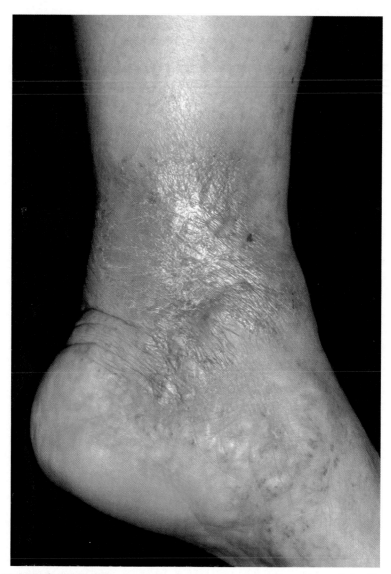

Figure 17-6 Stasis dermatitis *A plaque of eczematous dermatitis on the medial ankle overlying a venous varicosity.*

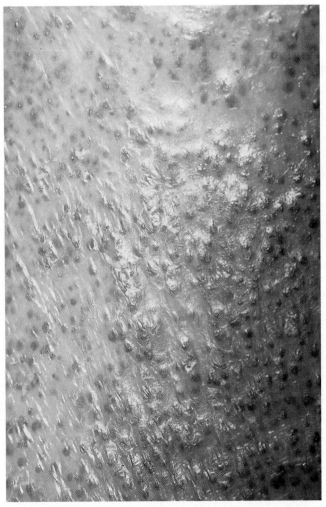

Figure 17-7 Atrophie blanche   *Dermal sclerosis with ivory-white skin stippled with dilated abnormal vasculature in an individual with chronic venous insufficiency (same individual as Figure 17-8).*

Management

Atrophie Blanche   Avoid trauma to area involved. Intralesional triamcinolone into painful lesions.

Varicose Veins

INJECTION SCLEROTHERAPY   A sclerosing agent such as tetradecyl sulfate is injected into varicosities, followed by prolonged compression. Used mainly to treat minor branch varicosities not associated with saphenous incompetence and new branch vein varicosities developing after surgery. Recurrence is very common within 5 years.

VASCULAR SURGERY   Incompetent perforating veins are identified, ligated, and divided, followed by stripping out of the main trunk of long and/or short saphenous veins. Residual perforating veins are the main cause of recurrences after surgery. In patients with combined arterial and CVI, bypass or angioplasty may prove beneficial.

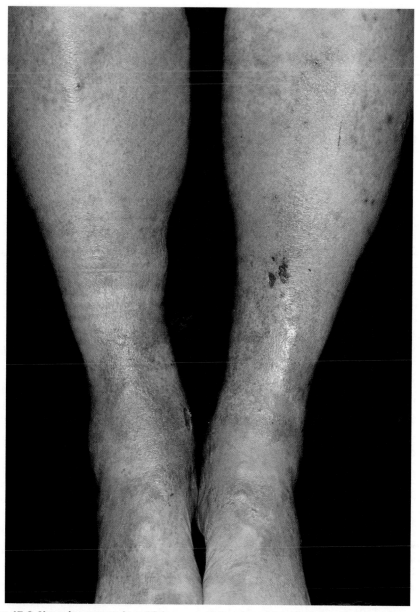

Figure 17-8 Chronic venous insufficiency and lipodermatosclerosis *The ankles are thin and the upper calves edematous creating a "champagne bottle" or "piano leg" appearance. An ulcer is present over the medial malleolus and atrophy blanche (see Figure 17-7 for close-up) is extensive on the lower legs. The patient has a history of deep vein thromboses, pulmonary embolization, and inferior vena cava ligation.*

LEG ULCERS

Leg ulcers occur relatively commonly in late middle and old age, arising in association with chronic venous insufficiency, chronic arterial insufficiency, or peripheral sensory neuropathy; in some patients, a combination of these factors is in play. Leg ulcers are associated with significant long-term morbidity and often do not heal unless the underlying problem(s) is corrected.

Epidemiology and Etiology

Sex   Venous ulcers: females > males

Age   Venous ulcers: middle-aged and elderly. Arterial ulcer: >45 years.

Etiology   In developed countries, most common causes include chronic venous insufficiency (80 % of cases), arterial insufficiency (5 % to 10 %), neuropathy, diabetes mellitus; in many cases, several of these factors are in play.

Prevalence   500,000 to 600,000 cases in the United States. The incidence of deep vein thrombosis appears to be decreasing. Arterial insufficiency is becoming more common in an aging population.

Risk Factors   Venous ulcers: minor injury, malnutrition, sedentary lifestyle

Inheritance   Half of patients have a family history of leg ulcers (presumably related to inheritance of valvular defects).

History

History

VENOUS ULCERS   Aching and swelling of legs that is exacerbated by dependency and relieved by elevation of leg. Stasis dermatitis associated with pruritus and weeping; "id" or autosensitization reaction associated with palmar vesicles resembling dyshidrotic eczema.

ARTERIAL ULCERS   Intermittent claudication and pain, even at rest, as disease progresses. Characteristically, painful at night. Pain often quite severe; may be worse when legs elevated, improving on dependency. Risk factors: cigarette smoking, diabetes mellitus.

NEUROPATHIC ULCERS   Most commonly associated with diabetes of many years' duration. Early symptoms of neuropathy include paresthesia, pain, anesthesia of leg and foot. Patients are often unaware of prior trauma that commonly precedes ulcerations of heel, plantar metatarsal area, or great toe.

Systems Review   See Chronic Venous Insufficiency (page 480) and Atherosclerosis, Atheroembolization, and Arterial Insufficiency (page 474).

Physical Examination

ULCERS ASSOCIATED WITH CHRONIC VENOUS INSUFFICIENCY

Skin Lesions   Venous ulcers arise in the setting of edema, induration, and/or lipodermatosclerosis. Varicose veins are best evaluated with the patient standing.

TYPES   *Edema* Eczematous (stasis) dermatitis. Lipodermatosclerosis (sclerosing panniculitis): induration and fibrosis of dermis and subcutaneous tissue; may precede venous ulceration. Chronic lymphedema may be associated with epidermal hyperplasia, termed *elephantiasis nostras verrucosa*.
Venous Ulcers Ulceration preceded by ischemia that presents as a red or blue-red patch. Minor trauma to this site often precipitates ulceration. Ulcers are usually punched out with irregular shaggy borders (Figure 17-9). Cellulitis may complicate stasis dermatitis or venous ulcers; repeated episodes cause additional damage to lymphatic drainage, thus compounding chronic lymphedema, lipodermatosclerosis, and pigmentation. Immobility of ankle joint results in fibrous or bony ankylosis.

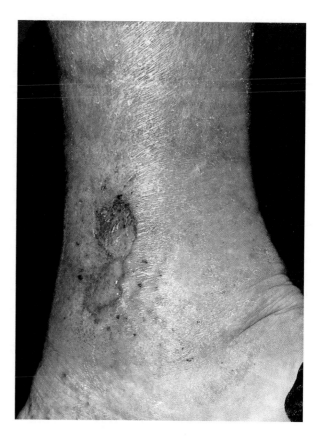

Figure 17-9 Ulcers associated with chronic venous insufficiency *Two ulcers over the medial malleolus (same patient as Figures 17-7 and 17-8).*

COLOR   Brown or brown-red (Figure 17-9)

DISTRIBUTION   Ulcers commonly develop on the medial lower aspect of the calf (Figure 17-9), especially over malleolus (lateral as well as medial), in the area supplied by incompetent perforating veins. In developed countries where shoes are worn, venous ulcers rarely occur on the feet. Stasis ulcers also can develop in the most dependent parts of a pendulous abdominal panniculus in a massively obese individual.

ULCERS ASSOCIATED WITH CHRONIC ARTERIAL INSUFFICIENCY

Skin Lesions

TYPES   Ulcer(s): punched out, sharply demarcated borders. A tissue slough is often present at the base, through which tendons can be seen. Exudation minimal. Associated findings of ischemia: loss of hair on feet and lower legs; shiny atrophic skin. Stasis pigmentation and lipodermatosclerosis are absent (Figure 17-10).

COLOR   Base: dry, gray or black

PALPATION   Pulse diminished or absent; painful

ARRANGEMENT   Ulceration may have the pattern of skin supplied by the involved artery.

DISTRIBUTION   Occur over sites of pressure or trauma: bony prominences (pretibial), supramalleolar (Figure 17-10) distal points such as toes

ULCERS ASSOCIATED WITH HYPERTENSION (MARTORELL'S ULCER)

Skin Lesions

TYPES   Ulcer(s): punched out, sharply demarcated borders, with surrounding halo of erythema

COLOR   Erythematous halo

PALPATION   Very painful. Pain relieved by placing leg in dependent position.

DISTRIBUTION   Anterior external aspect of leg (Figure 17-11) between middle and lower third of limb.

NEUROPATHIC AND DIABETIC ULCERS

Skin Lesions   The typical diabetic neuropathic foot is numb, warm, and dry, with palpable pulses.

TYPES   Ulcers: commonly surrounded by thick callus. Other findings include Charcot's arthropathy and neuropathic edema

COLOR   Base: dry, gray or black

PALPATION   Initially, change is loss of sensation of light touch of great toe and then foot; subsequently, ankle jerk reflex is lost; then joint position sense.

DISTRIBUTION   Ulcers usually occur at points of high-pressure loading, especially on the soles or at sites of deformity. Occur over sites of pressure or trauma: heel, metatarsal head, great toe.

General Findings

CARDIOVASCULAR SYSTEM   Cardiac function and peripheral pulses should be evaluated in all patients with leg ulcers. Measure systolic blood pressure at ankle.

NERVOUS SYSTEM   Neurologic findings should be evaluated in all patients with leg ulcers.

Differential Diagnosis

Leg Ulcer(s)   Vasculitis (polyarteritis nodosa), erythema induratum, calciphylaxis, neoplasia (SCC, BCC, lymphoma), infection (ecthyma, cutaneous tuberculosis, Buruli ulcer, *Mycobacterium marinum* infection, leprosy, invasive fungal infection, chronic HSV ulcer, chronic VZV infection, leishmaniasis, syphilis, yaws), trauma, pressure ulcer, extravasation of intravenous fluid, injecting drug user (skin popping), radiodermatitis, sickle cell anemia, pyoderma gangrenosum, necrobiosis lipoidica with ulceration, prolidase deficiency, factitia

Laboratory and Special Examinations

Hematology   CBC and differential. ESR. Rule out sickle cell anemia.

Chemistry   Blood glucose

Serology   ANA, STS when indicated

Cultures   Rule out secondary bacterial infection: *Staphylococcus aureus,* group A streptococcus. Uncommonly, *Pseudomonas aeruginosa, Candida.*

Patch Testing   Rule out associated allergic contact dermatitis when leg ulcers are associated with surrounding eczematous dermatitis to commonly used topical agents such as neomycin, parabens, lanolin, nitrofurazone, bacitracin, or formaldehyde.

Vascular Blood Flow Studies   Measure systolic blood pressure at ankle. Doppler flowmeter can be used to detect arterial pulsations over dorsalis pedis and posterior tibial arteries in those with imperceptible or barely perceptible pulses. Arteriography indicated in those with impaired arterial blood flow to assess feasibility of surgical repair.

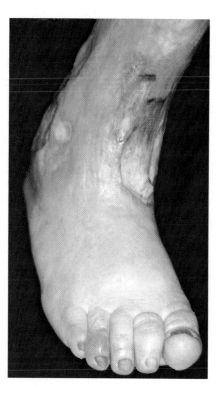

Figure 17-10 Ulcers associated with chronic arterial insufficiency *Large, painful, well-demarcated ulcers on the lower leg, ankle, and foot; the extemity was pulseless and cold, and the distal foot had a porcelain-white color.*

Imaging Rule out underlying osteomyelitis by x-ray examination. When indicated, additional studies such as CT scan, bone scan, gallium scan, or bone biopsy can be performed. Charcot's arthropathy occurs in diabetics, involving the metatarsotarsal joints.

Dermatopathology Biopsy of ulcer margin indicated if ulcer(s) has not improved after 3 months of therapy. Rule out vasculitis or inflammatory/infectious etiology; rule out underlying malignancy or malignant transformation (SCC).

Diagnosis

History and clinical findings (varicose veins, lipodermatosclerosis) confirmed by appropriate laboratory examinations

Pathophysiology

Venous Ulcers In half of patients venous ulcers are associated with prior venous thrombosis; in the remaining half with incompetence of superficial or communicating veins. Calf muscle pump dysfunction may occur because of deep venous insufficiency or obstruction, perforator incompetence, superficial venous insufficiency, arterial fistulas, neuromuscular dysfunction; commonly, a combination of these factors is in play. High venous pressure associated with capillary tortuousity and increased capillary permeability to large molecules results in deposition of a pericapillary fibrin layer. This layer is a barrier to diffusion of oxygen and other nutrients, resulting in ischemia and necrosis. Factors precipitating epidermal necrosis include minor trauma (scratch, knock) or contact dermatitis.

Arterial Ulcers See Atherosclerosis (page 474).

Neuropathic Ulcers Foot ulcers in diabetics are usually associated with both sensory neuropathy and ischemia, often complicated by infection. Pressure over prominences of foot leads progressively to callosity formation, autolysis, and finally ulceration.

Course and Prognosis

With correction of underlying causes, ulcers heal with initial formation of pink granulation tissue at the base, which is reepithelialized by epithelium from residual skin appendages or surrounding epidermis.

Infection Ulcers provide an easy portal of entry for infection, which should be suspected if pain appears or increases in intensity. Infection can occur relatively superficially in ulcer base or be more invasive with cellulitis and possible lymphangitis or bacteremia.

Eczematous Dermatitis Can be either stasis dermatitis, irritant dermatitis, or allergic contact dermatitis to one of many medicaments used in topical treatments

Neoplasia Ulcers can heal with a pseudoepitheliomatous epidermal hyperplasia within the scar, mimicking squamous cell carcinoma. Squamous cell carcinoma and, less commonly, basal cell carcinoma arise at sites of chronic (years) ulceration.

Venous Ulcers Heal with adequate management. Invariably recur, usually on multiple occasions, unless underlying causes are corrected.

Leg Ulcers in Diabetics Diabetics are particularly predisposed to leg ulcers and frequently have several etiologic factors in play, i.e., peripheral vascular disease, neuropathy, infection, and impaired healing.

Neurotrophic Ulcers Rule out underlying osteomyelitis in patients with prolonged purulent drain from ulcers.

Management

In general, factors such as anemia and malnutrition should be corrected to facilitate healing. Control hypertension. Weight reduction in the obese. Exercise; mobilize patient. Correct edema caused by cardiac, renal, or hepatic dysfunction. Depression is common, associated with chronic debilitation. Secondary infection should be treated with effective antibiotics.

Venous Ulcers Ulceration tends to be recurrent unless underlying risk factors are corrected, i.e., corrective surgery and/or elastic stockings worn on a daily basis.

REDUCE VENOUS HYPERTENSION Leg elevation. Elastic support stockings; beware of excess compression in patients with underlying arterial occlusion. Unna boot; replace weekly. Intermittent pneumatic compression.

TREAT UNDERLYING ECZEMATOUS DERMATITIS Whether atopic, stasis, or allergic contact eczematous dermatitis, should be treated initially with moist dressings for the acute exudative phase and subsequently with moderate to potent corticosteroid ointment for a limited time. Hydrated petrolatum for xerosis.

DEBRIDEMENT Moist saline dressings, changed frequently. Surgical debridement to remove necrotic tissue.

SYSTEMIC ANTIMICROBIAL AGENTS Treat secondarily infected ulcer or complications of lymphangitis or cellulitis.

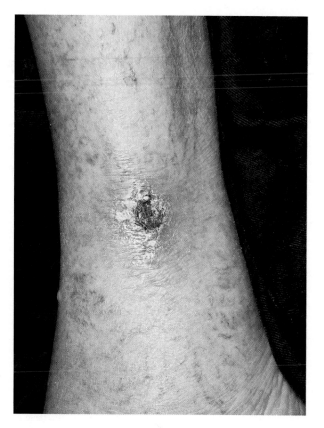

Figure 17-11 Ulcer associated with hypertension *Painful, crusted ulcer on the lower leg of an individual with uncontrolled hypertension.*

SKIN GRAFTING Large ulcers with healthy granulation tissue in the base can be grafted by pinch or split-thickness methods. The patient's own epidermis can be cultured in vitro and used for grafting.

Arterial Ulcers

SYMPTOMATIC Analgesics for ischemic pain

INCREASE LOCAL BLOOD FLOW Stop smoking. Control hypertension, diabetes. Exercise to increase collateral circulation. Elevate head of bed. Keep legs and feet warm.

DEBRIDEMENT Moist saline dressings, changed frequently. Surgery is usually contraindicated.

SYSTEMIC ANTIMICROBIAL AGENTS Treat secondarily infected ulcer or complications of lymphangitis or cellulitis.

ARTERIAL RECONSTRUCTION Endarterectomy to remove localized atheromatous plaques; reconstruction/bypass of occluded areas. Consider in patients with pain at rest or failure of ulcer to heal.

Neuropathic Ulcers

PREVENTION Distribute weight off pressure points by special shoes.

TREATMENT Debride callus around ulcer margin. Total-contact plaster casting removes pressure from ulcer site.

PRESSURE ULCERS

Pressure ulcers develop at body-support interfaces over bony prominences as a result of external compression of the skin, shear forces, and friction, which produce ischemic tissue necrosis. Pressure ulcers occur in patients who are obtunded mentally or have diminished sensation (as in spinal cord disease) in the affected region. Secondary infection results in localized cellulitis, which can extend locally into bone or muscle or into the bloodstream with resultant bacteremia and sepsis.
Synonyms: Pressure sore, bed sore, decubitus ulcer.

Epidemiology and Etiology

Age Any age. Risk factors for pressure ulcers are more common in the elderly. In many individuals, risk factors persist for the life of the patient. The greatest prevalence of pressure ulcers is in elderly, chronically bedridden patients.

Prevalence Acute care hospital setting, 3 % to 14 %; long-term care settings, 15 % to 25 %; home-care settings, 7 % to 12 %; spinal cord units, 20 % to 30 %.

Sex Equally prevalent in both sexes

Pathogenesis External compression of the epidermis, dermis, and hypodermis leads to ischemic tissue damage and necrosis. Risk factors for developing pressure ulcers: inadequate nursing care, diminished sensation/immobility (obtunded mental status, spinal cord disease), hypotension, fecal or urinary incontinence, presence of fracture, hypoalbuminemia, and poor nutritional status.

History

Onset Ulcers often develop within the first 2 weeks of acute hospitalization and more rapidly if the patient experiences significant immobilization.

Symptoms Painful unless there is altered sensorium

Physical Examination

Skin Lesions

CLINICAL CATEGORIES OF PRESSURE ULCERS
Early change (before ulcer formation): localized erythema that blanches on pressure

Stage I: Nonblanching erythema of intact skin

Stage II: Ulceration, superficial or partial-thickness skin loss involving the epidermis and/or dermis (Figure 17-12). Abrasions, vesicles, bullae, or shallow ulcers may be present.

Stage III: Deep crateriform ulceration with dermal involvement and full-thickness skin loss; damage or necrosis can extend down to, but not through, fascia.

Stage IV: Full-thickness ulceration (Figure 17-13) with extensive damage/necrosis to muscle, bone, or supporting structures

Well-established pressure ulcers are widest at the base and taper to a cone shape at the level of skin. Ulcers with devitalized tissue at the base (eschar) have a higher chance of secondary infection. Purulent exudate and erythema surrounding the ulcer suggest infection. Foul odor suggests anaerobic infection.

SIZE May enlarge to many centimeters.

PALPATION May or may not be tender. Borders may be undermined.

DISTRIBUTION Occur over bony prominences: sacrum (60 %) (Figure 17-13) >ischial tuberosities (Figure 17-12), greater trochanter, heel >elbow, knee, ankle, occiput.

General Examination Fever, chills, or increased pain of ulcer suggests possible cellulitis or osteomyelitis.

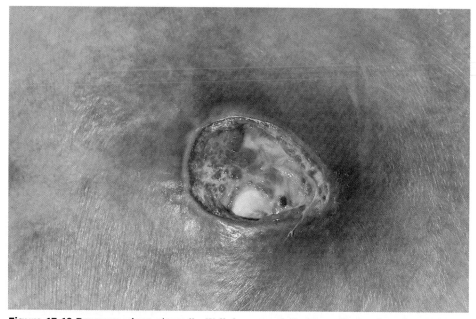

Figure 17-12 Pressure ulcer, stage II   *Well-demarcated ulcer extending to the subcutaneous fat overlying the ischial tuberosity.*

Differential Diagnosis

Infectious ulcer (actinomycotic infection, deep fungal infection, chronic herpetic ulcer), vasculitis ulcer, thermal burn, malignant ulcer (cutaneous lymphoma, basal cell or squamous cell carcinoma), pyoderma gangrenosum, rectocutaneous fistula

Laboratory and Special Examinations

Hematologic Studies   Elevated white blood cell count and erythrocyte sedimentation rate suggest infection (osteomyelitis or bacteremia).

Wound Culture

BACTERIAL CULTURE   Infection must be differentiated from colonization. Culture of the ulcer base detects only surface bacteria. Optimal culture technique: Deep portion of punch biopsy specimen obtained from the ulcer base is minced and cultured for aerobic and anaerobic bacteria. Most infections are polymicrobial and difficult to diagnose. Commonly cultured pathogens include: *Staphylococcus aureus,* methicillin-resistant *S. aureus,* group A streptococcus, enterococcus, *Proteus mirabilis, Pseudomonas aeruginosa, Haemophilus influenzae* (scalp ulcers), anaerobes, *Bacillus fragilis.*

VIRAL CULTURE   Rule out chronic herpes simplex virus ulcer.

Blood Culture Bacteremia often follows manipulation of ulcer (within 1 to 20 minutes of beginning the debridement); resolves within 30 to 60 minutes. Anaerobes are commonly present; frequently polymicrobial.

Biopsy

SKIN BIOPSY Epidermal necrosis with eccrine duct and gland necrosis. Variable infiltrate of neutrophils and mononuclear cells around necrotic eccrine glands. Deep ulcers show wedge-shaped infarcts of the subcutaneous tissue, obstruction of the capillaries with microthrombi, and endothelial cell swelling followed by endothelial cell necrosis and secondary inflammation.

BONE BIOPSY Is essential for diagnosing continuous osteomyelitis; specimen is examined histologically and microbiologically.

Imaging It is difficult to distinguish osteomyelitis from chronic pressure-related changes by radiogram or scan.

Diagnosis

Usually made clinically. Complications are assessed with data on cultures, biopsies, and imaging. Osteomyelitis occurs in nonhealing pressure ulcers; combination of elevated erythrocyte sedimentation rate, leukocytosis, and x-ray examination leads to diagnosis with 90 % sensitivity and specificity.

Pathophysiology

The mean skin capillary pressure is approximately 25 mmHg. External compression with pressures >30 mmHg will occlude the blood vessels so that the surrounding tissues become anoxic. Amount of damage is proportional to extent and duration of pressure. Healthy individuals can tolerate higher pressures. Repositioning the patient every 1 or 2 hours prevents the interface skin over a bony prominence from becoming ischemic, with subsequent ulcer formation. Secondary bacterial infection can enlarge the ulcer rapidly, extend to underlying structures (as in osteomyelitis), and invade the bloodstream, with bacteremia and septicemia. Infection also impairs or prevents healing.

Course and Prognosis

If pressure is relieved, some changes are reversible; intermittent periods of pressure relief will increase resistance to compression. Osteomyelitis occurs in nonhealing pressure ulcers (32 % to 81 %). Cellulitis and osteomyelitis require antibiotic treatment and prolong healing of ulcers. Septicemia is associated with a high mortality rate. Overall, patients with pressure ulcers have a fourfold risk of prolonged hospitalization and of dying when compared with patients without ulcers. With proper treatment, stages I and II ulcers will heal in 1 to 2 weeks and stages III and IV ulcers will heal in 6 to 12 weeks. Manipulation of pressure ulcers can cause bacteremia.

Management

Prophylaxis in At-Risk Patients Reposition patient every 2 hours (more often if possible); massage areas prone to pressure ulcers while changing position of patient; inspect for areas of skin breakdown over pressure points.

- Use interface air mattress to reduce compression.
- Minimize friction and shear forces by using proper positioning, transferring, and turning techniques.
- Clean with mild cleansing agents, keeping skin free of urine and feces.
- Minimize skin exposure to excessive moisture from incontinence, perspiration, or wound drainage.
- Maintain head of the bed at a relatively low angle of elevation (<30 degrees).
- Evaluate and correct nutritional status; consider supplements of vitamin C and zinc.
- Mobilize patients as soon as possible.

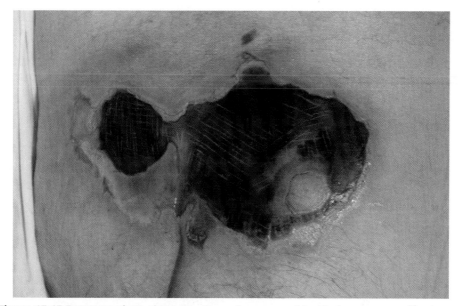

Figure 17-13 Pressure ulcer, stage IV *Huge ulcers covered by black eschar extending into the underlying fascia overlying the sacrum and surrounding tissues.*

Stages I and II Ulcers Topical antibiotics (preferably not neomycin) under moist sterile gauze may be sufficient for early erosions. Normal saline wet-to-dry dressings may be needed for debridement. If ulcer does not heal by 30 % within 2 weeks, consider hydrogels or hydrocolloid dressings.

Stages III and IV Ulcers Surgical management includes: debridement of necrotic tissue, bony prominence removal, flaps and skin grafts.

Infectious Complications

CONTINUOUS OSTEOMYELITIS Prolonged course of antimicrobial agent depending on sensitivities, with or without surgical debridement of necrotic bone

TRANSIENT BACTEREMIA Treatment is usually not indicated.

SEPSIS Marked by elevated temperature, chills, hypotension, and tachycardia and/or tachypnea

Section 18

THE NAILS AS CLUES TO MULTISYSTEM DISEASE*

The nails are rarely scrutinized during the physical examination unless there are prominent and obvious abnormalities. It is therefore important to examine the nails carefully for signs of multisystem disease.

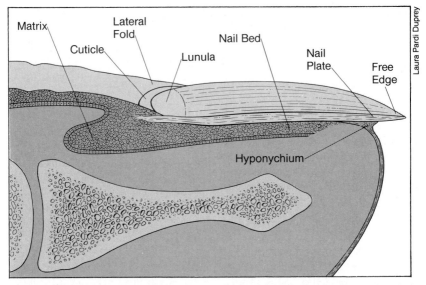

Figure 18-1 Normal nail   *The nail has several distinct anatomic areas. The hard nail plate emerges from a matrix of specialized epithelial cells. The matrix begins 7 to 8 mm under the proximal nail fold, and its distal end is the white crescent called the* lunula. *The richly vascularized nail bed lies directly beneath the plate to provide adherence and support and is the basis of the characteristic pink color. The proximal and lateral nail folds surround the plate on three sides, and the cuticle, an outgrowth of the proximal fold, provides a seal between the fold and the nail plate.*

*Modified from Kvedar JC, Fitzpatrick TB: A look at the nail for some clues to multisystem disease. *Current Challenges in Dermatology.* New York, Special Programs Division of HP Publishing Company. Summer, 1990.

Figure 18-2 Muehrcke's nails *Muehrcke's nails are characterized by paired narrow horizontal white bands, separated by normal color, that remain immobile as the nail grows. Muehrcke's nails are seen most often in patients with hypoalbuminemia associated with nephrotic syndrome, and their presence correlates with low serum albumin levels. The pathogenesis of this nail abnormality is not known.*

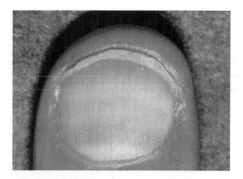

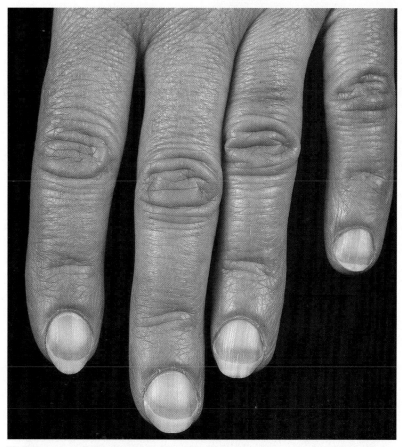

Figure 18-3 Terry's nail/"Half-and-Half" nail *The proximal two-thirds of the nail plate is white, whereas the distal third shows the red color of the nail bed. The dramatic color changes of Terry's nails are rare occurrences, but they may be a manifestation of congestive heart failure or hypoalbuminemia associated with hepatic cirrhosis. In the classic presentation of the half-and-half nail, the distal half is pink or brown and is sharply demarcated from the proximal half, which is dull and white and obliterates the lunula. The difference between half-and-half and Terry's nails is unclear and debatable. Half-and-half nails are found in 10 % of patients with the uremia of chronic renal failure. The color change does not correlate with the severity of renal disease.*

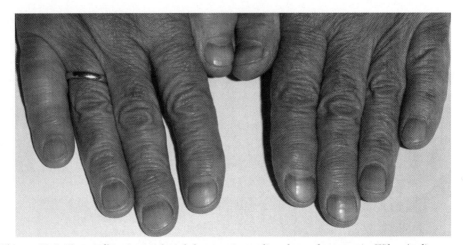

Figure 18-4 Blue nails *Antimalarial drugs, minocycline, hemochromatosis, Wilson's disease, ochronosis, and exposure to silver nitrate may be associated with blue or blue-gray nails. Wilson's disease is an autosomal recessive disorder that results in toxic accumulations of copper in the liver, brain, and other organs. The first clinical signs are often neurologic (resting and intention tremors, spasticity, rigidity, chorea), while Kayser-Fleischer rings (deposits of copper in the cornea) and a blue discoloration of the lunulae appear later. Ochronosis is an autosomal recessive defect of homogentisic acid metabolism, in which deposits of polymerized homogentisic acid appear as a blue pigmentation of the sclerae, as blue macules on the outer ear, and as a diffuse blue-gray pigmentation of the nail bed. Prolonged ingestion, injection, or mucosal absorption of silver nitrate produces* argyria—*a diffuse gray-blue pigmentation of the skin and bluish discoloration of the lunulae similar to that seen in Wilson's disease.*

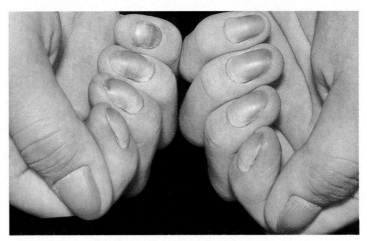

Figure 18-5 Yellow nail syndrome *A clinical triad characterizes the yellow nail syndrome: opaque yellow and dystrophic nails, lymphatic abnormalities (aplasia, ectasia, lymphedema, lymphangitis); and systemic illness, usually pulmonary disease (bronchiectasis, pleural effusion) or cancer (Hodgkin's lymphoma, endometrial carcinoma, malignant melanoma, lymphoma). Changes include a diffuse yellow-to-green color of the fingernails and toenails, nail thickening, slowed growth, and excessive curvature from side to side. There may be concomitant edema of the fingertips and ankles and on occasion very severe edema of the face. Even when severe, edema may be associated with normal lymph nodes on lymphangiography.*

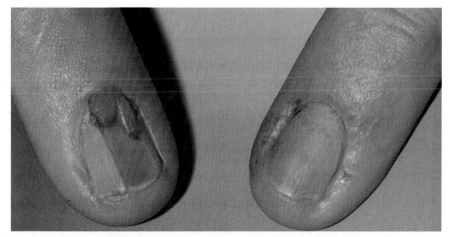

Figure 18-6 Periungual fibroma   *The appearance of periungual fibroma in any patient should prompt a careful family history, cutaneous examination, and neurologic workup (including imaging of the skull) for tuberous sclerosis. This inherited disorder has both cutaneous and neurologic manifestations. The degree of neurologic dysfunction varies, however, and in some patients a minor cutaneous finding such as periungual fibroma may be the only sign of the disease. These fibromas are asymptomatic but can produce a longitudinal groove in the nail plate when located in the proximal nail fold. There is no treatment for tuberous sclerosis; however, it is important to recognize the disease so that the patient and parents can receive genetic counseling.*

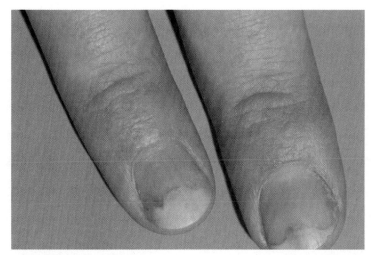

Figure 18-7 Onycholysis   *Onycholysis is a separation of the nail plate from the nail bed. The separated portion is white and opaque, in contrast to the pink translucence of the attached portion. Onycholysis may be a sign of hyperthyroidism (Plummer's nail), especially when it affects only the ring finger. In most cases of hyperthyroidism, the skin of the fingers is warm and moist with a velvety texture, and the palm is erythematous. Onycholysis is, however, a very common nail abnormality that also accompanies onychomycosis, trauma, chemical exposure, and psoriasis.*

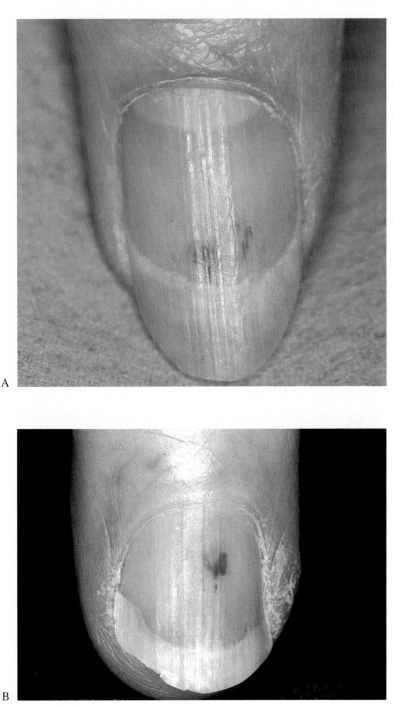

A

B

Figure 18-8 Splinter hemorrhages *The brown or red streaks that represent splinter hemor-rhages most often result from trauma to the nail and arise distally in the nail bed* (A). *They may, however, be a sign of infection endocarditis and arise in the midportion of the nail bed* (B).

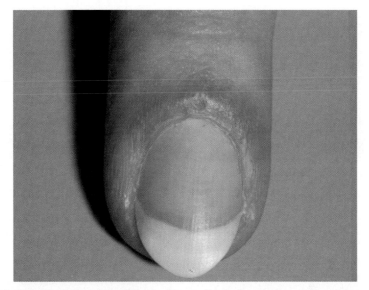

Figure 18-9 Nail fold telangiectasia *In this condition, the capillary loops of the proximal nail fold become tortuous and dilated, presumably as a result of injury from repeated bouts of microangiitis and immune-complex deposition. Nail fold telangiectasia occurs with varying degrees of severity. It is a characteristic feature of dermatomyositis but is also seen in systemic lupus erythematosus and rarely in progressive systemic sclerosis. Some believe a diagnosis of connective tissue disease can be made reliably on the basis of the nail fold abnormality.*

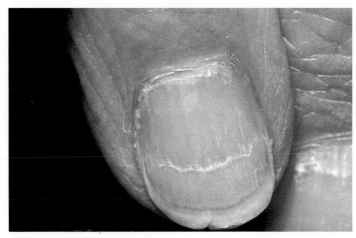

Figure 18-10 Beau's lines *The horizontal depressions across the nail plate that constitute Beau's lines are caused by a transient arrest in nail growth. A temporary growth arrest can occur during acute stress (e.g., high fever, circulatory shock, myocardial infarction, pulmonary embolism) and will manifest as Beau's lines as the nail grows out. It is therefore possible to pinpoint the date of the illness by the distance of the furrow from the proximal nail fold. Depending on the age of the patient, the nail plate takes 3 to 4 months to grow from its base to its distal edge. In a variation of Beau's lines, white transverse bands (Mee's lines) mark the stressful event.*

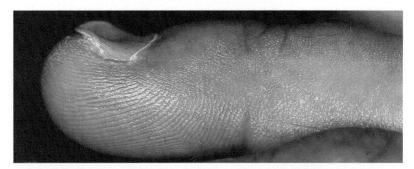

Figure 18-11 Koilonychia *Commonly called* spoon nails, *koilonychia is caused by softening and thinning of the nail plate that results in concave or spoon-shaped nails. Spoon nails are seen in patients with long-standing iron-deficiency anemia or Plummer-Vinson syndrome (a combination of koilonychia, dysphagia, and glossitis that primarily affects middle-aged women). Other causes include Raynaud's syndrome, hemochromatosis, and physical or chemical trauma. Koilonychia also may be inherited as an autosomal dominant disorder.*

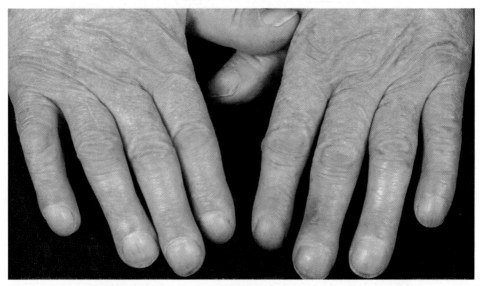

Figure 18-12 Clubbed fingers *Also known as* Hippocratic fingers, *clubbing appears as a bulbous enlargement and broadening of the fingertips. The angle made by the proximal nail fold and the nail plate (Lovibond's angle) exceeds 180 degrees. The tissue between the nail and underlying bone has a spongy quality that gives a "floating" sensation when pressure is applied downward and forward at the junction between the plate and proximal fold.*

Clubbed fingers are the result of hyperplasia of the fibrovascular tissue between the nail matrix and the bony phalanx. The pathogenesis is unknown, but an increased blood supply to the fingers is seen on arteriography. The hypervascularity is thought to be related to opening of the arteriovenous anastomosis by an unknown humoral vasodilating substance.

Clubbed fingers may be inherited as an autosomal dominant trait and are not associated with systemic disease. When acquired, clubbed fingers are most commonly indicative of cardiac disease (cyanotic heart disease, bacterial endocarditis), pulmonary disease (primary and metastatic cancer, bronchiectasis, lung abscess, mesothelioma), or gastrointestinal disease (regional enteritis, ulcerative colitis, and hepatic cirrhosis).

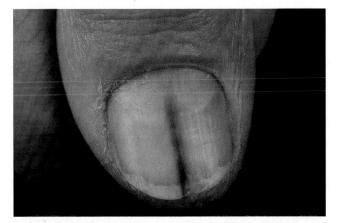

Figure 18-13 Brown nails *Abnormal pigmentation may affect the nail plate and nail bed individually or together. Brown nails occur in Addison's disease (plate), in hemochromatosis (plate), with gold therapy (plate), with arsenic intoxication (plate), and in malignant melanoma (plate, bed, fold). In white patients with multiple brown nails, important considerations in the differential diagnosis are Addison's disease and Nelson's syndrome (an ACTH-producing pituitary tumor that develops after bilateral adrenalectomy in patients with Cushing's syndrome).*

Brown linear bands or streaks are a common and normal finding in black- or brown-skinned persons. In white persons, a single pigmented streak may be a melanocytic nevus. However, when the proximal nail fold is also involved (Hutchinson's sign; Figure 9-19), malignant melanoma must be suspected. Hutchinson's sign may include brown-black discoloration of the proximal and lateral nail folds and brown-black pigmentation of the nail matrix, bed, and plate (obliterating the lunula). The nail plate also may show dystrophic changes.

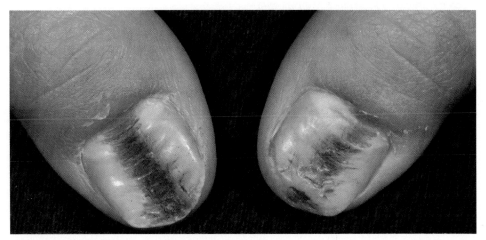

Figure 18-14 Onychodystrophia mediana canaliformis Synonyms: *Median canaliform dystrophy of the nails, tic habit. This striking morphologic change in the nail plate results from a compulsive habit of picking at the nail fold; this repeated injury damages the nail matrix, and the nail grows out in an abnormal form.*

Section 19

SKIN SIGNS OF SYSTEMIC CANCERS

MUCOCUTANEOUS SIGNS OF SYSTEMIC CANCER

Mucocutaneous findings may suggest systemic cancers in several ways: associations of heritable mucocutaneous disorders with systemic cancers, by action at a distance, i.e., paraneoplastic syndromes, or spread to skin or mucosal sites by direct, lymphatic, or hematogenous extension (cutaneous metastasis).

Classification

Heritable Disorders Cowden's syndrome, Peutz-Jeghers syndrome, Muir-Torre syndrome, Gardner's syndrome, von Recklinghausen's disease

Paraneoplastic Syndromes

STRONG ASSOCIATION WITH UNDERLYING CANCER Malignant acanthosis nigricans, Bazex's syndrome, carcinoid syndrome, erythema gyratum repens, hypertrichosis lanuginosa, ectopic ACTH syndrome, glucagonoma syndrome, neutrophilic dermatoses (Sweet's syndrome, pyoderma gangrenosum), mammary Paget's disease, paraneoplastic pemphigus

STATISTICAL ASSOCIATION WITH UNDERLYING CANCER Extramammary Paget's disease, Bowen's disease, exfoliative dermatitis, mycosis fungoides, pruritus, palmar keratoses, porphyria cutanea tarda, pityriasis rotunda, migratory phlebitis (Trousseau's syndrome)

POSSIBLE ASSOCIATION WITH UNDERLYING CANCER Arsenical keratoses, acquired ichthyosis, polymyositis, tripe palms, vasculitis

Cutaneous Metastases

DIRECT EXTENSION Paget's disease, extramammary Paget's disease

METASTASIS Persistent tumor, lymphatic extension, hematogenous spread

ACANTHOSIS NIGRICANS

Acanthosis nigricans (AN) is a diffuse, velvety thickening and hyperpigmentation of the skin, chiefly in axillae and other body folds, the etiology of which may be related to factors of heredity, associated endocrine disorders, obesity, drug administration, and in one form, malignancy.

Epidemiology and Etiology

Classification

Type 1: Hereditary benign AN. No associated endocrine disorder

Type 2: Benign AN. Various endocrine disorders associated with insulin resistance: insulin-resistant diabetes mellitus, hyperandrogenic states, acromegaly/gigantism, Cushing's disease, hypogonadal syndromes with insulin resistance, Addison's disease, hypothyroidism

Type 3: Pseudo-AN. Complication of obesity; more commonly seen in patients with darker pigmentation. Obesity produces insulin resistance.

Type 4: Drug-induced AN. Nicotinic acid in high dosage, stilbestrol in young males, glucocorticoid therapy, diethylstilbestrol/oral contraceptive, growth hormone therapy

Type 5: Malignant AN. Paraneoplastic, usually adenocarcinoma of GI or GU tract; less commonly, lymphoma

Age Type 1: onset during childhood or puberty

Etiology Dependent on associated disorder

History

Usually insidious onset; first visible change is darkening of pigmentation.

Physical Examination

Skin Lesions

TYPES All types of AN Darkening of pigmentation, skin appears dirty (Figures 19-1 and 19-2). As skin thickens, appears velvety; skin line further accentuated; surface becomes rugose, mammillated. Type 3 AN: velvety patch on inner, upper thigh at site of chafing; often has many skin tags in body folds, especially axillae, groins, neck. Type 5 AN: hyperkeratosis and hyperpigmentation more pronounced. Hyperkeratosis of palms/soles, involvement of oral mucosa and vermilion border of lips (Figure 19-2).

COLOR Accentuation of normal pigmentation

PALPATION Velvety feel

DISTRIBUTION Most commonly, axillae, neck (back, sides) (Figure 19-1); also, groins, anogenitalia (Figure 19-2), antecubital fossae, knuckles, submammary, umbilicus

Mucous Membranes Oral mucosa: velvety texture with delicate furrows. Type 5: Mucous membranes and mucocutaneous junctions commonly involved; warty papillomatous thickenings periorbitally, periorally (Figure 19-1).

General Examination Examine for underlying endocrine disorder in benign AN, and search for malignancy in malignant AN.

Differential Diagnosis

Dark Thickened Flexural Skin Confluent and reticulated papillomatosis (Gougerot-Carteaud syndrome), pityriasis versicolor, X-linked ichthyosis, retention hyperkeratosis, nicotinic acid ingestion

Laboratory and Special Examinations

Chemistry Rule out diabetes mellitus.

Dermatopathology Papillomatosis, hyperkeratosis; epidermis thrown into irregular folds, showing varying degrees of acanthosis

Imaging   Rule out associated carcinoma.

Endoscopy   Rule out associated carcinoma.

Diagnosis

Clinical findings

Pathophysiology

Epidermal changes may be caused by hypersecretion of pituitary peptide or nonspecific growth-promoting effect of hyperinsulinemia.

Course and Prognosis

Type 1: Accentuated at puberty and, at times, regresses when older. *Type 2:* Depending on underlying disturbance *Type 3:* May regress subsequent to significant weight loss. *Type 4:* Resolves when causative drug is discontinued. *Type 5:* AN may precede other symptoms of malignancy by 5 years; removal of malignancy may be followed by regression of AN.

Management

Symptomatic
Treat associated disorder. Pseudoacanthosis nigricans may regress with weight loss.

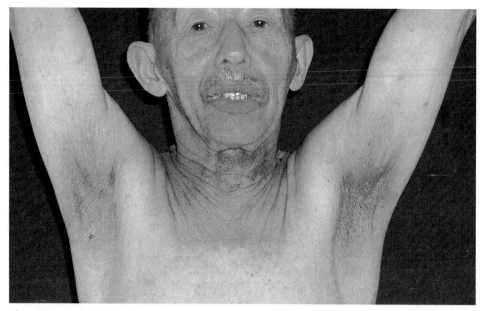

Figure 19-1 Malignant acanthosis nigricans (type 5) *The skin of the neck and axillae shows the typical velvety-textured, brown, hyperkeratotic and verrucous changes. Note also that the vermilion border of the lips is transformed into a velvety raspberry-like tissue. (Courtesy of F. Gschnait, M.D.)*

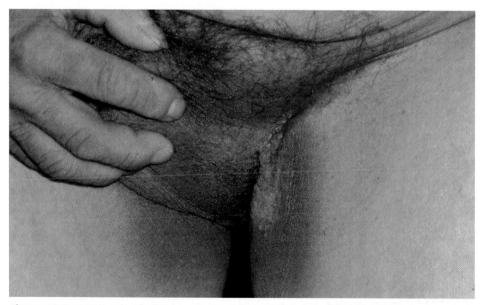

Figure 19-2 Acanthosis nigricans *Poorly defined, velvety, verrucous and papillomatous, dark-chocolate-brown plaques on the medial thighs and scrotum. Similar changes were also present in the axillae and neck.*

COWDEN'S SYNDROME

Cowden's syndrome (named after the propositus) is a heritable cancer syndrome with variable expressivity in a number of systems in the form of multiple hamartomatous neoplasms of ectodermal, mesodermal, and endodermal origin. There is a special susceptibility for breast and thyroid cancers, and the skin lesions, which are special adnexal tumors (tricholemmomas), are important markers because they portend the onset of the breast and thyroid cancers.

Synonym: Multiple hamartoma syndrome.

Epidemiology

Inheritance Autosomal dominant

Gene Locus Unknown

Incidence There are fewer than 100 patients reported to date, but the disease is probably more common than the published reports would indicate.

Age at Onset 4 to 75 years (median age 40 years)

Race Mostly whites, but there are reports in Japanese and in blacks.

Sex Males > females

History

History The skin lesions, which may appear first in childhood but develop over time, are tricholemmomas and are important because they often precede the onset of breast cancers in females.

Systems Review In addition to breast cancer (20 %), which is often bilateral, and thyroid cancer (8 %), there are various internal hamartomas: thyroid goiter, fibrocystic disease of the breast, GI polyposis, and rarely, carcinoma of the colon, prostate, and uterus. The CNS may be involved: mental retardation, seizures, neuromas, ganglioneuromas, and meningiomas of the ear canal.

Family History Autosomal dominant

Physical Examination

Skin

TYPES OF LESIONS

Tricholemmomas, skin-colored, pink (Figure 19-3), or brown papules having the appearance of flat warts or benign appendage tumors. These occur on the central area of the face, perioral areas, lips near the angles of the mouth, and the ears. Tricholemmomas may be quite extensive and disfiguring.

Translucent punctate keratoses of the palms and soles

Hyperkeratotic, flat-topped papules on the dorsa of the hands and forearms

Lipomas and angiomas (rare)

Mucous Membranes These lesions are important and quite characteristic: papules of the gingival, labial, and palatal surfaces; they are whiter than the surrounding mucosa and often coalesce, giving a "cobblestone" appearance (Figure 19-4). Papillomas of the buccal mucosa and the tongue. Squamous cell carcinoma of the tongue and basal cell carcinoma of the anal area may occur.

Systemic Findings

BREASTS Fibrocystic disease, fibroadenomas, adenocarcinoma; gynecomastia in males

THYROID Goiter, adenomas, thyroglossal duct cysts, follicular adenocarcinoma

GI TRACT Hamartomatous polyps throughout, but increased in large bowel; adenocarcinoma arising in polyp

FEMALE GENITAL TRACT Ovarian cysts, menstrual abnormalities

MUSCULOSKELETAL Craniomegaly, kyphoscoliosis, "adenoid" facies, high-arched palate

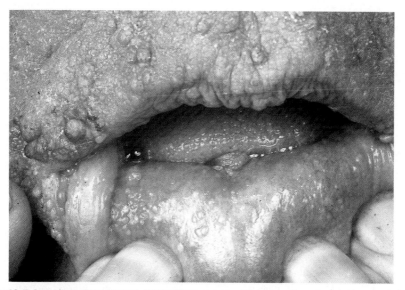

Figure 19-3 Cowden's syndrome: tricholemmonas *Multiple skin-colored warty papules on the face, as well as the mucosa of the lower lip.*

Differential Diagnosis

Tricholemmomas Multiple syringomas, multiple angiofibromas ±tuberous sclerosis, multiple trichoepitheliomas, flat warts (verruca plana), Muir-Torre syndrome,

Laboratory and Special Examinations

Dermatopathology Tricholemmomas show evidence of differentiation toward the outer root sheath cells of the hair follicles. Multiple biopsies may be necessary to obtain the characteristic histology. In one series, only 29 of 53 facial lesions (54 %) were diagnostic of tricholemmoma. The oral lesions are relatively acellular fibromas.

Imaging Mammography to rule out breast cancer. Thyroid scan.

Diagnosis

History and clinical findings with confirmation of tricholemmoma by lesional skin biopsy

Significance

It is important to establish the diagnosis of Cowden's syndrome so that these patients can be followed carefully to detect breast and thyroid cancers.

Course

Tumors may continue to develop throughout life.

Management

Prevention Genetic counseling. Individuals should be followed closely for development of breast and/or thyroid cancer. Because of the high risk of breast cancer (20 %), some female patients may prefer prophylactic bilateral mastectomy.

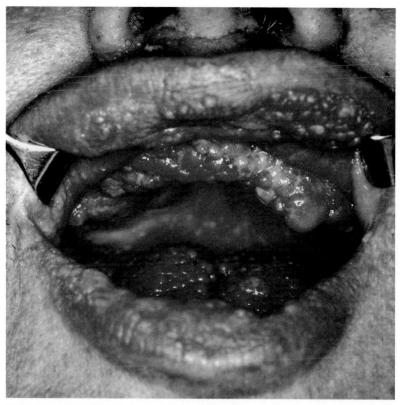

Figure 19-4 Cowden's syndrome: mucosal papillomas *Multiple skin-colored papules that simulate warts on the lips, gingiva, and tongue; clusters of aggregated papules were also present on the palates and buccal mucosae.*

GLUCAGONOMA SYNDROME

Glucagonoma syndrome is a rare but well-described clinical entity caused by excessive production of glucagon in an alpha cell tumor of the pancreas, characterized by superficial migratory necrolytic erythema (MNE) with erosions that crust and heal with hyperpigmentation, a beefy-red tongue, and angular cheilitis.

Epidemiology and Etiology

Age   Middle-aged to elderly

Etiology   Most cases associated with hyper-glucagonemia, but pathogenesis of MNE is not known.

History

Rash unresponsive to conventional therapy. Weight loss, abdominal pain.

Physical Examination

Skin Lesions

TYPES   Inflammatory plaques enlarge with central clearing, resulting in geographic areas that become confluent. Borders show vesiculation to bulla formation, crusting, and scaling (Figures 19-5 and 19-6).

ARRANGEMENT   Gyrate, circinate, arcuate, annular

DISTRIBUTION   Flexures, intertriginous areas perioral (Figure 19-5), perigenital (Figure 19-6). Fingertips red, shining, erosive.

Mucous Membranes   Glossitis, angular cheilitis, blepharitis

General Examination   Wasting, malnutrition

Differential Diagnosis

Moist Red Plaque(s)   Acrodermatitis enteropathica, zinc deficiency, pustular psoriasis, mucocutaneous candidiasis, Hailey-Hailey disease (familial pemphigus)

Laboratory and Special Examinations

Chemistry   Fasting plasma glucagon levels to >1000 ng/liter (normal 50 to 250 ng/liter) makes the diagnosis. Hyperglycemia, reduced glucose tolerance. Associated findings: severe malabsorption, gross hypoaminoacidemia, low serum zinc.

Dermatopathology   Early skin lesions show bandlike upper epidermal necrosis with retention of pyknotic nuclei and pale keratinocyte cytoplasm (electron microscopy shows vacuolar degeneration and lysis of organelles).

CT Scan, Angiography   Locates tumor within pancreas

Diagnosis

Clinical findings confirmed by skin biopsy and serum glucagon levels

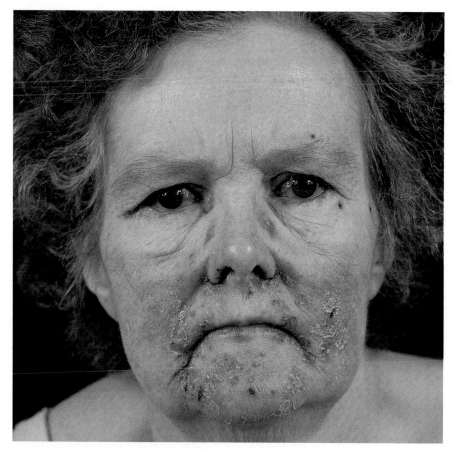

Figure 19-5 Glucagonoma syndrome: migratory necrolytic erythema   *Inflammatory dermatosis with angular cheilitis, inflammatory, scaly, and erosive plaques around the nose, mouth, and medial aspects of the eyes.*

Pathogenesis

Most cases are associated with glucagon production by a pancreatic glucagonoma. Pathogenesis of cutaneous findings is unknown; may be related to nutritional deficiency. MNE may respond to oral zinc or intravenous amino acid therapy. Isolated cases have been reported of MNE associated with advanced hepatic cirrhosis and a bronchial carcinoma.

Course and Prognosis

Depends on the aggressiveness of the glucagonoma. Hepatic metastases have occurred in 75 % of patients at the time of diagnosis. In that tumor is slow-growing, patients may have prolonged survival, even with metastatic disease.

Management

MNE Responds poorly to all types of therapy. Some cases have responded partially to zinc replacement.

Surgery Surgical excision of glucagonoma achieves cure in only 30 % of cases because of persistent metastases (usually liver). Surgery also reduces tumor masses and associated symptoms. MNE resolves or improves after tumor excision.

Chemotherapy Response usually poor

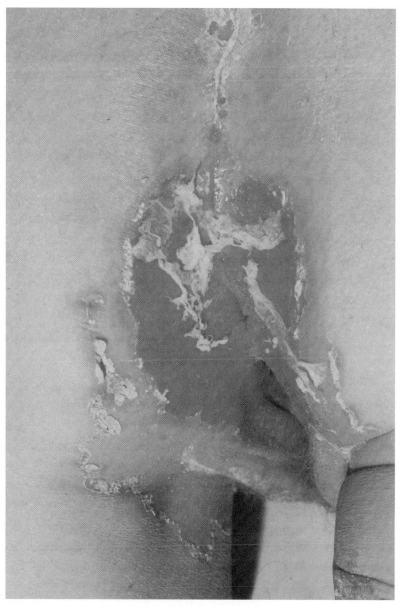

Figure 19-6 Glucagonoma syndrome: migratory necrolytic erythema *Polycyclic erosions in the anogenital region with necrotic flaccid epidermis still covering part of these erosions.*

PEUTZ-JEGHERS SYNDROME

Peutz-Jeghers syndrome (PJS) is a familial polyposis characterized by many congenital, small, pigmented macules (lentigines) on the lips and oral mucous membranes (periorificial lentiginosis). There are usually, but not always, multiple hamartomatous polyps in the small bowel, as well as in the large bowel and stomach, that cause abdominal symptoms and signs.

Epidemiology

Inheritance Autosomal dominant. Spontaneous mutations about 40 %.

Gene Locus Unknown

Age of Onset Pigmented macules: infancy and early childhood. Polyps: late childhood or before age 30.

Sex Equal incidence

History

Duration of Lesions The pigmented macules are congenital or may develop during infancy and early childhood. The macules may disappear over time on the lips, but the pigmentation of the mouth does not disappear and is therefore the *sine qua non* for the diagnosis. *The lentigines occur in some patients who never have abdominal lesions.*

Systems Review Abdominal symptoms (recurrent attacks of abdominal pain) occur first around age 10 and up to age 30, although rarely are first noted in older adults. Abdominal pain, GI bleeding, anemia. Increased incidence of breast, ovarian, and pancreatic cancer.

Family History Other individuals with similar findings

Physical Examination

Skin Lesions

TYPE Macule.

Color Dark brown or black
Size 2 to 5.0 mm; the lentigines on the face are smaller than those on the palms and soles and in the mouth.

SHAPE OF INDIVIDUAL LESION Round or oval

ARRANGEMENT OF MULTIPLE LESIONS The lesions occur on the lips (Figure 19-7) (especially the lower lip) in closely set clusters around the mouth and the bridge of the nose.

DISTRIBUTION Lips, buccal mucosa (Figure 19-8) and periorificial skin, nose, chin, palms and soles, dorsa of hands

Mucous Membranes These are the *sine qua non;* the lesions are dark brown, black, or bluish black. They are irregularly distributed on the gums, buccal mucosae, and hard palate.

Nails Pigmented streaks or diffuse involvement of the nail bed (rare)

GI Tract Hamartomatous polyps: small intestine > large intestine; may cause intussusception, obstruction. Adenocarcinoma may develop within polyp.

Differential Diagnosis

Cutaneous Lentigenes Freckles (lighter than lentigenes of PJS), solar lentigines, LEOPARD syndrome (more widely distributed than PJS), Cronkhite-Canada syndrome, Addison's disease, Gardner's syndrome

Mucosal Pigmentation Racial pigmentation in darkly pigmented individuals, amalgam tattoo, zidovudine pigmentation

Laboratory and Special Examinations

Pathology

LENTIGENES Increased epidermal melanin synthesis. Those on palms/soles may have block in the melanin transfer to ker-

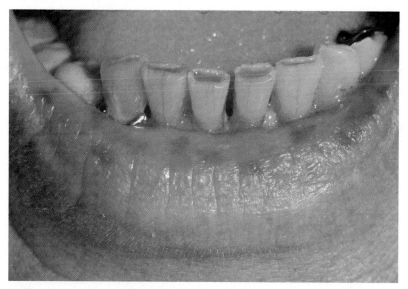

Figure 19-7 Peutz-Jeghers syndrome *Multiple, dark-brown lentigines on the vermilion border of the lip.*

atinocytes. Increased pigmentation occurs in the melanocytes and in the basal cells.

GI POLYPS Hamartomas, with mixture of glands and smooth muscle

Hematology Anemia from blood loss may be present.

Blood in Stool Check for occult bleeding.

Imaging Study of the GI tract is important in patients with the clinical presentation of pigmented macules.

Diagnosis

By history, clinical findings, and detection of GI polyps

Course and Prognosis

There is a normal life expectancy unless carcinoma develops in the GI tract and is unrecognized. Malignant neoplasms may be more frequent in the Japanese with this syndrome, and prophylactic colectomy has been recommended for these patients.

Management

Pigmented Macules Can be removed by laser surgery if a cosmetic concern to patient.

Polyps Patients should be followed by gastroenterologist or surgeon. Symptomatic polyps and those >1.5 cm should be removed. Should be seen every 1 to 2 years.

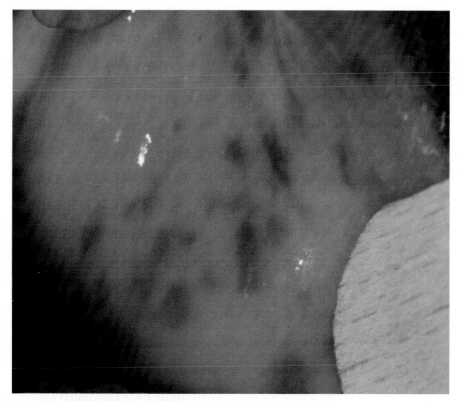

Figure 19-8 Peutz-Jeghers syndrome *Multiple, dark-brown macules that show some clustering on the buccal mucosa.*

METASTATIC CANCER TO THE SKIN

Metastatic cancer to skin is characterized by solitary or multiple dermal or subcutaneous nodules, occurring as cells from a distant noncontiguous primary malignant neoplasm, that are transported to and deposited within the skin or subcutaneous tissue by hematogenous or lymphatic routes or across the peritoneal cavity.

Epidemiology and Etiology

Age   Any age, but usually older

Sex   Frequency of primary tumors varies with sex.

FEMALES   Breast (69 %), large intestine (9 %), melanoma (5 %), lung (4 %), ovary (4 %), sarcoma (2 %), uterine cervix (2 %), pancreas (2 %), SCC of oral cavity (1 %), bladder (1 %)

MALES   Lung (24 %), large intestine (19 %), melanoma (13 %), SCC of oral cavity (12 %), kidney (6 %), stomach (6 %), urinary bladder (2 %), salivary glands (2 %), breast (2 %), 1 % each in prostate, thyroid, liver, SCC of skin

Incidence   0.7 % to 9 % of all patients with cancer

Variants

CANCER EN CUIRASSE   Usually local extension of breast cancer occurring in the presternal region, which resembles a metal breastplate of a cuirassier. Also occurs with primary of lung, GI tract, kidney.

PAGET'S DISEASE   Epidermal extension of breast cancer onto the areola, appearing as an eczematous patch

CARCINOMA ERYSIPELATODES   Inflammatory carcinoma resembling erysipelas, presenting as an erythematous plaque. Breast most common primary, but occurs with others as well (pancreas, parotid, tonsils, colon, stomach, rectum, melanoma, pelvic organs, ovary, uterus, prostate, lung).

CARCINOMA TELANGIECTATICUM   Breast cancer appearing as pinpoint telangiectases with dilated capillaries

SISTER MARY JOSEPH NODULE   Metastatic cancer to umbilicus

History

Prior history of primary internal cancer or may be first sign of visceral cancer. In one series, underlying cancer had been undiagnosed in 60 % of patients with lung cancer, in 53 % with renal cancer, in 40 % with ovarian cancer. Of patients with cutaneous metastases, skin lesion(s) was presenting sign in 37 % of men but only 6 % of women.

History of cancer chemotherapy

Physical Examination

Skin Lesions

TYPES   Nodule (Figure 19-9A and 19-9B), raised plaque, thickened fibrotic area. First detected when >5 mm. Fibrotic area may resemble morphea; occurring on scalp may produce alopecia. Initially, epidermis is intact, stretched over nodule; in time, surface may become ulcerated or hyperkeratotic (Figure 19-10).

COLOR   May appear inflammatory, i.e., pink to red (Figure 19-9B). Metastatic melanoma to dermis: blue to gray to black dermal nodules (Figure 19-12).

PALPATION   Firm to indurated

ARRANGEMENT   May be solitary, few, or multiple

DISTRIBUTION   Lung cancer to trunk, scalp. Hypernephroma to scalp, operative scar.

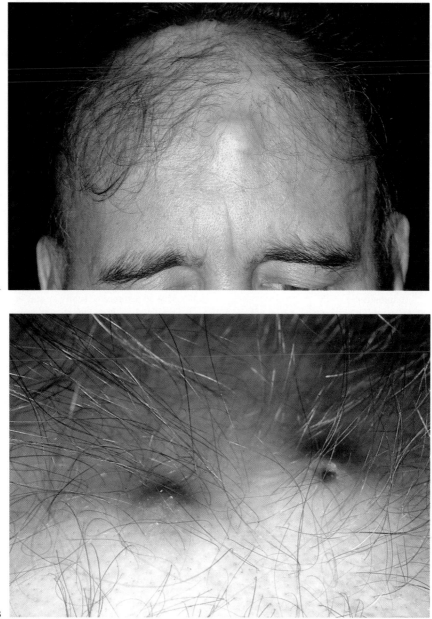

Figure 19-9 Metastatic cancer to the skin: bronchogenic cancer A. *Three dermal nodules on the scalp of a patient undergoing chemotherapy for metastatic lung cancer; the nodules were only apparent following loss of hair during chemotherapy. The anterior nodule is asymptomatic, noninflamed.* B. *Close-up of posterior lesions: erythematous nodules; crust at a biopsy site.*

Clinical Variants

Breast cancer may spread within lymphatics to skin of involved breast, resulting in inflammatory plaques resembling cellulitis (erysipelas) or in firm, flatter, telangiectatic plaques or papules and nodules (Figure 19-11).

PATTERNS OF CUTANEOUS INVOLVEMENT

Inflammatory metastatic carcinoma: erythematous patch or plaque with an active spreading border (carcinoma erysipeloides) (Figure 19-11)

En cuirasse metastatic carcinoma: diffuse morphea-like induration of skin. Begins as scattered, firm, lenticular papulonodules overlying erythematous or red-blue smooth cutaneous surface. Papulonodules coalesce into sclerodermoid plaque with no associated inflammation.

Telangiectatic metastatic carcinoma: violaceous papulovesicles resembling lymphangioma circumscriptum (Figure 19-11) where it is associated with carcinoma erysipeloides.

Nodular metastatic carcinoma: multiple firm papulonodules or nodules. Usually multiple, may be solitary. May have keratotic core resembling keratoacanthoma (Figure 19-10).

Alopecia neoplastica: occurs via hematogenous spread. On scalp, areas of hair loss resembling alopecia areata; well-demarcated, red-pink, smooth surface.

Paget's disease: sharply demarcated plaque or patch of erythema and scaling occurring on nipple or areola associated with underlying breast cancer (Figures 19-13 and 19-14).

Breast carcinoma of inframammary crease: cutaneous exophytic nodule resembling primary SCC or BCC of skin.

MISCELLANEOUS PATTERNS
With dilatation of lymphatics and superficial hemorrhage, may resemble lymphangioma. With lymph stasis and dermal edema, resembles pigskin or orange peel. May metastasize hematogenously to scalp, forming many subcutaneous nodules with "bag of marbles" feel to scalp.

Large intestines: Often presents on skin of abdomen or perineal regions; also, scalp or face. Most originate in rectum. May present with metastatic inflammatory carcinoma of inguinal region, supraclavicular area, or face and neck. Less commonly, sessile or pedunculated nodules on buttocks, grouped vascular nodules of groin or scrotum, or facial tumor. Rarely, cutaneous fistula after appendectomy or resembling hidradenitis suppurativa.

Lung carcinoma may produce a large number of metastatic nodules within a short period. Most commonly, reddish nodule(s) (Figure 19-9). Trunk/scalp; symmetric; along direction of intercostal vessels, may be zosteriform; in scar (thoracotomy site or needle aspiration tract).

Hypernephroma can produce solitary lesion; also widespread. Usually appear vascular, ±pulsatile, ±pedunculated; can resemble pyogenic granuloma. Most common on head and neck; also trunk and extremities.

Malignant melanoma may spread from primary cutaneous site to distant cutaneous site by lymphatic vessels (Figure 19-12). Primary sites also can be noncutaneous: eye, cervix, oral cavity. Cutaneous metastases of unknown primary also occur. Nodules, single or multiple. Usually deeply pigmented; amelanotic variants occur.

Sister Mary Joseph nodule is metastatic carcinoma to umbilicus from intraabdominal carcinoma, most commonly stomach, colon, ovary, pancreas; however, primary may be in breast. Easier to detect by palpation than by visual detection. Can be firm to indurated nodules, ±fissuring, ±ulceration, ±vascular appearance, ±discharge. In 15 % may be initial presentation of primary malignancy.

Carcinoma of bladder, ovary can spread contiguously to abdominal and inguinal skin similarly to breast cancer, as described above, and look like erysipelas.

General Examination Look for primary tumor.

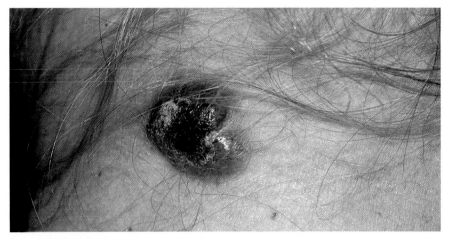

Figure 19-10 Metastatic cancer to the skin: breast cancer *Large, hyperkeratotic nodule on the posterior neck in a 40-year-old woman with metastatic breast cancer, present for 6 months; became ulcerated; similar but smaller lesions were present on the scalp and back.*

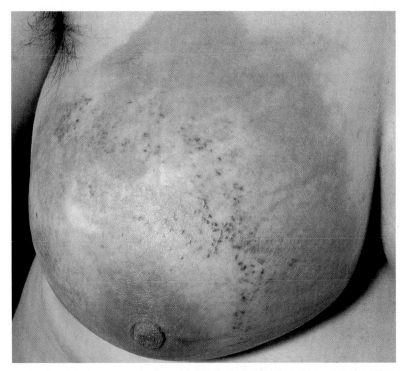

Figure 19-11 Metastatic cancer to the skin: inflammatory breast cancer (carcinoma erysipelatoides) *The breast is enlarged with an inflammatory, erythematous plaque resembling cellulitis or erysipelas on most of the surface; the cancer has spread via the cutaneous lymphatics. In addition, the breast is studded with numerous small, papular, erythematous telangiectases (telangiectetic carcinoma).*

Differential Diagnosis

"Blueberry muffin baby": neuroblastoma, congenital leukemia

Multiple cylindroma-like lesions: prostate adenocarcinoma, lung cancer, breast cancer

Epidermal inclusion or pilar cyst-like lesions: cancer of prostate, colon, breast

Kaposi's sarcoma-like lesions: cancer of kidney

Pyogenic granuloma-like lesions: amelanotic melanoma, renal cancer

Alopecia areata-like lesions: breast cancer

Lymphangioma-like lesions: cancer of breast, lung, cervix, ovary

Morphea-like lesions: cancer of breast, stomach, lung, mixed tumors, lacrimal gland

Laboratory and Special Examinations

Dermatopathology Carcinomatous deposits tend to spread in dermal lymphatic vessels, with resultant "Indian file" appearance of strands of cells. At times, cell differentiation sufficient to predict primary site; however, many times cells anaplastic. ±Dilatation of lymphatics secondary to carcinomatous lymphatic obstruction. Hypernephroma produces marked vascular proliferation.

Imaging Look for primary tumor.

Diagnosis

Clinical history of internal cancer suggests diagnosis, confirmed by skin biopsy.

Pathogenesis

Includes detachment of cancer cells from primary tumor, invasion, intravasation into blood or lymphatic vessel, circulation, stasis within vessel, extravasation, invasion into tissue, proliferation at metastatic site. Three patterns of metastases are observed: mechanical tumor stasis (anatomic proximity and lymphatic draining), site-specific (selective attachment of tumor cells to specific organ), nonselective (independent of mechanical or organ-specific factors). Cutaneous metastases may represent secondary metastases, i.e., metastases from lung and liver.

Course and Prognosis

In individuals with known cancer, cutaneous metastases are indicative of a poor prognosis. Average survival after detection of cutaneous metastasis only 3 months except for contiguous spread of breast cancer, which may last for years. With Paget's disease of breasts, prognosis better if no tumor palpable or no adenopathy.

Management

With solitary or few lesions and if patient not terminal, excision may be indicated.

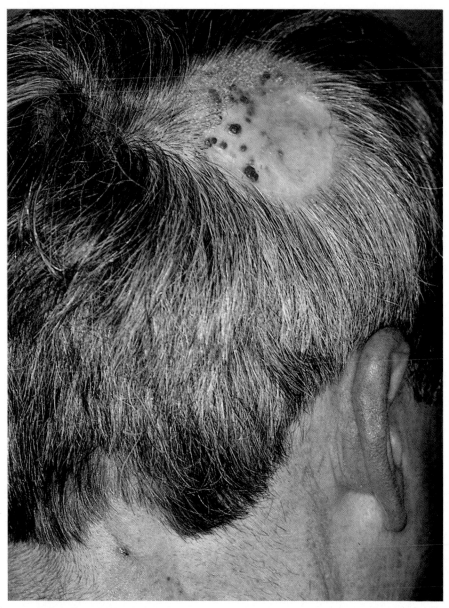

Figure 19-12 Recurrent melanoma *The primary melanoma had been excised from the scalp 2 years previously and the excision site grafted. The first recurrences were noted 6 months previously; the site was reexcised and a regional lymph node dissection performed. Melanoma recurring as red-purple dermal papules are seen at the grafted site and on the neck, along the surgical scar.*

MAMMARY PAGET'S DISEASE

Mammary Paget's disease (MPD) is a malignant neoplasm that unilaterally involves the nipple or areola and simulates a chronic eczematous dermatitis; it is associated with underlying intraductal carcinoma of the breast.

Epidemiology

Age 56 years (mean)

Sex Females, with rare examples in males

Incidence 1 % to 4 % of all breast cancers

History

Duration of Lesions Insidious onset over several months or years

Skin Symptoms May be asymptomatic. Pruritus, pain, burning. Discharge, bleeding, ulceration, nipple invagination.

Physical Examination

Skin Lesions

TYPE Scaling plaque, rather sharply marginated (Figure 19-13), and when scale is removed, the surface is moist and oozing (see Figure 19-14). Lesions range in size from 0.3 to 15 cm (mean 2.8 cm). An underlying breast mass is palpable in less than half of patients.

COLOR Faintly red

PALPATION In early stages there is no induration, but later, induration and infiltration develop, and nodules may be palpated.

SHAPE Oval with irregular borders

DISTRIBUTION Single lesion localized to one nipple and areola. May uncommonly occur bilaterally. May also develop in ectopic breast tissue in females and males.

Breast Intraductal carcinoma is present but palpable as a mass in less than half of patients with MPD.

Regional Lymph Nodes Lymph node metastases occur more often when MPD is associated with an underlying palpable mass.

Differential Diagnosis

Red Areolar/Periareolar Plaque Eczematous dermatitis, psoriasis, benign ductal papilloma, nipple-areola retention hyperkeratosis, impetigo, pityriasis versicolor, SCC *in situ,* familial pemphigus

Eczematous dermatitis of the nipples is usually bilateral; it is without any induration and responds rapidly to topical corticosteroids. Nevertheless, be suspicious of Paget's disease if "eczema" persists for longer than 3 weeks.

Laboratory and Special Examinations

Dermatopathology Neoplastic cells in epidermis. Typical large rounded cells with a large nucleus and without intercellular bridges (Paget's cells) that stain much lighter than surrounding keratinocytes.

Mammography Define underlying intraductal carcinoma.

Diagnosis

Clinical findings confirmed by biopsy findings

Course and Prognosis

When breast mass is not palpable, 92 % of pa-

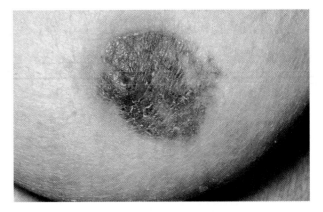

Figure 19-13 Mammary Paget's disease *A sharply demarcated scaling plaque mimicking eczema on the nipple, areola, and surrounding skin. The plaque is slightly indurated. The nipple has been partially resorbed.*

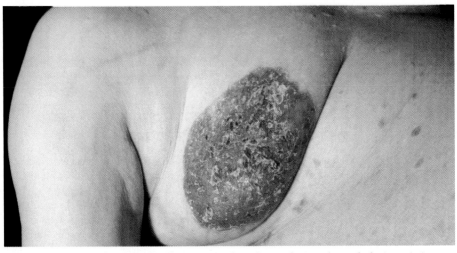

Figure 19-14 Mammary Paget's disease *In this advanced case, the scaly lesion mimics a plaque of psoriasis and has completely obliterated the nipple and the areola. Note the erosion and crusting, features not seen in psoriasis.*

tients survive 5 years; 82 %, 10 years. When breast mass is palpable, 38 % survive 5 years; 22 %, 10 years. Prognosis better if no palpable tumor is detected or no lymphadenopathy.

Management

Surgery, radiotherapy, and/or chemotherapy as in any other breast carcinomas. Lymph node dissection if regional nodes are palpable.

EXTRAMAMMARY PAGET'S DISEASE

Extramammary Paget's disease (EPD) is a neoplasm of the anogenital and axillary skin, histologically and clinically similar to Paget's disease of the breast, and often represents an intraepidermal extension of a primary adenocarcinoma of underlying apocrine glands or of the lower gastrointestinal, urinary, or female genital tracts.

Epidemiology and Etiology

Age >40 years

Sex Women>men

Etiology Unknown

Classification of Extramammary Paget's Disease

- Unassociated with underlying cancer
- Associated with underlying cancer, adjacent apocrine cancer, or eccrine gland carcinoma
- Associated with another type of cancer, usually of GI or GU tract

History

Skin Symptoms ±Itching

Physical Examination

Skin Lesions

TYPES Erythematous plaque, ±scaling, ±crusting, ±exudation; eczematous-appearing lesions. Borders sharply defined (Figures 19-15 and 19-16), geographic configuration.

COLOR Pink to red

DISTRIBUTION Most commonly anogenital region [vulva, scrotum (Figure 19-15), penis, perianal (Figure 19-16), perineal skin]; also, axilla, external ear canal, eyelids, umbilicus, pubic area. Rarely, more than one site involved simultaneously.

General Examination Rectum, urethra, cervix should be examined for primary adenocarcinoma. *Proctoscopy.* Careful examination of the anorectum must be performed, looking for a primary tumor.

Differential Diagnosis

Red Plaque Eczematous dermatitis, lichen simplex chronicus, lichen sclerosus et atrophicus, lichen planus, inverse pattern psoriasis, intertriginous, *Candida* intertrigo, SCC *in situ* (erythroplasia of Queyrat), human papillomavirus–induced SCC *in situ,* (amelanotic) superficial spreading melanoma

Laboratory and Special Examinations

Dermatopathology Characteristic Paget cells are dispersed between keratinocytes, occur in clusters, extend down into adnexal structures (hair follicles, eccrine ducts). Adnexal adenocarcinoma is often found when carefully searched for. Dermis shows chronic inflammatory reaction. In later stages, epidermis may be eroded/atrophic. Paget cells are characterized by clear, abundant cytoplasm and do not form intercellular bridges with adjacent keratinocytes. Both the cells and their nuclei are rounded; nuclei are vesicular or hyperchromatic. Cytoplasm PAS-positive, diastase-resistant, supporting glandular origin.

Rectal Examination, Sigmoidoscopy, Barium Enema For perineal/perianal EPD, searching for underlying carcinoma

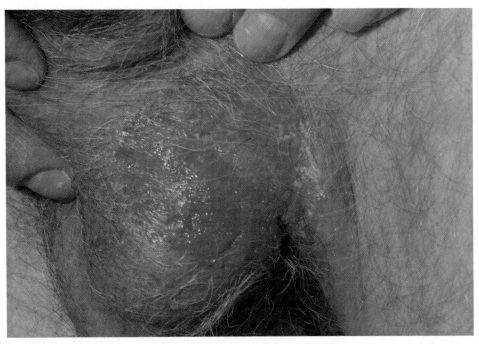

Figure 19-15 Extramammary Paget's disease *Moist, fairly well-demarcated, eroded, oozing, erythematous plaque on the scrotum and inguinal fold in an older male. The lesion is commonly mistaken for* Candida *intertrigo.*

Cystoscopy, Intravenous Pyelogram For genital EPD, searching for underlying carcinoma

Pelvic Examination For vulvar EPD, searching for underlying carcinoma

Diagnosis

Clinical suspicion confirmed by skin biopsy

Pathophysiology

The histogenesis of EPD is uncertain. Paget cells in the epidermis may occur as an *in situ* upward extension of an *in situ* adenocarcinoma within deeper glands. Alternatively, EPD may have a multifocal primary origin within the epidermis and its related appendages and does not represent an epidermotropic spread or metastasis from an underlying sweat gland carcinoma. Approximately 25 % of EPD can be shown to arise from a primary adenocarcinoma of underlying secretory glands. The primary tumor and Paget cells are usually mucus-secreting. Primary tumors in the anorectum can arise within the rectal mucosa or intramuscular glands.

Course and Prognosis

EPD remains *in situ* in the epidermis and adnexal epithelium in >65 % of cases. Prognosis related to existence of underlying adenocarcinoma. When no underlying neoplasm is present, there is a high recurrence rate, even after apparently adequate excision; this is due to the multifocal origin within epidermis and adnexal structures.

Management

EPD is usually much larger than is apparent clinically. Surgical excision must be controlled histologically (Mohs' microscopic surgery). If Paget cells are in dermis and regional lymph nodes are palpable, lymph node dissection may improve prognosis.

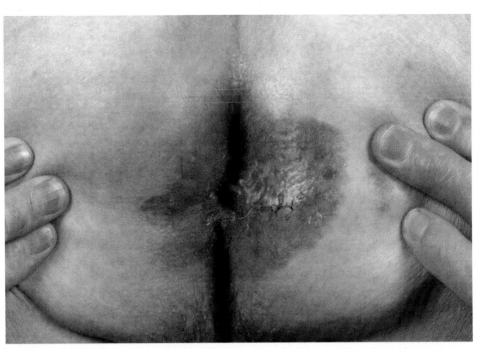

Figure 19-16 Extramammary Paget's disease *Sharply demarcated, scaly, erythematous plaque surrounds the anus and extends onto the buttocks. The lesion is commonly mistaken for eczema, psoriasis, or* Candida *intertrigo.*

SKIN SIGNS OF HEMATOLOGIC DISEASES

THROMBOCYTOPENIC PURPURA

Thrombocytopenic purpura is characterized by cutaneous hemorrhages occurring in association with a reduced platelet count, clinically usually small (petechiae) but at times larger (ecchymoses), which occur at sites of minor trauma/pressure (platelet count $<40,000/\mu$l) or spontaneously (platelet count $<10,000/\mu$l).

Epidemiology and Etiology

Age Acute idiopathic thrombocytopenic purpura (ITP)—children

Sex HIV-associated thrombocytopenic purpura—homosexual men

Etiology

DECREASED PLATELET PRODUCTION Direct injury to bone marrow, drugs (cytosine arabinoside, daunorubicin, cyclophosphamide, busulfan, methotrexate, 6-mercaptopurine, vinca alkaloids, thiazide diuretics, ethanol, estrogens), replacement of bone marrow, aplastic anemia, vitamin deficiencies, Wiskott-Aldrich syndrome

SPLENIC SEQUESTRATION Splenomegaly, hypothermia

INCREASED PLATELET DESTRUCTION *Immunologic* Autoimmune ITP, drug hypersensitivity (sulfonamides, quinine, quinidine, carbamazepine, digitoxin, methyldopa), after transfusion
Nonimmunologic Infection, prosthetic heart valves, disseminated intravascular coagulation (generalized stimulus; localized stimulus, Kasabach-Merritt syndrome), thrombotic thrombocytopenic purpura

History

Systems Review Usually sudden appearance of asymptomatic hemorrhagic skin and/or mucosal lesions

Physical Examination

Skin Lesions

TYPES *Petechiae*—small (pinpoint to pinhead) red nonblanching macules (Figures 20-1 and 20-2). *Ecchymoses*—black-and-blue spots; larger area or hemorrhage. *Vibices*—linear hemorrhages, often due to trauma.

COLOR Fresh areas of hemorrhage—red to dark brown. Older lesions—yellowish-green tinge.

PALPATION Nonpalpable. Lesions do not blanch with pressure.

ARRANGEMENT OF MULTIPLE LESIONS Possible linear lesion at sites of trauma

DISTRIBUTION Upper trunk, legs

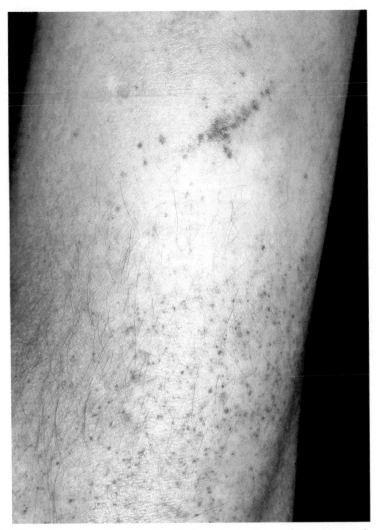

Figure 20-1 Thrombocytopenic purpura *Myriads of petechiae on the upper arm of an HIV-infected 25-year-old male was the presenting manifestation of his disease. A linear arrangement of petechiae (koebnerization or isomorphic phenomenon) with an ecchymosis at the site of minor trauma.*

Mucous Membranes   Petechiae (Figure 20-2), gingival bleeding

General Examination   Possible CNS hemorrhage

Differential Diagnosis

Nonhemorrhagic Blanching Vascular Lesions   Telangiectasia/erythema

True Hemorrhagic Lesions   Bateman's (actinic or senile) purpura, purpura of scurvy, progressive pigmentary purpura (Schamberg's disease), purpura following severe Valsalva maneuver (tussive, vomiting/retching), traumatic purpura, factitial or iatrogenic purpura, Gardner-Diamond syndrome (autoerythrocyte sensitization syndrome), palpable nonblanching purpura, i.e., vasculitis.

Laboratory and Special Examinations

Hematology   Thrombocytopenia

Bone Marrow Aspiration   Defines state of platelet production

Serology   Rule out HIV disease.

Lesional Skin Biopsy   May be contraindicated due to postoperative hemorrhage; however, usually can be controlled by suturing biopsied site.

Diagnosis

Clinical suspicion confirmed by platelet count

Pathophysiology

Platelet plugs by themselves effectively stop bleeding from capillaries and small blood vessels but are incapable of stopping hemorrhage from larger vessels. Platelet defects produce problems with small-vessel hemostasis, small hemorrhages in the skin or in the CNS.

Course and Prognosis

Varies with the etiology

Management

Identify underlying cause and correct if possible. If platelet count is very low ($<10,000/\mu l$), bed rest to reduce risk of hemorrhage.

Corticosteroids   For ITP, possible course of oral corticosteroid

High-Dose Immunoglobulin

Platelet Transfusions   If platelet count $<10,000/\mu l$, platelet transfusion may be indicated.

Chronic ITP   Splenectomy may be indicated.

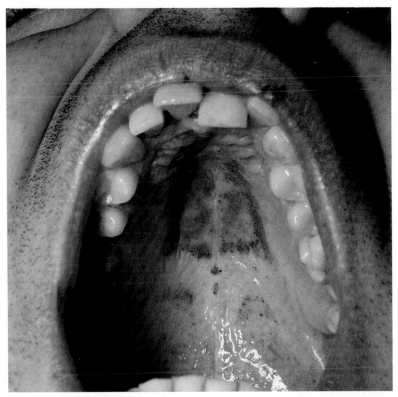

Figure 20-2 Thrombocytopenic purpura *Multiple, petechial hemorrhages on the palate.*

DISSEMINATED INTRAVASCULAR COAGULATION

Disseminated intravascular coagulation (DIC) is a widespread blood clotting disorder occurring within blood vessels, associated with a wide range of clinical circumstances (bacterial sepsis, obstetrical complications, disseminated malignancy, massive trauma), and manifested by purpura fulminans (cutaneous infarctions and/or acral gangrene) or bleeding from multiple sites. The spectrum of clinical symptoms associated with DIC ranges from relatively mild and subclinical to explosive and a life-threatening bleeding disorder.

Synonyms: Purpura fulminans, consumption coagulopathy, defibrination syndrome, coagulation-fibrinolytic syndrome.

Epidemiology and Etiology

Age Purpura fulminans most commonly in children

Etiology

EVENTS THAT INITIATE DIC *Massive Tissue Destruction* Tumor products, crushing trauma, extensive surgery, severe intracranial damage; retained contraception products, placental abruption, amniotic fluid embolism; certain snake bites; hemolytic transfusion reaction; acute promyelocytic leukemia; burn injuries

Extensive Destruction of Endothelial Surfaces, Exposure to Foreign Surfaces Vasculitis (Rocky Mountain spotted fever, meningococcemia, or occasionally gram-negative septicemia); heat stroke, malignant hyperthermia; extensive pump oxygenation (repair of aortic aneurysm); eclampsia, preeclampsia; giant hemangioma (Kasabach-Merritt syndrome); immune complexes; postvaricella purpura gangrenosa

EVENTS THAT COMPLICATE AND PROPAGATE DIC Shock, complement pathway activation

History

Duration of Lesion Hours to days; rapid evolution

History Complication developing during convalescence from etiologic circumstances. Fever, chills associated with onset of hemorrhagic lesions.

Physical Examination

Skin Lesions

TYPES

Hemorrhage from multiple cutaneous sites, i.e., surgical incisions, venipuncture or catheter sites

Preinfarction: peripheral acrocyanosis

Infarction (purpura fulminans) (Figures 20-3 and 20-4): massive ecchymoses with sharp, irregular ("geographic") borders and erythematous halos, ± evolution to hemorrhagic bullae and blue to black gangrene; peripheral gangrene on hands, feet, tip of nose with subsequent autoamputation if patient survives

COLOR Infarctive lesions are deep purple to black.

ARRANGEMENT OF MULTIPLE LESIONS Often symmetric

DISTRIBUTION Infarctive lesions: distal extremities; areas of pressure; lips, ears, nose, trunk

Mucous Membranes Hemorrhage from gingiva

General Examination High fever, ±shock. Multitude of findings depending on the associated medical/surgical problem

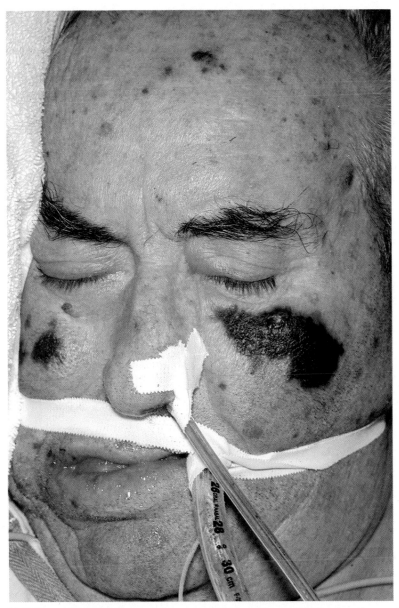

Figure 20-3 Disseminated intravascular coagulation: purpura fulminans *Geographic cutaneous infarctions on the cheeks with smaller lesions on the forehead; lesions were also present on the hands, elbows, thighs, and feet. The patient was a diabetic with* S. aureus *sepsis and died within 24 hours after onset of the purpuric lesions.*

Differential Diagnosis

Large Cutaneous Infarctions Necrosis following initiation of warfarin therapy, heparin necrosis, calciphylaxis, atheroembolization

Laboratory and Special Examinations

Dermatopathology Occlusion of arterioles with fibrin thrombi. Dense PMN infiltrate around infarct and massive hemorrhage

Hematologic Studies

CBC Schistocytes (fragmented RBCs), arising from RBC entrapment and damage within fibrin thrombi, seen on blood smear; platelet count low

COAGULATION STUDIES Reduced plasma fibrinogen; elevated fibrin degradation products; prolonged PT, PTT, and thrombin time

Diagnosis

Clinical suspicion confirmed by coagulation studies

Pathophysiology

Uncontrolled activation of coagulation results in thrombosis and consumption of platelets/clotting factors II, V, VIII. If the activation occurs slowly, excess activated products produced, predisposing to vascular infarctions/venous thrombosis. If the onset is acute, hemorrhage surrounding wound sites and IV lines/catheters or bleeding into deep tissues is usually seen.

Course and Prognosis

Mortality rate is high. Surviving patients require skin grafts or amputation for gangrenous tissue. Common complications: severe bleeding, thrombosis, tissue ischemia/necrosis, hemolysis, organ failure.

Management

Correct reversible cause.
Control bleeding or thrombosis: heparin, pentoxyphyllin.
Prevent recurrence in chronic DIC.

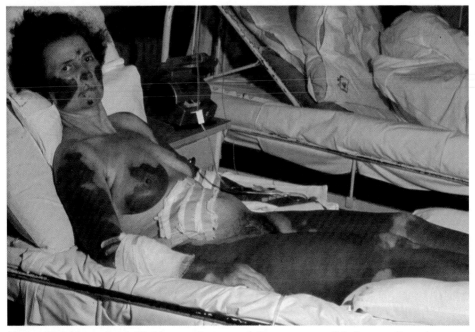

Figure 20-4 Disseminated intravascular coagulation: purpura fulminans *Extensive geographic areas of cutaneous infarction with hemorrhage involving the face, breast, and extremities; although the patient looked alert, she died within several days.*

Section 21

CUTANEOUS LYMPHOMAS, LEUKEMIAS, HISTIOCYTOSES, MASTOCYTOSIS, AND LYMPHOMATOID PAPULOSIS

ADULT T-CELL LEUKEMIA/LYMPHOMA

Adult T-cell leukemia/lymphoma (ATL/L) is a neoplasm of CD4+ T cells, caused by human T-cell lymphotrophic virus I (HTLV-I), manifested by skin infiltrates, hypercalcemia, visceral involvement, lytic bone lesions, and abnormal lymphocytes on the peripheral smears.

Epidemiology and Etiology

Age   Average age of onset 35 to 55 years

Sex   Males > females

Race   Japanese, blacks

Etiology   HTLV-I, a human retrovirus. Malignant cells are activated CD4+ T cells with an increased expression of the alpha chain of the interleukin-2 receptor. Infection by the virus usually does not cause disease, which suggests that other environmental factors are involved. Immortalization of some infected CD4 T cells, increased mitotic activity, genetic instability, and impairment of cellular immunity can all occur after infection with HTLV-I. These events may increase the probability of additional genetic changes which, by chance, may lead to the development of leukemia in some people (>5 %). Most of these effects have been attributed to the HTLV–I–encoded protein tax.

Transmission   Sexual intercourse; perinatally; exposure to blood or blood products (same as HIV). Leukemia develops 20 to 40 years after infection.

Geography   Southwestern Japan (Kyushu), Africa, Caribbean Islands, southeastern United States

Classification   Four main categories. In the relatively indolent smoldering and chronic forms, the median survival is 2 years or more. In the acute and lymphomatous forms, it ranges from 4 to 6 months.

History

Systems Review   Fever, weight loss, abdominal pain, diarrhea, pleural effusion, ascites, cough, sputum

Physical Examination

Skin Lesions

TYPES   Lesions occur in 50 % of ATL/L. Single to multiple papules (Figure 21-2), ±purpura; nodules (Figure 21-1); large plaques, ±ulceration; generalized erythroderma; poikiloderma; papulosquamous lesions; diffuse alopecia.

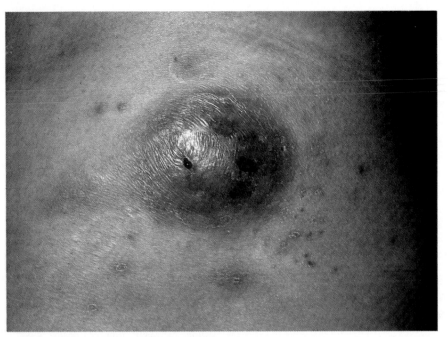

Figure 21-1 Acute T-cell leukemia/lymphoma *Large, red-violet tumor with surrounding red papules and nodules.*

COLOR   Erythematous, violaceous, brown

PALPATION   Firm lesions

DISTRIBUTION   Trunk > face > extremities

General Examination

ABDOMEN   Hepatomegaly (50 %), spleno-megaly (25 %)

LYMPH NODES   Lymphadenopathy (75 %) sparing mediastinal lymph nodes

Differential Diagnosis

Multiple Cutaneous Nodules   Cutaneous T-cell lymphoma (mycosis fungoides), Sézary's syndrome

Laboratory and Special Examinations

Hematology   WBC ranges from normal to 500,000/μl. Peripheral blood smear—polylobulated lymphocytic nuclei, resembling Sézary cells.

Dermatopathology   Perivascular and/or diffuse infiltrates with large abnormal lymphocytes in the upper to middle dermis; epidermis often spared. Alternatively, dense intradermal infiltration and Pautrier's microabscesses, composed of many large abnormal lymphocytes, ±giant cells.

Chemistry   Hypercalcemia: 25 % at time of diagnosis of ATL/L; > 50 % during clinical course

Serology   Seropositive (ELISA, Western blot) to HTLV-I; in IVDU, up to 30 % have dual retroviral infection with both HTLV-I and HIV.

Diagnosis

Characteristic clinical findings, seropositivity to HTLV-I, confirmation of integration of HTLV-I proviral DNA in the cellular DNA of the ATL/L cells

Pathophysiology

Hypercalcemia felt to be due to osteoclastic bone resorption

Course and Prognosis

Course may be smoldering or chronic for prolonged period (abnormal lymphocytosis, skin infiltrates, modest bone marrow involvement) or massive lymphoma. Mean survival with acute crisis in hypercalcemic patients 12.5 weeks (range 2 weeks to 1 year); if normocalcemic, 50 weeks. Cause of death: opportunistic infections, disseminated intravascular coagulation.

Management

Various regimens of cytotoxic chemotherapy; the rates of complete response are <30 %, and responses lack durability. The acute and lymphomatous forms resist conventional cytotoxic chemotherapy. Recently, excellent results have been obtained with the combination of oral zidovudine and subcutaneous interferon-alpha. Obtain HTLV-I serology of family members, sexual partners. If seropositive, should not donate blood.

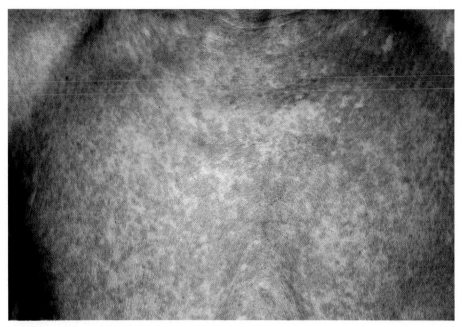

Figure 21-2 Acute T-cell leukemia/lymphoma *Disseminated, red-violet papules becoming confluent on the chest.*

CUTANEOUS T-CELL LYMPHOMA

Cutaneous T-cell lymphoma (CTCL) is a term that applies to T-cell lymphoma first manifested in the skin, but since the neoplastic process involves the entire lymphoreticular system, the lymph nodes and internal organs become involved in the course of the disease. CTCL is a malignancy of helper T cells (CD4+).

Synonym: Mycosis fungoides.

Epidemiology and Etiology

Age 50 years (range 5 to 70 years)

Sex Male : female ratio 2 : 1

Incidence Uncommon but not rare

Etiology Human T-lymphotrophic virus (HTLV) in some patients

History

Onset of Lesions Months to years, often preceded by various diagnoses such as psoriasis, nummular dermatitis, and "large plaque" parapsoriasis

Skin Symptoms Pruritus, often intractable, but may be none

Systems Review Negative except in late stages with visceral organ involvement

Physical Findings

Skin Lesions

TYPES

Plaques, scaling (Figures 21-3 to 21-5) or not scaling, large (>3.0 cm), at first superficial, much like "eczema" or psoriasis or mimicking a "mycosis," and later becoming thicker or "infiltrated"

Nodules and tumors (Figure 21-6) with or without ulcers

Poikiloderma (Figure 21-3) with or without plaques and nodules. Extensive infiltration can cause leonine facies (Figure 21-7).

COLOR Different shades of red

SHAPE Round, oval, arciform, annular, concentric, bizarre

ARRANGEMENT Randomly distributed discrete plaques, nodules, and tumors or diffuse involvement with erythroderma (Sézary's syndrome) and palmoplantar keratoderma

DISTRIBUTION Often spares exposed areas (in early stages). No typical distribution pattern, random localization. Leonine facies (Figure 21-7).

General Examination Careful examination for lymphadenopathy

Sézary's Syndrome This is a leukemic form of CTCL consisting of (1) erythroderma, (2) lymphadenopathy, (3) elevated WBC (>20,000/μl) with a high proportion of so-called Sézary cells, (4) hair loss, and (5) pruritus.

Differential Diagnosis

Scaling Plaques High index of suspicion is needed in patients with atypical or refractory "psoriasis," "eczema," and poikiloderma atrophicans vasculare. Repeated biopsies are necessary. CTCL often mimics psoriasis in being a scaly plaque and disappearing with sunlight exposure.

Laboratory and Special Examinations

Repeated and multiple biopsies often are necessary to finally establish the diagnosis.

Dermatopathology

SITE Epidermis and dermis

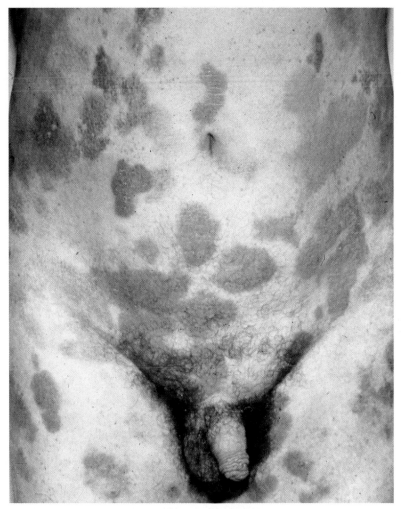

Figure 21-3 Cutaneous T-cell lymphoma (mycosis fungoides): patch stage *Generalized, flat, reddish-to-brownish plaques with some scaling, mimicking psoriasis.*

Diagnostic Checklist

1. History
2. Lymph nodes, axillary and inguinal, and biopsy of nodes if palpable
3. Skin biopsy with 1-μm sections
4. Chest radiograph
5. Complete blood count with differential
6. CT scan of abdomen (usually peripheral nodes involved first)
7. Buffy coat

1. Mycosis cells (Lutzner cells): T cells with hyperchromatic, irregularly shaped (cerebriform) nuclei. Mitoses vary from rare to frequent.
2. Microabscesses in the epidermis containing mycosis cells (Pautrier's microabscesses)
3. Bandlike and patchy infiltrate in upper dermis of atypical lymphocytes (mycosis cells) extending to skin appendages. Abnormal T cells can be identified by electron microscopy (and by experienced investigators sometimes even by light microscopy): typically convoluted nucleus.
4. Monoclonal antibody techniques: Mycosis cells are activated CD4+ cells; T-cell receptor rearrangement studies: monoclonal.

Hematology Eosinophilia, 6 % to 12 %, could increase to 50 %. Buffy coat: abnormal circulating T cells (Sézary type) and increased WBC ($20,000/\mu l$). Bone marrow examination is not helpful.

Chemistry Lactic dehydrogenase isoenzymes 1, 2, and 3 increased in erythrodermic stage

Chest X-Ray Search for hilar lymphadenopathy.

Imaging In stage I and stage II disease, diagnostic imaging (CT, gallium scintigraphy, liver-spleen scan, and lymphangiography) does not provide more information than biopsies of lymph nodes.

CT Scan With more advanced diseases to search for retroperitoneal nodes in patients with extensive skin involvement, lymphadenopathy, or tumors in the skin

Liver-Spleen Scan To identify any focal areas

Diagnosis

In the early stages the diagnosis of CTCL is a problem. Clinical lesions may be typical, but histologic confirmation may not be possible for years despite repeated biopsies. One-micron-thick sections may be helpful. For early diagnosis, cytophotometry (estimation of aneuploidy and polyploidy) and estimation of the indentation of pathologic cells (nucleocontour index) are helpful. Fresh tissue should be sent for immunophenotyping of infiltrating T cells by use of monoclonal antibodies and T-cell receptor rearrangement studies. Lymphadenopathy and the detection of abnormal circulating T cells in the blood appear to correlate well with *internal* organ involvement. See TNM classification and staging (Tables 21-A and 21-B).

Course and Prognosis

The course is quite unpredictable until a histologic diagnosis is made; i.e., a clinical diagnosis of suspicious CTCL (pre-CTCL) may be present for years. Once histologic diagnosis is made, the course of the disease varies with the source of the patient material studied. At the National Institutes of Health in the United States there was a median survival rate of 5 years from the time of the histologic diagnosis, while in Europe a less malignant course is seen. Similarly, it would appear that in office practice there is a prolonged course (sometimes 10 to 15 years). After histologic diagnosis is made, everyone agrees that prognosis is much worse when (1) tumors are present (mean survival 2.5 years), (2) there is lymphadenopathy (mean survival 3 years), (3) > 10 % of the skin surface is involved with pretumor-stage CTCL, and (4) there is a generalized erythroderma. Patients <50 years of age have twice the survival rate of patients >60 years.

Management (See Table 21-B)

If the pre-CTCL stage, in which the histologic diagnosis is not established, PUVA photochemotherapy is the most effective treatment. For histologically proven plaque-stage disease with no lymphadenopathy and no abnormal circulating T cells, PUVA photochemotherapy is

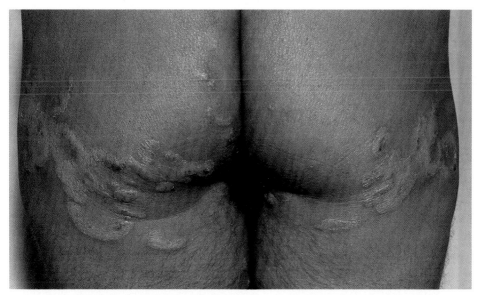

Figure 21-4 Cutaneous T-cell lymphoma (mycosis fungoides): plaque stage *Multiple annular and circinate plaques, some with psoriasiform scale on the buttocks.*

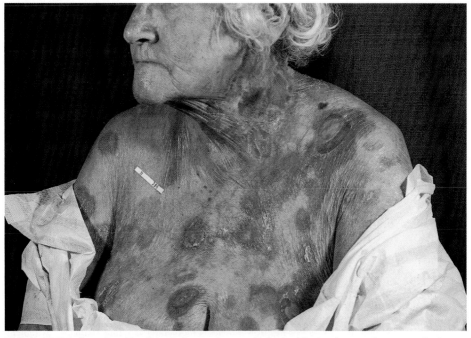

Figure 21-5 Cutaneous T-cell lymphoma (mycosis fungoides): plaque stage *Multiple annular and circinate plaques, some with psoriasiform scale, some with erosion, indurated upon palpation.*

TABLE 21-A TNM CLASSIFICATION OF MYCOSIS FUNGOIDES (MF) AS ADOPTED FOR THE U.S. NATIONAL CANCER INSTITUTE WORKSHOP ON CUTANEOUS T-CELL LYMPHOMAS (1979)

T: Skin	T_0	Clinically and/or histologically suspicious lesions
	T_1	Limited plaques, papules, or eczematous patches covering less than 10 % of the skin surface
	T_2	Generalized plaques, papules, or erythematous patches covering more than 10 % of the skin surface
	T_3	Tumors (1 or more)
	T_4	Generalized erythroderma (Sézary's)
N: Lymph nodes	N_0	No clinically abnormal peripheral nodes, pathology negative for MF
	N_1	Clinically abnormal peripheral lymph nodes, pathology negative for MF
	N_2	No clinically abnormal peripheral lymph nodes, pathology positive for MF
	N_3	Clinically abnormal peripheral lymph nodes, pathology positive for MF
B: Blood	B_0	Less than 5 % atypical circulating lymphocytes
	B_1	Greater than 5 % atypical circulating lymphocytes (Sézary's)
M: Visceral organs	M_0	No visceral organ involvement
	M_1	Histologically proven visceral involvement

TABLE 21-B STAGING SYSTEM FOR CUTANEOUS T-CELL LYMPHOMA

Stages	T	N	M
IA	T_1	N_0	M_0
IB	T_2	N_0	M_0
IIA	T_{1-2}	N_1	M_0
IIB	T_3	N_{0-1}	M_0
III	T_4	N_{0-1}	M_0
IVA	T_{1-4}	N_{2-3}	M_0
IVB	T_{1-4}	N_{0-3}	M_1

also the method of choice. Also used at this stage are topical chemotherapy with nitrogen mustard in an ointment base (10 mg %) and total electron-beam therapy, singly or in combination. If isolated tumors should develop, these should be treated with local x-ray or electron-beam therapy. For extensive plaque stage with multiple tumors or in patients with lymph- adenopathy or abnormal circulating T cells, electron-beam plus chemotherapy is probably the best combination for now; randomized, controlled studies of various combinations are in progress. Also, extracorporeal PUVA photochemotherapy is being evaluated in patients with Sézary's syndrome.

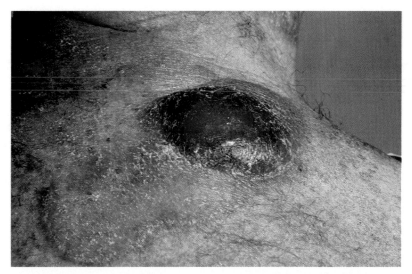

Figure 21-6 Cutaneous T-cell lymphoma (mycosis fungoides): tumor stage *A fleshy, tomato-like, partially eroded nodule arising from a larger, slightly elevated, psoriasiform plaque with scaling and central atrophy.*

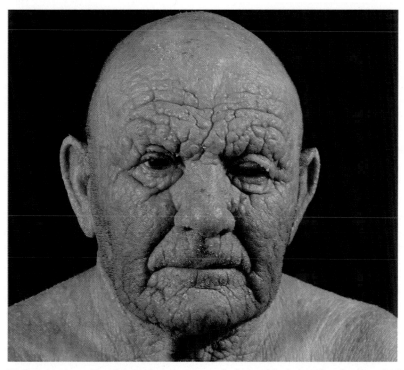

Figure 21-7 Cutaneous T-cell lymphoma (mycosis fungoides): leonine facies *Diffuse in-filtration of the skin has caused a coarsening of the facial features, with thickening of the brows and glabella; the neck and trunk are also involved.*

SÉZARY'S SYNDROME

This syndrome is a rare special variant of cutaneous T-cell lymphoma (CTCL) (mycosis fungoides) characterized by generalized or universal erythroderma, peripheral lymphadenopathy, and cellular infiltrates of atypical lymphocytes (Sézary cells) in the skin and in the blood.

Epidemiology

Age Over 60 years

Sex Males > females

History

Duration of Lesions The disease may arise *de novo* or, less commonly, result from extension of a preexisting circumscribed CTCL.

Skin Symptoms Pruritus, intense and generalized

Physical Examination

Appearance of Patient Sick, shivering, and scared

Skin Lesions Confluent erythematous scaling dermatitis

COLOR Red; the syndrome has been called the "red man syndrome" (Figure 21-8)

DISTRIBUTION Generalized or involving the entire skin surface (universal) (Figures 21-8 and 13-1)

Palms and Soles Diffuse hyperkeratosis

Hair Alopecia

General Examination Generalized lymphadenopathy

Differential Diagnosis

Erythroderma Exfoliative dermatitis of unknown etiology can mimic Sézary's syndrome and can even have elevation of Sézary cells in the buffy coat. Adult T-cell leukemia/lymphoma (see page 540).

Laboratory Examinations

Dermatopathology

LIGHT MICROSCOPY *Site* Epidermis and dermis
Process Cell proliferation
Cell Types In the upper dermis there is a dense infiltration of lymphocytes, histiocytes, and varying numbers of Sézary cells. The Sézary cell is virtually indistinguishable from the so-called mycosis cell when viewed by either light microscopy or electron microscopy. In the epidermis there are Pautrier's microabscesses, containing Sézary cells, and other mononuclear cells. The lymph nodes may contain nonspecific inflammatory cells (dermatopathic lymphadenopathy), or there can be a complete replacement of the nodal pattern by Sézary cells. The cell infiltrates in the viscera in CTCL are the same as are present in the skin. However, Sézary cells are not absolutely specific for Sézary's syndrome, since these atypical lymphocytes can occur in nonspecific exfoliative dermatitis. Immunophenotyping: CD4+ cells; T-cell receptor rearrangement: monoclonal process.

EM TECHNIQUES The Sézary cells contain many infoldings of the nuclear membrane, with finger-like projections in the nucleoplasm.

Laboratory Examination of Blood

HEMATOLOGY There may be a moderate leukocytosis or a normal WBC. The buffy coat contains from 15 % to 30 % atypical lymphocytes (Sézary cells).

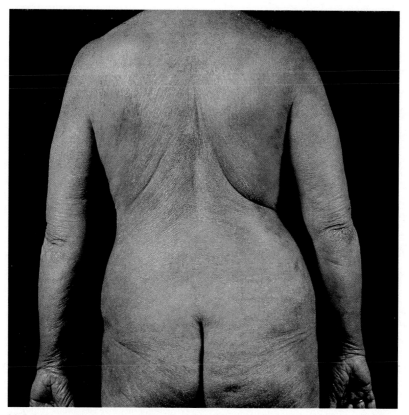

Figure 21-8 Cutaneous T-cell lymphoma: Sézary syndrome *Generalized erythema, scaling, and thickening of the skin (erythroderma); the palms are hyperkeratotic. Generalized lymphadenopathy was present. The buffy coat contained 45 % atypical lymphocytes (Sézary cells).*

Diagnosis

The three features are erythroderma, generalized lymphadenopathy, and presence of increased numbers of atypical lymphocytes in the buffy coat.

Course and Prognosis

The course without treatment is progressive, and patients die from opportunistic infections.

Management

Systemic Chemotherapy is effective in some patients.

Phototherapy PUVA photochemotherapy with and without systemic retinoids (e.g., 13-retinoic acid) is effective for the erythroderma but does not induce remission of lymph node involvement. Extracorporeal PUVA photochemotherapy is the most recent promising treatment, but its efficacy in remission induction and maintenance is not yet known because there has not been long-term follow-up.

CUTANEOUS B-CELL LYMPHOMA

A clonal proliferation of B-lymphocytes can be confined to the skin or more often is associated with systemic B-cell lymphoma.

Epidemiology and Etiology

Age of Onset > 50 years

Sex   Similar to cutaneous T-cell lymphoma

Incidence   Rare

Etiology   Unknown

History

Eruption of crops of asymptomatic nodules and plaques, usually localized

Systems Review   Negative except in cases with systemic involvement

Physical Examination

Skin Lesions

TYPES   Indurated plaques or nodules (Figures 21-9 and 21-10) with a smooth surface

COLOR   Different shades of red to plum color

ARRANGEMENT   Single or multiple, widespread or localized, asymmetric

CONSISTENCY   Firm, nontender, cutaneous or fixed subcutaneous masses

General Examination   Careful examination for lymphadenopathy or extracutaneous involvement

Differential Diagnosis

Skin Nodule(s)/Tumor(s)   Cutaneous T-cell lymphoma, leukemia cutis, leprosy, granuloma faciale, atypical mycobacterial infections, sarcoidosis

Dermatopathology

A dense nodular or diffuse monomorphous infiltrate of lymphocytes usually separated from the epidermis by a zone of normal collagen. B-cell–specific monoclonal antibody studies facilitate differentiation of cutaneous B-cell lymphoma from pseudolymphoma and cutaneous T-cell lymphoma and permit more accurate classification of the cell type. Most cases will react with CD19, 20, 22, and 28. Gene typing studies confirm diagnosis employing immunoglobulin gene rearrangement.

Diagnosis

In the early stages, cutaneous B-cell lymphoma can mimic any nodular infiltrate occurring in the skin, including cutaneous T-cell lymphoma. Patients should be investigated thoroughly for extracutaneous disease, and if found, bone marrow, lymph node, and peripheral blood studies will show morphologic cytochemical and immunologic features similar to those of the cutaneous infiltrates.

Management

X-ray therapy to localized lesions and chemotherapy for systemic disease

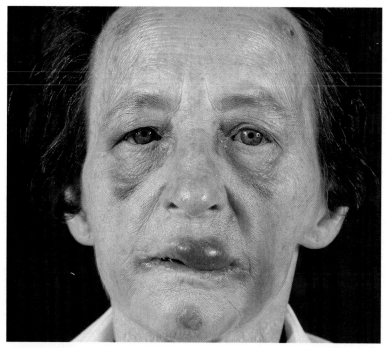

Figure 21-9 Cutaneous B-cell lymphoma *Multiple, well-defined, red-to-brownish and -bluish nodules on the face with associated edema.*

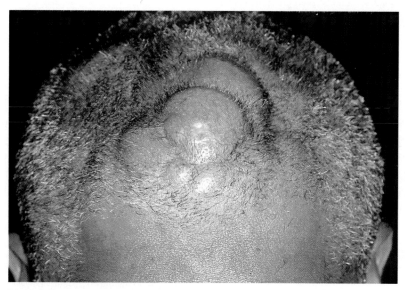

Figure 21-10 Cutaneous B-cell lymphoma *Multiple, skin-colored dermal tumors on the scalp.*

ANGIOCENTRIC LYMPHOMA

Angiocentric lymphoma (AL) is a multisystem disease involving predominantly the skin, lungs, CNS, and kidneys, with characteristics of both inflammatory and neoplastic processes, combining the angiodestructive and granulomatous features of Wegener's granulomatosis with the cellular atypicality of lymphoma.

Synonym: Lymphomatoid granulomatosis.

Epidemiology and Etiology

Age Peak incidence third to sixth decade

Sex Males > females

Etiology Considered to be a pleomorphic T-cell lymphoma

History

Cough, dyspnea, chest pain, ±hemoptysis

Physical Examination

Skin Lesions Present in 40 % to 50 % of cases

TYPES Macules, papules, nodules (Figure 21-11), plaques, annular plaques with central clearing, vesicles. Ulcerations. Ichthyosis, alopecia, necrobiosis lipoidica–like lesions.

COLOR Initially, erythematous

PALPATION Soft to firm ulcers with soggy borders

DISTRIBUTION Gluteal areas, lower legs, head and neck. In the face AL presents as lethal midline granuloma with massive destruction of soft tissue (Figure 21-11).

General Examination Should include chest x-ray, endoscopy of upper digestive and respiratory tracts, CT scan and MRI of CNS.

Differential Diagnosis

Wegener's granulomatosis

Laboratory and Special Examinations

Chest X-Ray Transient alveolar or interstitial infiltrates and effusions; progress to nodular, masslike densities, ±cavitation of nodules

ECG Myocardial ischemia

Dermatopathology Angiocentric and angiodestructive granulomatous infiltrate with pleomorphic and highly atypical lymphoreticular cells having immunophenotypical markers of T cells; often massive necrosis

Diagnosis

Clinical suspicion confirmed by biopsy findings

Pathophysiology

There is increasing evidence that AL is a malignant T-cell lymphoma.

Course and Prognosis

Frequently, AL presents in skin before clinically manifesting in other organ systems (20 % of cases). Skin most common site (40 % to 50 %) of extrapulmonary involvement, followed by brain and kidneys. Prognosis: poor, with 65 % to 90 % mortality reported.

Management

Early treatment of AL with prednisone and cyclophosphamide may transiently halt progression.

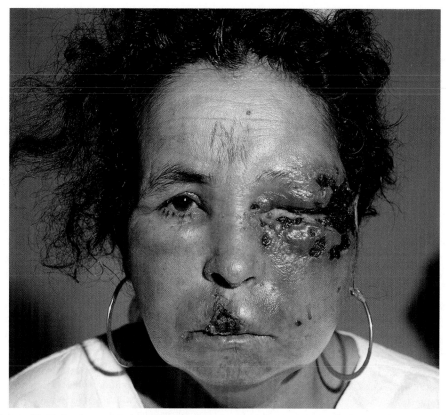

Figure 21-11 Angiocentric lymphoma *Papules, nodules, tumors, and ulcers with associated facial edema. The markings on the forehead are a tribal tatoo of this North African woman.*

LANGERHANS CELL HISTIOCYTOSIS

Langerhans cell histiocytosis (LCH) is an idiopathic group of disorders characterized histologically by proliferation and infiltration of tissue by Langerhans cell–type histiocytes that fuse into multinucleated giant cells and form granulomas with eosinophils. LCH is characterized clinically by lytic bony lesions and cutaneous findings that range from soft tissue swelling to eczema- and seborrheic dermatitis–like changes and ulceration.

Synonyms: Type II histiocytosis, nonlipid reticuloendotheliosis, eosinophilic granuloma, Hand-Schüller-Christian disease, Letterer-Siwe disease.

Classification

The disorders of xanthohistiocytic proliferation involving histiocytes, foam cells, and mixed inflammatory cells are divided into Langerhans cell (histiocytic X) (LCH) and non-Langerhans cell (nonhistiocytic X) histiocytoses. The staging of LCH is presented in Table 21-C.

Unifocal LCH Most commonly manifested by a single osteolytic bony lesion. Skin and soft tissue lesions not so uncommon (known as *eosinophilic granuloma*).

Multifocal LCH Similar to unifocal LCH; however, bony lesions are multiple and interfere with function of neighboring structures. Multifocal LCH involves bones, skin (second most frequently involved organ), soft tissue, lymph nodes, lungs, and pituitary glands.

Letterer-Siwe Syndrome (LSS) The most aggressive of multifocal LCH forms, with skin involvement and infiltration of various organs causing organomegaly, thrombocytopenia

Epidemiology and Etiology

Age

UNIFOCAL LCH Most commonly, childhood and early adulthood

MULTIFOCAL LCH Most commonly, childhood

LSS More commonly, first few years; also, adult form occurs.

Sex Males > females

Etiology Unknown

Incidence Rare

History

Unifocal LCH Systemic symptoms uncommon. Pain and/or swelling over underlying bony lesion. Disruption of teeth with mandibular disease, fracture, otitis media due to mastoid involvement; recalcitrant ulcer on oral mucosa or genital region. Often, lesions are asymptomatic and diagnosed on radiographs for unrelated disorders.

Multifocal LCH Erosive lesions are exudative, pruritic, or painful, with poor response to local treatments. Moist scalp and intertriginous lesions may have offensive odor. Associated disorders include otitis media caused by destruction of temporal and mastoid bones, proptosis due to orbital masses, loose teeth with infiltration of maxilla or mandible, anterior and/or pituitary dysfunction with involvement of sella

TABLE 21-C STAGING OF LCH[1]

A. Localized LCH
  1. Bone (one or two adjacent lesions)
  2. Lymph node
  3. Skin
B. Disseminated LCH
  1. Bone, multifocal
  2. Bone and soft tissue or soft tissues alone (except skin and isolated lymph node)
  3. Organ dysfunction (liver, lungs, hemopoietic system)

[1]Histiocyte Society.

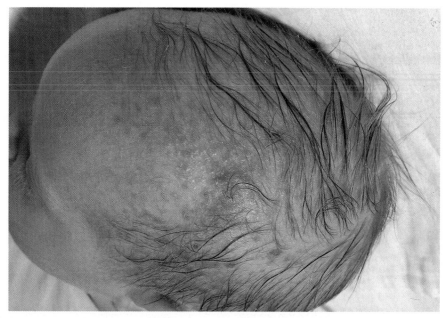

Figure 21-12 Langerhans cell histiocytosis *Small, yellow-pink papules with a greasy scale on the scalp in this infant.*

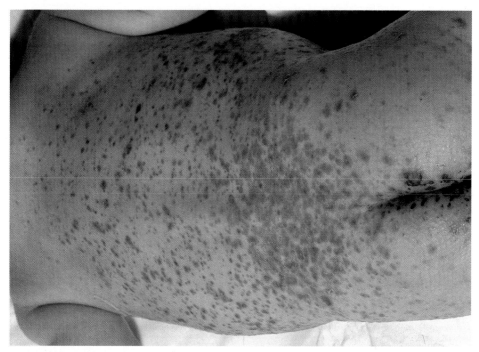

Figure 21-13 Langerhans cell histiocytosis: Letterer-Siwe syndrome *Erythematous papules and nodules with purpura, crusting, and ulceration, becoming confluent on the trunk of a young child.*

turcica. Sellar involvement associated with growth retardation. Diabetes insipidus occurs secondary to hypothalamic or pituitary involvement. Triad of lytic skull lesions, proptosis, and diabetes insipidus: *Hand-Schüller-Christian disease.* Lung involvement associated with chronic cough, pneumothorax.

LSS Child is systemically ill with a course that resembles a systemic infection or malignancy. Hepatomegaly, petechiae and purpura, generalized skin eruption.

Physical Examination

Skin Lesions

UNIFOCAL LCH   *Type*

1. Swelling over bony lesion, over long or flat bone, tender

2. Cutaneous/subcutaneous nodule, yellowish, may be tender and break down, occurring anywhere

3. Sharply marginated ulcer, usually in genital and perigenital region or oral mucous membrane (gingiva, hard palate). Necrotic base, draining, tender (Figure 21-15).

MULTIFOCAL LCH   *Type*   As in unifocal LCH; in addition, regionally localized (head) or generalized eruptions. Papulosquamous, seborrheic dermatitis-like, eczematous dermatitis-like lesions (Figure 21-12); sometimes vesicular; lesions may be purpuric (Figure 21-13), necrotic; areas may coalesce with loss of epidermis; may become heavily crusted. Intertriginous lesions (Figure 21-14) may be exudative and become secondarily infected and ulcerate. Mandibular and maxillary bone involvement may result in loss of teeth (Figure 21-15). Ulceration of vulva. *Palpation* Area overlying bony lesions may be tender; papulosquamous eruption usually rough due to crusting; removal of crusts occurs easily and leaves erosions and punched-out, flat ulcers. *Distribution* Tumorous swelling: calvarium, sphenoid bone, sella turcica, mandible, long bones of upper extremities. Papulosquamous eruptions on scalp

(Figure 21-12), face, and trunk, particularly abdomen and buttocks (Figure 21-13). Skin lesions can be discrete and localized or disseminated and generalized. Ulcers: vulva, gingiva. Eczema- and seborrhea-like changes seen on scalp and in intertriginous areas; erosions occur in groin, axillae, anogenital region (Figure 21-1), retroauricular, neck.

General Findings

UNIFOCAL LCH   Pain and swelling over affected bony lesion, painful ulcer

MULTIFOCAL LCH   Bony lesions occur in calvarium, sphenoid bone, sella turcica, mandible, long bones of upper extremities, and vertebrae.

LSS   Hepatosplenomegaly, lymphadenopathy, involvement of lungs and other organs, bone marrow; thrombocytopenia

Differential Diagnosis

Unifocal LCH   Rule out other causes of lytic bony lesion.

Multifocal LCH   Infectious and neoplastic disorders

LSS   Infectious and neoplastic disorders

Laboratory and Special Examinations

Radiographic Findings

UNIFOCAL LCH   Single osteolytic lesion in a long or flat bone (in children, calvarium, femur; in adults, rib)

MULTIFOCAL LCH   Osteolytic lesions in calvarium, sphenoid bone, sella turcica, mandible, vertebrae, and/or long bones of upper extremities. Chest: diffuse micronodular and interstitial infiltrate in midzones and bases of lungs with sparing of costophrenic angles; later, honeycomb appearance, pneumothorax. Extent of osseous involvement established by bone scanning.

LSS   Scans show organomegaly.

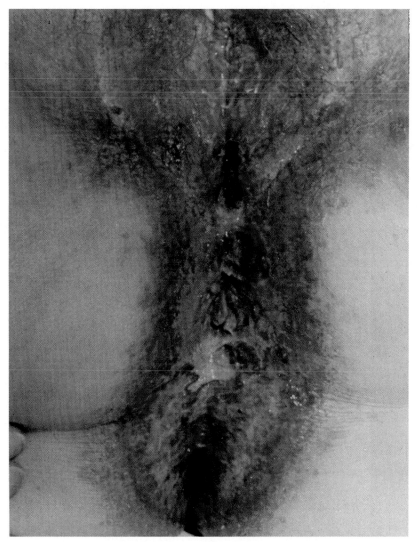

Figure 21-14 Langerhans cell histiocytosis: Letterer-Siwe syndrome *Confluent erythematous papules with hemorrhage, necrosis, scaling, and ulceration in the anogenital and perineal region.*

Histopathology Constant histologic feature of LCH is proliferation of Langerhans cells that have abundant pale eosinophilic cytoplasm with indistinct cell borders, a folded, indented, kidney-shaped nucleus with finely dispersed chromatin, and small, inconspicuous nucleoli. For diagnostic purposes, Langerhans cells in LCH have to be recognized by morphologic, ultrastructural (Birbeck granules), histochemical, and immunehistochemical markers (see Table 21-D).

Diagnosis

All forms of LCH require confirmation of diagnosis by biopsy (skin, bone, or soft tissue/internal organs). Since skin is the organ most frequently involved after bone, skin biopsies have great diagnostic significance (see Histopathology, above).

Pathophysiology

The proliferating Langerhans cell appears to be primarily responsible for the clinical manifestation. The stimulus for the proliferation is unknown.

Course and Prognosis

Unifocal LCH Benign course with excellent prognosis for spontaneous resolution

Multifocal LCH Spontaneous remissions possible. Prognosis poorer at extremes of age and with extrapulmonary involvement.

LSS Commonly fulminant and fatal. Spontaneous remissions uncommon. Current staging on scoring systems for evaluation of prognosis are based on number of organs involved, presence or absence of organ dysfunction, and age. The worst prognosis is in the very young with multifocal LCH and organ dysfunction.

Management

Unifocal LCH Curettage with or without bony chip packing. Low-dose (300 to 600 rad) radiotherapy. Extraosseous soft tissue lesions: surgical excision or low-dose radiotherapy.

Multifocal LCH Diabetes insipidus and growth retardation treated with vasopressin and human growth hormone. Low-dose radiotherapy to bony lesions. Systemic treatment with corticosteroids or vinblastine, mercaptopurine, and methotrexate given as single agents or in combination also with epipodophyllotoxin (etoposide) for prevention and treatment of diabetes insipidus. Topical corticosteroids for discrete cutaneous lesions. Cutaneous lesions respond best to PUVA or topical nitrogen mustard.

LSS Only a few controlled studies of chemotherapy exist. The use of vinblastine results in complete or partial remission in 55 %; combination chemotherapy in 70 %.

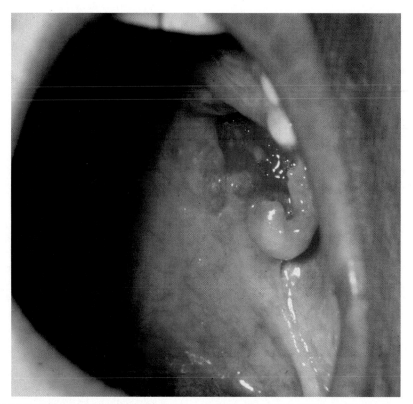

Figure 21-15 Langerhans cell histiocytosis: eosinophilic granuloma *Solitary, ulcerated nodule with loss of teeth on the gingival ridge near the palate, associated with involvement of the maxillary bone.*

TABLE 21-D   DIAGNOSIS IN LCH[1]

Presumptive diagnosis
   Clinical histopathologic
Diagnosis (two or more criteria)
   ATPase+
   S-100 protein+
   Alpha-D mannosidase+
   Peanut agglutinin+
Definite diagnosis
   CD1a+
   Birbeck granules

[1]Histiocyte Society.

MASTOCYTOSIS SYNDROMES

Mastocytosis is associated with an abnormal accumulation of mast cells within the skin and at various systemic sites, which, because of pharmacologically active substances, is manifested clinically by local cutaneous and systemic symptoms.

Epidemiology and Etiology

Classification
Generalized cutaneous mastocytosis Urticaria pigmentosa (UP), telangiectasia macularis eruptiva perstans (TMEP), diffuse cutaneous mastocytosis (DCM)
Mastocytoma (MC) Often solitary
Systemic mastocytosis (SM)
Mast cell "leukemia" Malignant mastocytosis

Age MC and UP: onset between birth and 2 years of age (55 %); infancy-onset UP rarely associated with SM

History

History Stroking lesion causes it to itch. Various drugs are capable of causing mast cell degranulation and release of pharmacologically active substances that exacerbate symptoms: alcohol, dextran, polymyxin B, morphine, codeine. Flushing episode may be accompanied by headache, dyspnea/wheezing, diarrhea, syncope.

Systems Review Tachycardia, hypotension, syncope. Headaches, nausea, vomiting, diarrhea (±alcohol exacerbated); malabsorption; portal hypertension. Bone pain. Neuropsychiatric symptoms (malaise, irritability). Rhinorrhea, wheezing. _Systemic mastocytosis: Up to half of patients may not have any skin findings;_ weight loss, weakness, episodes of flushing, headache, diarrhea.

Physical Examination

Skin Lesions

TYPES **_MC_** Macular to papular to nodular lesions (Figures 21-16 and 21-17), yellow to tan-pink, which become raised and erythematous (urticate) when stroked (Darier's sign); in some patients, lesions become bullous. Often solitary; may be multiple.

_UP_ Skin color to slightly tan macules to slightly raised papules/nodules (Figure 21-16). Darier's sign: wheal develops in the lesion after rubbing with the rounded end of a pen, which causes degranulation of the mast cells. In infants, urticating wheals may become bullous. Dermographism. Bright-red flushing occurring spontaneously, following rubbing skin, after ingestion of alcohol or mast cell degranulation agents.

TMEP At first glance, freckle-like macules (Figure 21-18) with fine telangiectasia in long-standing lesion; urticate with gentle stroking. Dermographism.

DCM Yellowish, thickened appearance of skin; "doughy." Smooth with scattered elevation, resembling leather, "pseudoxanthomatous mastocytosis"; skin folds exaggerated, especially in axilla/groin. Large bullae may occur following trauma or spontaneously. DCM may present as erythroderma (Figure 21-19).

COLOR Skin color to tan

DISTRIBUTION **_UP_** < 10 to > 100, widespread symmetric distribution
TMEP Hundreds of lesions, centripetal, trunk > extremities; lesions may be confluent.

Differential Diagnosis

Mastocytoma Juvenile xanthogranuloma, Spitz nevus

Flushing Carcinoid syndrome

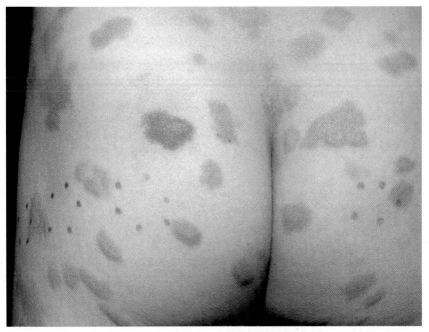

Figure 21-16 Mastocytosis: generalized urticaria pigmentosa *Multiple, flat-topped papules and small plaques of brownish color on the buttocks of a child. Rubbing a lesion has resulted in urtication and an axon flare, a positive Darier's sign.*

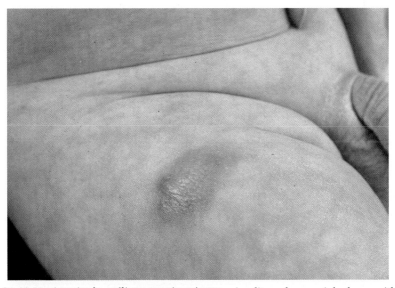

Figure 21-17 Mastocytosis: solitary mastocytoma *A solitary, brown-pink plaque with poorly demarcated borders on the thigh of young child; the lesion was a tan macule prior to stoking (positive Darier's sign).*

UP, DCM, TMEP Histiocytosis X, secondary syphilis, papular sarcoid, generalized eruptive histiocytoma, non-X histiocytosis of childhood

Laboratory and Special Examinations

CBC Systemic mastocytosis: anemia, leukocytosis, eosinophilia

Urine Patients with extensive cutaneous involvement may have increased 24-hour urinary histamine excretion two to three times normal (36 ± 15 μg).

Bone Scan and Imaging Define bone involvement (lytic bone lesions, osteoporosis or osteosclerosis) and small bowel involvement. Small bowel "follow-through" to detect lesions in the small intestine.

Dermatopathology Epidermis is normal. Accumulation of normal-looking mast cells in dermis. Mast cell infiltrates may be sparse (spindle-shaped mast cells) or densely aggregated (cuboidal shape) and have a perivascular or nodular distribution. Mast cells have metachromatically stained (Giemsa's or toluidine blue) granules either intracytoplasmic or extracellular. Pigmentation due to increased melanin in basal layer.

Diagnosis

Clinical suspicion, positive Darier's sign, confirmed by skin biopsy

Pathophysiology

Mast cells contain several pharmacologically active substances that are associated with the clinical findings in mastocytosis: histamine (urticaria, GI symptoms), prostaglandin D_2 (flush, cardiovascular symptoms, GI symptoms), heparin (bleeding into lesion at biopsy site), neutral protease/acid hydrolases (patchy hepatic fibrosis, bone lesions).

Course and Prognosis

Most cases of solitary mastocytoma and generalized UP in children resolve spontaneously. Adults with onset of UP or TMEP with extensive cutaneous involvement have a higher risk for development of systemic mastocytosis than do infants, in whom SM is rare. In young children, acute and extensive degranulation may be life-threatening (shock).

Management

Avoidance of drugs that may cause mast cell degranulation and histamine release: alcohol, dextran, polymyxin B, morphine, codeine, scopolamine, D-tubocurarine, nonsteroidal anti-inflammatory agents.

Antihistamines, both H_1 and H_2. Disodium cromoglycate 200 mg q.i.d. may ameliorate pruritus, whealing, flushing, diarrhea, abdominal pain, and disorders of cognitive function. PUVA treatment is effective for skin lesions but recurrence is common.

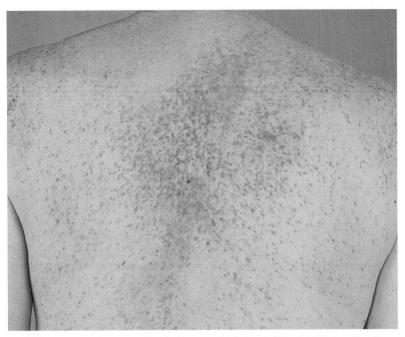

Figure 21-18 Mastocytosis: telangiectasia macularis eruptiva perstans *Small, tan-pink macules and telangiectases on the back.*

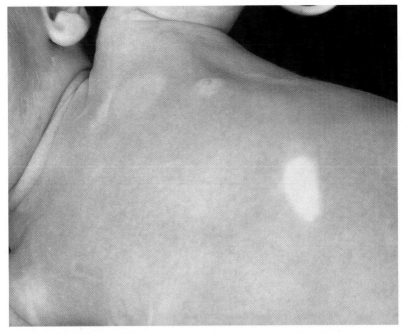

Figure 21-19 Mastocytosis: diffuse cutaneous mastocytosis *The skin of this infant is uniformly erythrodermous secondary to infiltrating mast cells with several spared, white areas of normal skin.*

LEUKEMIA CUTIS

Leukemia cutis (LC) is a localized or disseminated skin infiltration by leukemic cells. It is usually a sign of dissemination of systemic disease or relapse of existing leukemia.

Epidemiology

Incidence Uncommon overall; reported incidence varies from $< 5\%$ to 50%, depending on the type of leukemia.

Age Any age; more common in people over age 50

Sex No predilection, but a slightly higher number of cases involving men have been reported.

Associated Diseases Both acute and chronic leukemias, including the leukemic phase of non-Hodgkin's lymphoma and hairy cell leukemias. Most commonly occurs with acute monocytic leukemia M5 and acute myelomonocytic leukemia M4.

History

Most commonly after or concurrent with diagnosis of hematologic malignancy. However, the lesions occasionally precede the onset of systemic leukemia and its symptoms.

Skin Symptoms Usually absent. Uncommonly, infiltrates are pruritic, tender, or painful. Onset is often sudden, with many lesions arising over several days.

Systemic Review Leukemic patients often will display concurrent systemic symptoms from their disease, either at the time of the initial diagnosis or during a relapse.

Physical Examination

Skin Lesions Pattern of presentation of LC is variable and may have features that overlap with other inflammatory reactions.

TYPES Most common lesions are small (2 to 5 mm) papules (Figure 21-20), nodules (Figures 21-21 and 21-22), or plaques. Similar lesional morphologies occur with different types of leukemia, and vice versa; a specific type of leukemia may present with a variety of morphologies. Inflammatory disorders occurring in patients with leukemia are modified by the participation of leukemic cells in the infiltrate, resulting in less common findings such as ecchymoses, palpable purpura, ulcerative lesions, erythroderma, bullous lesions, gingival hypertrophy, arciform lesions, and lesions that resemble pyoderma gangrenosum, urticaria, urticaria pigmentosa, or psoriasis guttata.

COLOR Depends on the color of the patient's skin. LC lesions are usually somewhat more pink, violaceous, or darker than normal skin. Skin-colored to brown and violaceous. In patients with thrombocytopenia, lesions can have a hemorrhagic component.

PALPATION Lesions are always palpable; they feel indurated and often firm. Tenderness is uncommon. The elevated nature of the lesions is usually best observed by side lighting.

DISTRIBUTION LC may occur at any site. Localized or disseminated; usually on trunk, extremities (Figures 21-20 and 21-21), and face. Leukemic gingival infiltration (hypertrophy) occurs with acute monocytic leukemia.

General Examination Systemic signs associated with hematologic malignancies are often present. Not infrequently, cutaneous manifestation may be the initial presenting symptom and may contribute importantly to the diagnosis.

Differential Diagnosis

The differential diagnosis is large because of the broad clinical manifestations of LC and the many nonspecific inflammatory reactions that are common in leukemic patients. It is most im-

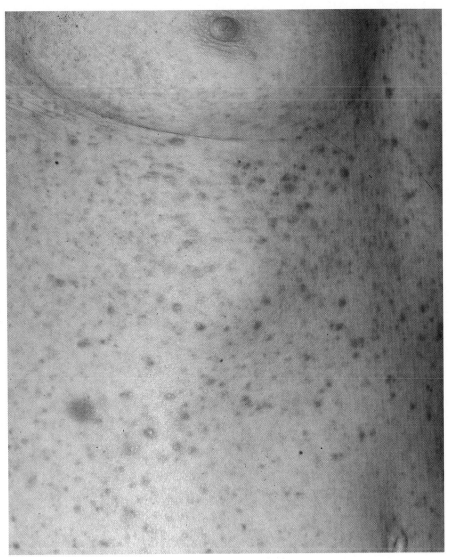

Figure 21-20 Leukemia cutis *Hundreds of tan-pink papules and a nodule on the trunk of a female with acute myelogenous leukemia arose during a one-week interval.*

portant to differentiate LC from a wide variety of disseminated infections occurring in the immunocompromised, neutropenic host, including bacterial sepsis (*Staphylococcus aureus, Pseudomonas aeruginosa*), fungemia (*Candida, Aspergillus*), and disseminated viral infections (herpes simplex virus, varicella-zoster virus). Inflammatory disorders that must be ruled out include neutrophilic dermatoses (Sweet's syndrome, pyoderma gangrenosum), adverse cutaneous drug reactions, transfusion-associated graft-versus-host disease, vasculitis, and erythema multiforme.

Laboratory Examinations

Hematology Leukemic cells are usually visible in the smear of peripheral blood, but they are absent in aleukemic leukemia.

Bone Marrow Aspirate Confirms the diagnosis and defines the type

Dermatopathology Dermis, subcutaneous large perivascular, periadnexal, or diffuse. Myeloblasts, atypical myelocytes

Immunophenotyping Conforms with type of leukemia

Diagnosis

Hematologic studies with complete analysis of bone marrow aspirate and peripheral blood smear and cutaneous histology and immunophenotyping are needed to make the diagnosis. If cutaneous findings precede any systemic disease, careful assessment of peripheral blood smears and bone marrow biopsies must be made. In an emergency, a touch preparation from a skin biopsy along with the clinical findings may be sufficient to suggest the diagnosis of LC.

Course and Prognosis

The prognosis for the LC is directly related to the prognosis for the systemic disease.

Management

Therapy is usually directed at the leukemia itself. However, systemic chemotherapy sufficient for bone marrow remission may not treat the cutaneous lesions effectively. Thus a combination of systemic chemotherapy and local electron-beam therapy or PUVA may be necessary for chemotherapy-resistant LC lesions.

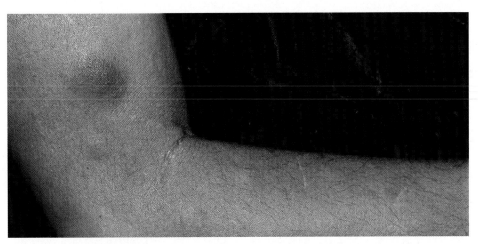

Figure 21-21 Leukemia cutis *A large, dark-brown nodule and a smaller papule on the upper arm of a male with acute myelogenous leukemia; six similar nodules were also present on the trunk.*

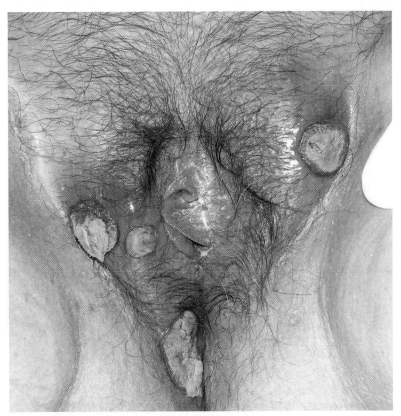

Figure 21-22 Leukemia cutis: chloroma *Large, ulcerated, green-hued tumors (chloromas) in the inguinal and perineal regions of a female with acute myelogenous leukemia; similar lesions were also present in the axillae and on the tongue.*

LYMPHOMATOID PAPULOSIS

Lymphomatoid papulosis is an asymptomatic, chronic, self-healing, polymorphous eruption characterized by recurrent crops of lesions that regress spontaneously, with histologic features suggestive of lymphocytic atypia and a low but real risk of malignant transformation.

Epidemiology

Incidence 1.2 to 1.9 cases per million

Age Childhood to elderly; average age 40 years

Sex Both sexes

Inheritance None; occurs sporadically

History

Usually asymptomatic; occasionally, lesions are pruritic, tender, or painful. Negative history of weight loss, anorexia, fever, sweating. If these are present, pursue workup for systemic lymphoma.

Physical Examination

Skin Lesions Lesions appear in crops of recurrent, self-healing eruptions. Lesions may resolve spontaneously at any point in their evolution, and only those which progress to later stages produce scarring. Individual lesions evolve over a 2- to 8-week period.

TYPES Primary lesions include papules (Figure 21-23), nodules, and uncommonly, tumors. Lesions are initially smooth, hemorrhagic, hyperkeratotic, but central necrosis, crusting (Figure 21-24), and ulceration may evolve. Diameter ranges from 2 to 30 mm. Number of lesions: few to hundreds. With healing, atrophic scars remain, at times with postinflammatory hyper- or hypopigmentation.

COLOR Erythematous to red-brown, central hemorrhage and necrosis black

ARRANGEMENT Usually random but often grouped; occasionally, folliculocentric

DISTRIBUTION Primarily trunk and extremities; rarely, oral or genital mucosa

Other Organ Systems Uninvolved

Differential Diagnosis

Multiple Papules/Nodules in Various Stages of Development *Pityriasis lichenoides et varioliformis acuta (Mucha-Habermann disease)*—clinically similar without histologic atypia. *Lymphoma cutis, Hodgkin's or non-Hodgkin's type*—clinically progressive, histologically malignant. *Large-cell anaplastic T-cell lymphoma,* regressing atypical histiocytosis; mycosis fungoides: papular—broader, less wedge-shaped infiltrate, no vasculitis, few extravasated erythrocytes, more epidermotropic. Also histiocytosis X, lymphocytoma cutis, papular drug eruption, papular urticaria, scabies, viral exanthem.

Laboratory Examinations

Dermatopathology Superficial or deep, perivascular or interstitial mixed-cell infiltrate, wedge-shaped, sometimes interstitial. Epidermis: focal spongiosis, mild exocytosis, necrotic keratinocytes, necrosis, or ulceration. Frequent extravasated erythrocytes. Small-vessel lymphocytic vasculitis in 10 %. Cytologically, atypical cells may comprise 50 % of infiltrate.

TYPE A Large, atypical histiocytic lymphocytes with abundant cytoplasm, convoluted nucleus with occasional binucleation, multipolar mitosis, and Reed-Sternberg-like cells

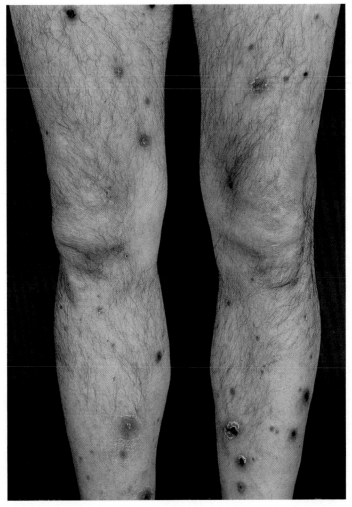

Figure 21-23 Lymphomatoid papulosis *Multiple, brown-red papules and nodules of varying size with hemorrhage, central necrosis, ulceration, and crusting.*

TYPE B Smaller, atypical lymphocytes with cerebriform nuclei, epidermotropism, and occasional mitosis

Immunohistochemistry Predominantly activated, interleukin-2 receptor–positive, HLA-DR–positive, Ki-1 (CD30)–positive; T-helper cells (CD4). Southern blot hybridization: clonal T-cell population in 50 %.

Other Negative workup for systemic involvement

Diagnosis

Based on typical histology and immunohistochemistry, lack of systemic involvement by history and physical examination. May necessitate periodic biopsy to rule out blastic transformation, especially with tumor formation. No reliable histologic, immunohistochemical, or genotypic test available for prediction of risk of progression to lymphoma.

Etiology and Pathogenesis

Unknown; considered to be either a low-grade lymphoma controlled by host mechanisms or a true pseudolymphoma involving T-helper lymphocytes without systemic involvement. Antigens shared with and occasional progression to Hodgkin's disease or cutaneous T-cell lymphoma suggest a low-grade lymphoma, perhaps induced by chronic antigenic stimulation, while low incidence of progression to true malignancy suggests pseudolymphoma. Lymphomatoid papulosis may begin as a chronic, reactive, polyclonal lymphoproliferative phenomenon that sporadically overwhelms host immune defenses and evolves into a clonal, antigen-independent, true lymphoid malignancy. Belongs in the spectrum of primary cutaneous Ki-1+ lymphoproliferative disorders, including pseudo-Hodgkin's disease of the skin, regressing atypical histiocytosis, Hodgkin's lymphoma, and Ki-1+ large cell lymphoma.

Significance

Chronic atypical eruption of low but real malignant potential may prove emotionally and diagnostically challenging for physician and patient alike.

Course and Prognosis

May remit in 3 weeks or continue for decades. Patients may experience periods without lesions or have continuous, repetitive outbreaks. In 10 % to 20 % of patients lymphomatoid papulosis is preceded by, associated with, or followed by another type of lymphoma: mycosis fungoides, Hodgkin's disease, or CD30 large cell lymphoma. May persist despite systemic chemotherapy for concurrent lymphoma.

Management

No treatments have proved consistently effective, as is evidenced by the multiple reported therapies. Topical agents include corticosteroids and carmustine (BCNU). Electron-beam irradiation has been employed as well. PUVA may control the disease but does not affect the long-term prognosis. Tetracyclines, sulfones, and systemic corticosteroids have been reported as effective by some researchers. A wide spectrum of systemic agents has been used, including retinoids, methotrexate, chlorambucil, cyclophosphamide, cyclosporine, and interferon-alpha-2b

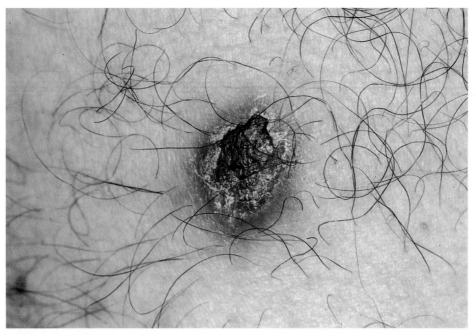

Figure 21-24 Lymphomatoid papulosis *A typical brown-red nodule with central necrosis and crusting.*

Section 22

ADVERSE CUTANEOUS DRUG REACTIONS

INTRODUCTION

Adverse cutaneous drug reactions (ACDRs) are common, occurring in 2 % to 3 % of hospitalized patients. Complications of drug therapy, overall, are the most common adverse event for hospitalized individuals, accounting for 19 % of such events. ACDR in an ambulatory practice occurs frequently, many commonly used drugs having reaction rates of greater than 1 %. The majority of reactions are mild, accompanied by pruritus, resolving promptly after the offending drug is discontinued. However, severe, life-threatening ACDRs do occur and are unpredictable. Drug eruptions can mimic virtually all the morphologic expressions in dermatology and must be first on the differential diagnosis in the appearance of a sudden symmetric eruption. Drug eruptions are caused by immunologic or nonimmunologic mechanisms and are provoked by systemic or topical administration of a drug. The majority are based on a hypersensitivity mechanism and may be of types I, II, III, or IV.

Classification

Type I: Immediate-Type Immunologic Reactions IgE-mediated. Drug (penicillin). Manifested by urticaria and angioedema of skin or mucosa and edema of other organs and fall in blood pressure (anaphylactic shock). Occur more commonly if drug (antigen) is administered intravenously than by mouth.

Type II: Cytotoxic Reactions Drug (penicillin, cephalosporins, sulfonamides, rifampin) plus cytotoxic antibodies causes lysis of cells such as platelets or leukocytes. Alternatively, drug (quinine, quinidine, salicylamide, isoniazid, chlorpromazine, sulfonamides, sulfonylureas) plus antibodies (immune complexes form) causes lysis or phagocytosis.

Type III: Serum Sickness, Drug-Induced Vasculitis IgG or, less commonly, IgM antibodies formed against drug. Mediated by deposition of *immune complexes* in small vessels, activated by complement and recruitment of granulocytes. Onset of reaction: 5 to 7 days between introduction of drug and appearance of reaction. Manifested by vasculitis, urticaria-like lesions, arthritis, nephritis, alveolitis, hemolytic anemia, thrombocytopenia, agranulocytosis.

Type IV: Morbilliform (Exanthematous) Reactions Cell-mediated immune reaction. Sensitized lymphocytes react with drug, liberating cytokines, which trigger cutaneous inflammatory response.

Immunologic hypersensitivity reactions are manifested by a variety of distinct clinical patterns:

• Exanthematous reactions	Type IV, type III(?)
• Urticaria, angioedema	Type I, type III
• Fixed drug eruption	Type III(?), type IV(?)
• Bullous eruptions	Type IV(?)

- Stevens-Johnson syndrome/toxic epidermal necrolysis — Type III, type IV(?)
- Vasculitis — Type III
- Lichenoid eruptions — Type IV(?)
- Photoallergic reactions — Type IV

The nonimmunologic drug eruptions are caused by (1) idiosyncrasy *sensu strictiori*—reactions due to hereditary enzyme deficiencies; (2) cumulation, such as melanosis due to gold or amiodarone; (3) irritancy of a topically applied drug; (4) an individual idiosyncrasy to a topical or systemic drug; (5) mechanisms not yet known; and (6) reactions due to the combination of a drug with ultraviolet irradiation (photosensitivity). These may have a toxic (T) or immunologic (allergic) (A) pathology.

Guidelines for Assessment of Possible Adverse Drug Reactions*

- Alternative causes should be excluded, especially infections, in that many infections (especially viral) are difficult to distinguish clinically from the adverse effects of drugs used to treat infections.
- The interval between introduction of a drug and onset of the reaction should be examined.
- Any improvement after drug withdrawal should be noted.
- The caregiver should determine whether similar reactions have been associated with the same compound.
- Any reaction on readministration of the drug should be noted.

Findings Indicating Possible Life-Threatening ACDR*

Clinical Findings

CUTANEOUS

Confluent erythema
Facial edema or central facial involvement
Skin pain
Palpable purpura
Skin necrosis
Blisters of epidermal detachment
Positive Nikolsky's sign (epidermis separates readily from dermis with lateral pressure)
Mucous membrane erosions
Urticaria
Swelling of the tongue

GENERAL

High fever (temperature >40°C)
Enlarged lymph nodes
Arthralgias or arthritis
Shortness of breath, wheezing, hypotension

Laboratory Results

HEMATOLOGY Eosinophil count >1000/μl. Lymphocytosis with atypical lymphocytes.

CHEMISTRY Abnormal results of liver function tests

Diagnosis

Usually made on clinical findings. Lesional skin biopsy is helpful in defining the type of reaction pattern occurring but does not help in identifying the offending drug. Skin tests and radioallergosorbent tests are helpful in diagnosing IgE-mediated type I hypersensitivity reactions, more specifically to penicillins.

* Roujeau JC, Stern RS: Severe adverse cutaneous reactions to drugs. *N Engl J Med* 1994; 331:1272–1285.

EXANTHEMATOUS DRUG ERUPTION

An exanthematous drug eruption is an adverse hypersensitivity reaction to an ingested or parenterally administered drug characterized by a cutaneous eruption that mimics a measles-like viral exanthem; systemic involvement is minimal.

Synonyms: Morbilliform drug eruption, maculopapular drug eruption.

Epidemiology and Etiology

Incidence   Most common type of cutaneous drug reaction

Age   Less common in the very young

Etiology   *Drugs with a high probability of reaction* (3 % to 5 %): penicillin and related antibiotics, carbamazepine, allopurinol, gold salts (10 % to 20 %). *Medium probability:* sulfonamides (bacteriostatic, antidiabetic, diuretic), NSAIDs, hydantoin derivatives, isoniazid, chloramphenicol, erythromycin, streptomycin. *Low probability* (1 % or less): barbiturates, benzodiazepines, phenothiazines, tetracyclines.

History

Mononucleosis   Up to 100 % of patients with Epstein-Barr virus (EBV) or cytomegalovirus (CMV) mononucleosis syndrome given ampicillin or amoxicillin develop an exanthematous drug eruption.

HIV Infection   50 % to 60 % of HIV-infected patients who receive sulfa drugs (i.e., trimethoprim-sulfamethoxazole) develop eruption.

Drug History   Increased incidence of reactions in patients on allopurinol given ampicillin/amoxicillin

Prior Drug Sensitization   Patients with prior history of exanthematous drug eruption will most likely develop a similar reaction if rechallenged with same drug. About 10 % of patients sensitive to penicillins given cephalosporins will exhibit cross-drug sensitivity and develop eruption. Patients sensitized to one sulfa-based drug (bacteriostatic, antidiabetic, diuretic) may crossreact with another category of the drug in 20 % of cases.

Onset   *Early reaction:* In a previously sensitized patient, eruption starts within 2 or 3 days after administration of drug. *Late reaction:* Sensitization occurs during administration or after completing course of drug; peak incidence at ninth day after administration. However, drug eruption may occur at any time between the first day and 3 weeks after the beginning of treatment. Reaction to penicillin can begin 2 or more weeks after drug is discontinued.

Systems Review   ±Fever. Usually quite pruritic.

Physical Examination

Vital Signs   ±Elevated temperature (drug fever)

Skin Lesions

TYPE   Macules and/or papules, a few millimeters to 1 cm in size (Figure 22-1). Purpura may be seen in lesions of lower legs. In individuals with thrombocytopenia, exanthematous eruptions can mimic vasculitis because of intralesional hemorrhage. *May progress to generalized exfoliative dermatitis, especially if drug not discontinued.* Scaling and/or desquamation may occur with healing; also, erythema multiforme-like.

COLOR   Bright or *"drug" red.* Resolving lesions have hues of tan and purple.

ARRANGEMENT OF MULTIPLE LESIONS   Macules and papules frequently become confluent (Figure 22-1).

DISTRIBUTION   Symmetric (Figure 22-1). Almost always on trunk and extremities. Confluent lesions in intertriginous areas, i.e., axilla, groin, inframammary area. Palms and soles variably involved. In children, may be limited to face and extremities. Eruption may be accentuated in striae. May spare face, nipple,

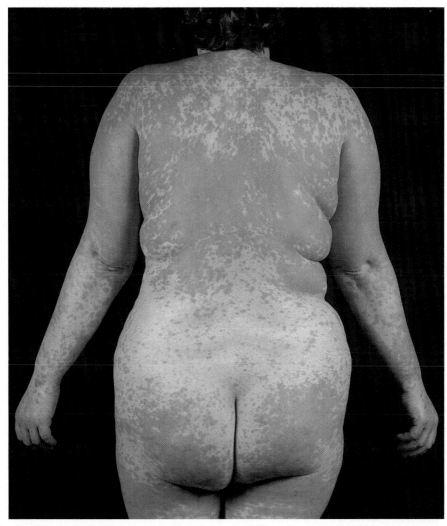

Figure 22-1 Exanthematous drug eruption: ampicillin *Symmetrically arranged, brightly erythematous macules and papules, discrete in some areas and confluent in others on the back and extremities.*

periareolar area, surgical scar. Reactions to ampicillin usually appear initially on the elbows, knees, and trunk, extending symmetrically to most areas of body.

Mucous Membranes ±Enanthem on buccal mucosa

Reactions to Specific Drugs

AMPICILLIN, AMOXICILLIN   Up to 100 % of patients with Epstein-Barr or cytomegalovirus mononucleosis syndrome (primary infection) given ampicillin, amoxicillin developed drug eruptions.

NSAIDS   Incidence: 1 % to 3 %. Site: trunk, pressure areas. Onset: 1 to 2 weeks after beginning therapy.

BARBITURATES   Morphology: macular or maculopapular; scarlatiniform. Site: face, trunk. Onset: few days after initiation of therapy. Crossreactivity with other barbiturates: not universal.

NITROFURANTOIN   Associated findings: fever, peripheral eosinophilia, pulmonary edema, chest pain, dyspnea. Onset: 2 weeks after initiation of therapy; within hours if previously sensitized.

HYDANTOIN DERIVATIVES   Morphology: macular or confluent erythema. Site: begins on face, spreading to trunk and extremities (see Drug Hypersensitivity Syndrome, page 584). Onset: 2 weeks after initiation of therapy. Associated findings: fever, peripheral eosinophilia; facial edema; lymphadenopathy (can mimic lymphoma histologically).

ISONIAZID   Morphology: morbilliform; may evolve to exfoliative dermatitis. Associated findings: fever; hepatitis.

BENZODIAZEPINES   Incidence: very low. Onset: few days after initiation of therapy. Rechallenge: frequently rash does not occur.

PHENOTHIAZINES   Site: begins on face, spreading to trunk (mainly back) and extremities. Onset: between first and third weeks after initiation of therapy. Associated findings:

periorbital edema. Rechallenge: rash may not occur. Crossreactivity: common.

CARBAMAZEPINE   Morphology: diffuse erythema; severe erythroderma may follow. Site: begins on face, spreading rapidly to all areas; may occur in photodistribution. Onset: 2 weeks after initiation of therapy. Associated findings: facial edema.

SULFONAMIDES   Incidence: common up to 50 % to 60 % in HIV-infected patients. Morphology: morbilliform, erythema multiforme-like.

ALLOPURINOL   Incidence: 5 %. Morphology: morbilliform. Site: begins on face, spreading rapidly to all areas; may occur in photodistribution. Onset: 2 to 3 weeks after initiation of therapy. Associated findings: facial edema; systemic vasculitis, especially involving kidneys. Rash may fade in spite of continued administration.

GOLD SALTS   Incidence: 10 % to 20 % of patients; dose-related. Morphology: diffuse erythema; exfoliative dermatitis, lichenoid, hemorrhagic, bullous, or pityriasis rosea-like eruptions may follow.

General Examination   Findings associated with the indication for drug administration

Differential Diagnosis

Exanthematous Eruption   Viral exanthem, secondary syphilis, atypical pityriasis rosea, early widespread allergic contact dermatitis

Laboratory and Special Examinations

Hemogram   ±Peripheral eosinophilia

Dermatopathology   Perivascular lymphocytes and eosinophils

Diagnosis

Clinical diagnosis, at times confirmed by histologic findings

Pathophysiology

Exact mechanism unknown. Probably delayed hypersensitivity. Rash with EBV and CMV mononucleosis probably not allergic.

Course and Prognosis

After discontinuation of drug, rash usually fades; however, it may worsen for a few days. Occasionally fades even though drug is continued. Eruption usually recurs with rechallenge, although not always. In some cases of exanthematous penicillin reactions, readministration of the drug does not cause the eruption. Duration of ampicillin eruption following discontinuation of drug: 3 to 5 days.

Of more concern, a morbilliform eruption may be the initial presentation of a more serious eruption, i.e., toxic epidermal necrolysis, Stevens-Johnson syndrome, hypersensitivity syndrome, or serum sickness.

Management

The definitive step in management is to identify the offending drug and discontinue it.

Indications for Discontinuation of Drug   Urticaria (concern for anaphylaxis), facial edema, blisters, mucosal involvement, ulcers, palpable or extensive purpura, fever, lymphadenopathy

Symptomatic Treatment   Oral antihistamine to alleviate pruritus

Corticosteroids

POTENT TOPICAL CORTICOSTEROID PREPARATION May help speed resolution of eruption, especially if secondary changes of eczematous dermatitis have occurred due to scratching

ORAL OR IV CORTICOSTEROIDS   Usually not indicated or helpful if the offending drug has been discontinued. If the drug cannot be substituted or omitted, systemic corticosteroids can be administered to treat the ACDR; also, to induce more rapid remission.

Prevention   The patient must be aware of his or her specific drug hypersensitivity and that other drugs of the same class can crossreact. Although an exanthematous drug eruption may not recur if the drug is given again, readministration is best avoided by using a different agent. Wearing a medical alert bracelet is advised.

DRUG-INDUCED ACUTE URTICARIA, ANGIOEDEMA, EDEMA, AND ANAPHYLAXIS

Drug-induced urticaria and angioedema occur due to a variety of mechanisms and are characterized clinically by transient wheals and larger edematous areas that involve the dermis and subcutaneous tissue (angioedema). In some cases, cutaneous urticaria/angioedema is associated with systemic anaphylaxis, which is manifested by respiratory distress, vascular collapse, and/or shock. *Synonym:* Angioneurotic edema.

Epidemiology and Etiology

Classification

IMMUNE-MEDIATED (ALLERGIC) URTICARIA/ANGIOEDEMA *IgE-Mediated* Antibiotics (especially penicillins), radiographic contrast agents.

Complement-Mediated By way of immune complexes activating complement and releasing anaphylatoxins that induce mast cell degranulation. Serum sickness, administration of whole blood, immunoglobulins.

Immune Complex-Mediated Reactions resemble serum sickness, penicillin.

NONALLERGIC URTICARIA (ANAPHYLACTOID REACTIONS) *Analgesics/Anti-inflammatory Drugs (NSAIDs)* Drugs inhibit or block cyclooxygenase enzyme in prostaglandin synthesis. Also associated with rhinosinusitis and asthma.

Radiographic Contrast Media Most reactions are nonallergic; rarely, allergic.

Angiotensin-Converting Enzyme (ACE) Inhibitors In 0.1 % to 0.2 % of patients, ACE inhibitors induce a rapid swelling in the nose, throat, mouth, glottis, larynx, lips, and/or tongue. May be due to inhibition of kinin metabolism. Not dose-related; nearly always develops within the first week of therapy, usually within the first few hours after the initial dose. Individuals undergoing hemodialysis with high-flux dialysis membranes (increases bradykinin production) at much higher risk (up to 35 %)

Calcium-Channel Blockers Nifedipine produces peripheral edema in 10 % to 30 % of treated patients. The edema is localized to the lower legs and feet and probably occurs secondary to vasodilation of dependent arterioles and small blood vessels rather than to generalized fluid retention.

Drugs Releasing Histamine See below.

Drugs Causing Urticaria/Angioedema/Anaphylaxis

ANTIBIOTICS AND CHEMOTHERAPEUTIC AGENTS Penicillins: ampicillin, amoxicillin, dicloxacillin, mezlocillin, penicillin G, penicillin V, ticarcillin. Cephalosporins, including third generation. Sulfonamides and derivatives.

CVS DRUGS Amiodarone, procainamide.

IMMUNOTHERAPEUTICS, VACCINES Antilymphocyte serum, levamisole, horse serum

CYTOSTATIC AGENTS L-Asparaginase, bleomycin, cisplatin, daunorubicin, 5-fluorouracil, procarbazine, thiotepa

ACE INHIBITORS Captopril, enalopril, lininopril

CALCIUM-CHANNEL BLOCKERS Nifedipine, diltiazem, verapramil

DRUGS RELEASING HISTAMINE Centrally acting drugs (morphine, meperidine, atropine, codeine, papaverine, propanidid, alfaxalone); muscle relaxants (D-turbocurarine, succinylcholine); sympathomimetics (amphetamine, tyramine); hypotensive agents (hydralazine, tolazoline, trimethaphan camsylate); antimicrobial agents (pentamidine, propamidine, stilbamidine, quinine, vancomycin); others (radiographic contrast media).

Incidence Angioedema occurs in 1 per 10,000 courses of penicillin and leads to death

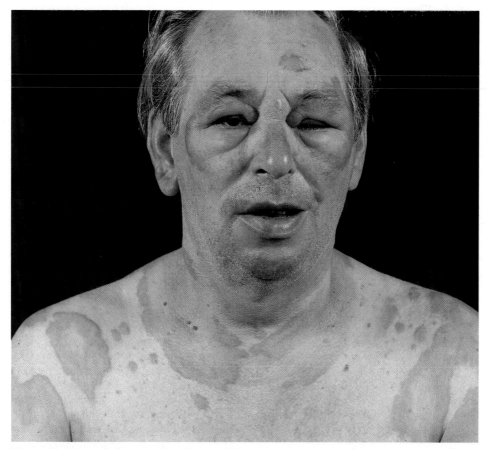

Figure 22-2 Drug-induced urticaria: penicillin *Large, urticarial wheals on the face, neck, and trunk with angioedema in the periorbital region.*

in 1 to 5 per 100,000 courses. Angioedema associated with angiotensin-converting enzyme (ACE) inhibitors occurs in 2 to 10 per 10,000 new users.

History

Time from Initial Drug Exposure to Appearance of Urticaria

IgE-MEDIATED Initial sensitization, usually 7 to 14 days; urticaria may occur while the drug is still being administered or after it is discontinued. In previously sensitized individuals, usually within minutes or hours.

IMMUNE COMPLEX-MEDIATED Initial sensitization, usually 7 to 10 days, but as long as 28 days; in previously sensitized individuals, symptoms appear 12 to 36 hours after drug readministered.

ANALGESICS/ANTI-INFLAMMATORY DRUGS Occurs following administration of drug by 20 to 30 minutes (up to 4 hours).

Prior Drug Exposure

RADIOGRAPHIC CONTRAST MEDIA 25 % to 35 % probability of repeat reaction in individuals with history of prior reaction to contrast media

Duration of Lesions Hours

Skin Symptoms Pruritus, burning of palms/soles, auditory canal. With airway edema, difficulty breathing.

Constitutional Symptoms IgE-mediated: flushing, sudden fatigue, yawning, headache, weakness, dizziness; numbness of tongue, sneezing, bronchospasm, substernal pressure, palpitations; nausea, vomiting, crampy abdominal pain, diarrhea

Systems Review Arthralgia

Physical Examination

Skin Lesions

TYPE

Large wheals (Figure 22-2), which appear and resolve within a few hours, spontaneously or with therapy; reappear

Angioedema: extensive tissue swelling with involvement of deep dermal and subcutaneous tissues. Often pronounced on face with skin-colored enlargement of portion of face (eyelids, lips, tongue) (Figures 22-2 and 22-3).

COLOR   Pink with larger lesions having white central area surrounded by an erythematous halo (Figure 22-2)

SHAPE   Oval, arciform, annular, polycyclic, serpiginous, and bizarre patterns

ARRANGEMENT   Annular, arciform, linear, target, and iris lesions occur. Initial part of lesion resolves as the newer portions advance centrifugally, at times merging with other lesions.

DURATION   Transient, hours

DISTRIBUTION   Localized, regional (Figure 22-3), or generalized (Figure 22-2). Angioedema: genitalia, or any site. Mucosa: upper airway with possible obstruction of breathing

General Findings

IGE-MEDIATED REACTIONS   Hypotension. Bronchospasm, laryngeal edema

Differential Diagnosis

Acute Edematous Red Pruritic Plaque(s)
Allergic contact dermatitis (poison ivy, poison oak dermatitis), cellulitis, insect bite(s)

Laboratory and Special Examinations

Dermatopathology   Edema of the dermis or subcutaneous tissue, dilation of venules, mild perivascular infiltrate, mast cell degranulation.

Complement Studies   Decreased in serum sickness

Ultrasonography   For early diagnosis of bowel involvement; if abdominal pain is present, this may indicate edema of the bowel.

Diagnosis

Clinical diagnosis, at times confirmed by histologic findings

Pathophysiology

IgE-mediated urticaria: Lesions result from antigen-induced release of biologically active molecules (leukotrienes, prostaglandins) from mast cells or basophilic leukocytes sensitized with specific IgE antibodies (type I, anaphylactic hypersensitivity). Mediators released increase venular permeability, modulate the release of biologically active materials from other cell types. In sensitized individuals, a very small amount of drug can trigger a serious reaction. Parenteral administration of the drug in a sensitized individual is much more likely to trigger anaphylaxis than oral administration. Urticaria can be immediate or accelerated, depending on whether IgE molecules are present before drug exposure or are formed during exposure.

In complement-mediated urticaria, complement is activated by immune complexes, which results in the release of anaphylatoxins, which, in turn, induce mast cell degranulation. Intolerance to salicylates is presumably mediated by abnormalities of the arachidonic acid pathway.

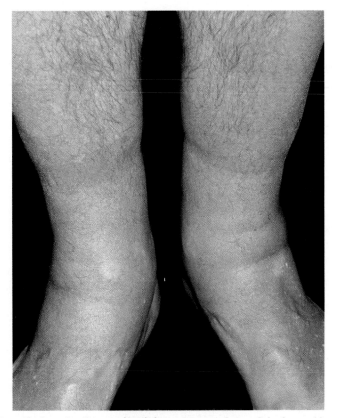

Figure 22-3 Drug-induced edema: nifedipine *Pitting edema of the leg, ankle, and foot (note pitting caused by the stocking elastic) occurred following increased dosing of nifedipine, due to increased vascular permeability.*

Course and Prognosis

Drug-induced urticaria/angioedema usually resolves within hours to days to weeks after the causative drug is withdrawn.

Management

The offending drug should be identified and withdrawn as soon as possible.

Prevention

PREVIOUSLY SENSITIZED INDIVIDUALS   The patient should carry information listing drug sensitivities (wallet card, bracelet).

RADIOGRAPHIC CONTRAST MEDIA   Avoid use of contrast media known to have caused prior reaction. If not possible, pretreat patient with antihistamine and prednisone (1 mg/kg) 30 to 60 minutes prior to contrast media exposure.

Treatment of Acute Severe Urticaria/Anaphylaxis

EPINEPHRINE   (0.3 to 0.5 ml of a 1:1000 dilution) subcutaneously, repeating in 15 to 20 minutes. Maintain airway. Intravenous access.

Antihistamines H_1 blockers or H_2 blockers or combination

Systemic Corticosteroids

INTRAVENOUS   Hydrocortisone or methylprednisolone for severe symptoms

ORAL   Prednisone 70 mg, tapering by 10 or 5 mg daily over 1 to 2 weeks, is usually adequate.

DRUG HYPERSENSITIVITY SYNDROME

Hypersensitivity syndrome refers to a specific severe systemic idiosyncratic adverse drug reaction characterized by rash, fever, often with hepatitis, arthralgias, lymphadenopathy, or hematologic abnormalities.

Epidemiology and Etiology

Age Any age

Race Reactions to antiepileptic drugs may be higher in black individuals.

Etiology Antiepileptic drugs (phenytoin, carbamazepine, phenobarbital) and sulfonamides are the most frequent cause. Other drugs: allopurinol, gold salts, dapsone, sorbinil

History

Onset 2 to 6 weeks after drug is initially used, and later than most other serious skin reactions

Prodrome Fever, rash

Systems Review Fever

Physical Examination

Vital Signs ±Elevated temperature (drug fever)

Skin Lesions

TYPES Early: exanthematous eruption (Figure 22-4). May progress to generalized exfoliative dermatitis, especially if drug not discontinued. Scaling and/or desquamation may occur with healing.

COLOR Bright or *"drug" red.* Resolving lesions have hues of tan and purple.

ARRANGEMENT OF MULTIPLE LESIONS Randomly scattered macules and papules frequently become confluent.

DISTRIBUTION Symmetric. Almost always on trunk and extremities. Lesions may become confluent and generalized.

Mucous Membranes ±Oral exanthem

General Examination

LYMPH NODES Lymphadenopathy usually due to benign lymphoid hyperplasia.

OTHER Involvement of heart, lungs, thyroid, liver, brain also occurs

Differential Diagnosis

Early That of morbilliform eruptions. Can mimic early measles or rubella.

Later Serum sickness, drug-induced vasculitis, Henoch-Schönlein purpura, cryoglobulin-associated vasculitis, vasculitis associated with infection and collagen vascular diseases

Rash Plus Lymphadenopathy Rubella, primary EBV or CMV mononucleosis syndrome

Laboratory and Special Examinations

Hemogram Peripheral eosinophilia (30 % of cases). Mononucleosis-like atypical lymphocytes.

Chemistries Hepatitis

Histology

SKIN Perivascular lymphocytes and eosinophils

LYMPH NODES Benign lymphoid hyperplasia. Uncommonly, atypical lymphoid hyperplasia, pseudolymphoma.

KIDNEY Interstitial nephritis

Diagnosis

Clinical diagnosis confirmed by histology of organ(s) involved

Pathophysiology

Some patients have a genetically determined in-

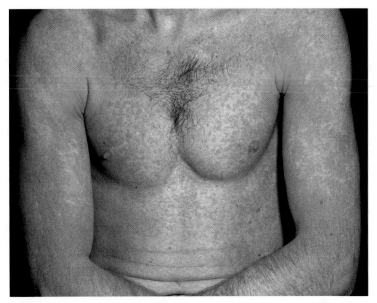

Figure 22-4 Drug hypersensitivity syndrome: phenytoin *Symmetrical, bright-red, exanthematous eruption, confluent in some sites; the patient had associated lymphadenopathy.*

ability to detoxify the toxic arene oxide metabolic products of anticonvulsant agents. Slow *N*-acetylation of sulfonamide and increased susceptibility of leukocytes to toxic hydroxylamine metabolites are associated with higher risk of hypersensitivity syndrome.

Course and Prognosis

Cutaneous reactions associated with anticonvulsant agents characterized by facial swelling, exfoliative dermatitis, and bullous or purpuric lesions and associated with fever, lymphadenopathy, eosinophilia, arthritis, and/or hepatitis, which begins >2 weeks after therapy is initiated and has a much higher risk of developing severe hypersensitivity syndrome. Rarely, patients die from systemic hypersensitivity such as with eosinophilic myocarditis.

Rash and hepatitis may persist for weeks after drug is discontinued. In patients treated with systemic corticosteroids, rash and hepatitis may recur as corticosteroids are tapered. Lymphadenopathy usually resolves when drug is withdrawn; however, rare progression to lymphoma has been reported.

Management

Identify and discontinue the offending drug.

Symptomatic Treatment Oral antihistamine to alleviate pruritus

Corticosteroids

TOPICAL CORTICOSTEROIDS High-potency topical corticosteroids applied b.i.d. are usually helpful in relieving cutaneous symptoms of pruritus but do not alter systemic hypersensitivity.

SYSTEMIC CORTICOSTEROIDS Prednisone (≥0.5 mg/kg/day) usually results in rapid improvement of symptoms and laboratory parameters.

Future Drug Therapy Cross-sensitivity between various aromatic antiepileptic drugs occurs, making it difficult to select alternative anticonvulsant therapy.

Prevention The individual must be aware of his or her specific drug hypersensitivity and that other drugs of the same class can crossreact. These drugs must never be readministered. Patient should wear a medical alert bracelet.

FIXED DRUG ERUPTION

A fixed drug eruption (FDE) is an adverse cutaneous reaction to an ingested drug, characterized by the formation of a solitary, but at times multiple, plaque, bulla, or erosion; if the patient is rechallenged with the offending drug, the FDE occurs repeatedly at the identical skin site (i.e., fixed) within hours of ingestion.

Epidemiology and Etiology

Age Rare in children

Etiology

Drugs most commonly implicated:

  Phenolphthalein
  Antimicrobial agents
    Tetracyclines (tetracycline, minocycline)
    Sulfonamides, including "nonabsorbable" drugs; crossreactions with antidiabetic and diuretic sulfa drug may occur.
    Metronidazole
    Nystatin
  Anti-inflammatory agents
    Salicylates
    NSAIDs
    Phenylbutazone
    Phenacetin
  Psychoactive agents
    Barbiturates, including Fiorinal
    Quaalude, Doriden
  Oral contraceptives
  Quinine (including quinine in tonic water), quinidine.
  Many other commonly used drugs also have been reported to cause FDE.

Food: peas, beans, lentils have been implicated.
Food coloring: in food or medications

History

Drug History Patients frequently give a history of identical lesion(s) occurring at the identical location. FDEs may be associated with a headache for which the patient takes a barbiturate containing analgesic, with constipation for which the patient takes a phenolphthalein-containing laxative, or with a cold for which the patient takes an over-the-counter medication containing a yellow dye. The offending "drug" in food dye-induced FDE may be difficult to identify, i.e., yellow dye in Galliano liqueur or phenolphthalein in maraschino cherries; quinine in tonic water.

Skin Symptoms Usually asymptomatic. May be pruritic or burning. Painful when eroded. Patients note a residual area of postinflammatory hyperpigmentation between attacks.

Time to Onset of Lesion(s) Occur from 30 minutes to 8 hours after ingestion of drug in previously sensitized individual.

Duration of Lesion(s) Lesions persist if drug is continued. Resolve days to few weeks after drug is discontinued.

Physical Examination

Skin Lesions

TYPE The characteristic early lesion is a sharply demarcated macule (Figure 22-5), round or oval in shape, occurring within hours after ingestion of the offending drug. Most commonly, lesions are solitary (Figure 22-6), but they may be multiple (Figure 22-7). Size varies from a few millimeters up to 10 to 20 cm in diameter. Within a few hours the lesion becomes edematous, thus forming a plaque, which may evolve to become a bulla and then an erosion.

COLOR Initially, erythema, then dusky red to violaceous. After healing, dark brown with violet hue postinflammatory hyperpigmentation.

PALPATION Eroded lesions, especially on genital or oral mucosa, are quite painful (Figures 22-5 and 22-6).

ARRANGEMENT Single lesions most common.

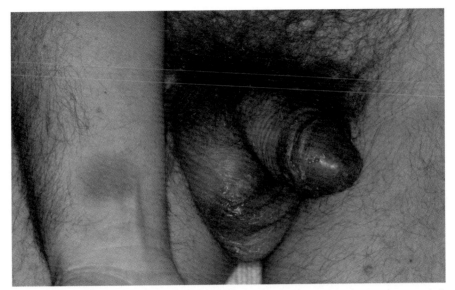

Figure 22-5 Fixed drug eruption: phenolphthalein *A violet plaque on the wrist, eroded plaques on the glans penis and scrotum, associated with extensive intraoral erosions. This was the fourth such episode and followed ingestion of a phenolphthalein-containing laxative.*

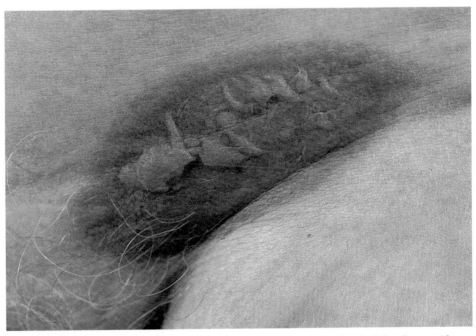

Figure 22-6 Fixed drug eruption: phenylbutazone *A large, oval, red-violet plaque with central bulla formation on the lower abdomen and inguinal region.*

When multiple, random. A great number of lesions may simulate toxic epidermal necrolysis (Figure 22-7).

DISTRIBUTION The genital skin is the most commonly involved site, but any site may be involved. Face: perioral, periorbital.

Mucous Membranes FDEs may occur within the mouth or on the conjunctivae. May simulate herpes simplex, conjunctivitis, or urethritis.

Differential Diagnosis

Solitary Genital Erosion Recurrent herpetic lesion

Multiple Erosions Stevens-Johnson syndrome, toxic epidermal necrolysis

Oral Erosion(s) Aphthous stomatitis, primary herpetic gingivostomatitis, erythema multiforme

Laboratory and Special Examinations

Patch Test The suspected drug can be placed as a patch test at a previously involved site; an inflammatory response occurs in 30 % of cases.

Dermatopathology Similar to findings in erythema multiforme: individual keratinocyte necrosis, basal vacuolization, dermal edema, perivascular and interstitial lymphohistiocytic infiltrate, at times with eosinophils. Subepidermal vesicles and bullae with overlying epidermal necrosis. Between outbreaks, the site of FDE shows marked pigmentary incontinence with melanin in macrophages in upper dermis.

Diagnosis

Made on clinical grounds. Readministration of the drug confirms diagnosis but should be avoided.

Pathogenesis

Unknown

Course and Prognosis

FDE resolves within a few weeks of withdrawing the drug. Recurs within hours following ingestion of a single dose of the drug.

Management

Treatment of Lesion(s) Identify and withhold the offending drug. A newly erupted lesion of FDE presents as an inflammatory plaque, with or without erosion. Noneroded lesions can be treated with a potent topical corticosteroid ointment. Eroded cutaneous lesions can be treated with bacitracin or Silvadene ointment and a dressing until the site is reepithelialized. Postinflammatory hyperpigmentation (dermal melanin) may persist at the site of an FDE for months or years and does not respond to hydroquinone therapy.

Prevention Identify and withhold the offending drug. Various types of sulfa drugs may crossreact.

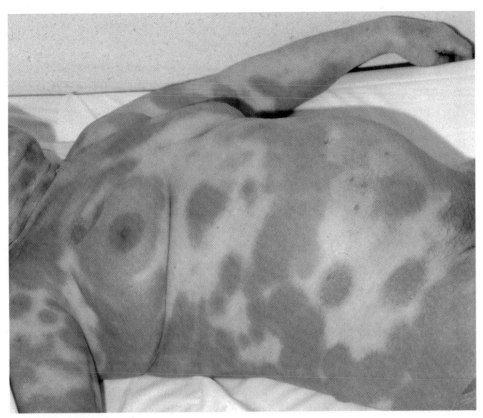

Figure 22-7 Generalized fixed drug eruption: tetracycline *Multiple, confluent, violaceous-red, oval erythematous areas, some of which later became bullous. The eruption may be difficult to distinguish from toxic epidermal necrolysis.*

STEVENS-JOHNSON SYNDROME AND TOXIC EPIDERMAL NECROLYSIS

Stevens-Johnson syndrome (SJS) and toxic epidermal necrolysis (TEN) are mucocutaneous drug-induced or idiopathic reaction patterns characterized by skin tenderness and erythema of skin and mucosa, followed by extensive cutaneous and mucosal exfoliation, and are potentially life-threatening due to multisystem involvement.
Synonym: TEN: Lyell's syndrome.

Epidemiology and Etiology

Age Any age, but most common in adults >40 years

Sex Equal incidence

Incidence *TEN:* 0.4 to 1.2 per million person-years. *SJS:* 1.2 to 6 per million person-years

Risk Factors Systemic lupus erythematosus, HLA-B12, HIV disease

Etiology *TEN:* 80 % of cases have strong association with specific medication; <5 % of patients report no drug use. Also: chemicals, *Mycoplasma* pneumonia, viral infections, immunization. *SJS:* 50 % are associated with drug exposure; etiology often not clear-cut.

DRUGS MOST FREQUENTLY IMPLICATED Sulfa drugs (sulfadoxine, sulfadiazine, sulfasalazine, cotrimazole), allopurinol, hydantoins, carbamazepine, phenylbutazone, piroxicam, chlormezanone, amithiozone, amino-penicillins

DRUGS ALSO IMPLICATED Cephalosporins, fluoroquinolones, vancomycin, rifampin, ethambutol, fenbufen, tonoxicam, tiaprofenic acid, diclofenac, sulindac, ibuprofen, ketoprofen, naproxen, thiabendazole

Definition of SJS and TEN Not clearly defined. SJS is considered by most a maximal variant of erythema multiforme (major) and TEN a maximal variant of SJS. Both can start with target-like lesions; however, about 50 % of TEN do not, and in these the condition evolves from diffuse erythema and immediate necrosis and detachment.

SJS <10 % epidermal detachment

SJS/TEN OVERLAP 10 % to 30 % epidermal detachment

TEN >30 % epidermal detachment

History

Time from First Drug Exposure to Onset of Symptoms 1 to 3 weeks. Occurs more rapidly with rechallenge

Prodrome Fever, influenza-like symptoms 1 to 3 days prior to mucocutaneous lesions. Mild to moderate skin tenderness, conjunctival burning or itching

Skin Symptoms Skin pain, burning sensation, tenderness, paresthesia.

Mucous Membrane Symptoms Mouth lesions are painful, tender.

General Symptoms Impaired alimentation, photophobia, painful micturition, anxiety

Drug Ingestion Occurs after days of ingestion of the drug; newly added drug is most suspect.

Physical Examination

Skin Lesions

TYPES *Prodromal Rash* Morbilliform, erythema multiforme-like; diffuse erythema
  Early Necrotic epidermis first appears as macular areas (Figures 22-8 and 22-9) with crinkled surface that enlarge and coalesce.
  Later Sheet-like loss of epidermis. Raised flaccid blisters (Figures 22-8 and 22-9) that spread with lateral pressure (Nikolsky's sign) on erythematous areas. With trauma, full-thickness epidermal detach-

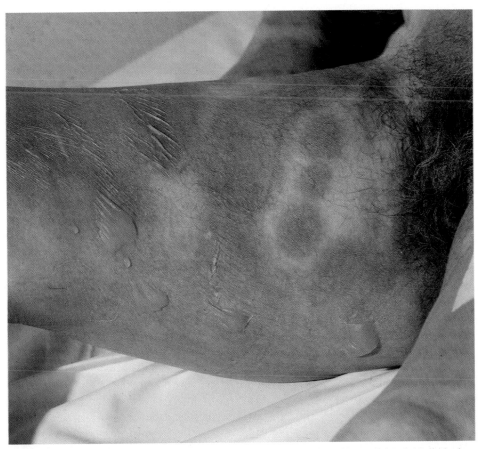

Figure 22-8 Stevens-Johnson syndrome *Generalized eruption of lesions that initially had a target-like appearance but then became confluent, brightly erythematous, and bullous. The patient had extensive mucous membrane involvement and tracheobronchitis.*

ment yields exposed, red, oozing dermis (Figure 22-10).

Recovery Regrowth of epidermis begins within days; completed in 3 weeks. Pressure points and periorificial sites exhibit delayed healing. Skin that is not denuded acutely is shed in sheets, especially palms/soles. Nails may shed.

COLOR Very early lesions pink-red (Figure 22-9). Later, dusky cyanotic (Figure 22-8). Red and glistening following epidermal sloughing (Figure 22-10).

PALPATION Even early lesions are tender.

DISTRIBUTION Initial erythema on face, extremities, becoming confluent over a few hours or days. Epidermal sloughing may be generalized, resulting in large denuded areas, resembling a second-degree thermal burn. Denudation most pronounced over pressure points. Scalp, palms, soles may be less severely involved or spared. *SJS:* widely distributed with prominent involvement of trunk and face. TEN: generalized, universal (Figure 22-10)

Mucous Membranes 90 % of patients have mucosal lesions, i.e., erythema, painful erosions: lips, buccal mucosa, conjunctiva, genital and anal skin.

EYES 85 % have conjunctival lesions: hyperemia, pseudomembrane formation; synechiae between eyelids and conjunctiva; keratitis, corneal erosions.

SEQUELAE *Skin* Scarring, irregular pigmentation, eruptive nevomelanocytic nevi, abnormal regrowth of nails
Eyes Common, including Sjögren-like sicca syndrome with deficiency of mucin in tears; entropion, trichiasis squamous metaplasia, neovascularization of conjunctiva and cornea; symblepharon, punctate keratitis, corneal scarring; persistent photophobia, burning eyes, visual impairment, blindness
Anogenitalia Phimosis, vaginal synechiae

General Findings Fever usually higher in TEN (>38°C) than in SJS. Usually mentally alert. In distress due to severe pain. Tubular necrosis. Acute renal failure; erosions in lower respiratory tract, gut. Epithelial erosions of trachea, bronchi, GI tract.

Differential Diagnosis

Early Exanthematous or pustular drug eruptions, erythema multiforme (EM) major, scarlet fever, phototoxic eruptions, toxic shock syndrome, graft-versus-host disease (GVHD)

Fully Evolved EM major (see typical target lesions, predominantly on extremities), GVHD (may mimic TEN; less mucosal involvement), thermal burns, phototoxic reactions, staphylococcal scalded-skin syndrome (in young children, rare in adults), generalized bullous fixed drug eruption, exfoliative dermatitis

Laboratory and Special Examinations

Hematology Anemia, lymphopenia; eosinophilia uncommon. Neutropenia correlates with poor prognosis.

Dermatopathology

EARLY Vacuolization/necrosis of basal keratinocytes and individual cell necrosis throughout the epidermis

LATE Full-thickness epidermal necrosis and detachment with formation of subepidermal split above basement membrane. Little or no inflammatory infiltrate in dermis. Immunofluorescence studies unremarkable, ruling out other blistering disorders.

Diagnosis

Clinical findings confirmed by biopsy

Pathophysiology

Pathogenesis unknown but consistent with immunologic mechanisms, i.e., cell-mediated cytotoxic reaction against epidermal cells. Epidermis infiltrated by activated lymphocytes, mainly CD8 cells, and macrophages. Cytokines produced by activated mononuclear cells and keratinocytes probably contribute to local cell death, fever, and malaise.

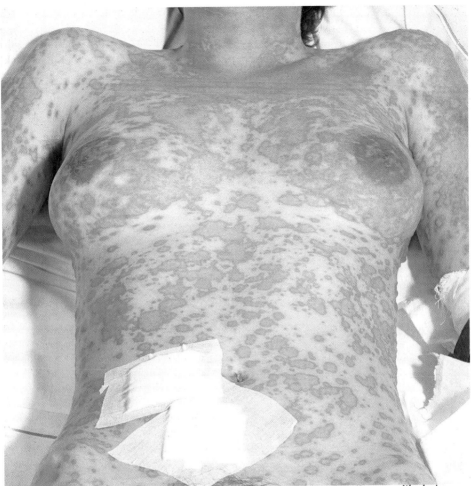

Figure 22-9 Toxic epidermal necrolysis *Generalized rash of originally target-like lesions which coalesced and became vesicular and eventually eroded note bullous lesions in sternoclavicular region; oral conjunctival, nasal, and vulvar erosions were also present and there was shedding of cilia and nails.*

Course and Prognosis

Average duration of progression is <4 days. Course similar to that of extensive thermal burns. Prognosis related to extent of skin necrosis. Transcutaneous fluid loss large and varies with area of denudation; associated electrolyte abnormalities. Prerenal azotemia common. Bacterial colonization common, and associated with sepsis. Other complications include hypermetabolic state and diffuse interstitial pneumonitis. Mortality rate for TEN 30 %, mainly in elderly; for SJS, <5 %. Mortality related to sepsis, GI hemorrhage, fluid/electrolyte imbalance.

If the patient survives the first episode of SJS or TEN, reexposure to the causative drug may be followed by recurrence within hours to days, more severe than the initial episode.

Management

Acute SJS/TEN

- Early diagnosis and withdrawal of suspected drug(s) are very important.
- Patients are best cared for in a burn or intensive care unit.
- Manage replacement of IV fluids and electrolytes as for patient with a third-degree thermal burn.
- Systemic corticosteroids are probably *not* helpful in reducing morbidity or mortality but this has not been proven. Some claim beneficial effects particularly if corticosteroids are given in high doses and early.
- Pentoxiphyllin IV by continuous drip early on in the eruption has been anecdotally reported to be beneficial.
- Conjunctival erythromycin ointment
- Suction frequently with oropharyngeal involvement to prevent aspiration pneumonitis.
- Debride only frankly necrotic skin.
- Diagnose and treat complicating infections, including sepsis (fever, hypotension, change in mental status).

Prevention The patient must be aware of the likely offending drug and that other drugs of the same class can crossreact. These drugs must never be readministered. Patient should wear a medical alert bracelet.

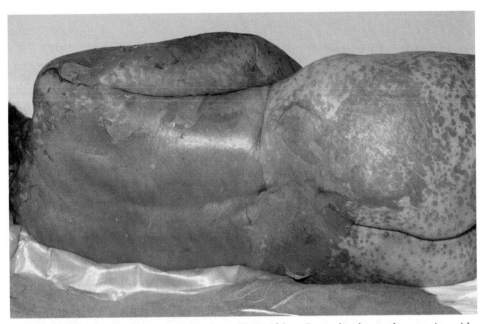

Figure 22-10 Toxic epidermal necrolysis: sulfonamide *Generalized, macular eruption with some target-like lesions which rapidly developed epidermal necrosis, positive Nikolsky's sign, bulla formation, and denuded erosive areas.*

DRUG-INDUCED PIGMENTATION

Drug-induced alterations in pigmentation are relatively common, resulting from a variety of endogenous and exogenous pigments, and can be of significant cosmetic concern to the patient.

Etiology

The following drugs are capable of inducing hyperpigmentation of skin and/or mucosa:

Antiarrhythmic: amiodarone

Antimalarials: chloroquine, quinacrine, quinine

Antimicrobial: minocycline, clofazimine, zidovudine

Antiseizure: hydantoins

Cytostatic: bleomycin, cyclophosphamide, doxorubicin, daunorubicin, busulfan, 5-fluorouracil, dactinomycin

Heavy metals: silver, gold, mercury

Hormones: adrenocorticotropic hormone (ACTH), estrogen/progesterone

Psychiatric: chlorpromazine

Pathogenesis

Increase in melanin: ACTH, phenytoin, estrogen/progesterone

Increase in hemosiderin: minocycline

Increase in exogenous pigment: minocycline (metabolite of minocycline)

Physical Examination

Skin Findings

AMIODARONE *Incidence* >75 % of patients after 40-g cumulative dose after >4 months of therapy. More common in skin phototypes I and II.

Pigment Lipofuscin type pigment deposited in macrophages and endothelial cells

Mechanism A low-grade or minimal photosensitivity; limited to the light-exposed areas in a small number (8 %) of patients.

Discoloration Dusky-red erythema and, later, blue-gray dermal melanosis (ceru-loderma) (Figure 22-11) in exposed areas (face and hands); "phototoxic" type erythema (rare).

Other Side Effects Pulmonary fibrosis, pneumonitis, hepatotoxicity, thyroid disturbances, neuropathy, and myopathy

Course The low-grade photosensitivity disappears in 12 to 24 months after the drug is discontinued. The long period results from the gradual elimination of the photoactive drug from the lysosomal membranes. The pigmentation also disappeared after 33 months in one patient who was followed carefully.

MINOCYCLINE Onset delayed, usually after total dose of >50 g, but may occur after a small dose.

Pigment Not melanin but an iron-containing brown pigment, located in the dermal macrophages.

Discoloration Blue-gray or slate-gray pigmentation (Figure 22-12).

Arrangement Stippled or diffuse.

Distribution Extensor legs, ankles, dorsa of feet, face, especially around eyes; sites of trauma or inflammation such as acne scars, contusions, abrasions; hard palate, teeth; nails

Internal Sites Bones, cartilage, thyroid ("black thyroid")

Course Discoloration gradually disappears over a period of months after drug is discontinued.

CLOFAZIMINE *Discoloration* Reddish brown (range, pink to black)

Distribution Light-exposed areas; conjunctivae; accompanied by red sweat, urine, feces. Subcutaneous fat is orange.

ZIDOVUDINE *Discoloration* Brown

Distribution Brown macules on lips or oral mucosa; longitudinal brown bands in nails

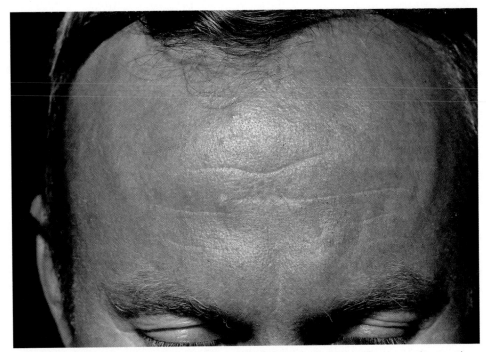

Figure 22-11 Drug-induced pigmentation: amiodarone *A striking slate-gray pigmentation in a photodistribution of the face. The blue color (ceruloderma) is due to the deposition of melanin and lipofuscin contained in macrophages and endothelial cells in the dermis. The pigmentation is reversible but it may take up to a year to complete resolution.*

ANTIMALARIALS [CHLOROQUINE, HYDROXY-CHLOROQUINE (PLAQUENIL), QUINACRINE (ATABRINE)] *Incidence* Occurs in 25 % of individuals who take the drug for >4 months.

Discoloration Brownish, gray-brown, and/ or blue-black, due to melanin, hemo-siderin, as well as quinacrine-containing complexes. *Quinacrine:* yellow, yellow-green

Distribution Over shins; face, nape of neck; hard palate (sharp line of demarca-tion at soft palate); under finger- and toe-nails; also may occur in cornea and retina. *Quinacrine:* skin and sclerae (resembling icterus); yellow-green fluorescence of nail bed with Wood's lamp

Course Discoloration disappears within a few months of discontinuing drug. *Quinacrine:* can fade after 2 to 6 months even though drug is continued

PHENYTOIN *Dose* High over a long period of time (>1 year)

Discoloration Spotty, resembling melasma, in light-exposed areas

Pigment Melanin

BLEOMYCIN *Mechanism* Unknown

Discoloration Tan to brown to black

Distribution Increase in epidermal melanin occurs at sites of minor inflammation, i.e., parallel linear streaks at sites of dermatographism induced by excoria-tion ("flagellate" pigmentation), most commonly on the back, elbows, small joints, nails.

CYCLOPHOSPHAMIDE (CYTOXAN) *Discoloration* Brown
Arrangement Diffuse or discrete macules
Distribution Elbows; palms with addisonian pigmentation and macules

BUSULFAN (MYLERAN) *Incidence* Occurs in 5 % of treated patients
Discoloration Addisonian-like pigmentation
Distribution Face, axillae, chest, abdomen, oral mucous membranes

ACTH *Discoloration* Addisonian pigmentation of skin and oral mucosa
Mechanism First 13 amino acids of ACTH are identical to alpha-melanocyte–stimulating hormone (MSH).

ESTROGENS/PROGESTERONE Caused by endogenous and exogenous estrogen combined with progesterone, i.e., during pregnancy or with oral contraceptive therapy. Sunlight causes marked darkening of pigmentation.
Discoloration Tan/brown (melasma or chloasma)
Distribution Face, especially forehead, cheeks, and perioral area; also occurs on linea alba, nipples/areolae, vulva.
Course Discoloration may persist despite discontinuation of drug (see page 589).

CHLORPROMAZINE AND OTHER PHENOTHIAZINES
Dose Occurs following long-term (>6 months), high-dose (>500 mg/day) therapy.
Mechanism Phototoxic reaction
Discoloration Slate-gray, blue-gray, or brownish

Distribution Areas exposed to light, i.e., chin and cheeks
Course After discontinuation of drug, discoloration usually fades slowly.

SILVER (ARGYRIA OR ARGYROSIS) *Source* Silver nitrate nose drops; silver sulfadiazine applied as an ointment (Silvadene)
Pigment Silver sulfide (silver nitrate is converted into silver sulfide by light, as in photographic film).
Discoloration Blue-gray
Site Primarily areas exposed to light, i.e., face, dorsa of hands, nails (see Figure 18-4), conjunctiva; also diffuse

GOLD (CHRYSIASIS) *Source* Organic colloidal gold preparations used in therapy of rheumatoid arthritis
Incidence 5 % to 25 % of all treated patients and is dose-dependent
Dose In high-dose therapy, appears in a short time; with lower dose, occurs after months
Discoloration Blue-gray to purple
Distribution Light-exposed areas; sclerae
Course Persists long after drug discontinued

IRON *Source* IM iron injections; multiple blood transfusions
Discoloration Brown or blue-gray
Distribution Generalized; also, local deposits at site of injection

CAROTENE *Source* Ingestion of large quantities of beta-carotene–containing vegetables; beta-carotene tablets (Lumitene)
Discoloration Yellow-orange
Distribution Most apparent on palms and soles

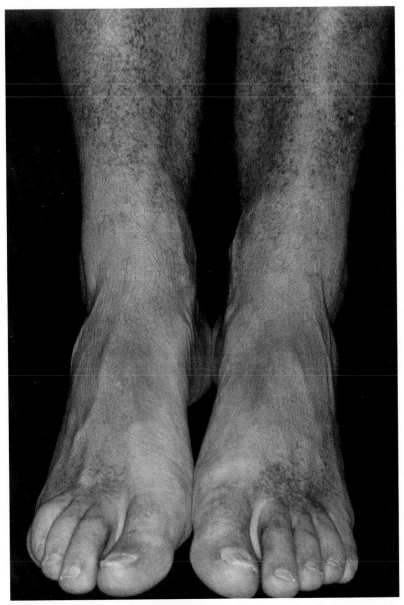

Figure 22-12 Drug-induced pigmentation: minocycline *Stippled, blue-gray macular pigmentation on the legs and dorsum of the feet occurs only after long-term drug ingestion. The brown pigment is iron-containing and is not melanin.*

NECROSIS FROM WARFARIN

Skin necrosis from warfarin is a rare reaction usually occurring between the third and fifth days of anticoagulation therapy with the warfarin derivatives, manifested by sharply demarcated, purpuric cutaneous infarction.

Epidemiology and Etiology

Incidence 1 in 10,000 warfarin-treated individuals

Age Middle-aged to elderly

Sex Females >> males, especially if obese

Etiology Warfarin derivatives, indandione compounds

Risk Factors Higher initial dosing, obesity, female sex. Individuals with hereditary deficiency of protein C, a natural anticoagulant protein, are at highest risk. Also, protein S or antithrombin III deficiency.

History

Lag Time Reaction appears within 3 to 5 days after initiation of warfarin therapy.

Systems Review Indications for warfarin use: history of venous thrombosis, atrial fibrillation ± embolization, prophylaxis and treatment of pulmonary embolism

Physical Examination

Skin Lesions

TYPES Lesions vary with severity of reaction: petechiae to ecchymoses to hemorrhagic infarcts to extensive necrosis. *Early:* large indurated dermal plaque(s). *Later:* quickly evolve to well-demarcated, deep purple to black, geographic areas of necrosis (Figure 22-13). Hemorrhagic bullae, large erosions may complicate infarcts. Later, deep tissue sloughing and ulceration if lesions are not debrided and grafted.

COLOR *Early:* red. *Later:* violaceous to near-black.

PALPATION Lesions are quite tender and *painful.*

SHAPE OF INDIVIDUAL LESION Usually geographic

ARRANGEMENT OF MULTIPLE LESIONS Often single. Many present as two lesions, one on either breast.

DISTRIBUTION Areas of abundant subcutaneous fat: breasts, buttocks, abdomen, thighs, calves. Acral areas are spared.

General Examination Findings for indications for warfarin administration. Obesity. Otherwise, unremarkable.

Differential Diagnosis

Cutaneous Necrosis Purpura fulminans (disseminated intravascular coagulation), hematoma/ecchymosis in overly anticoagulated patient, necrotizing soft tissue infection, vasculitis, rare necrosis after vasopressin treatment, brown recluse spider bite.

Heparin Necrosis Associated with vessel thrombosis and fibrin injection (Figure 22-14), at distal skin sites, and in other organs. Coagulation studies: levels of fibrinogen and fibrin split products usually normal, platelet counts often depressed

Laboratory and Special Examinations

Dermatopathology Epidermal necrosis, thrombosis and occlusion of most blood vessels, scanty inflammatory response

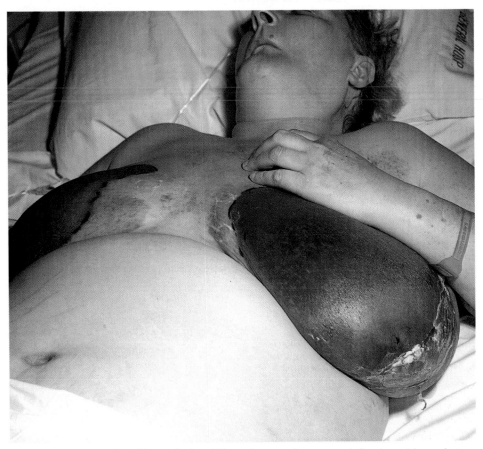

Figure 22-13 Necrosis with warfarin *Bilateral areas of cutaneous infarction with purple-to-black coloration of the breast surrounded by an area of erythema, occurred on the fifth day of warfarin therapy.*

Coagulation Studies Usually within normal limits. May be associated with hereditary or acquired protein C deficiency.

Diagnosis

Clinical diagnosis

Pathogenesis

Idiosyncratic reaction. In individuals with hereditary deficiency of protein C, a natural anticoagulant protein, warfarin greatly depresses protein C levels before decreasing other vitamin K-dependent coagulation factors, inducing a transient hypercoagulable state and thrombus formation.

Course and Prognosis

Depending on severity of reaction, lesions may subside, heal by granulation, or require surgical intervention. If area of necrosis is large in an elderly, debilitated patient, may be life-threatening. If warfarin is inadvertently readministered, reaction recurs.

Management

Early Management Early diagnosis is key.

- Warfarin should be discontinued.
- Administer vitamin K to reverse the effect of warfarin.
- Substitute heparin as an anticoagulant.
- Administer monoclonal antibody-purified protein C concentrate to protein C-deficient patients.

Later Management

- Treat necrotic tissue as a third-degree burn.
- Debride necrotic tissue.
- Graft debrided site.

Prevention The patient should be aware that the reaction will recur whenever warfarin or its derivatives are readministered. Wearing a medical alert bracelet is advised.

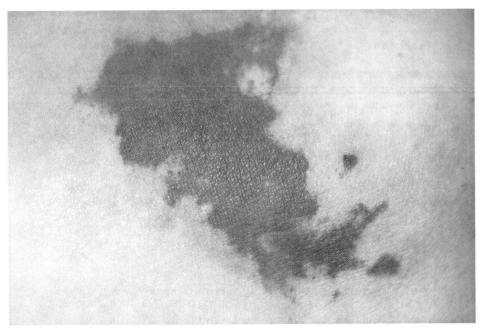

Figure 22-14 Heparin necrosis *An irregularly configured but sharply defined area of hemorrhagic infarction at the site of heparin administration.*

CUTANEOUS BACTERIAL INFECTIONS

IMPETIGO AND ECTHYMA

Staphylococcus aureus and *Streptococcus pyogenes* are capable of causing superficial infections involving the epidermis (impetigo) or extending into the dermis (ecthyma), characterized by crusted erosions or ulcers. The infections may arise as primary infections in minor superficial breaks in the skin or as secondary infections of preexisting dermatoses (impetiginization or secondary infection).

Epidemiology and Etiology

Etiology In the 1990s, *S. aureus* most commonly; also, group A beta-hemolytic *Streptococcus pyogenes* (GAS); or mixed *S. aureus* and GAS. Bullous impetigo: 80 % caused by phage 2 staphylococci (60 % of these of type 71), which produce exotoxins and which also cause staphylococcal scalded-skin syndrome.

Age Primary infections more common in children. Secondary infections, any age. Bullous impetigo: children, young adults.

Incidence Impetigo accounts for 10 % of skin problems in general dermatology clinics.

Predisposing Factors Colonization of the skin by *S. aureus* and GAS is promoted by warm ambient temperature, high humidity, presence of skin disease (especially atopic dermatitis), age of patient, prior antibiotic therapy, poor hygiene, crowded living conditions, and neglected minor trauma. Topical corticosteroids have little effect on the microflora of the skin, except in those with atopic dermatitis; topical corticosteroids applied to atopic dermatitis usually reduce the density of *S. aureus*. Impetiginization or secondary infection also occurs in lesions of eczema and scabies. Ecthyma: lesion of neglect—develops in excoriations; insect bites; minor trauma in diabetics, elderly patients, soldiers, and alcoholics.

Portal of Entry

PRIMARY IMPETIGO Arises at minor breaks in the skin

SECONDARY IMPETIGINIZATION Arises in a variety of underlying dermatoses and traumatic breaks in the integrity of the epidermis: *Underlying Dermatoses*

- Inflammatory dermatoses: atopic dermatitis, contact dermatitis, stasis dermatitis, psori-

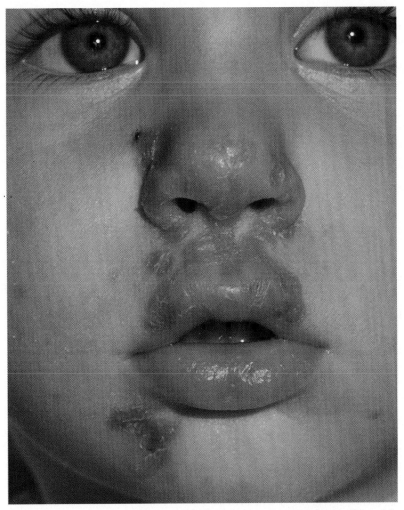

Figure 23-1 Impetigo: Group A beta-hemolytic *Streptococcus pyogenes* *Crusted (golden-yellow, stuck-on) erosions becoming confluent on the nose, cheek, lips, and chin; clinical lesions are preceded by nasal colonization with* S. aureus.

asis vulgaris, chronic cutaneous lupus erythematosus, pyoderma gangrenosum
- Bullous disease: pemphigus vulgaris, bullous pemphigoid, sunburn, porphyria cutanea tarda
- Ulcers: pressure, stasis
- Chronic lymphedema
- Umbilical stump
- Herpes simplex, varicella, herpes zoster
- Dermatophytosis: tinea pedis, tinea capitis

Trauma

- Abrasion
- Laceration
- Puncture
- Bites: human, animal, insect
- Burns

History

Duration of Lesions Impetigo: days to weeks. Ecthyma: weeks to months.

Symptoms Impetigo: variable pruritus, especially associated with atopic dermatitis. Ecthyma: pain, tenderness.

Physical Examination

Skin Lesions

TYPE *Nonbullous Impetigo* Transient superficial small *vesicles* or *pustules,* rupture resulting in *erosions,* which in turn become surmounted by a *crust* (Figure 23-1)
  Bullous Impetigo *Vesicles* (Figure 23-2) and *bullae* (Figure 23-3) containing clear yellow or slightly turbid fluid without surrounding erythema, arising on normal-appearing skin. With rupture, bullous lesions decompress. If roof of bulla is removed, shallow moist *erosion* forms.
  Ecthyma *Ulceration* with a thick adherent *crust* (Figure 23-4)

COLOR Nonbullous impetigo: golden-yellow crust (Figure 23-1); bullous impetigo: gray to brownish, hemorrhagic crusts; at times, an erythematous halo. Ecthyma: hemorrhagic crust.

SIZE AND SHAPE 1.0 to 3.0 cm; round or oval;

central healing. Ecthyma: larger lesions; round or oval. (Figure 23-4).

PALPATION Ecthyma: may be tender, indurated

ARRANGEMENT Scattered, discrete lesions; some large, confluent lesions; satellite lesions occur by autoinoculation.

DISTRIBUTION Face, arms, legs, buttocks. Bullous impetigo: trunk, face, hands, intertriginous sites. Ecthyma: ankles, dorsa of feet, thighs, buttocks.

Miscellaneous Physical Findings At times, regional lymphadenopathy

Differential Diagnosis

Nonbullous Impetigo Excoriation, perioral dermatitis, seborrheic dermatitis, allergic contact dermatitis, herpes simplex, dermatophytosis (tinea facialis, tinea corporis, tinea capitis), scabies

Bullous Impetigo Allergic contact dermatitis, herpes simplex, herpes zoster, bacterial folliculitis, thermal burns, bullous pemphigoid, dermatitis herpetiformis

Ecthyma Chronic herpetic ulcers, excoriated insect bites, neurotic excoriations, cutaneous diphtheria, porphyria cutanea tarda (dorsa of hands), venous (stasis) and atherosclerotic ulcers (legs).

Laboratory and Special Examinations

Gram's Stain Gram-positive cocci, in chains or clusters, within neutrophils

Culture *S. aureus,* commonly; GAS (especially from older lesions). Failure of oral antibiotic may be indication of infection by methicillin-resistant *S. aureus* (MRSA).

Hematology ±Leukocytosis

Serology Anti-DNAse beta detects prior GAS infection.

Dermatopathology Impetigo: vesicle formation in the subcorneal or granular region,

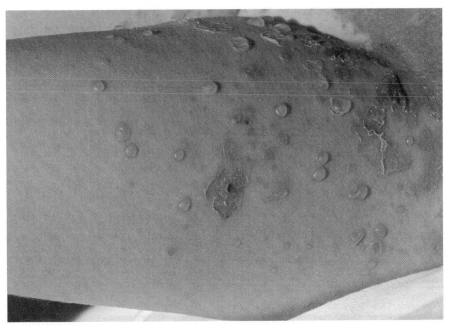

Figure 23-2 Bullous impetigo: S. aureus *Scattered, discrete, thin-walled vesicles and bullae that easily rupture and form erosions.*

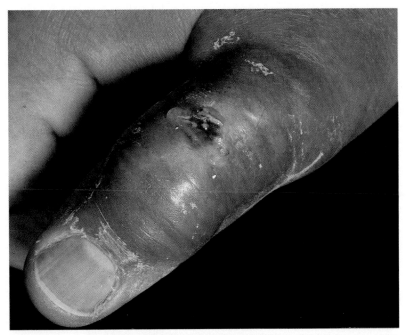

Figure 23-3 Bullous impetigo: S. aureus *A large, single bulla with surrounding erythema and edema on the thumb of a child; the bulla has ruptured and clear serum exudes from it.*

acantholytic cells, spongiosis, dermal perivascular infiltrate of lymphocytes and neutrophils; gram-positive cocci in blister fluid and within neutrophils

Diagnosis

Clinical findings, at times confirmed by Gram's stain or culture

Pathogenesis

Between 20 % and 40 % of normal adults are persistent nasal carriers of S. aureus; 20 % of adults are colonized on the perineum or axillae. S. aureus can be isolated from 90 % of individuals with atopic dermatitis in involved skin and 70 % from nonlesional skin. GAS usually colonizes the skin first and subsequently the nasopharynx. An intact stratum corneum is the most important defense against invasion of pathogenic bacteria. Teichoic acid moieties on S. aureus and GABHS bind to fibronectin receptors on nonintact epidermis.

Course and Prognosis

Untreated, lesions progress for several weeks, in some cases forming ecthyma; the latter usually occurs with poor hygiene (e.g., in the homeless, under boots of soldiers in maneuvers); in most cases, spontaneous resolution. With adequate treatment, prompt resolution. Lesions can progress to invasive infection with lymphangitis, suppurative lymphadenitis, cellulitis or erysipelas, bacteremia, septicemia. Nonsuppurative complications of GAS infection include guttate psoriasis, scarlet fever, and glomerulonephritis. Recurrence may occur because of failure to eradicate organism or reinfection from a family member. Ecthyma often heals with scar.

Management

Prevention Benzoyl peroxide wash (soap bar). Check family members for signs of impetigo. Between 20 % and 25 % of individuals are nasal carriers of S. aureus.

Topical Treatment Mupirocin (pseudomonic acid) ointment is a topical antibiotic preparation, highly effective in eliminating both GAS and S. aureus, including MRSA. Apply three times daily to involved skin and to nares for 7 to 10 days.

Systemic Treatment

GAS

> Penicillin VK: 250 mg q.i.d. for 10 days. If compliance is a problem, benzathine penicillin 600,000 units IM in children 6 years or younger, 1.2 million units if 7 years or older.
> Erythromycin: 250 to 500 mg (adults) q.i.d. for 10 days
> Cephalexin: 250 to 500 mg (adults) q.i.d. for 10 days

S. AUREUS

> Dicloxacillin: 250 to 500 mg (adults) q.i.d. for 10 days
> Cephalexin: 250 to 500 mg (adults) q.i.d. for 10 days; 40 to 50 mg/kg/day (children) for 10 days
> Amoxicillin plus clavulanic acid (beta-lactamase inhibitor): 20 mg/kg/day given t.i.d. for 10 days
> Macrolides (for penicillin-allergic individuals): If S. aureus is sensitive:
>
>> Erythromycin ethylsuccinate: 1 to 2 g/day (adults) in four divided doses for 10 days; 40 mg/kg/day (children) q.i.d. for 10 days
>> Clarithromycin: 250 to 500 mg b.i.d. for 10 days
>> Azithromycin: 250 mg q.d. for 5 to 7 days
>
> Clindamycin: 150 to 300 mg (adults) q.i.d. for 10 days; 15 mg/kg/day (children) q.i.d. for 10 days

Methicillin-Resistant S. aureus

Mupirocin ointment
Minocycline: 100 mg b.i.d. for 10 days
Trimethoprim-sulfamethoxazole: 160 mg TMPS + 800 mg SMZ b.i.d.
Ciprofloxacin: 500 mg b.i.d. for 7 days

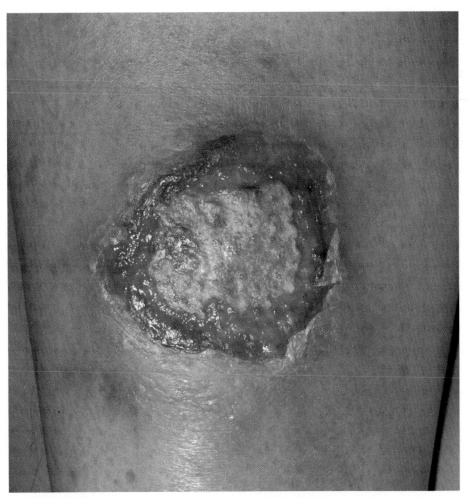

Figure 23-4 Ecthyma *A large, circumscribed ulcer with a necrotic base and surrounding erythema in the pretibial region.*

ABSCESS, FURUNCLE, AND CARBUNCLE

An *abscess* is a circumscribed collection of pus appearing as an acute or chronic localized infection and associated with tissue destruction. A *furuncle* is an acute, deep-seated, red, hot, tender nodule or abscess that evolves from a staphylococcal folliculitis. A *carbuncle* is a deeper infection comprised of interconnecting abscesses usually arising in several contiguous hair follicles.

Epidemiology and Etiology

Age   Children, adolescents, and young adults

Sex   More common in boys

Etiology   *Staphylococcus aureus.* Much less commonly, other organisms. Abscesses can be sterile, a response to a foreign body, such as a ruptured inclusion cyst. Dental abscesses can point anywhere on the face, even at sites distant from their origin. Sterile or infected abscesses can occur at injection sites.

Predisposing Factors   Chronic staphylococcal carrier state in nares, axillae, perineum, or bowel. Diabetes, obesity, poor hygiene, bactericidal defects (e.g., in chronic granulomatosis), defects in chemotaxis, and hyper-IgE syndrome (Job's syndrome)

Pathogenesis

Folliculitis, furuncles, and carbuncles represent a continuum of severity of staphylococcal infection. These cutaneous infections arise in chronic *S. aureus* carriers. Control/eradication of carrier state treats/prevents folliculitis, furuncle, and carbuncle formation.

History

Duration of Lesions   Days

Skin Symptoms   Throbbing pain and invariably exquisite tenderness

Constitutional Symptoms   Carbuncles may be accompanied by low-grade fever and malaise.

Physical Examination

Skin Lesions

TYPE   *Abscess*   May arise in any organ or structure. Abscesses that present on the skin arise in the dermis (Figure 23-5), subcutaneous fat, muscle, or a variety of deeper structures. Initially, a tender nodule forms. In time (days to weeks), pus collects within a central space (Figure 23-6). A well-formed abscess is characterized by fluctuance of the central portion of the lesion.

Furuncle   Initially, a firm tender nodule, up to 1 to 2 cm in diameter (Figure 23-7) with a central necrotic plug. In many individuals, furuncles occur in setting of staphylococcal folliculitis in beard area or neck. Nodule becomes fluctuant with abscess formation below necrotic plug often topped by a central pustule. Following rupture or drainage of pustule and discharge of necrotic plug, a nodule with cavitation remains. A variable zone of cellulitis may surround the furuncle.

Carbuncle   Evolution is similar to that of furuncle. Comprised of several to multiple, adjacent, coalescing furuncles (Figure 23-8). Characterized by multiple loculated dermal and subcutaneous abscesses, superficial pustules, necrotic plugs, and sieve-like openings draining pus

COLOR   Bright red

PALPATION   Indurated, very painful

SHAPE   Round

ARRANGEMENT   Single or grouped

DISTRIBUTION   Isolated single lesions or a few multiple lesions

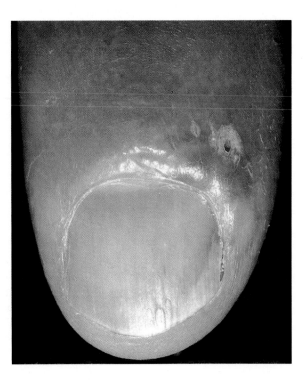

Figure 23-5 Abscess: S. aureus paronychia *A very tender paronychial abscess with surrounding cellulitis on the distal phalanx; an epidermal defect is present, the probable portal of entry.*

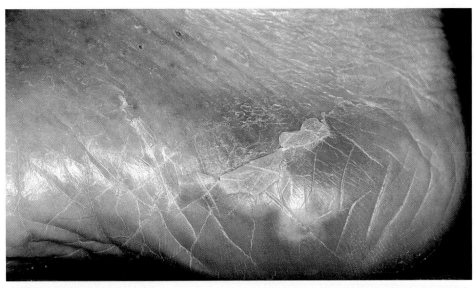

Figure 23-6 Abscess: S. aureus *A very tender abscess with surrounding erythema on the heel. The patient was a diabetic with neuropathy, and had a sewing needle lodge in the soft tissue, which had provided the portal of entry.*

SITES OF PREDILECTION *Abscesses* Any cutaneous region. At sites of puncture wounds (Figure 23-6). Upper trunk for abscesses in ruptured inclusion cysts.

  Furuncles, Carbuncles Hair-bearing regions: beard area, posterior neck and occipital scalp, axillae, buttocks

Differential Diagnosis

Painful Dermal/Subcutaneous Nodule Ruptured epidermoid or pilar cyst, hidradenitis suppurativa (axillae, groin, vulva), necrotizing HSV infection

Laboratory and Special Examinations

Gram's Strain Gram-positive cocci within PMN leukocytes and in extracellular space

Bacterial Culture

PUS Culture of pus isolates *S. aureus.* Sensitivities to antimicrobial agents may determine management.

BLOOD Culture if patient is febrile ± constitutional symptoms before beginning treatment.

ANTIBIOTIC SENSITIVITIES Identifies methicillin-resistant *S. aureus* (MRSA) and need for changing usual antibiotic therapy.

Dermatopathology Pyogenic infection arising in hair follicle and extending into deep dermis and subcutaneous tissue (furuncle) and with loculated abscesses (carbuncle)

Diagnosis

Clinical findings confirmed by findings on Gram's stain and culture

Course and Prognosis

Most cases resolve with incision and drainage and systemic antibiotic treatment. At times, however, furunculosis is complicated by bacteremia and possible hematogenous seeding of heart valves, joints, spine, long bones, and viscera (especially kidneys). *S. aureus* can hematogenously disseminate via venous drainage to cavernous sinus with resultant cavernous venous thromboses and meningitis. Some individuals are subject to recurrent furunculosis particularly in diabetes. The incidence of infection caused by MRSA is increasing.

Management

The treatment of an abscess, furuncle, or carbuncle is incision and drainage, usually accompanied by systemic antimicrobial therapy.

Prevention Individuals subject to repeated furuncle/carbuncle formation can reduce *S. aureus* carriage by use of an antibacterial soap while bathing. Mupirocin ointment is effective for eliminating nasal carriage.

Surgery Incision and drainage are often adequate for treatment of abscesses, furuncles, or carbuncles. Scissors or scalpel blade can be used to drain loculated pus in carbuncles; if this is not done, resolution of pain and infection can be delayed despite systemic antibiotic therapy. Dental abscesses are often associated with devitalized tooth pulp, which must be removed or the tooth extracted.

Adjunctive Therapy Application of heat to the lesion promotes localization/consolidation and aids early spontaneous drainage.

Systemic Antimicrobial Therapy In healthy individuals, incision and drainage are often adequate therapy. Systemic antibiotics speed resolution in healthy individuals and are mandatory in any individual at risk for bacteremia (e.g., immunosuppressed patients).

  Dicloxacillin 250 to 500 mg (adult dose) q.i.d. for 10 days
  Cephalexin 250 to 500 mg (adult dose) for 10 days; 40 to 50 mg/kg/day (children) for 10 days
  Amoxicillin Plus Clavulanic Acid (Beta-Lactamase Inhibitor) 20 mg/kg/day t.i.d. for 10 days

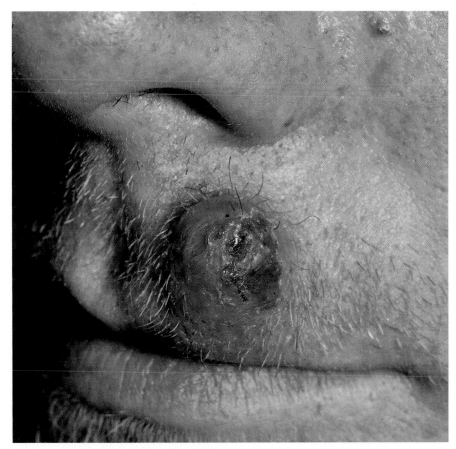

Figure 23-7 Furuncle: S. aureus *An extremely painful, inflammatory nodule with a central necrosis on the upper lip; the lesion arose from a site of folliculitis in the beard area.*

Macrolides (for Penicillin-Allergic Individuals) If *S. aureus* is sensitive:

Erythromycin ethylsuccinate: 40 mg/kg/day q.i.d. for 10 days; 1 to 2 g/day in four divided doses for 10 days (adult dose)

Clarithromycin: 250 to 500 mg b.i.d. for 10 days

Azithromycin: 250 mg q.d. for 5 to 7 days

Clindamycin 150 to 300 mg (adult dose) q.i.d. for 10 days; 15 mg/kg/day (children) q.i.d. for 10 days

Methicillin-Resistant *S. aureus* (MRSA)

Minocycline 100 mg b.i.d. for 10 days

Trimethoprim-Sulfamethoxazole 2 to 4 tabs/day; 1 to 2 DS/day

Ciprofloxacin 500 b.i.d. for 7 days

Vancomycin Intravenous administration for severe infections

Recurrent Furunculosis Usually related to persistent *S. aureus* in the nares, perineum, and body folds.

Topical Therapy Shower with providone-iodine soap or benzoyl peroxide (bar or wash). Apply mupirocin ointment daily to the inside of nares and other sites of *S. aureus* carriage. Appropriate antibiotic treatment is continued until all lesions have resolved and then may be given as a once-a-day prophylactic dose for many months.

Rifampin 600 mg PO for 7 to 10 days for eradication of carrier state

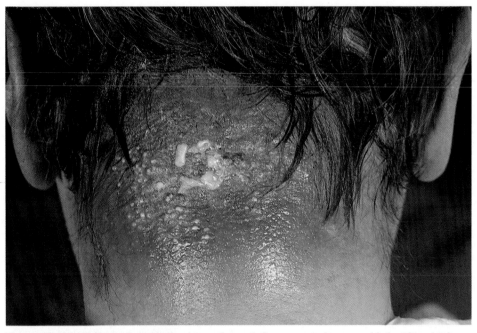

Figure 23-8 Carbuncle: S. aureus *A very large, inflammatory plaque studded with multiple pustules, some of which have ruptured draining pus, on the nape of the neck. This very painful area is surrounded by erythema and edema (cellulitis), extends down to fascia, and has formed from a confluence of many furuncles.*

ERYTHRASMA

Erythrasma (Greek: "red spot") is a chronic bacterial infection caused by *Corynebacterium minutissimum* affecting the intertriginous areas of the toes, groins, and axillae, which mimics epidermal dermatophyte infections.

Epidemiology and Etiology

Age   Adults

Etiology   *C. minutissimum,* gram-positive rod (diphtheroid), part of normal skin flora, which causes superficial infection under certain conditions

Predisposing Factors   Diabetes; warm, humid climate. Prolonged occlusion of skin, maceration.

History

Duration of Lesions   Months, years

Skin Symptoms   Usually asymptomatic. Occasionally, burning sensation, pruritus.

Physical Examination

Skin Lesions

TYPE   Macule, usually large, slightly scaling, sharply marginated (see Figure 23-9)

COLOR   Red or brownish red

INTERDIGITAL   Erosive with collarette-like scale

ARRANGEMENT   Confluent patches, scattered, discrete lesions

SITES OF PREDILECTION   Groin folds (Figure 23-9), axillae, subpanniculus, intergluteal, inframammary, toe web spaces (Figure 23-10)

Differential Diagnosis

Well-Demarcated Intertriginous Plaque
Dermatophytosis, cutaneous candidiasis, pityriasis versicolor, inverse-pattern psoriasis, seborrheic dermatitis, pitted keratolysis (toe web spaces, caused by *Micrococcus sedentarius*)

Laboratory and Special Examinations

Direct Microscopic   Negative for fungal forms on KOH preparation of scales

Wood's Lamp   Characteristic coral-red fluorescence. May not be present if patient has bathed recently.

Bacterial Culture   Rule out *Staphylococcus aureus* or group A streptococcal infection

Diagnosis

Clinical findings, absence of fungi on direct microscopy, positive Wood's lamp examination

Course

Relapses occur if predisposing causes are not corrected.

Management

Prevention   Wash with benzoyl peroxide (bar or wash).

Topical Therapy   Benzoyl peroxide (2.5 %) gel daily for 7 days. Topical erythromycin solution b.i.d. for 7 days.

Systemic Antibiotic Therapy   Erythromycin 250 mg q.i.d. for 14 days

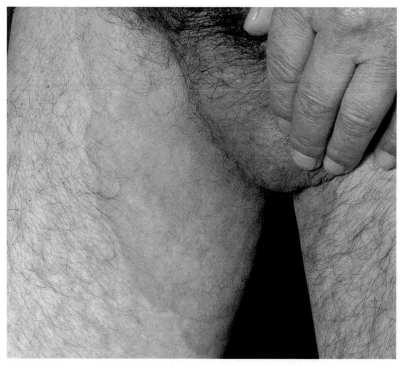

Figure 23-9 Erythrasma *Sharply marginated, brownish-red, slightly scaling macular patch on the inguinal area and medial thighs appears bright coral-red when examined with a Wood's lamp. KOH preparation was negative for hyphae.*

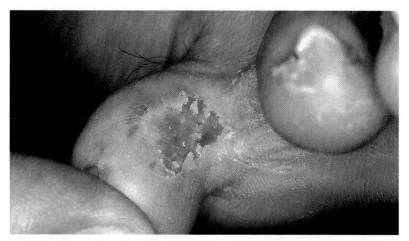

Figure 23-10 Erythrasma *This macerated and partially eroded interdigital webspace appeared a bright coral-red when examined with a Wood's lamp; KOH preparation was negative for hyphae. Epidermal dermatophytosis (note tinea unguium of fourth toenail) had previously been treated with a topical antifungal agent, but clinical findings failed to resolve.*

ERYSIPELOID

Erysipeloid is an acute but slowly evolving cellulitis occurring at sites of inoculation, most commonly the hands, and is often occupational, associated with handling fish, shellfish, meat, poultry, hides, bones.

Synonym: Crab dermatitis.

Epidemiology and Etiology

Sex   Males > females (3:1)

Occupation   Virtually restricted to persons who handle dead animal matter in their work, either nonedible (rendered products such as grease, fertilizer, bones, shells) or edible (meat, poultry, fish, shellfish). Fishermen, fish handlers, butchers, meat processing workers, poultry workers, farmers, veterinarians, abattoir workers, housewives, poachers.

Etiology   *Erysipelothrix rhusiopathiae,* a gram-positive rod. The organism is widespread in nature, capable of infecting both vertebrates (mammals, birds, fish) and invertebrates (shellfish, insects).

Transmission   Organism is primarily saprophytic. Human infection restricted to persons who handle dead animal matter. No vectors. Not contagious.

Season   Summer and early fall

Geography   Worldwide

History

Incubation Period   2 to 7 days

History   Occupational exposure

Skin Symptoms   Itching, burning, throbbing, pain

Systems Review   Systemic symptoms uncommon

Physical Examination

Skin Lesions

TYPES   Painful, swollen plaque with sharply defined irregular raised border, occurring at the site of inoculation (Figure 23-11). Enlarges peripherally with central fading. Vesiculation uncommon. Nonsuppurative. Edema nonpitting; may limit movement of interphalangeal joint. Central (older) site heals as lesion expands centrifugally (up to 1 cm/day).

COLOR   Purplish-red acutely. Brownish with resolution.

DISTRIBUTION   Finger or hand, distal to wrist; terminal phalanges usually spared

General Findings

LYMPH NODES   Occasional lymphangitis or lymphadenitis. Endocarditis: search for this.

Differential Diagnosis

Red, Painful Plaque on Hand   Other bacterial cellulites, including *Vibrio* cellulitis, allergic contact dermatitis

Laboratory and Special Examinations

Dermatopathology   Acute dermal inflammation: bacilli are extracellular, located deep in dermis.

Culture   Most successful from lesional biopsy specimen obtained from advancing border. Infected tissue also can be sampled by injecting nonbacteriostatic saline into advancing edge of lesion, aspiration, and culture of aspirate.

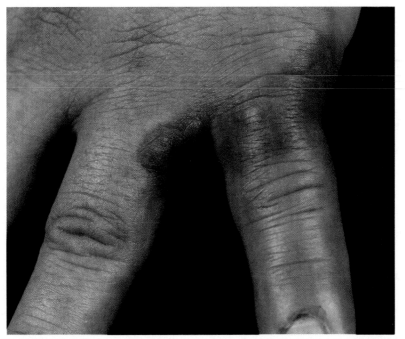

Figure 23-11 Erysipeloid *A well-demarcated, violaceous, cellulitic plaque (without epidermal changes of scale or vesiculation) on the dorsum of the hand and fingers; the site was somewhat painful, tender, and warm.*

Diagnosis

Clinical diagnosis by history of exposure and unique clinical appearance, confirmed by isolation of *E. rhusiopathiae* in lesional biopsy specimen

Pathophysiology

Infection follows an abrasion, scratch, or puncture wound while handling organic material containing the organism.

Course and Prognosis

Usually self-limited, subsiding spontaneously in about 3 weeks. Endocarditis or septic arthritis rarely may complicate bacteremia. Only a third of cases of bacteremia and endocarditis arise from clinically evident skin infection. Remaining two-thirds of cases attributed to subclinical cutaneous infection and ingestion of infected meat or fish. Despite adequate antibiotic therapy, mortality from endocarditis is 30% to 40%.

Management

Prevention Use of gloves by workers who are handling meat and fish

Antibiotic Therapy

> *Drug of choice:* penicillin G: 1.2 million units of benzathine penicillin (600,000 units into each buttock)
> *Alternative:* erythromycin 250 to 500 mg q.i.d. for 7 days

PITTED KERATOLYSIS

Pitted keratolysis (PK) presents as defects in the thickly keratinized skin of the plantar foot with sculpted pits of variable depth, depending on the thickness of the stratum corneum, usually associated with pedal hyperhidrosis, caused by *Micrococcus sedentarius.*

Epidemiology and Etiology

Age   Young adulthood

Sex   Males >> females

Predisposing Factors   Hyperhidrosis of the feet

Etiology   *M. sedentarius*

History

History   Often history of misdiagnosis of tinea pedia

Skin Symptoms   Usually asymptomatic. Foot odor. Uncommonly, itching, burning, tenderness.

Physical Examination

Skin Lesions

TYPE   Pits in stratum corneum, 1 to 8 mm in diameter (Figure 23-12). Pits can remain discrete or, more often, become confluent, forming large areas of eroded stratum corneum.

COLOR   Involved areas are white when stratum corneum is fully hydrated.

SHAPE   Round to oval

ARRANGEMENT   Symmetric or asymmetric involvement of both feet

DISTRIBUTION   Toe webs. Ball or heel of foot in contact with shoe.

Differential Diagnosis

White Plaques on Feet   Tinea pedis, *Candida* intertrigo, erythrasma, gram-negative web space infection

Laboratory and Special Examinations

KOH Preparation   Negative for hyphae

Wood's Lamp Examination   Negative for bright coral-red fluorescence (erythrasma)

Culture   In some cases, rule out *Staphylococcus aureus,* group A streptococcus, or *Pseudomonas aeruginosa* infection

Diagnosis

Clinical diagnosis ruling out other causes

Pathophysiology

High local humidity and hyperhidrosis facilitate growth of *M. sedentarius.*

Course and Prognosis

Persists and recurs until the underlying predisposing factors are corrected.

Management

Prophylaxis   Wash with lather from benzoyl peroxide soap bar. Reduce sweating with agents such as aluminum chloride, powders such as Zeasorb.

Treatment   Daily applications of agents such as benzoyl peroxide preparations or topical antibiotics such as erythromycin are usually effective.

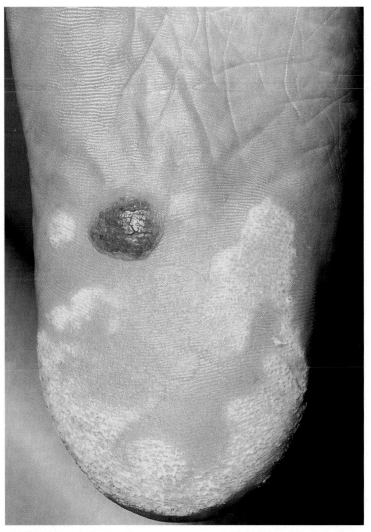

Figure 23-12 Pitted keratolysis *The stratum corneum of the plantar heel is macerated (saturated with water), within which are multiple, confluent erosions (defects in the stratum corneum or "pits"). A congenital nevomelanocytic nevus is also present.*

Section 24

SYSTEMIC BACTERIAL INFECTIONS

INFECTIVE ENDOCARDITIS

Infective endocarditis (IE) is a microbial infection implanted on a heart valve or on the mural endocardium; it is characterized by fever, valvular destruction, and peripheral embolization (Table 24-A).

Epidemiology and Etiology

Classification

ACUTE BACTERIAL ENDOCARDITIS (ABE) Caused by more invasive organisms. Can attack normal valve or mural endocardium. Agents: *Staphylococcus aureus, Streptococcus pneumoniae* (alcoholics with pneumonia), group A streptococcus, *Neisseria gonorrhoeae, Salmonella, Pseudomonas aeruginosa* (intravenous drug users, IVDUs)

SUBACUTE BACTERIAL ENDOCARDITIS (SBE) Defined as duration of more than 6 weeks. Caused by a variety of less virulent bacteria. Commonly, bacteria are members of the indigenous flora. Characteristically, infection is on deformed valves. Agents: streptococci of oral cavity, GI and GU tracts; *Hemophilus* organisms, *S. epidermidis.*

Etiology Most common is bacterial: (1) *S. viridans,* enterococci, and other streptococci account for about 50 %, (2) *S. aureus, S. epidermidis* 20 %, (3) in 15 % to 20 % no causative agent can be isolated, (4) remainder uncommon bacterial and fungal organisms. Staphylococcal, fungal, gramnegative bacterial agents common in IVDUs, as well as polymicrobial IE. *S. aureus* most common cause with a normal valve. Also, fungi (*Candida albicans*), rickettsiae, chlamydiae.

Transmission Circumstances that result in transient bacteremia: dental procedures, intravenous drug use, various infections, induced abortions, intrauterine contraceptive devices, temporary transvenous pacemakers, prolonged IV infusions, endoscopic procedures. Estimated risk for IE in IVDUs in the United States: 2 % to 5 % per year.

Risk Factors

UNDERLYING HEART DISEASE (1) Acquired heart disease—70 % (rheumatic valvular disease, calcific stenosis, "floppy" mitral or aortic valves, prolapsing mitral valve leaflet, i.e., "click-murmur" syndrome, idiopathic hypertrophic subaortic stenosis, calcified mitral annulus. (2) Congenital heart disease (interventricular septal defect, patent ductus arteriosus, pulmonic valve in tetralogy of Fallot).

PROSTHETIC MATERIAL Prosthetic heart valves, xenografts, intracardiac "patches," vascular prostheses

IVDU Increasingly common risk factor for IE

History

History

SBE Fever, sweats, weakness, myalgias, arthralgias, malaise, fatigability, anorexia, chilly

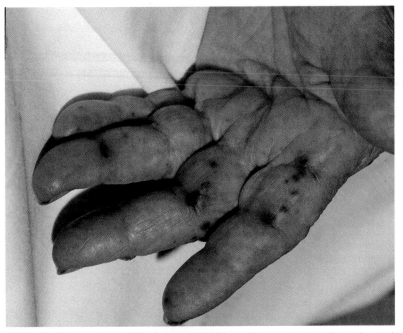

Figure 24-1 Infective endocarditis: Janeway lesions *Hemorrhagic, infarcted macules and papules on the volar fingers in a patient with* S. aureus *endocarditis.*

sensations, cough. Recent history of dental extraction or scaling, cystoscopy, rectal surgery, tonsillectomy. Fever, weight loss, cerebrovascular accident, arthralgia, arthritis, diffuse myalgias.

ABE Onset abrupt with high fever and rigors, rapid downhill course

IV Drug Use Occurs in 0.2 % to 2 % of users annually. Right-sided IE more common than left-sided. *S. aureus* in >50 %; 5 % polymicrobial. Septic emboli common.

Physical Examination

Consider IE in any patient with fever and heart murmur.

Skin Lesions (see Table 24-A)

TYPES *Janeway Lesions Nonpainful,* small, erythematous or hemorrhagic macules or nodules of palms (Figure 24-1) or soles. More common in ABE but occur in SBE.

Osler's Nodes Tender to painful, purplish, split pea–sized, subcutaneous nodules in the pulp of the fingers and/or toes and thenar and hypothenar eminences (Figure 24-2). Transient, disappearing within several days (5% of patients). In ABE, associated with minute infective emboli; aspiration may reveal the causative organism, i.e., *S. aureus.* In SBE, associated with immune complexes and small-vessel arteritis of skin.

Subungual Splinter Hemorrhages Linear in the *middle* of the nail bed (IE) (see Section 18). (IE). *Distal hemorrhages are traumatic.*

Petechial Lesions Small, nonblanching, reddish brown macules. Occur on extremities, upper chest, mucous membrane [conjunctivae (Figure 24-3), palate]. Occur in crops. Fade after a few days. 20 % to 40 %

Clubbing of Fingers Seen after prolonged course of untreated SBE (15%)

Gangrene of Extremities Secondary to embolization

Pustular Petechiae, Purulent Purpura With *S. aureus*

General Examination

HEART   SBE 90% have murmurs; ABE only two-thirds have murmur, which may change, heart failure.

EYE   Petechial and flame-shaped hemorrhages in retina, cotton-wool exudates in fundus, Roth's spots (oval or boat-shaped white areas in the retina that are surrounded by a zone of hemorrhage), endophthalmitis

SPLEEN   Splenomegaly (25 % to 60 %), splenic abscess

LIVER   Hepatomegaly

JOINTS   Septic arthritis with ABE

THROMBOEMBOLIC PHENOMENA   Significant embolic episodes occur in one-third of patients, resulting in stroke, seizures, monocular blindness, mesenteric artery occlusion with abdominal pain, ileus, melena, splenic infarction, pulmonary infarction, gangrene of extremities, mycotic aneurysms.

Differential Diagnosis

ABE   Meningococcemia, disseminated intravascular coagulation

SBE   Acute rheumatic fever, marantic endocarditis, collagen vascular diseases (SLE with cardiac involvement, systemic vasculitis), dysproteinemia, atrial myxoma, organizing left atrial thrombus, atheromatous embolism, cytomegalovirus infection following cardiac surgery (postperfusion syndrome)

Laboratory and Special Examinations

Dermatopathology   Osler's node in subacute IE shows aseptic necrotizing vasculitis.

Blood   Anemia, elevated ESR, leukocytosis in ABE but often WBC normal with SBE, depressed serum complement, immune complexes (90 %), rheumatoid factor (50 % with SBE)

HIV Serology   Commonly positive in IVDUs

Blood Cultures   Establish the diagnosis; usually no more than six are required.

Urinalysis   Hematuria, pyuria

Imaging   Echo-Doppler study demonstrates vegetations, acute severe mitral or aortic regurgitation. Evidence of septic pulmonary emboli suggests tricuspid valve IE. Systemic embolization can occur from aortic or mitral valve.

Diagnosis

Confirmed by isolating infecting organism with four to six blood cultures before antibiotic therapy.

Pathophysiology

Subacute IE   Requires a previously damaged cardiac valve, sterile platelet-fibrin thrombus, bacteremia, and high titer of agglutinating antibody for the infecting organisms. During transient bacteremia, organisms adhere to the valve or mural endocardium or to overlying fibrin-platelet aggregate. Cutaneous findings caused by circulating immune complexes.

Acute IE   Presence of sterile platelet-fibrin thrombus may not be necessary. Skin manifestations (Osler's nodes) result from septic embolism in most cases.

Course and Prognosis

Varies with the underlying cardiac disease and baseline health of the patient, as well as with the complications that occur. Complications: congestive heart failure, stroke, other systemic embolizations, septic pulmonary embolization. Aortic valve involvement has higher risk of death or need for surgery.

Management

Antimicrobial Therapy   Appropriate IV antibiotic therapy depending on the sensitivities of the infecting organism

Surgery   Most common indication, congestive heart failure. Valve replacement.

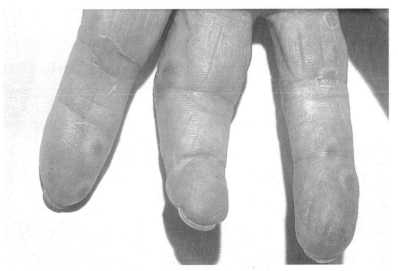

Figure 24-2 Infective endocarditis: Osler's nodes *Violaceous, tender nodules on the volar fingers associated with minute infective emboli or immune complex deposition.*

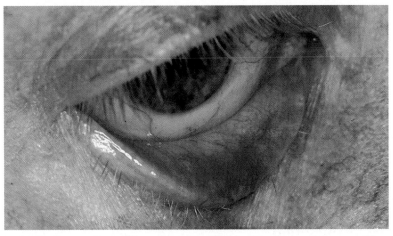

Figure 24-3 Infective endocarditis: subconjunctival hemorrhage *Submucosal hemorrhage of the lower eyelid in an elderly diabetic with enterococcal endocarditis; splinter hemorrhages in the midportion of the nail bed (see Figure 18-8) and Janeway lesions were also present.*

TABLE 24-A CUTANEOUS MANIFESTATIONS AND CHARACTERISTICS OF INFECTIVE ENDOCARDITIS

Cutaneous Manifestations	Palpation	Morphologic Findings
Osler's node	Tender	Erythematous papules and nodules with white centers; may necrose
Janeway's lesions	Nontender	Hemorrhagic papules
Splinter hemorrhages	Nontender	Subungual hemorrhagic streaks

GRAM-POSITIVE INFECTIONS

STAPHYLOCOCCAL SCALDED-SKIN SYNDROME

Staphylococcal scalded-skin syndrome (SSSS) is a toxin-mediated epidermolytic disease characterized by erythema, widespread detachment of the superficial layers of the epidermis, resembling scalding, and occurring mainly in newborns and infants under 2 years of age. Severity ranges from a localized form, bullous impetigo, to a generalized form with extensive epidermolysis and desquamation. The clinical spectrum of SSSS includes: (1) bullous impetigo, (2) bullous impetigo with generalization, (3) scarlatiniform syndrome, (4) generalized scalded-skin syndrome. *Synonyms:* Ritter's disease.

Epidemiology and Etiology

Age Most common in neonates during first 3 months of life. Infants and young children. Rare in adults.

Etiology *Staphylococcus aureus* of phage group II, mostly type 71, which elaborate two distinct exotoxins, epidermolytic or exfoliatin toxins A and B
   Site of toxin production: purulent conjunctivitis, otitis media, occult nasopharyngeal infection; bullous impetigo

History

Immune Status Adults with immunosuppression or renal insufficiency subject to SSSS

Skin Symptoms SSSS: early erythematous areas are very tender.

Physical Examination

Skin Lesions

TYPES **Localized Form** See Section 23 (bullous impetigo): intact flaccid purulent bullae, clustered. Rupture of the bullae results in moist red and/or crusted erosive lesions.
   Generalized Form
   Exotoxin-induced changes: micromacular scarlatiniform rash (staphylococcal scarlet fever syndrome) or diffuse, ill-defined erythema (Figure 24-4) and a fine, stippled, sandpaper appearance occur initially.

In 24 hours, erythema deepens in color and involved skin becomes *tender.* With epidermolysis, epidermis appears wrinkled and can be removed by gentle pressure (skin resembles wet tissue paper) (Figure 24-4). In some infants, flaccid bullae occur. Unroofed epidermis forms erosions with red, moist base.

PALPATION Gentle lateral pressure causes shearing off of superficial epidermis (Nikolsky's sign). Children are difficult to hold because of skin tenderness.

ARRANGEMENT In bullous impetigo, lesions often are clustered in an intertriginous area.

DISTRIBUTION Bullous impetigo: intertriginous areas. SSSS: *Initially* periorificially on face, neck, axillae, groins; becoming more widespread in 24 to 48 hours. Initial erythema and later sloughing of epidermis are most pronounced periorificially on face (Figure 24-5) and in flexural areas on neck, axillae, groins, antecubital area, back (pressure points). Condition becomes generalized, resembling scalding (Figure 24-5).

MUCOUS MEMBRANES Uninvolved

General Examination Possible low-grade fever. Irritable child.

Differential Diagnosis

Drug-induced toxic epidermal necrolysis, toxic shock syndrome, Kawasaki's syndrome, eczema herpeticum

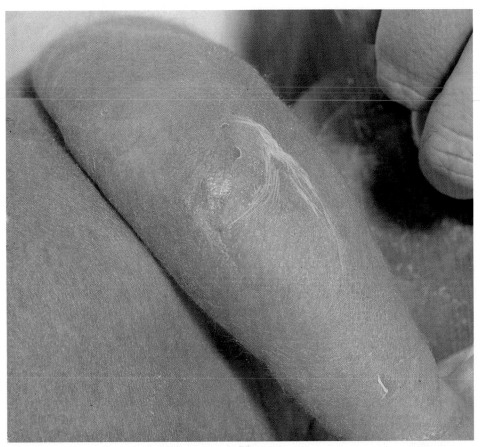

Figure 24-4 Staphylococcal scalded-skin syndrome *The skin of this infant is diffusely erythematous; gentle pressure to the skin of the arm has sheared off the epidermis, which folds like tissue paper.*

Laboratory and Special Examinations

Gram's Stain Bullous impetigo: pus in bullae, clumps of gram-positive cocci within PMN. SSSS: gram-positive cocci only at colonized site, not in areas of epidermolysis.

Bacterial Culture Bullous impetigo: *S. aureus* isolated from involved site. SSSS: *S. aureus only at site of infection* (i.e., site of toxin production), i.e., umbilical stump, ala nasi, nasopharynx, conjunctivae, external ear canal, stool. *S. aureus is not recovered from sites of sloughing skin or bullae.*

Dermatopathology Intraepidermal cleavage with splitting occurring beneath and within stratum granulosum

Diagnosis

Clinical findings confirmed by bacterial cultures

Pathophysiology

In newborns and infants, *S. aureus* colonizes nose, conjunctivae, or umbilical stump without causing clinically apparent infection, producing an exotoxin (exfoliatin, epidermolysin) that is transported hematogenously to the skin. In bullous impetigo exotoxin is produced in impetigo lesion. Specific antistaphylococcal antibody, metabolic differences, or greater ability to localize, metabolize, and excrete in individuals >10 years of age probably accounts for decreased incidence of SSSS with older age. At times purulent conjunctivitis, otitis media, or occult nasopharyngeal infection occurs at site of toxin production. The exfoliative toxin causes acantholysis and intraepidermal cleavage within the stratum granulosum. The few cases of SSSS reported in adults were associated with immunodeficiency or renal insufficiency. Local effects of the toxin result in bullous impetigo, but with absorption of the toxin,

a mild scarlatiniform rash accompanying the bullous lesions may be seen. Conversely, local effects of the toxin may be absent, with systemic absorption resulting in a staphylococcal scarlet fever syndrome. More extensive epidermal damage is characterized by sloughing of superficial epidermis in SSSS. Healing spontaneously occurs in 5 to 7 days.

Course and Prognosis

In late phases of SSSS, and in an accelerated manner, following adequate antibiotic treatment, the superficially denuded areas heal in 3 to 5 days associated with generalized desquamation in large sheets of skin; there is no scarring. Death can occur in neonates with extensive disease.

Management

General Care Hospitalization is recommended for neonates and young children, especially if skin sloughing is extensive and parental compliance questionable. Discharge home when significant improvement is apparent. If case is mild and home care reliable, children can be treated with oral antibiotic.

Topical Therapy Baths or compresses for debridement of necrotic superficial epidermis. Topical antimicrobial agents for impetigo lesions: mupirocin ointment, bacitracin, or silver sulfadiazine ointment. Avoid triple antibiotic ointment containing neomycin, which is a frequent allergen, causing contact dermatitis.

Systemic Antimicrobial Therapy (See Section 23)

> *Oxacillin:* IV in divided doses every 4 hours for those who are severely ill or have extensive skin involvement
> *Dicloxacillin:* PO after significant improvement with IV antibiotic or for children with mild disease and reliable parents

Adjunctive Therapy Replace significant water and electrolyte loss intravenously in severe cases.

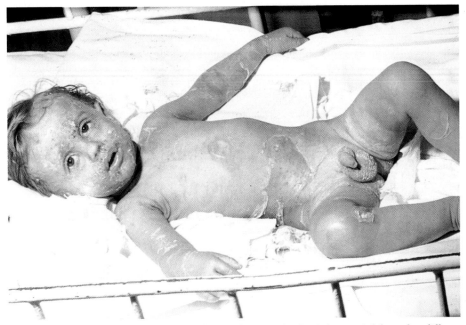

Figure 24-5 Staphylococcal scalded-skin syndrome *In this infant, painful, tender, diffuse erythema was followed by generalized epidermal sloughing.* S. aureus *had colonized the nares with perioral impetigo, the site of exotoxin production.*

TOXIC SHOCK SYNDROME

Toxic shock syndrome (TSS) is an acute toxin-mediated illness caused by toxin-producing *Staphylococcus aureus,* characterized by rapid onset of fever, hypotension, generalized skin and mucosal erythema, and multisystem failure, occurring in menstrual (MTSS) and nonmenstrual (NMTSS) patterns.

Epidemiology and Etiology

Age In the United States, MTSS: 23 years (mean age); NMTSS: 27 years (mean age)

Sex In the United States prior to 1984, more than 99 % of cases were in females; after 1984, 55 % in females.

Race In the United States, 97 % of MTSS in whites; 87 % of NMTSS in whites

Etiology *S. aureus* producing TSS toxin 1 (TSST-1); other factors. Severe group A streptococcal infections also can cause a TSS-like syndrome.

Risk Factors

MTSS Use of vaginal tampon of greater absorbency

NMTSS Nonsurgical wounds (burns, skin ulcers, cutaneous and ocular injuries), surgical wounds, nasal packs, postpartum infections, vaginal nonmenstrual origin (contraceptive sponge, contraceptive diaphragm). Influenza.

STREPTOCOCCAL TSS Diabetes mellitus, peripheral vascular disease

Underlying Disorders NMTSS can occur secondary to a wide variety of primary *S. aureus* infections as well as secondary infection of underlying dermatoses.

History

Incubation Period Shorter in NMTSS. Following surgical procedure, <4 days.

History Recurrent symptoms in MTSS in untreated cases; tampon use. Sudden onset of fever, hypotension. Tingling sensation, hands and feet. Maculopapular eruption, pruritic.

Systems Review Generalized myalgias, muscle tenderness and weakness; headache, confusion, disorientation, seizures; profuse diarrhea; dyspnea

Physical Examination

Skin Lesions

TYPES Generalized scarlatiniform erythroderma, most intense around infected area. Macular eruption (see scarlet fever, page 644). Petechiae, bullae, uncommonly. Edema, extensive generalized nonpitting. Subsequent desquamation of palms, soles (Figure 24-6).
NMTSS Look for cutaneous site of infection.
Streptococcal TSS Cellulitis, necrotizing fasciitis, puerperal sepsis, varicella in children, and rarely asymptomatic streptococcal pharyngitis

DISTRIBUTION Edema most marked on face, hands, feet

MUCOUS MEMBRANES Look for forgotten or retained vaginal tampon. Intense erythema and injection of bulbar conjunctivae and mucous membranes of mouth, tongue, pharynx, vagina, tympanic membranes. Strawberry tongue. Subconjunctival hemorrhages. Ulcerations of mouth, vagina, esophagus, bladder.

General Findings Fever, hypotension, multiorgan system failure. Renal and CNS complications more common in NMTSS.

Differential Diagnosis

Toxin-Mediated Infections Staphylococcal scalded-skin syndrome, scarlet fever, group A streptococcal TSS, gastroenteritis

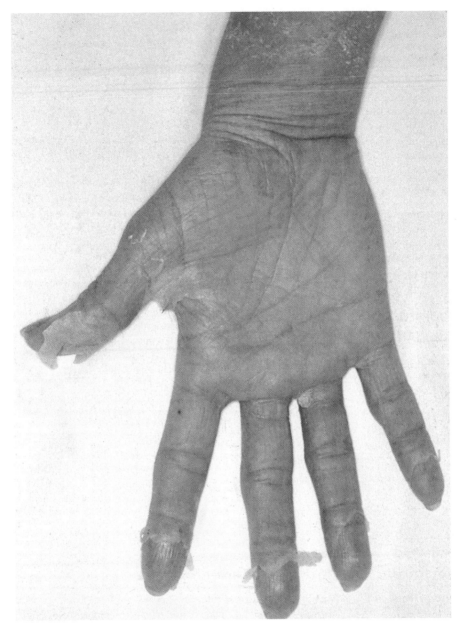

Figure 24-6 Toxic shock syndrome: desquamation   *The epidermis is desquamating on the wrist and volar hand in a female with menstrual TSS; 7 days previously, the skin was diffusely erythematous.*

Localized Infections with Abdominal Pain and Shock Urinary tract infection, pelvic inflammatory disease, septic abortion, gastroenteritis

Multisystem Infection Septic shock with localized infection (meningococcus, gonococcus, pneumococcus, *Hemophilus influenzae* type B), leptospirosis, measles, Rocky Mountain spotted fever, tick-borne typhus, viral syndrome (adenoviruses, enteroviruses), Legionnaires' disease, toxoplasmosis

Multisystem Illness, Possibly of Infectious Etiology Kawasaki's syndrome

Noninfectious Diseases Systemic lupus erythematosus, acute rheumatic fever, adverse cutaneous drug reactions (erythema multiforme, Stevens-Johnson syndrome), juvenile rheumatoid arthritis

Laboratory and Special Examinations

Gram's Stain Vaginal, wound exudate: many leukocytes and gram-positive cocci in clusters

Culture Vaginal, wound exudate, foreign body: TSST-1–producing *S. aureus*. Streptococcal TSS: GAS recovered from blood or primary site of infection.

Biopsy Confluent epidermal necrosis, vacuolar alteration of dermal-epidermal junction, subepidermal vesiculation, little or no inflammatory infiltrate in dermis

Diagnosis

TSS clinical case definition (CDC):
> *Fever* Temperature $\geq 38.9°C$
> *Rash* Diffuse macular erythroderma
> *Desquamation* 1 to 2 weeks after onset of illness, particularly of palms, soles, fingers, toes
> *Hypotension* Systolic blood pressure ≤ 90 mm Hg for adults. For children, >5th percentile by age <16 years of age. Orthostatic syncope or orthostatic dizziness.
> *Involvement of Three or More of the Following Organ Systems (see Table 24-B)*

Pathophysiology

S. aureus multiplies in foreign body or minor wound infection, elaborating the TSST-1, which is absorbed and causes the clinical changes. TSST-1 causes decrease in vasomotor tone and leakage of intravascular fluid. Rapid onset of hypotension followed by tissue ischemia and multisystem organ failure.

Course and Prognosis

Diagnosis of NMTSS is often delayed because of the wide variety of clinical settings and associated symptomatology. Complications: refractory hypotension, adult respiratory distress syndrome, cardiomyopathy, arrhythmias, encephalopathy, acute renal failure, metabolic aci-

TABLE 24-B

Organ Systems	Clinical and Laboratory Findings
Gastrointestinal	Vomiting or diarrhea at onset of illness
Muscular	Severe myalgia or creatinine phosphokinase more than twice upper limit of normal
Mucous membranes	Vaginal, oropharyngeal, or conjunctival hyperemia
Renal	BUN or serum creatinine more than twice upper limit of normal, or 5 WBCs per HPF in the absence of urinary tract infection
Hepatic	Total bilirubin, SGOT, or SGPT more than twice upper limit of normal
Hematologic	Platelets $\leq 100,000/\mu l$
CNS	Disorientation or alterations in consciousness without focal neurologic signs when fever and hypotension are absent

dosis, liver necrosis, disseminated intravascular coagulation. Recurrence of untreated, menses-associated TSS is high. Antibiotic therapy and discontinuance of tampons significantly reduce risk. Recurrences after nonmenstrual TSS are rare. The mortality of NMTSS is higher than that of MTSS. *Streptococcal TSS:* associated with mortality of 25 % to 50 %.

Management

Usually patients are managed best in intensive care facility.

Local Infection Remove potentially foreign bodies. Drain and irrigate infected sites.

Systemic Antimicrobial Therapy IV antistaphylococcal antibiotic

Adjunctive Therapy Aggressive monitoring and management of specific organ system failure (i.e., management of fluid, electrolyte, metabolic, and nutritional needs). Methylprednisolone for severe cases.

SOFT TISSUE INFECTIONS: ERYSIPELAS AND CELLULITIS

Cellulitis is an acute, spreading infection of dermal and subcutaneous tissues, characterized by a red, hot, tender area of skin, often at the site of bacterial entry, caused most frequently by group A beta-hemolytic streptococci (erysipelas) or *Staphylococcus aureus.*

Epidemiology and Etiology

Age   Any age. Children <3 years; older individuals.

Etiology

MOST COMMON   ***Adults***   *S. aureus,* group A beta-hemolytic *Streptococcus pyogenes* (GAS)
Children   *Hemophilus influenzae,* GAS, *S. aureus*

UNCOMMON   ***Adults***   *H. influenzae* type b (Hib), group B streptococci (GBS), pneumococci. In diabetics or in patients with impaired immunity: *Escherichia coli, Proteus mirabilis, Acinetobacter, Enterobacter, Pseudomonas aeruginosa, Pasteurella multocida, Vibrio vulnificus; Mycobacterium fortuitum* complex; *Cryptococcus neoformans.*
Children   Pneumococci, *Neisseria meningitidis* group B (periorbital)

Portals of Entry   Cellulitis can arise via a portal of entry through any mucocutaneous site or, less commonly, spread hematogenously to soft tissue. Blood-borne pathogens causing cellulitis include *S. pneumoniae, V. vulnificus,* and *C. neoformans.*

Underlying dermatoses

- Bullous disease: pemphigus vulgaris, bullous pemphigoid, sunburn, porphyria cutanea tarda
- Chronic lymphedema
- Dermatophytosis: tinea pedis, tinea capitis, tinea barbae
- Viral infections: herpes simplex, varicella, herpes zoster
- Inflammatory dermatoses: atopic dermatitis, contact dermatitis, stasis dermatitis, psoriasis, chronic cutaneous lupus erythematosus, pyoderma gangrenosum
- Superficial pyoderma: impetigo, folliculitis, furunculosis, carbuncle, ecthyma
- Ulcers: pressure, chronic venous insufficiency, ischemic, neuropathic
- Umbilical stump

Trauma

- Abrasion
- Bites: human, animal, insect
- Burns
- Laceration
- Puncture

Surgical wound

- Surgical incisions
- Venous access devices

Mucosal infection

- Oropharynx, nasal mucosa
- Middle ear

Risk Factors   Drug and alcohol abuse, cancer and cancer chemotherapy, chronic lymphedema (postmastectomy, postcoronary artery grafting, previous episode of cellulitis), cirrhosis, diabetes mellitus, iatrogenic immunosuppression (neutropenia), immunodeficiency syndromes, malnutrition, neutropenia, renal failure, systemic atherosclerosis

History

Incubation Period   Few days

Prodrome   Occurs less often than commonly thought. Malaise, anorexia; fever, chills can develop rapidly, before cellulitis is apparent clin-

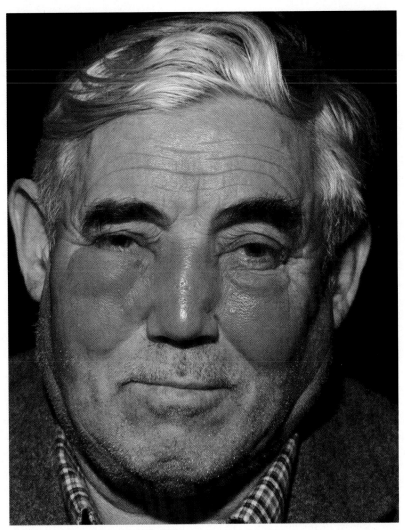

Figure 24-7 Erysipelas: group A streptococcus *Painful, shiny, erythematous, edematous plaques involving eyelids, cheeks, and the nose of an elderly febrile male. On palpation the skin is hot and tender.*

ically. Higher fever (38.5°C) and chills usually associated with GAS.

Previous Treatment   Prior episode(s) of cellulitis in an area of lymphedema

Drug Ingestion   IVDU

Immune Status   Immunocompromised patients susceptible to infection with bacteria of low pathogenicity

History   Local pain and tenderness. Necrotizing infections associated with more local pain and systemic symptoms.

Physical Examination

Skin Lesions

TYPE   *Portals of Entry*   Breaks in skin, ulcers, chronic dermatosis
  Plaque   Red, hot, edematous and shiny, and very tender area of skin of varying size (Figures 24-7 and 24-8); borders usually sharply defined, irregular, and slightly elevated; bluish purple color with *H. Influenzae*. Vesicles, bullae, erosions, abscesses, hemorrhage, and necrosis may form in plaque. Lymphangitis.

DISTRIBUTION   *Adults*   Lower leg: most common site, following interdigital tinea (Figure 24-8). Arm: in young male, consider IV drug use; in female; postmastectomy. Trunk: operative wound site (Figure 24-9). Face: following rhinitis, conjunctivitis (Figure 24-7)
  Children   Cheek, periorbital area, head, neck most common: usually *H. Influenzae* (Figure 24-10). Extremities: *S. aureus,* group A streptococci.

LYMPH NODES   Can be enlarged and tender, regionally

Variants

S. *AUREUS* CELLULITIS   Often a portal of entry is apparent; usually a focal infection. Most common pathogen in injection drug user. Toxin syndromes (scalded-skin syndrome, toxic shock syndrome) may occur. Endocarditis may follow bacteremia.

ERYSIPELAS   Usually caused by GAS. Most common cause of virulent soft tissue infection in a healthy host sometimes without evident portal of entry. Superficial type of cellulitis involving lymphatics. Margin of lesion is raised, sharply demarcated from adjacent normal skin, often painful (Figures 24-7 and 24-8). Sites of predilection: face, lower legs, areas of preexisting lymphedema, umbilical stump.

GBS   Colonizes anogenital region. Causes anogenital cellulitis, which may extend into pelvic tissues. Following childbirth, known as *puerperal sepsis.*

STREPTOCOCCUS   PNEUMONIAE   CELLULITIS   Occurs more commonly in individuals with systemic lupus erythematosus with complement deficiency, HIV disease, corticosteroid therapy, drug or alcohol abuse. Infected sites show bulla formation, brawny erythema, violaceous hue.

ERYSIPELOID   *Erysipelothrix   rhusiopathiae* cellulitis on hand, especially finger after handling saltwater fish, shellfish, meat, hides, poultry. Violaceous erythema. Spreads slowly. Usually no systemic symptoms. Uncommonly, associated with bacteremia and aortic valvulitis (see Section 23, page 618 and Figure 23-11).

ECTHYMA GANGRENOSUM   *P. aeruginosa* most common etiology. Usually neutropenic. Site very painful. Inflammatory area shows necrosis related to septic vasculitis; epidermis sloughs with large eroded/ulcerated areas (Figure 24-19). Most common sites: anogenital, axilla. Extends rapidly. Bacteremia common.

H. *INFLUENZAE* CELLULITIS   Occurs mainly in young children <2 years of age. Cheek, periorbital area, head, neck most common sites (Figure 24-10). Clinically, swelling, characteristic violaceous erythema hue. Use of Hib vaccine has dramatically reduced incidence.

V. *VULNIFICUS* CELLULITIS   Underlying disorders: cirrhosis, diabetes, immunosuppres-

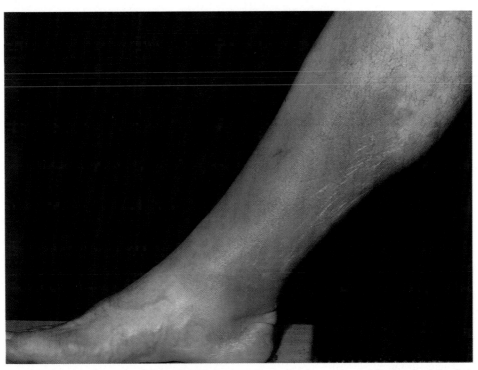

Figure 24-8 Erysipelas: group A steptococcus *Extensive, brawny, painful, sharply defined, erythematous edema of the leg and ankle; the portal of entry was erosive interdigital tinea pedis.*

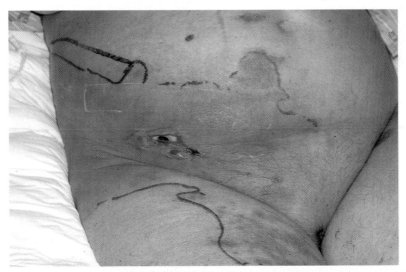

Figure 24-9 Cellulitis at operative site: E. coli *Following a lymph node biopsy in an elderly female with lymphoma, bright erythema and edema arose at the operative site, extending centrifugally rapidly, associated with high fever. The blue ink outlines the maximal extent of erythema prior to initiation of antibiotic therapy.*

sion. Follows ingestion of raw/undercooked seafood, gastroenteritis, bacteremia with seeding of skin; also exposure of skin to sea water. Characterized by bulla formation, necrotizing vasculitis (Figure 24-11). Usually on the extremities; often bilateral.

A. HYDROPHILA CELLULITIS Exposure to fresh water; preexisting wound. Lower leg. NSI

CAPNOCYTOPHAGA CANIMORSUS Immunosuppression or asplenia; exposure to a dog

PASTEURELLA MULTOCIDA Follows cat bite

CLOSTRIDIAL SPECIES CELLULITIS Associated with trauma, contamination by soil or feces, malignant intestinal tumor. Infection may be characterized by gas, marked systemic toxicity.

M. CHELONEI–M. FORTUITUM COMPLEX CELLULITIS History of recent surgery, injection, penetrating wound. Low-grade cellulitis. Systemic findings lacking.

CRYPTOCOCCAL CELLULITIS Patient always immunocompromised. Red, hot, tender, edematous plaque on extremity. Rarely multiple noncontiguous sites.

NECROTIZING SOFT TISSUE INFECTIONS (NSI) Differ from other variants because of significant tissue necrosis (Figure 24-12), lack of response to antimicrobial treatment alone, and need for surgical debridement of devitalized tissues. Starts with erythema and painful induration of underlying soft tissues; rapid development of black eschar which transforms into liquefied black and malodorous necrotic mass. Divided into three categories: *necrotizing cellulitis, necrotizing fasciitis, myonecrosis.* In that presence of fascial necrosis can be determined only by surgical exploration and histopathologic examination of involved tissue, necrotizing cellulitis cannot be differentiated from necrotizing fasciitis on clinical grounds alone. NSI in the genital area is called Fournier's gangrene.

Differential Diagnosis

Erysipelas/Cellulitis Deep vein thrombosis/thrombophlebitis, stasis dermatitis, early contact dermatitis, giant urticaria, fixed drug eruption, erythema nodosum, erythema migrans (Lyme borreliosis), prevesicular herpes zoster, eosinophilic cellulitis, erysipelas-like lesion of familial Mediterranean fever

Necrotizing Soft Tissue Infections Vasculitis, embolism with infarction of skin, peripheral vascular disease, purpura fulminans, calciphylaxis, warfarin necrosis, traumatic injury, brown recluse spider bite

Laboratory and Special Examinations

Hematology WBC and ESR may be elevated.

Smears Gram's stain of exudate, pus, bulla fluid, aspirate, or touch preparation may show bacteria. GAS: chains of gram-positive cocci. *S. aureus:* clusters of gram-positive cocci. Clostridia: gram-negative rods, few neutrophils.

"Touch" Preparation Lesional skin biopsy specimen touched to microscope slide. Potassium hydroxide applied; examined for yeast and mycelial forms of fungus; detects *Candida, Cryptococcus, Mucor.* Gram's stain: detects bacteria.

Cultures Primary lesion, aspirate or biopsy of leading edge of inflammation, blood; positive in only one-quarter of cases. Fungal and mycobacterial cultures indicated in atypical case. Needle aspiration may be helpful. Culture of lesional biopsy specimen.

Dermatopathology Helpful in ruling out noninfectious inflammatory dermatoses. Histology of excised tissue defines presence and extent of NSI. Helpful with cryptococcal cellulitis. Immunofluorescent staining with polyclonal and monoclonal antibodies to organisms such as GAS may demonstrate GAS in the reticular dermis.

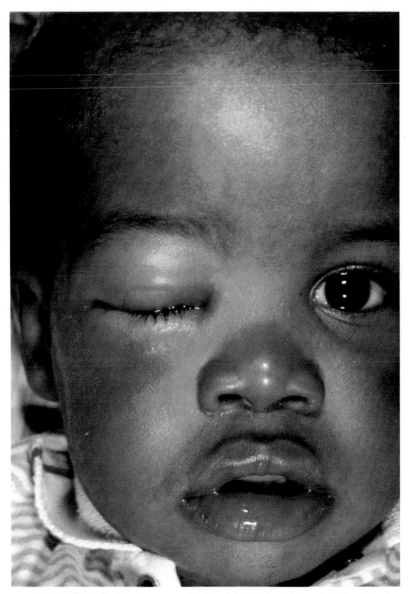

Figure 24-10 Cellulitis: H. influenzae *Erythema and edema of the right side of the face of a young child. (Courtesy of Arthur R. Rhodes, M.D.)*

Imaging MRI may be helpful in diagnosis of severe acute infectious cellulitis, distinguishing pyomyositis, necrotizing fasciitis, and infectious cellulitis with or without subcutaneous abscess formation. X-ray examination of involved sites helpful in identifying soft tissue gas and extensive soft tissue involvement.

Diagnosis

Clinical diagnosis. Confirmed by culture in only 25 % of cases in immunocompetent patients. Suspicion of necrotizing fasciitis requires immediate deep biopsy and frozen-section histopathology.

Pathogenesis

Following entry, infection spreads to tissue spaces and cleavage planes as hyaluronidases break down polysaccharide ground substances, fibrinolysins digest fibrin barriers, lecithinases destroy cell membranes. Local tissue devitalization, e.g., trauma, is usually required to allow for significant anaerobic bacterial infection. The number of infecting organisms is usually small, suggesting that cellulitis may be more a reaction to bacterial superantigens than to overwhelming tissue infection.

Course and Prognosis

Dissemination of infection (lymphatics, hematogenously) with metastatic sites of infection oc-curs if treatment is delayed. Abnormal or synthetic heart valve may be colonized and infected. In preantibiotic era, mortality was very high. Without surgical debridement, necrotizing fasciitis is fatal. If neutropenia exists, prognosis depends on recovery of neutrophil count.

Management

Prophylaxis

INDIVIDUALS WITH PRIOR EPISODES OF CELLULITIS Especially in sites of chronic lymphedema: support stockings, antiseptics to skin, chronic secondary antimicrobial prophylaxis (penicillin G, dicloxacillin, or erythromycin, 500 mg daily)

STATUS POST SAPHENOUS VEIN HARVEST Especially with tinea pedis: Wash with benzoyl peroxide bar daily, followed by application of topical antifungal cream.

PNEUMOCOCCUS Immunize those at risk.

HIB Chemoprophylaxis for household contacts <4 years of age if unimmunized

VIBRIO SPECIES Diabetics, alcoholics, cirrhotics should avoid eating undercooked seafood.

Supportive Rest, immobilization, elevation, moist heat, analgesia

Antimicrobial Therapy (see Table 24-C)

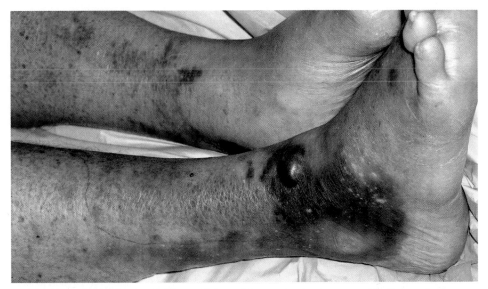

Figure 24-11 Cellulitis: V. vulnificus *Bilateral hemorrhagic plaques and bullae on the legs, ankles, and feet of an older diabetic with cirrhosis. Unlike other types of cellulitis in which microorganisms enter the skin locally, that caused by* V. vulnificus *usually follows a primary enteritis with bacteremia and dissemination to the skin.*

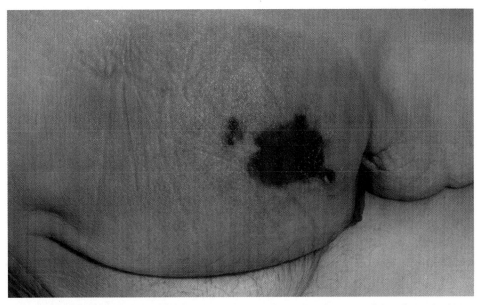

Figure 24-12 Necrotizing fasciitis *Erythematous, edematous plaque involving the entire buttock with rapidly progressive central area of necrosis in an obtunded patient.*

TABLE 24-C ANTIMICROBIAL THERAPY OF CELLULITIS

Infecting Organisms	Drugs of First Choice	Alternative Drugs
Staphylococcus aureus or *epidermidis*		
non-penicillinase-producing	Penicillin G or V	A cephalosporin, vancomycin, imipenem, clindamycin, a fluoroquinolone
Penicillinase-producing	A penicillinase-resistant penicillin	A cephalosporin, vancomycin, amoxicillin/clavulanic acid, ticarcillin/clavulanic acid, piperacillin/tazobactam, ampicillin/sulbactam, imipenem, clindamycin, a fluoroquinolone
Methicillin-resistant	Vancomycin± gentamicin ± rifampin	Trimethoprim-sulfamethoxazole, minocycline, a fluoroquinolone
Streptococcus pyogenes (group A) and groups C and G	Penicillin G or V	An erythromycin, a cephalosporin, vancomycin, clarithromycin, azithromycin, clindamycin
Streptococcus, group B	Penicillin G or ampicillin	A cephalosporin, vancomycin, an erythromycin
Streptococcus pneumoniae	Penicillin G or V	An erythromycin, a cephalosporin, vancomycin, rifampin, trimethoprim-sulfamethoxazole, azithromycin, clarithromycin, clindamycin, chloramphenicol
Hemophilus influenzae	Cefotaxime or ceftriazone	Cefuroxime, chloramphenicol

TABLE 24-C ANTIMICROBIAL THERAPY OF CELLULITIS

Infecting Organisms	Drugs of First Choice	Alternative Drugs
Pseudomonas aeruginosa	Ticarcillin, mezlocillin, or piperacillin + tobramycin, gentamicin, or amikacin	Ceftazidime, imipenem, or aztreonam + tobramycin, gentamicin, or amikacin; a fluoroquinolone
Vibrio vulnificus	A tetracycline	Trimethoprim-sulfamethoxazole, a fluoroquinolone
Aeromonas	Trimethoprim-sulfamethoxazole	Gentamicin or tobramycin, imipenem, a fluoroquinolone
Clostridium perfringens	Penicillin G	Metronidazole, clindamycin, imipenem, a tetracycline, chloramphenicol
Mycobacterium fortuitum (complex)	Amikacin+ doxycycline	Cefoxitin, rifampin, a sulfonamide
Cryptococcus neoformans	Amphotericin B 0.3–0.6 mg/kg intravenously, ±flucytosine	Fluconazole 400 mg orally, daily; itraconazole 200 mg orally, twice daily; amphotericin B 0.5–1 mg/kg intravenously, weekly
Mucormycosis	Amphotericin B 1–1.5 mg/kg/day intravenously	No dependable alternative

SOURCES: The choice of antibacterial drugs. *Med Lett* 1994;36:53–60; Systemic antifungal drugs. *Med Lett* 1994;36:16–18.

SCARLET FEVER

Scarlet fever is an acute infection of the tonsils, skin, or other sites by an erythrogenic exotoxin-producing strain of group A *Streptococcus,* associated with a characteristic toxigenic exanthem.

Epidemiology and Etiology

Age   Children

Etiology   Usually group A beta-hemolytic *Streptococcus pyogenes* (GAS). Uncommonly, exotoxin-producing *Staphylococcus aureus.*

History

Incubation Period   Rash appears within 1 to 3 days after onset of infection.

Exposure   Household member(s) may be a streptococcal carrier.

Physical Examination

Skin Lesions

TYPES   *Site of GAS Infection*   Pharyngitis; tonsillitis. Infected surgical or other wound. Impetiginous skin lesion.

Exanthem   Finely punctate erythema is first noted on the upper part of the trunk. Face becomes flushed but with a perioral pallor. Initial punctate lesions become confluently erythematous, i.e., scarlatiniform. Linear petechiae (Pastia's sign) (Figure 24-13) occur in body folds. Intensity of the exanthem varies from mild to moderate erythema confined to the trunk to an extensive purpuric eruption.

Petechiae   Scattered petechiae occur (Rumpel-Leede test for capillary fragility positive).

Desquamation   Exanthem fades within 4 to 5 days and is followed by brawny desquamation on the body and extremities and by sheetlike exfoliation on the palms (Figure 24-14) and soles. In subclinical or mild infections, exanthem and pharyngi-

tis may pass unnoticed. In this case patient may seek medical advice only when exfoliation on the palms and soles is noted.

COLOR   Pink to scarlet, which is difficult to detect in dark-skinned individuals. Circumoral pallor.

PALPATION   Sandpaper feel as desquamation begins

ARRANGEMENT   Erythema may be accentuated in skin folds such as neck, axillae, groin, antecubital and popliteal fossae (Pastia's lines).

DISTRIBUTION   Erythema first noted on trunk. Spreads to extremities. Erythema accentuated at pressure points and in body folds. Pastia's signs noted in antecubital and axillary folds. Palms/soles usually spared.

MUCOUS MEMBRANES   *Site of GAS Infection* Acute follicular or membranous tonsillitis. May be asymptomatic or mild and go undetected.

Enanthem   Pharynx beefy red. Tongue initially is white with scattered red, swollen papillae (white strawberry tongue). By the fourth or fifth day, the hyperkeratotic membrane is sloughed, and the lingular mucosa appears bright red (red strawberry tongue) (Figure 24-15). Punctate erythema and petechiae may occur in the palate.

Variant   Toxic strep syndrome: toxemia, organ failure, and a scarlatiniform rash associated with GAS cellulitis

General Examination   Patient may appear acutely ill with high fever, headache, nausea, vomiting. Anterior cervical lymphadenitis associated with pharyngitis/tonsillitis.

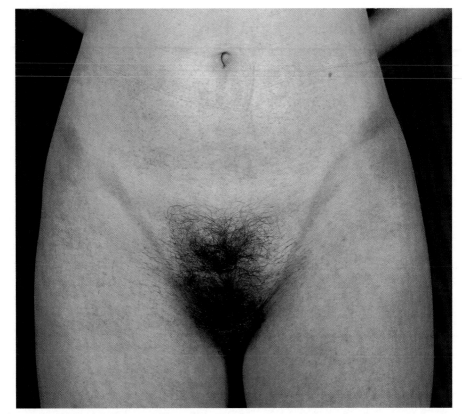

Figure 24-13 Scarlet fever: Pastia's sign *Finely punctate erythema has become confluent (scarlatiniform) on the lower trunk and thighs with petechiae having a linear configuration in the inguinal regions.*

Differential Diagnosis

Generalized Exanthem Staphylococcal scarlet fever (pharyngitis, tonsillitis, strawberry tongue, and palatal enanthem not seen), staphylococcal or streptococcal toxic shock syndrome, Kawasaki's syndrome, viral exanthem, drug eruption

Laboratory and Special Examinations

Gram's Stain Gram-positive cocci in chains (GAS) or clusters (*S. aureus*) identified in smear from infected wound or impetiginized skin lesion

Rapid Direct Antigen Tests (DATs) Used to detect GAS antigens in throat swab specimens

Culture Isolate GAS or *S. aureus* on culture of specimen from throat or wound.

Serology Serologic tests detect immune responses to extracellular products (streptolysin O, hyaluronidase, DNase B, NADase, and streptokinase) and cellular components (M protein, group A antigen) of GAS. Useful in demonstrating antecedent streptococcal infection in individuals who lack documentation of recent GAS infection but who present with nonsuppurative sequelae (rheumatic fever, glomeru-lonephritis).

Test of Historic Interest   Schultz-Carlton re-action: intradermal injection of erythrogenic antitoxin into scarlet fever exanthem causes blanching of rash. Dick test: intradermal injec-tion of erythrogenic toxin produces local ery-thema (positive test, patient lacks erythrogenic antitoxic antibody).

Diagnosis

Clinical findings confirmed by detecting strep-tococcal antigen in a rapid test and/or culturing GAS from throat or wound

Pathophysiology

Erythrogenic toxin production depends on the presence of a temperate bacteriophage. Patients with prior exposure to the erythrogenic toxin have antitoxin immunity and neutralize the toxin. The scarlet fever syndrome therefore does not develop in these patients. Since several ery-throgenic strains of beta-hemolytic *Streptococ-cus* cause infection, it is theoretically possible to have a second episode of scarlet fever. Strains of *S. aureus* can synthesize an erythrogenic ex-otoxin producing a scarlatiniform exanthem.

Course and Prognosis

Production of erythrogenic toxin does not alter the course of the GAS infection. In some cases, GAS may enter the bloodstream with resultant high fever and marked systemic toxicity (toxic scarlet fever) and consequent metastatic foci of infection. Suppurative complications of GAS

infection include peritonsillar cellulitis, peri-tonsillar abscess, retropharyngeal abscess; oti-tis media, acute sinusitis; suppurative cervical lymphadenitis.

Nonsupportive sequelae of streptococcal infec-tions, i.e., acute rheumatic fever, acute glomeru-lonephritis, and erythema nodosum, may follow if the infection goes untreated. The incidence of acute rheumatic fever had markedly decreased during the past two decades but is currently on the rise.

Management

Symptomatic Therapy   Aspirin or acetamino-phen for fever and/or pain

Systemic Antimicrobial Therapy   The goal of therapy is to eradicate GAS throat carriage to prevent rheumatic fever.

DRUG OF CHOICE   Penicillin because of its ef-ficacy in prevention of rheumatic fever.

Penicillin G benzathine: 1.2 million units IM (adults); 600,000 units IM (children <60 lb)
Penicillin V: 250 mg PO q.i.d. for 10 days

PENICILLIN-ALLERGIC PATIENTS

Erythromycin estolate: 20 to 40 mg/kg/day
or
Erythromycin ethylsuccinate: 40 mg/kg/day
Azithromycin, clarithromycin
Cephalosporin (for those who cannot toler-ate oral erythromycin)

Follow-Up   Reculture of throat recommended for individuals with history of rheumatic fever or if a family member has history of rheumatic fever.

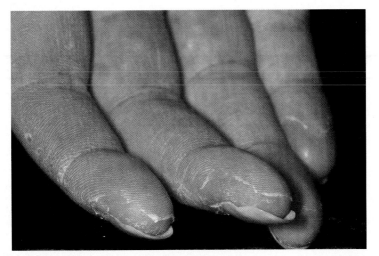

Figure 24-14 Scarlet fever: desquamation *Desquamation of the volar fingertips occurring 10 days after onset of group A streptococcal pharyngitis in an adult female.*

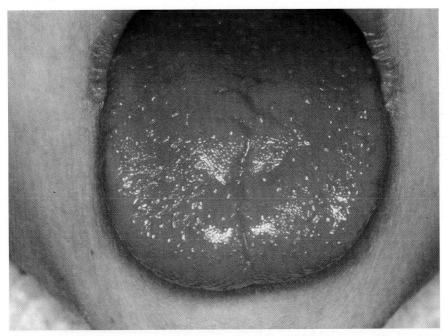

Figure 24-15 Scarlet fever: red strawberry tongue *Bright-red tongue with prominent papillae on the fifth day after onset of group A streptococcal pharyngitis in a child.*

GRAM-NEGATIVE INFECTIONS

MENINGOCOCCEMIA

Meningococcemia is meningococcal bacteremia seeding from the nasopharynx, occurring as acute meningococcal septicemia that may be fulminant (Waterhouse-Friderichsen syndrome), meningococcal meningitis, or chronic meningococcemia, and characterized by fever, petechial or purpuric lesions, hypotension, signs of meningitis, with high morbidity and mortality.

Epidemiology

Age Highest incidence in children aged 6 months to 1 year; lowest in persons over 20 years

Risk Groups Absence of spleen. Alcoholic. Complement deficiency, especially C5 to C8.

Etiology *Neisseria meningitidis,* meningococcus, a gram-negative coccus. Nasopharyngeal carrier rate: 5 % to 15 %.

Transmission Person-to-person through inhalation of droplets of aerosolized infected nasopharyngeal secretions

Season Highest incidence in midwinter, early spring; lowest in midsummer

Geography Worldwide. Occurs in epidemics or sporadically.

History

Prodrome Cough, headache, sore throat, nausea/vomiting. May be very short.

Systems Review

ACUTE MENINGOCOCCEMIA Spiking fever, chills, arthralgia, myalgia. Stupor, hemorrhagic lesions, hypotension may be evident within a few hours of onset of symptoms in fulminant meningococcemia.

CHRONIC MENINGOCOCCEMIA Intermittent fever, rash, myalgia, arthralgia, headache, anorexia

Physical Examination

Appearance Patient appears acutely ill with marked prostration.

Vital Signs High fever, tachypnea, tachycardia, mild hypotension

Skin Lesions

TYPE Characteristically, petechial—small, irregular, "smudged," often raised with pale grayish vesicular centers. Transient urticarial, macular/papular lesions. Discrete pink macules/papules/petechiae (1 to 3 mm) (Figure 24-16) in 75 % of cases. Sparse. May have lighter halo. Fulminant: purpura, ecchymosis and confluent, often bizarre-shaped grayish to black necrosis associated with disseminated intravascular coagulation in fulminant disease (Figure 24-17). Identical to purpura fulminans.

DISTRIBUTION Most commonly, trunk, extremities, but can be anywhere, including palms/soles

MUCOUS MEMBRANES Petechiae on palate

CHRONIC MENINGOCOCCEMIA Intermittent appearance of lesions. Macular and papular lesions, usually distributed about one or more painful joints or pressure points. Erythema nodosum-like lesions on calves. Petechiae, which may evolve to vesicles or pustules. Minute hemorrhage with paler areola. Purpuric areas with pale blue-gray centers; hemorrhagic tender nodules.

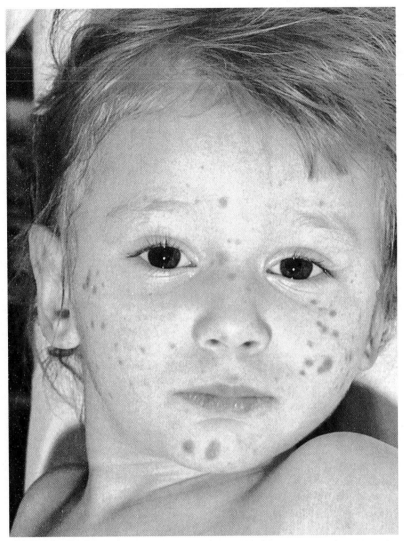

Figure 24-16 Acute meningococcemia *Discrete, pink-to-purple macules and papules as well as purpura on the face of this young child. These lesions represent early disseminated intravascular coagulation with its cutaneous manifestation purpura fulminans.*

General Examination

Meningitis 50 % to 88 % of patients with meningococcemia develop meningitis. Signs of meningeal irritation, altered consciousness. Agitated, maniacal behavior. Signs of increased intracranial pressure.

Rarely Septic arthritis, purulent pericarditis, bacterial endocarditis

Variants Fulminant meningococcemia with adrenal hemorrhage (Waterhouse-Friderichsen syndrome)

Chronic Meningococcemia Intermittent fever, arthritis/arthralgia

Differential Diagnosis

Acute Meningococcemia and Meningitis Acute bacteremias and endocarditis, acute "hypersensitivity" vasculitis, enteroviral infections, Rocky Mountain spotted fever, toxic shock syndrome

Chronic Meningococcemia Subacute bacterial endocarditis, acute rheumatic fever, Henoch-Schönlein purpura, rat-bite fever, erythema multiforme, gonococcemia

Laboratory and Special Examinations

Dermatopathology In chronic meningococcemia, no bacteria demonstrable. Mononuclear perivascular infiltrate. Lesions probably immune-mediated.

Gram's Stain Scrapings from nodular lesions show gram-negative diplococci.

Laboratory Examination of Blood Polymorphous leukocytosis

Cultures Blood culture: acute meningococcemia, meningococcus in nearly 100 %; meningitis one-third positive. CSF culture: usually positive. Skin biopsy culture: up to 85 %.

Diagnosis

Clinical impression confirmed by cultures

Pathophysiology

Primary focus is usually a subclinical nasopharynx infection. Hematogenous dissemination seeds the skin and meninges. Endotoxin felt to be involved in hypotension and vascular collapse. Disseminated intravascular coagulation seen in fulminant meningococcemia similar to Schwartzman reaction. Meningococci are found within endothelial and PMN cells. Local endothelial damage, thrombosis, and necrosis of the vessel walls occur. Edema, infarction of overlying skin, and extravasation of RBC are responsible for the characteristic macular, papular, petechial, hemorrhagic, and bullous lesions. Similar vascular lesions occur in the meninges and in other tissues. The frequency of hemorrhagic cutaneous manifestations in meningococcal infections, compared with infections with other gram-negative organisms, may be due to increased potency and/or unique properties of meningococcal endotoxins for the dermal reaction. On the other hand, lipopolysaccharide (LPS) endotoxins from meningococci and *Escherichia coli* are equally potent producers of the generalized Schwartzman reaction and lethality in mice. In chronic meningococcemia, usually during periodic fevers, rash, and joint manifestations, meningococci can be isolated from the blood; unusual host-parasite relationship is central to this persistent infection.

Course and Prognosis

Acute Meningococcemia Untreated, ends fatally. Adequately treated, recovery rate for meningitis or meningococcemia is >90 %. Mortality for severe disease or Waterhouse-Friderichsen syndrome remains very high. Prognosis is poor when purpura/ecchymosis is present at time of diagnosis.

Chronic Meningococcemia Untreated, may recur over a few weeks to 8 months; average

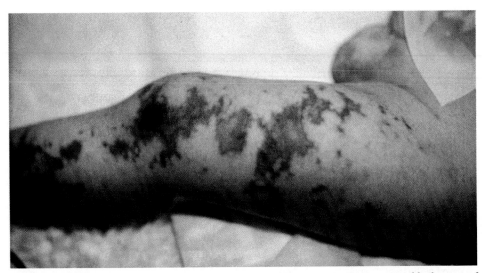

Figure 24-17 Acute meningococcemia: purpura fulminans *Maplike, gray-to-black areas of cutaneous infarction of the leg in a child with* N. meningitidis *meningitis and disseminated intravascular coagulation.*

duration 6 to 8 weeks; may evolve into acute meningococcemia, meningitis, endocarditis; 100 % cure with antibiotics.

Management

Immunization <20 % of meningococcal isolates from associated disease belong to serogroups for which vaccines are available.

Prophylaxis of Contacts of Primary Cases of Meningococcemia

SULFADIAZINE Sulfonamide prophylaxis has been abandoned because of sulfa-resistant meningococcal strains.

RIFAMPIN 600 mg b.i.d. in adults, 10 mg/kg/day as two equal portions in children 1 to 12 years, or 5 mg/kg/day as two equal portions for newborns for 2 days. Alternatively, minocycline 100 mg b.i.d. for 5 days in adults. Ciprofloxacin is also effective.

Antimicrobial Therapy

PENICILLIN G 300,000 units/kg/day IV up to 24 million units/day. Alternatives: ceftriaxone, cefotaxime.

AMPICILLIN IV for 10 days

CHLORAMPHENICOL In penicillin-allergic individuals

CAT-SCRATCH DISEASE

Cat-scratch disease (CSD) is a benign, self-limiting zoonotic infection characterized by a primary skin or conjunctival lesion, following cat scratches or contact with a cat, and subsequent acute to subacute tender regional lymphadenopathy.

Synonyms: Cat-scratch fever, benign lymphoreticulosis, nonbacterial regional lymphadenitis.

Epidemiology and Etiology

Age   Majority of cases <21 years

Sex   More common in males than in females

Etiology   Several subspecies of *Bartonella henselae* (formerly *Rochalimaea henselae*). Uncommonly, *Afipia felis* (formerly cat-scratch disease bacillus).

Transmission   History of cat contact in 90 % of cases; of these individuals, 75 % have history of scratch, bite, or lick. Blood cultures of kittens frequently are positive for *B. henselae.* Adult cats are blood culture–negative but are *B. henselae*–seropositive. Familial cases may occur shortly after addition of a kitten to the household.

Season   Late fall, winter, or early spring in cooler climes; July and August in warmer climes

Geography   Worldwide

Incidence   20,000 cases annually in the United States, of whom 2000 are hospitalized.

History

Incubation Period   Primary lesion at bite/scratch site: 1 to 8 weeks. Regional lymphadenopathy: 5 to 50 days after primary lesion appears.

Duration of Lesions   A local primary lesion occurs within 2 weeks at the site of scratch or injury in about half of patients.

Prodrome   Mild fever and malaise occur in less than half the patients. Chills, general aching, and nausea are infrequently present.

Physical Examination

Skin Lesions

TYPE   Innocuous-looking, small (1.5 cm) papule, vesicle, or pustule at the inoculation site; may ulcerate. Residual linear cat scratch. Associated regional lymphadenitis (Figure 24-18).

COLOR   Skin color pink to red

PALPATION   Firm, at times tender

DISTRIBUTION   Primary lesion on exposed skin of head, neck, extremities

MUCOUS MEMBRANES   If portal of entry is the conjunctiva, 3- to 5-mm whitish yellow granulation on palpebral conjunctiva associated with tender preauricular and/or cervical lymphadenopathy; referred to as the *oculoglandular syndrome of Parinaud.*

OTHER SKIN FINDINGS   Urticaria, transient maculopapular eruption, vesiculopapular lesions, erythema nodosum

HIV-INFECTED PATIENTS   Many develop bacillary angiomatosis, cutaneous hemangiomas that resemble Kaposi's sarcoma. Lesions vary in number from a few scattered to hundreds of generalized lesions.

General Examination   Regional lymphadenopathy (Figure 24-18) evident within a few days to a few weeks after the primary lesion. Nodes are usually solitary, moderately tender, freely movable. Nodes may suppurate. Generalized lymphadenopathy or involvement of the lymph nodes of more than one region is unusual. Less common: encephalitis, pneumonitis, thrombocytopenia, osteomyelitis, hepatitis, abscesses in liver or spleen.

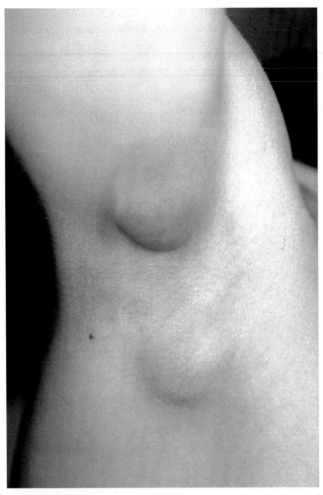

Figure 24-18 Cat-scratch disease *Acute, very tender, axillary lymphadenopathy in a child; cat scratches were present on the dorsum of the ipsilateral hand. (Courtesy of Howard Heller, M.D.)*

Differential Diagnosis

Regional Lymphadenopathy, ±Distal Cutaneous Lesion Suppurative bacterial lymphadenitis, atypical mycobacteria, sporotrichosis, tularemia, toxoplasmosis, infectious mononucleosis, tumors, sarcoidosis, lymphogranuloma venereum, coccidioidomycosis

Other Cat-Associated Infections *Pasteurella multocida* bite infection, *Capnocytophaga* (DF-2) spp. bite infection, sporotrichosis, *Microsporum canis* dermatophytosis, *Toxocara*

cata (larva migrans), *Dirofilaria repens* subcutaneous nodules

Laboratory and Special Examinations

Hematology WBC usually normal; ESR commonly elevated

Dermatopathology Primary lesion: mid-dermal, small areas of frank necrosis surrounded by necrobiosis and palisaded histiocytes; multinucleated giant cells and eosinophils also may be seen. Demonstration of small, pleomorphic bacilli in Warthin-Starry–stained sections of primary skin lesion, conjunctiva, or lymph nodes

Culture   Isolation of *B. henselae* from lymph node aspirates is seldom possible, perhaps because the strains of *Bartonella* causing CSD are more fastidious than those which cause bacteremia or because the lymph node aspirates contain few viable bacteria.

Serology   Antibodies to *B. henselae* usually positive ≥1:64

Polymerase Chain Reaction (PCR)   *B. henselae* DNA detected in aspirates of pus from involved lymph nodes in 96 % of cases

Diagnosis

The diagnosis of CSD is suggested by regional lymphadenopathy developing over a 2- to 3-week period in an individual with cat contact and a primary lesion at the site of contact and can be confirmed by identification of *B. henselae* from tissue or serodiagnosis

Course and Prognosis

Self-limiting, usually within 1 to 2 months. Uncommonly, prolonged morbidity with persistent high fever, suppurative lymphadenitis, severe systemic symptoms. Uncommonly, cat-scratch encephalopathy occurs. Antibiotic therapy has not been very effective in altering the course of the infection

Management

Symptomatic in most cases

Antimicrobial Therapy   In comparison with bacillary angiomatosis, which is also caused by *B. henselae,* specific antimicrobial therapies have not proved effective in treatment of CSD.

Surgery   Occasionally, surgical drainage of suppurative node is indicated.

ECTHYMA GANGRENOSUM AND CUTANEOUS *Pseudomonas aeruginosa* INFECTIONS

Ecthyma gangrenosum (EG) is a primary skin infection, most commonly caused by *Pseudomonas aeruginosa,* characterized by a cutaneous infarction progressing to large ulcerated gangrenous lesions. EG occurs most commonly in the setting of profound prolonged neutropenia and is often followed by *P. aeruginosa* bacteremia.

Epidemiology and Etiology

Etiology   Most commonly, the gram-negative bacillus *P. aeruginosa.* Also, *Staphylococcus aureus, Serratia marcescens, Escherichia coli, Neisseria meningitidis, Aeromonas hydrophilia,* and fungi of *Aspergillus* and *Rhyzopus* groups.

Transmission   Pseudomonal carriage increases with length of hospital stay and antibiotic administration. Entry sites for bacteremia at breaks in mucocutaneous barriers: sites of trauma, foreign bodies (IV or urinary catheter), aspiration/aerosolization into respiratory tract, decubitus or skin ulcers, thermal burns.

Risk Factors   Hospitalization; immunocompromise; neutropenia; use of cancer chemotherapy, corticosteroids, antibiotics (recently); catheters (IV, urethral); cancer; debilitation

History

Symptoms   High fever, chills

Immune Status   Often immunocompromised

Physical Findings

Skin Lesions

TYPE   *Ecthyma Gangrenosum*   Begins as erythematous macule (cutaneous ischemic lesion that quickly evolves to an infarction) (Figure 24-19A and 19B). The epidermis overlying the ischemic area forms a bulla. Epidermis eventually sloughs, forming an ulcer. EG usually occurs as solitary lesion but may occur as a few lesions.
   Other Lesions Associated with Pseudomonas Septicemia   "Rose" spotlike lesions: erythematous macules and/or papules on trunk as in typhoid fever; occur with *Pseudomonas* infection of GI tract, i.e., diarrhea, headache, high fever (Shanghai fever). Painful clustered vesicular to bullous lesions: multiple painful nodules representing small embolus type lesions.

GRAM-NEGATIVE WEBSPACE INFECTION   Intertrigo of toe webspaces: green color (Figure 24-20)

COLOR   Initially erythematous progressing to hemorrhagic bluish (so-called gunmetal gray). Fully evolved EG: blackish central necrosis with erythematous halo.

PALPATION   Frequently tender; may be painless

DISTRIBUTION   EG: axillae, groin, perianal; may occur anywhere, including lip and tongue

MUCOUS MEMBRANES   May occur intraorally

General Examination   Bacteremia from EG may be associated with septic shock

Differential Diagnosis

Ischemic/Infarcted Plaque(s)   Other conditions that produce skin lesions by direct involvement of blood vessels such as vasculitis, cryoglobulinemia, fixed drug eruption, pyoderma gangrenosum

Laboratory and Special Examinations

Cultures   In most cases, *P. aeruginosa* can be cultured from both blood and ecthymatous skin lesions. However, EG can remain a localized cutaneous infection, not accompanied by systemic

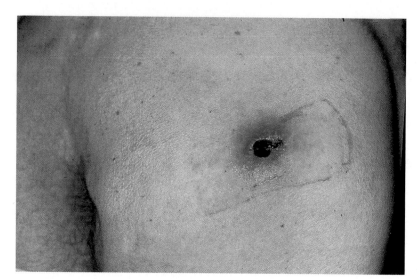

A

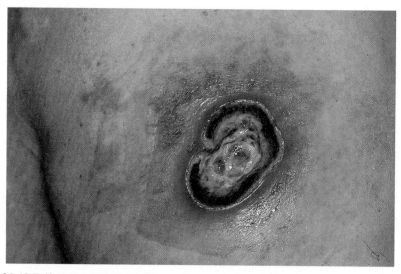

B

Figure 24-19 Ecthyma gangrenosum   A. *An extremely painful, infarcted area with surrounding erythema present for 5 days on the buttock of a neutropenic HIV-infected male. This primary cutaneous infection was associated with bacteremia.* B. *Two weeks later, the lesion had progressed to a large ulceration.*

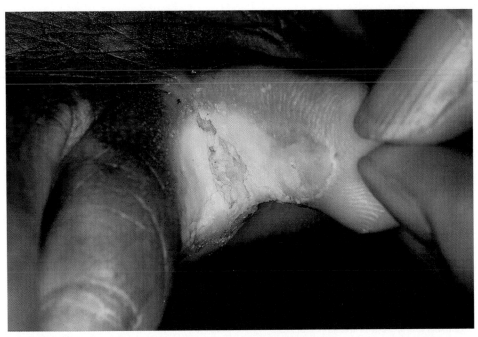

Figure 24-20 Gram-negative webspace infection: P. aeruginosa *Macerated hyperkeratotic, green skin in a webspace of the foot. KOH preparation was negative, as was Wood's lamp examination;* P. aeruginosa *was isolated on culture.*

infection; in this case, only culture of exudate or biopsy specimen from the lesion is positive for *P. aeruginosa.*

Dermatopathology Vasculitis without thrombosis. Paucity of neutrophils at site of infection. Bacilli found in media and adventitia, but usually not in intima, of vessel.

Diagnosis

Clinical suspicion confirmed by blood and skin exudate/biopsy specimen culture

Pathophysiology

EG is primarily a necrotizing cellulitis. Pseudomonal bacteremia/septicemia occurs following vascular invasion with seeding from cutaneous sites. EG follows an impaired immune function in the host rather than spread from individual to individual or increased pathogenicity.

Course and Prognosis

Prognosis depends on prompt restoration of altered immunity, usually on correction of neutropenia. When occurring as a local infection in the absence of bacteremia, prognosis is much more favorable.

Management

Antimicrobial Therapy Antibiotic and dosage are adjusted according to sensitivities and results of cultures.

Surgery Following control of infection, areas of infarction should be debrided.

MYCOBACTERIAL INFECTIONS

LEPROSY

Leprosy is a chronic granulomatous disease caused by *Mycobacterium leprae* and principally acquired during childhood or young adulthood. The skin, mucous membrane of the upper respiratory tract, and peripheral nerves are the major sites of involvement in all forms of leprosy. The clinical manifestations, natural history, and prognosis of leprosy are related to the host response, and the various types of leprosy (tuberculoid, lepromatous, etc.) represent the spectra of the host's immunologic response (cell-mediated immunity).
Synonym: Hansen's disease

Clinicopathologic Classification of Leprosy

(Based on clinical, immunologic, and bacteriologic findings.)

Tuberculoid (TL) Localized skin involvement and/or peripheral nerve involvement; few organisms are present in the skin biopsies.

Lepromatous (LL) Generalized involvement including skin, upper respiratory mucous membrane, the reticuloendothelial system, adrenal glands, and testes; many bacilli are present in tissue.

Borderline (or "Dimorphic") (BL) Has features of both tuberculoid and lepromatous leprosy. Usually many bacilli present, varied skin lesions: macules, plaques; progresses to tuberculoid or regresses to lepromatous.

Indeterminate and Transitional Forms (See Pathophysiology below.)

Epidemiology and Etiology

Etiology *M. leprae* is a slender, straight, or slightly curved, acid-fast rod, about 3.0 by 0.5 μm. The organism cannot be cultured in vitro.

Hosts Humans are the main reservoirs of *M. leprae.* Wild armadillos (Louisiana) as well as mangabey monkeys and the chimpanzee are naturally infected with *M. leprae*; armadillos can develop lepromatous lesions.

Transmission Mode of transmission of *M. leprae* is uncertain; however, human-to-human transmission is the norm. The main source of dissemination is individuals with multibacillary-type infection, shedding several millions of bacilli per day from nasal and upper respiratory tract secretions. Portals of entry of *M. leprae* are poorly understood but include ingestion of food or drink, inoculation into or through skin (bites, scratches, small wounds, tattoos), or inhalation into nasal passages or lungs.

Scope of Problem Worldwide (estimated 12 millions); approximately 5.5 million individuals are estimated to require or are receiving chemotherapy for leprosy, of whom 2 to 3 millions have significant disabilities. Fifty-three countries report endemic leprosy. India has approximately 4 million cases.

Geography At present, more prevalent in hot and humid climates (Africa, Southeast Asia, and South and Central America). New lesions may first appear or suddenly flare during the hot, rainy season. The disease is endemic in Texas, southern Louisiana, Hawaii, and California, and immigrants with leprosy are not uncommonly seen in Florida and New York City. There are approximately 2500 patients with leprosy in the continental United States.

Sex Males > females

Race There appears to be an inverse relationship between the skin color and the severity of the disease; in the black African, susceptibility is high, but there is a predominance of milder forms of the disease, i.e., tuberculoid vis-à-vis lepromatous.

Age Incidence rate peaks at 10 to 20 years; prevalence peaks at 30 to 50 years.

Predisposing or Risk Factors (1) Residence in an endemic area, (2) having a blood relative with leprosy, (3) poverty (malnutrition?), and (4) contact with affected armadillos

Pathophysiology

The clinical spectrum of leprosy depends exclusively on variable limitations in the host's capability to develop effective cell-mediated immunity (CMI) to *M. leprae*. The organism is capable of invading and multiplying within peripheral nerves and infecting and surviving within endothelial and phagocytic cells in many organs.

Subclinical infection with leprosy is common among residents in endemic areas. Presumably the subclinical infection is handled readily by the host's CMI response. Clinical expression of leprosy is the development of a granuloma, and the patient may develop a "reactional state," which may occur in some form in over 50 % of certain groups of patients. The granulomatous spectrum of leprosy consists of (1) a high-resistance tuberculid response (TT), (2) a low- or absent-resistance lepromatous pole (LL), (3) a dimorphic or borderline region (BB) and two intermediary regions: (4) borderline lepromatous (BL), and (5) borderline tuberculoid (BT). In order of decreasing resistance, the spectrum is TT, BT, BB, BL, LL.

Immunologic Responses Immune responses to *M. leprae* can produce several types of reactions associated with a sudden change in the clinical status.

LEPRA TYPE 1 REACTIONS (DOWNGRADING AND REVERSAL REACTIONS) Individuals with BT and BL develop inflammation within existing skin lesions: Downgrading reactions occur prior to therapy; reversal reactions occur in response to therapy. Type 1 reactions can be associated with low-grade fever, new

multiple small "satellite" skin maculopapular skin lesions, and/or neuritis.

LEPRA TYPE 2 REACTIONS (ERYTHEMA NODOSUM LEPROSUM) Seen in half of LL patients, usually occurring after initiation of antilepromatous therapy, generally within the first 2 years of treatment. Massive inflammation with erythema nodosum-like lesions (ENL)

LUCIO'S REACTION Individuals with diffuse LL develop shallow, large polygonal sloughing ulcerations on the legs. The reaction appears to be either a variant of erythema nodosum leprosum (ENL) or secondary to arteriolar occlusion. The ulcers heal poorly, recur frequently, and may occur in a generalized distribution. Generalized Lucio's reaction is frequently complicated by secondary bacterial infection and sepsis.

History

Onset Insidious and painless, first affects the peripheral nervous system with persistent or recurrent paresthesias and numbness without any visible clinical signs. At this stage there may be transient macular skin eruptions.

Systems Review Neural involvement leads to muscle weakness, muscle atrophy, severe neuritic pain, and contractures of the hands and feet.

LEPRA TYPE 1 REACTIONS Acute or insidious tenderness and pain along affected nerve(s), associated with loss of function

Physical Examination

Tuberculoid Leprosy

TYPE OF LESION A few well-defined hypopigmented anesthetic macules (Figure 24-21) with raised edges and varying in size from a few millimeters to very large lesions covering the entire trunk

COLOR OF LESION Erythematous or purple border and hypopigmented center

BORDER OF LESION Sharply defined, raised

SHAPE OF LESIONS Often annular

DISTRIBUTION OF LESIONS Any site including the face

NERVE INVOLVEMENT May be a thickened nerve on the edge of the lesion; large peripheral nerve enlargement frequent (ulnar)

Lepromatous Leprosy

TYPES OF LESIONS Small erythematous or hypopigmented macules that are anesthetic; later papules, plaques (Figure 24-22), nodules, and diffuse thickening of the skin, with loss of hair (eyebrows and eyelashes). Facies leonina (lion's face) due to thickening, nodules and plaques distort normal facial features.

COLOR OF LESIONS Normal skin color or erythematous or slightly hypopigmented

DISTRIBUTION OF LESIONS Bilaterally symmetric involving earlobes, face, arms, and buttocks, or less frequently the trunk and lower extremities

MUCOUS MEMBRANES Tongue: nodules, plaques, or fissures

Borderline Leprosy Lesions are intermediate between tuberculoid and lepromatous and comprised of macules, papules, and plaques. Anesthesia and decreased sweating are prominent in the lesions.

Reactional Phenomenon

LEPRA TYPE 1 REACTIONS Skin lesions become acutely inflamed associated with edema and pain; may ulcerate. Edema most severe on face, hands, and feet.

LEPRA TYPE 2 REACTIONS (ENL) Present as painful red skin nodules, arising superficially and deeply; lesions form abscesses or ulcerate. Lesions occur most commonly on face and extensor limbs.

LUCIO'S REACTION Presents as irregularly shaped erythematous plaques; lesions may resolve spontaneously or undergo necrosis with ulceration.

General Findings

EYE The anterior chamber can be invaded in LL with resultant glaucoma and cataract formation. Corneal damage can occur secondary to trichiasis and sensory neuropathy, secondary infection, and muscle paralysis. Uveitis occurs in some individuals with ENL.

TESTES May be involved in LL with resultant hypogonadism

Differential Diagnosis

Tuberculoid Leprosy Epidermal dermatophytosis (tinea corporis), pityriasis alba, pityriasis versicolor, seborrheic dermatitis, vitiligo, morphea, yaws, onchocerciasis, nutritional dyschromia

Lepromatous Leprosy Granuloma annulare, sarcoidosis, cutaneous tuberculosis, atypical mycobacterial infection, Wegener's granulomatosis, post-kala-azar dermal leishmaniasis, neurofibromatosis, necrobiosis lipoidica, Kaposi's sarcoma

Borderline Leprosy Late syphilis, lupus erythematosus, gyrate erythemas, cutaneous leishmaniasis, mycosis fungoides

Peripheral Neuropathy Peroneal muscular atrophy (Charcot-Marie-Tooth disease), Déjerine-Sottas disease (familial hypertrophic interstitial neuritis), primary amyloidosis of peripheral nerves, syringomyelia, tabes dorsalis, hereditary sensory radicular neuropathy, congenital indifference to pain, peripheral neuropathy of varied etiology

Many Acid-Fast Bacilli in Biopsy Specimens of Skin or Other Tissues *M. avium-intracellulare* complex infection in HIV-infected individuals

Laboratory and Special Examinations

Slit-Skin Smears A small skin incision is made; the site is then scraped in order to obtain tissue fluid, which is examined following Ziehl-Neelsen staining. Specimens are usually obtained from both earlobes and two other active lesions. The bacterial index (BI) is computed as shown in Table 24-D.

Negative BIs are seen in paucibacillary cases, treated cases, and cases examined by an inexperienced technician.

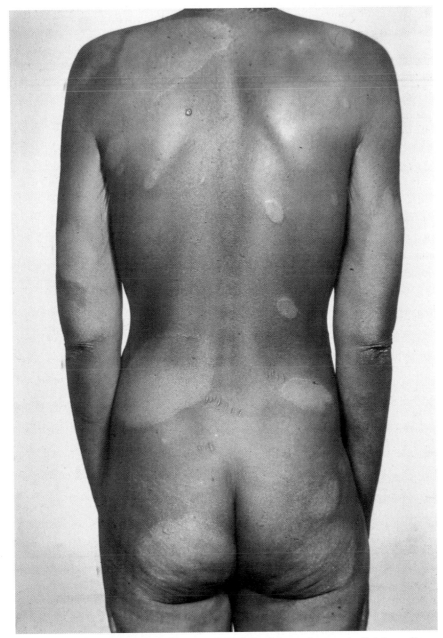

Figure 24-21 Leprosy: tuberculoid type *Well-defined, hypopigmented, slightly scaling, anesthetic macules and plaques.*

Nasal Smears or Scrapings No longer recommended

Culture *M. leprae* has not been cultured in vitro; however, it does grow when inoculated into the mouse foot pad. Routine bacterial cultures to rule out secondary infection.

PCR *M. leprae* DNA detected by this technique makes the diagnosis of early paucibacillary leprosy and identifies *M. leprae* following therapy.

Dermatopathology TL shows epithelioid cell granulomas forming around dermal nerves; AFBs are sparse or absent. LL shows an extensive cellular infiltrate separated from the epidermis by a narrow zone of normal collagen. Skin appendages are destroyed. Macrophages are filled with *M. leprae,* having abundant foamy or vacuolated cytoplasm (lepra cells or Virchow cells).

Diagnosis

Made if one or more of the cardinal findings are detected: skin lesions characteristic of leprosy with diminished or loss of sensation, enlarged peripheral nerves, finding of *M. leprae* in skin or, less commonly, other sites.

Course and Prognosis

After the first few years of drug therapy, the most difficult problem is management of the changes secondary to neurologic deficits—contractures and trophic changes in the hands and feet. This requires a team of health care professionals: orthopedic surgeons, hand surgeons, podiatrists, ophthalmologists, neurologists, physical medicine and rehabilitation professionals, etc. Uncommonly, secondary amyloidosis with renal failure can complicate long-standing leprosy. Lepra type 1 reactions last 2 to 4 months in individuals with BT and up to 9 months in those with BL. Lepra type 2 reactions (ENL) occur in 50 % of individuals with LL and 25 % of those with BL within the first 2 years of treatment. ENL may be complicated by uveitis, dactylitis, arthritis, neuritis, lymphadenitis, myositis, orchitis. Lucio's reaction or phenomenon occurs secondary to vasculitis with subsequent infarction.

Management

The two most widely used drugs are dapsone and rifampin, which are generally available. Clofazimine and thalidomide are available through the National Hansen's Disease Center in Carville, Louisiana.

General principles of management include: eradicate infection with antilepromatous therapy, prevent and treat reactions, reduce the risk of nerve damage, educate patient to deal with neuropathy and anesthesia, treat complications of nerve damage, rehabilitate patient into society.

Antilepromatous Therapy: Multidrug Regimens (Adult Doses)

PAUCIBACILLARY DISEASE (TT AND BT)

Monthly, supervised medication	Rifampin, 600 mg
Daily, unsupervised medication	Dapsone, 100 mg
Duration	6 months; all treatments then stop
Follow-up after stopping treatment	Minimum of 2 years with clinical examinations at least every 12 months

MULTIBACILLARY DISEASE (LL, BL, AND BB)

Monthly, supervised medication	Rifampin, 600 mg Clofazamine, 300 mg
Daily, unsupervised medication	Dapsone, 100 mg Clofazamine, 50 mg
Duration	A minimum of 2 years, but whenever possible until slit-skin smears are negative
Follow-up after stopping treatment	A minimum of 5 years with clinical and bacteriologic examinations at least every 12 months

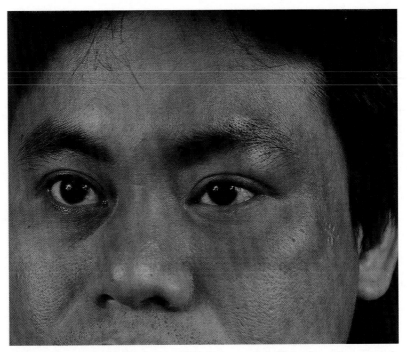

Figure 24-22 Leprosy: borderline type *Well-demarcated, infiltrated, erythematous plaque on the left periorbicular region. The initial diagnosis was erysipelas, which did not respond to antibiotic treatment.*

Therapy of Reactions

<small>LEPRA TYPE 1 REACTIONS</small>

Prednisone 40 to 60 mg daily; the dosage is gradually reduced over a 2- to 3-month period. Indication for prednisone: neuritis, lesions that threaten to ulcerate, lesions appearing at cosmetically important sites (face).

<small>LEPRA TYPE 2 REACTIONS (ENL)</small>

Prednisone 40 to 60 mg daily, tapered fairly rapidly

Thalidomide given for recurrent ENL; 100 to 300 mg h.s.

<small>LUCIO'S REACTION</small> Neither prednisone nor thalidomide is very effective. *Prednisone* 40 to 60 mg daily, tapered fairly rapidly.

Systemic Antimicrobial Agents Secondary infection of ulcerations should be identified and treated with appropriate antibiotics to prevent deeper infections such as osteomyelitis.

Orthopedic Care Splints should be supplied to prevent contractures of denervated regions. Careful attention to foot care to prevent neuropathic ulceration.

TABLE 24-D   BACTERIAL INDEX (BI)—RIDLEY'S LOGARITHMIC SCALE

0	No bacteria seen in 100 fields (oil-immersion)
1+	1–10 bacteria in 100 fields
2+	1–10 bacteria in 10 fields
3+	1–10 bacteria in an average field
4+	10–100 bacteria in an average field
5+	100–1000 bacteria in an average field
6+	Many clumps of bacteria (>1000) in an average field

CUTANEOUS TUBERCULOSIS

Cutaneous tuberculosis (CTb) is highly variable in its clinical presentation, depending on the immunologic status of the patient and the route of inoculation of mycobacteria into the skin.

Classification of Cutaneous Tuberculosis

Exogenous Infection

Primary inoculation tuberculosis (PITb): via percutaneous inoculation occurs at the inoculated site in a nonimmune host.

Tuberculosis verrucosa cutis (TbVC): via percutaneous inoculation occurs at the inoculated site in an individual with prior tuberculosis infection.

Endogenous Spread

Lupus vulgaris (LV)
Scrofuloderma (SD)
Metastatic tuberculosis abscess (MTbA)
Acute miliary tuberculosis (AMTb)
Orificial tuberculosis (OTb)

Tuberculosis due to BCG Immunization

Epidemiology and Etiology

Age AMTb more common in infants and adults with advanced immunodeficiency. PITb more common in infants. SD more common in adolescents, elderly. LV affects all ages.

Sex LV more common in females. TbVC more common in males.

Race Tuberculosis in blacks, in general, less favorable prognosis than in whites

Occupation TbVC: previously in physicians, medical students, and pathologists as verruca necrogenica, anatomist's wart, postmortem wart; in butchers and farmers from *Mycobacterium bovis*

Etiology The obligate human pathogenic mycobacteria: *M. tuberculosis, M. bovis,* and occasionally, bacillus Calmette-Guérin (BCG)

Incidence CTb has declined steadily worldwide, paralleling the decline of pulmonary tuberculosis. Always rare in the United States compared with Europe. Incidence of various types of CTb varies geographically; LV, SD most common types in Europe; LV, verrucous lesions more common in tropics; TbVC a common type in third world countries. Recently, the incidence of CTb has been increasing, often associated with AIDS.

Epidemiology Predisposing factors for tuberculosis include poverty, crowding, HIV infection. The type of clinical lesion depends on the route of cutaneous inoculation and the immunologic status of the host. Cutaneous inoculation results in a tuberculous chancre in the nonimmune host but TbVC in the immune host. Modes of endogenous spread to skin include: direct extension from underlying tuberculous infection, i.e., lymphadenitis or tuberculosis of bones and joints results in SD; lymphatic spread to skin results in LV; hematogenous dissemination results in either AMTb, LV, or MTbA.

Route of Cutaneous Infection May be exogenous, by autoinoculation, or endogenous

Tuberculosis in HIV Disease Tuberculosis is the most common opportunistic infection occurring in HIV-infected individuals who reside in developing nations. Cutaneous tuberculosis has been reported in these individuals. Tuberculosis is an emerging infection in HIV-infected individuals in developed nations; the problem of multidrug resistance is also common in these persons.

Physical Examination

Primary Inoculation Tuberculosis

TYPES OF LESIONS Initially, papule occurs at the inoculation site 2 to 4 weeks after the

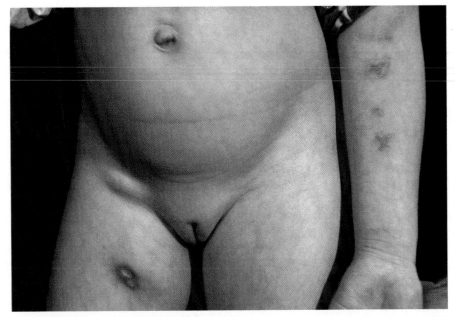

Figure 24-23 Primary inoculation tuberculosis *A large, ulcerated nodule at the site of* M. tuberculosis *inoculation on the right thigh associated with inguinal lymphadenopathy. A positive tuberculin test is demonstrated on the arm.*

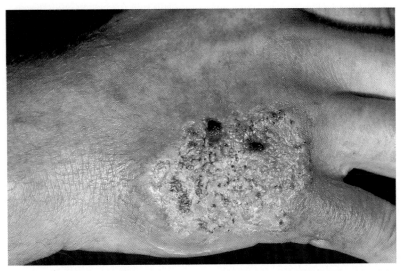

Figure 24-24 Tuberculosis verrucosa cutis *Crusted and hyperkeratotic plaque arising at the site of inoculation in an individual previously infected with* M. tuberculosis. *There is no associated axillary lymphadenopathy.*

wound. Lesion enlarges to a painless ulcer, i.e., a tuberculous chancre (up to 5 cm) (Figure 24-23), with shallow granular base and multiple tiny abscesses or, alternatively, may be covered by thick crust. Undermined margins; older ulcers become indurated with thick crusts. Deeper inoculation results in subcutaneous abscess. Intraoral inoculation results in ulcers on gingiva or palate. Regional lymphadenopathy occurs within 3 to 8 weeks (Figure 24-23).

COLOR OF LESIONS   Ulcer margins reddish blue

DISTRIBUTION OF LESIONS   Most common on exposed skin at sites of minor injuries. Oral lesions occur following ingestion of bovine bacilli in nonpasteurized milk; in the past, lesions in male babies have occurred on the penis after ritual circumcision.

Tuberculosis Verrucosa Cutis

TYPES OF LESIONS   Initial papule with violaceous halo. Evolves to hyperkeratotic, warty, firm plaque (Figure 24-24). Clefts and fissures occur from which pus and keratinous material can be expressed. Border often irregular. Lesions are usually single, but multiple lesions occur. No lymphadenopathy.

COLOR OR LESIONS   Base brownish red to purplish

DISTRIBUTION OF LESIONS   Most commonly on dorsolateral hands and fingers. In children, lower extremities, knees.

Lupus Vulgaris

TYPES OF LESIONS   Initial flat papule is ill-defined and soft and evolves into well-defined, irregular plaque (Figure 24-25). The consistency is characteristically soft; if the lesion is probed, the instrument breaks through the overlying epidermis. Surface is initially smooth or slightly scaly but may become hyperkeratotic. Hypertrophic forms result in soft tumorous nodules. Ulcerative forms present as punched-out, often serpiginous ulcers surrounded by soft, brownish infiltrate. Involvement of underlying cartilage but not bone results in its destruction (ears, nose). Scarring is prominent, and character-

istically, new brownish infiltrates occur within the atrophic scars.

COLOR OF LESIONS   Reddish brown. Diascopy (i.e., the use of a glass slide pressed against the skin) reveals an "apple jelly" (i.e., yellowish brown) color.

DISTRIBUTION OF LESIONS   Usually solitary, but several sites may occur. Most lesions on the head and neck, most often on nose and ears or scalp. Lesions on trunk and extremities rare. Disseminated lesions after severe viral infection (measles) (*lupus postexanthematicus*).

Scrofuloderma

TYPES OF LESIONS   Firm subcutaneous nodule that initially is freely movable; the lesion then becomes doughy and evolves into an irregular, deep-seated node or plaque that liquefies and perforates (Figure 24-26). Ulcers and irregular sinuses, usually of linear or serpiginous shape, discharge pus or caseous material. Edges are undermined, inverted, and dissecting subcutaneous pockets alternate with soft, fluctuating infiltrates and bridging scars.

COLOR OF LESIONS   Reddish blue, brownish

DISTRIBUTION OF LESIONS   SD most often occurs in the parotidal, submandibular, and supraclavicular regions; lateral neck; SD most often results from continuous spread from affected lymph nodes or tuberculous bones (phalanges, sternum, ribs) or joints.

Metastatic Tuberculosis Abscess

TYPES OF LESIONS   Also called *tuberculous gumma.* Subcutaneous abscess, nontender, "cold," fluctuant. Coalescing with overlying skin, breaking down and forming fistulas and ulcers.

COLOR OF LESIONS   Initially normal skin color, later reddish blue

DISTRIBUTION OF LESIONS   Single or multiple lesions, often at sites of previous trauma

Acute Miliary Tuberculosis

TYPES OF LESIONS   Exanthem. Disseminate lesions are minute macules and papules or pur-

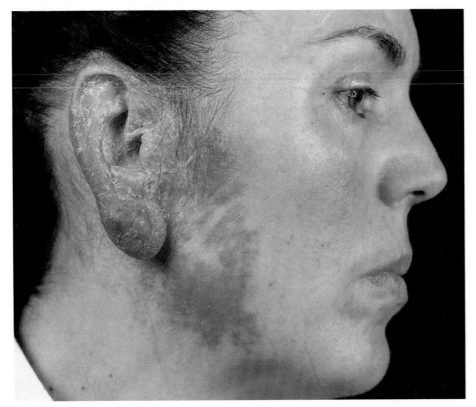

Figure 24-25 Lupus vulgaris *Reddish-brown plaque which on diascopy exhibits the diagnostic yellow-brown apple-jelly color. Note nodular infiltration of the earlobe, scaliness of the helix, and atrophic scarring in the center of the plaque.*

puric lesions. Sometimes vesicular and crusted. Removal of crust reveals umbilication.

COLOR OF LESIONS   Red or purpuric

DISTRIBUTION OF LESIONS   Disseminated on all parts of the body, particularly the trunk

Orificial Tuberculosis

TYPES OF LESIONS   Small yellowish nodule on mucosa breaks down to form painful circular or irregular ulcer (Figure 24-27) with undermined borders and pseudomembranous material, yellowish tubercles, and eroded vessels at its base. Surrounding mucosa swollen, edematous, and inflamed.

COLOR OF LESIONS   Initially yellowish; ulcer red, hemorrhagic, and purulent

DISTRIBUTION OF LESIONS   Since OTb results from autoinoculation of mycobacteria from progressive tuberculosis of internal organs, it is usually found on the oral, pharyngeal (pulmonary tuberculosis), vulvar (genitourinary tuberculosis), and anal (intestinal tuberculosis) mucous membranes. Lesions may be single or multiple, and in the mouth most often occur on the tongue, soft and hard palate, or lips. OTb may occur in a tooth socket following tooth extraction.

Differential Diagnosis

Primary Inoculation Tuberculosis   Chancriform syndrome: primary syphilis with chancre, cat-scratch disease, sporotrichosis, tularemia, *M. marinum* infection

Tuberculosis Verrucosa Cutis Verruca vulgaris, *M. marinum* infection, pyoderma, blastomycosis, chromomycosis, bromoderma, hypertrophic lichen planus, SCC

Lupus Vulgaris Sarcoidosis, lymphocytoma, lymphoma, chronic cutaneous lupus erythematosus, tertiary syphilis, leprosy, blastomycosis, lupoid leishmaniasis, pyodermas

Scrofuloderma Invasive fungal infections, sporotrichosis, nocardiosis, actinomycosis, tertiary syphilis, acne conglobata, hidradenitis suppurativa

Metastatic Tuberculosis Abscess Panniculitis, invasive fungal infections, hidradenitis, tertiary syphilis

Orificial Tuberculosis Aphthous ulcers, histoplasmosis, syphilis, SCC

Laboratory and Special Examinations

Dermatopathology PITb: initially nonspecific inflammation; after 3 to 6 weeks, epithelioid cells, Langhans giant cells, lymphocytes, caseation necrosis. AMTb: nonspecific inflammation and vasculitis. All other forms of CTb show more or less typical tuberculous histopathology; TbVC is characterized by massive pseudoepitheliomatous hyperplasia of epidermis and abscesses. Mycobacteria are found in PITb, SD, AMTb, MTbA, OTb, but only with difficulty or not at all in LV and TbVC.

Culture Yields mycobacteria also from lesions of LV and TbVC

PCR Can be used to identify *M. tuberculosis* DNA in tissue specimens

Skin Testing PITb: Patient converts from intradermal skin test negative to positive during the first weeks of the infection. AMTb: usually negative. SD, MTbA, and OTb: may be negative or positive depending on state of immunity. LV and TbVC: positive.

Diagnosis

Clinical, histologic findings, confirmed by isolation of *M. tuberculosis* on culture

Pathophysiology

The clinical lesions occurring in the skin depend on whether the host has had prior infection with *M. tuberculosis,* and therefore delayed hypersensitivity to the organism, and the inoculation route and mode of spread.

Course and Prognosis

The course of CTb is quite variable, depending on the type of cutaneous infection, amount of inoculum, extent of extracutaneous infection, age of the patient, immune status, and therapy. PITb: without treatment, usually resolves within 12 months, with some residual scarring. Rarely, LV develops at site of PITb. Tuberculosis due to BCG immunization: depends on general state of immunity. It may assume appearance and course of PITb, LV, or SD; in the immune compromised it may lead to MTbA or AMTb.

Management

Only PITb and TbVC limited to the skin. All other patterns of CTb are associated with systemic infection that has disseminated secondarily to the skin. As such, therapy should be aimed at achieving a cure, avoiding relapse, and preventing emergence of drug-resistant mutants.

Antituberculous Therapy Prolonged antituberculous therapy with at least two drugs is indicated for all cases of CTb except for TbVC that can be excised. Isoniazid and rifampin, supplemented with ethambutol, streptomycin or pyrizinamid in the initial phases. Isoniazid and rifampin for at least 9 months; can be shortened to 6 months if four drugs are given during the first 2 months.

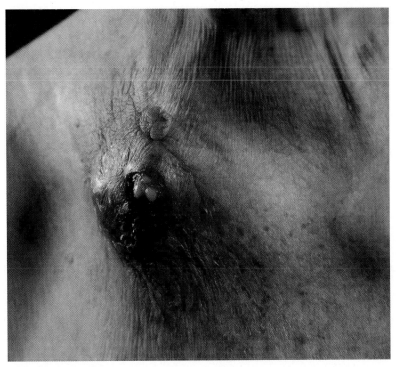

Figure 24-26 Scrofuloderma *Large abscess near the clavicular head, which upon pressure extrudes pus and caseous material. A tuberculous lymphadenitis undergoes necrosis with abscess formation, subsequently draining to the skin surface.*

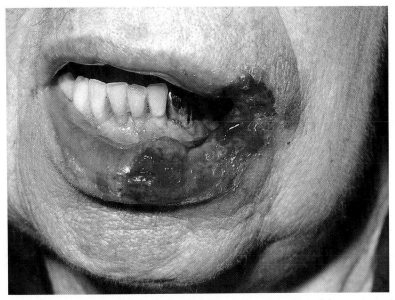

Figure 24-27 Orificial tuberculosis *A large, painful ulcer on the lips of this patient with advanced cavitary pulmonary tuberculosis.*

CUTANEOUS ATYPICAL MYCOBACTERIAL INFECTIONS

Mycobacteria other than *Mycobacterium tuberculosis* (MOTT) ("atypical" mycobacteria) are environmental mycobacteria, commonly found in water and soil, and have low-grade pathogenicity. Unlike tuberculosis and leprosy, infection is acquired from environmental exposure; person-to-person transmission does not occur. MOTT that most often cause cutaneous infection include *M. marinum, M. ulcerans,* and *M. fortuitum* complex.

Classification of MOTT

Group I	Photochromogens
	M. marinum
	M. kansasii
	M. simiae
Group II	Scotochromogens
	M. scrofulaceum
	M. flavescens
	M. szulgai
Group III	Nonchromogens
	M. ulcerans
	M. avium-intracellulare complex (MAC)
	M. gastrii
	M. terrae
	M. triviale
	M. xenopi
	M. haemophilum
	M. novum
	M. nonchromogenicum
Group IV	Rapid growers
	M. fortuitum complex
	M. fortuitum
	M. chelonae
	M. abscessus
	M. phlei
	M. vaccae
	M. smegmatis
	M. diernhoferi

Mycobacterium marinum INFECTION

M. marinum infections follow traumatic inoculation while the exposed skin is in an aqueous environment, whether a fish tank, swimming pool, or brackish water, and is characterized clinically by an inflammatory verrucous or crusted lesion at the inoculation site, and in some cases lymphangitic spread.
Synonyms: Swimming pool granuloma, fish tank granuloma.

Epidemiology and Etiology

Age   Second to fourth decades

Sex   Males>females

Etiology   *M. marinum*

Occupation   Occupation or avocation around water, maintenance of fish tank

Transmission   Traumatic inoculation into skin during aquatic activity

Season   Swimming pool granuloma usually begins in summertime. Fish tank granuloma, no seasonal variation.

History

Incubation Period   Very variable. Most commonly few weeks to few months following inoculation.

Duration of Lesions   Months to years

History   Lesion at site of injury while in aqueous environment. Most commonly, asymptomatic. Afebrile. Cosmetic inconvenience. Possible local tenderness; limitation of movement if lesion over a joint; itching; painful when bumped.

Physical Examination

Skin Lesions

TYPES   At site of inoculation, papule(s) enlarging to inflammatory nodule or plaque 1 to 4 cm in size. Surface of lesions may be scaling (hyperkeratotic) or verrucous (Figure 24-28). Lesions may become ulcerated and have a superficial crust, granulation tissue base, ±serosanguineous or purulent discharge. In some cases, small satellite papules, draining sinuses, fistulas may develop. Atrophic scarring follows spontaneous regression or successful therapy.

Sporotrichoid Pattern   Subcutaneous or intradermal cystlike swelling may occur, 1.5 to 2.0 cm in diameter, some distance proximal to the original lesions. Deep-seated nodules in a linear configuration on hand and forearm exhibit sporotrichoid spread. Boggy inflammatory reaction may mimic bursitis, synovitis, or arthritis about the elbow, wrist, or interphalangeal joints.

Disseminated Cutaneous Infection   Distinctly rare

COLOR   Inflammatory (red to red-brown).

ARRANGEMENT   Usually solitary lesions at sites of inoculation (trauma) such as over a knuckle on the hand. Linear arrangement with sporotrichoid pattern on forearm and upper arm.

DISTRIBUTION   Usually solitary, over bony prominence; may be multiple. Following trauma while swimming: most commonly on elbow, finger, knee; less commonly on ankle, toe or foot, leg, neck. Following aquarium exposure: most commonly on right hand.

General Examination

LYMPH NODES   Regional lymphadenopathy and lymphangitis

Differential Diagnosis

Solitary Verrucous or Ulcerated Lesion on Extremity   Verruca vulgaris, sporotrichosis, blastomycosis, erysipeloid, tularemia, *M. tuberculosis* (tuberculosis verrucosa cutis), nocardiosis, leishmaniasis, syphilis, yaws, iododerma, bromoderma, foreign-body response to sea urchin or barnacle, benign or malignant skin tumors

Sporotrichoid Lesion Staphylococcal or group A streptococcal lymphangiitis, sporotrichosis, tularemia, leishmanisis, nocardiosis, actinomycosis

Laboratory and Special Examinations

Skin Tests Intradermal testing with purified protein derivative standard (PPD-S) often positive.

Skin Biopsy Suggestive but not pathognomonic. Early: dermal inflammatory reaction with lymphocytes, polymorphonuclear cells, histiocytes. Epidermal hyperkeratosis and acanthosis may be seen. Older lesions: More typical tuberculoid architecture is developed with epithelioid cells and Langhans giant cells. No typical caseation necrosis. Acid-fast stain demonstrates *M. marinum* only in approximately 50 % of cases.

Smears of Exudate or Pus Acid-fast bacilli can be demonstrated in some cases.

Culture Culture at 32°C. Lesional biopsy specimen should be ground in saline solution with mortar and pestle or material secured by swab inoculated on Loewenstein-Jensen tubes and incubated at 32°C, 37°C, and at room temperature. *M. marinum will not grow at 37°C on primary isolation.* Grows out in 2 to 4 weeks; photochromogenic. Early lesions yield numerous colonies. Lesions 3 months or older generally yield few colonies.

Diagnosis

History of trauma in an aqueous environment, clinical findings, confirmed by isolation of *M. marinum* on culture

Course and Prognosis

Most usually benign and self-limited but can remain active for a prolonged period. Single papulonodular lesions resolve spontaneously within 3 months to 3 years, whereas sporotrichoid form can persist up to 45 years.

Management

Antibiotics

EMPIRICAL TREATMENT

> Drug of first choice: minocycline 100 mg b.i.d.
> Alternative drugs: trimethoprim-sulfamethoxazole, rifampin, clarithromycin

M. MARINUM ISOLATED AND SENSITIVITIES DETERMINED If sensitivities show drug resistance, then rifampin (600 mg q.i.d.) and ethambutol (800 mg q.i.d.) is an effective combination in 90 % of patients and should be given in sporotrichoid form of infection.

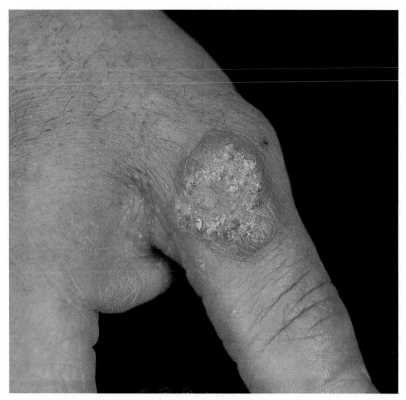

Figure 24-28 M. marinum infection ("fish-tank" granuloma) *A red-violet, verrucous plaque on the dorsum of the thumb of a fish tank hobbyist arose at the site of an abrasion.*

Mycobacterium ulcerans INFECTION

M. ulcerans infections occur at sites of traumatic inoculation, usually the legs, resulting in large to gigantic deep painless ulcerations, occurring in tropical regions of Africa and Australia.
Synonyms: Buruli ulcer (Africa), Bairnsdale ulcer (Australia).

Epidemiology and Etiology

Sex   Females > males

Age   Children, young adults

Etiology   *M. ulcerans.* An environmental habitat for the organism has not been established.

Transmission   Inoculation probably occurs via pricks and cuts from plants, occurring in wet, marshy, or swampy sites.

Geography   The tropics, most infections occurring in Africa and Australia

History

Incubation Period   Approximately 3 months

Symptoms   The early nodule at site of trauma and subsequent ulceration are usually painless.

Physical Examination

Skin Lesions

TYPE   A painless subcutaneous swelling occurs at the site of inoculation. Lesion enlarges and ulcerates. The ulcer extends into the subcutaneous fat, and its margin is deeply undermined (Figure 24-29). Ulcerations may enlarge to involve an entire extremity.

DISTRIBUTION   Legs more commonly involved (sites of trauma). Any site may be involved.

General Findings   Fever, constitutional findings are usually absent.

REGIONAL LYMPH NODES   Enlargement usually absent

Differential Diagnosis

Subcutaneous Induration   Panniculitis, phycomycosis, nodular vasculitis, pyomyositis

Large Cutaneous Ulceration   Blastomycosis, sporotrichosis, nocardiosis, actinomycosis, mycetoma, chromomycosis, pyoderma gangrenosum, basal cell carcinoma, squamous cell carcinoma, necrotizing soft tissue infections

Laboratory and Special Examinations

Bacterial Culture   Rule out secondary bacterial infection.

Mycobacterial Culture   *M. ulcerans* grows optimally at 32 to 33°C.

Dermatopathology   Necrosis originates in the interlobular septa of the subcutaneous fat. Ulceration is surrounded by granulation tissue with giant cells but no caseation necrosis or tubercles. Acid-fast bacilli are always demonstrable.

Diagnosis

Clinical findings confirmed by isolation of *M. ulcerans* from lesional skin biopsy specimen

Course and Prognosis

Ulcerations tend to persist for months to years. Spontaneous healing occurs eventually in many patients. Ulceration and healing can be complicated by scarring, contracture of the limb, and lymphedema. Secondary bacterial infection of the ulcer is an uncommon complication.

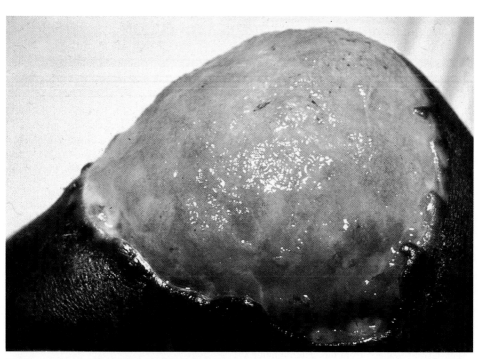

Figure 24-29 M. ulcerans infection (buruli ulcer) *A huge ulcer with a clean base and under-mined margins extends into the adipose tissue of a Ugandan child. (Courtesy of M. Dittrich, M.D.)*

Management

Heat In that *M. ulcerans* prefers cooler temperatures, application of heat to the involved site has been reported to be effective.

Surgery Excision of the infected tissue, usually followed by grafting, is effective.

Antimycobacterial Chemotherapy Usually responds poorly. Combinations of sulfamethe-moxazole, rifampin, and minocycline may be effective.

Mycobacterium fortuitum COMPLEX INFECTION

M. fortuitum complex (MFC) organisms cause infections at sites of inoculation, either surgical, injection, or traumatic, characterized by wound infections occurring several weeks after the insult.

Epidemiology and Etiology

Epidemiology   Cutaneous infection accounts for 60 % of MFC infections.

Sex   Females > males

Age   Children, young adults

Etiology   The MFC organisms are rapid growers and include *M. fortuitum, M. chelonae,* and *M. abscessus.*

Geography   *M. chelonae* is predominantly in Europe; *M. abscessus,* in the United States and Africa.

Natural Reservoirs   The organisms are widely distributed, being found in soil, dust, and water. Can be isolated from tap water, municipal water supplies, moist areas in hospitals, contaminated biologicals, aquariums, domestic animals, marine life.

Transmission   Inoculation occurs via traumatic puncture wounds (50 %) or surgical procedures/injections (50 %). Contaminated gentian violet used for skin marking has been the source.

History

Incubation Period   Usually within 1 month (range 1 week to 2 years)

History   Surgical wound infections follow augmentation mammaplasty, median sternotomy, and percutaneous catheterizations.

Symptoms   Infection presents as a painful traumatic or surgical wound infection.

Physical Examination

Skin Lesions

TYPES   Cold postinjection abscesses. Traumatic wound infections (Figure 24-30) present as dark red, infiltrated nodule, ±abscess formation, ±drainage of serous exudate. In immunocompromised individuals, infection can disseminate hematogenously to skin (multiple recurring abscesses on the extremities) and joints.

ARRANGEMENT   Linear lesions, commonly at incision sites

DISTRIBUTION   Traumatic infection occurs more commonly on the extremities. Surgical infections occur in scars of median sternotomy and augmentation mammaplasty.

General Findings   Other primary MFC infections include pneumonitis, osteomyelitis, lymphadenitis, postsurgical endocarditis.

Differential Diagnosis

Traumatic and Postoperative Wound Infection   *Staphylococcus aureus* and group A *Streptococcus* infections, various other bacteria, foreign-body reaction, allergic contact dermatitis to topically applied agent, *Candida albicans* infection, *Aspergillus* spp. infection

Laboratory and Special Examinations

Bacterial Culture   Rule out secondary bacterial infection.

Mycobacterial Culture   MFC organisms usually can be isolated on primary culture in 2 to 30 days; when recultured, the organisms grow well in 1 to 3 days.

Dermatopathology   Polymorphonuclear microabscesses and granuloma formation with foreign-body–type giant cells (dimorphic inflammatory response) are seen. Necrosis is often present without caseation. AFB can be seen within microabscesses.

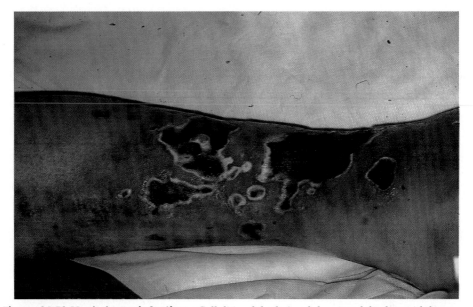

Figure 24-30 M. chelonae infection *Cellulitis of the leg and dorsum of the foot with large areas of necrosis. The infection occurred at surgical sites following venous harvesting and coronary artery bypass in a 40-year-old diabetic male, and eventually necessitated bilateral above-knee amputations.*

Diagnosis

Clinical findings confirmed by isolation of MFC from lesional skin biopsy specimen

Course and Prognosis

The infection becomes chronic unless treated with antimycobacterial therapy, ±surgical debridement.

Management

Antimycobacterial Chemotherapy MFC organisms are resistant to all antimycobacterial agents except amikacin and several newer agents such as fluoroquinolones and newer macrolides are frequently effective. Severe infection is usually treated with amikacin combined with another effective drug for 4 weeks, followed by 6 months of oral therapy. Mild to moderate infection is treated with an effective oral agent for 6 or more weeks.

Surgery Debridement with delayed closure is effective for localized infections.

LYME BORRELIOSIS

Lyme borreliosis (LB) is a spirochetal infectious disease transmitted to humans by the bite of an infected tick. Lyme disease (LD), the syndrome occurring early in the infection, is characterized by a pathognomonic eruption, erythema migrans (EM), followed by involvement of the joints, nervous system, and/or heart and lymphocytoma. Chronic cutaneous LB is manifested by acrodermatitis chronica atrophicans.

Epidemiology and Etiology

Age Children (<15 years), adults (20 to 45 years and older)

Sex In the United States, males and females equally affected, except those aged 10 to 19 years (males: 55 %) and those aged 30 to 39 (females: 56 %)

Etiology *Borrelia burgdorferi*

Incidence In 1994, 13,000 reported cases in the United States by 44 state health departments, a 58 % increase from the previous year

Risk for Exposure Strongly associated with prevalence of tick vectors and proportion of those ticks which carry *B. burgdorferi*. In the northeastern states with endemic disease, the infection rate of the nymphal *Ixodes scapularis* tick with *B. burgdorferi* is commonly 20% to 35 %.

Transmission Ticks cling to vegetation; are most numerous in brushy, wooded, or grassy habitats; not found on open sandy beaches. *B. burgdorferi* is transmitted to humans following biting and feeding of nymphs (Figure 24-31) or, less commonly, ticks.

Vector Ixodid ticks: *I. scapularis, I. pacificus, I. ricinus, I. persulcatus*

NORTH AMERICA Deer tick *I. scapularis* (black-legged tick) in northeastern and north-central regions of United States; *I. pacifica* (western black-legged tick) in Pacific coastal states

EUROPE Sheep tick *I. ricinus*

Season Late May through early fall (80 % of early LB begins in June and July) in the mid-western and eastern United States; January through May in the Northwest.

Geography

NORTH AMERICA Most cases reported from the northeastern and north-central regions. States with the highest incidence in 1994 were Connecticut (62 cases per 100,000), Rhode Island (47), New York (29), New Jersey (20), Delaware (16), Pennsylvania (12), Wisconsin (8), and Maryland (8); these states accounted for 88 % of nationally reported cases.

EUROPE Occurs widely throughout the continent and Great Britain. Cases also documented from Asia, Australia, northern Africa. Ixodid ticks are also indigenous to South America and other parts of Africa; not known if transmission of *B. burgdorferi* occurs in those areas.

Staging of LB

Stage I: Acute
  Systemic symptoms (fever, chills, myalgia, headaches, weakness, photophobia)
  Erythema migrans
  Lymphocytoma
Stage II: Intermediate
  Carditis
  Meningitis, cranial neuritis, radiculoneuropathy
  Arthralgia/myalgia
Stage III: Chronic
  Arthritis
  Acrodermatitis chronica atrophicans (ACA)
  Encephalomyelitis

History

Incubation Period Onset after tick bite: EM,

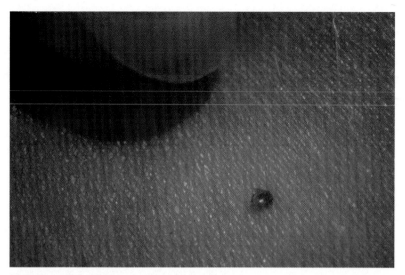

Figure 24-31 Deer tick (Ixodes scapularis) feeding *A blood-distended nymph with a finger for size comparison; transmission of* B. burgdorferi *usually occurs only after prolonged attachment and feeding (>18 hours).*

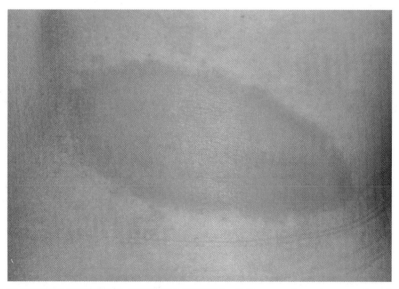

Figure 24-32 Lyme borreliosis: erythema migrans *Solitary erythematous annular plaque on the lateral trunk occurring at the site of an asymptomatic tick bite.*

7 to 12 days (range 1 to 180 days); neurologic: average 38 days (2 weeks to months); cardiac: 35 days (3 weeks to >5 months); joints: 67 days (4 days to 2 years)

Prodrome Malaise, fatigue, lethargy, headache, fever, chills, stiff neck, arthralgia, myalgia, backache, anorexia, sore throat, nausea, dysesthesia, vomiting, abdominal pain, photophobia

History Ixodid tick bites are asymptomatic. Only 14 % of LB patients are aware of a preceding tick bite. Removal of the pinhead-sized tick within 18 hours of attachment may preclude transmission. EM may be associated with burning sensation, itching, or pain. Only 75 % of patients with LB exhibit EM.

Physical Examination

Cutaneous Findings in Early LB

TYPES OF LESIONS *Erythema Migrans (EM)* Initial macule or papule enlarges within days to form an expanding annular lesion with a distinct red border and partially clearing middle (Figure 24-32), i.e., EM, at the bite site. Maximum median diameter is 15 cm (range 3 to 68 cm). Center may become indurated, vesicular, or necrotic. At times concentric rings form. When occurring on the scalp, only a linear streak may be evident on the face or neck. Multiple EM lesions are seen when multiple bite sites occur (Figure 24-33).

Secondary Lesions 17 % develop multiple annular secondary lesions, ranging in number from 2 to >100. Secondary lesions resemble EM but are smaller, migrate less, and lack central induration (Figure 24-34)

Lymphocytoma Cutis (LC) *Synonyms:* Lymphadenosis benigna cutis (LABC), pseudolymphoma of Spiegler and Fendt. Most often a solitary (may be grouped) nodule (Figure 24-35) or plaque; occasionally translucent; red to brown to purple in color; located on the head, especially earlobe, areola, scrotum, and extremities; 3 to 5 cm in diameter; usually asymptomatic.

Other Cutaneous Findings Malar rash, diffuse urticaria, subcutaneous nodules (panniculitis)

COLOR OF LESIONS EM: Erythematous evolving to violaceous

DISTRIBUTION OF LESIONS EM: Trunk and proximal extremities, especially the axillary and inguinal areas, most common sites. Secondary lesions: any site except the palms and soles; can become confluent.

MUCOUS MEMBRANES Red throat, conjunctivitis

LB may occur without EM or secondary lesions and present only with the late manifestations. Also, late manifestations may occur despite treatment (inadequate) of early LB with tetracycline.

Cutaneous Findings in Long-Standing LB

ACRODERMATITIS CHRONICA ATROPHICANS *Early Inflammatory Phase (Months to Years)* (Figure 24-36) Initially, diffuse or localized violaceous erythema, usually on one extremity, accompanied by mild to prominent edema, most commonly involving the extensor surfaces and periarticular areas. Asymptomatic dull-red infiltrated plaques arise on the extremities, more commonly on lower legs than forearms, which slowly extend centrifugally over several months to years, leaving central areas of atrophy.

End Stage Skin becomes atrophic, veins and subcutaneous tissue become prominent, easily lifted and pushed into fine accordion-like folds, i.e., "cigarette paper" or "tissue paper" skin (Figure 24-38). Lesions may be single or multiple.

Sclerotic or Fibrotic Plaques and Bands Localized fibromas and plaques are seen as subcutaneous nodules around the knees and elbows (Figure 24-37); may involve

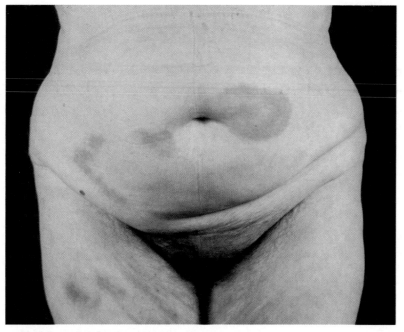

Figure 24-33 Lyme borreliosis: erythema migrans *Three erythematous plaques with central clearing on the lower abdomen and thigh arising at multiple tick-bite sites.*

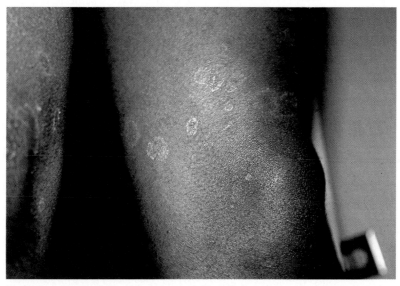

Figure 24-34 Lyme borreliosis: secondary lesions *Multiple, small, scaling lesions on the thighs. The lesions result from spirochetemia from the primary bite site (erythema migrans) with resultant disseminated infection. These lesions are analogous to the papulosquamous lesions that occur in secondary syphilis.*

the joint capsule with subsequent limitation of movement of joints in hand, feet, or shoulders. Fibrotic/sclerotic band along ulna is pathognomonic ("ulnar band").

General Findings

ACUTE OR PRIMARY MANIFESTATIONS   Fever: in adults, low-grade; in children, may be high and persistent. Regional lymphadenopathy, generalized lymphadenopathy, right upper quadrant tenderness, frank arthritis, splenomegaly, hepatomegaly, muscle tenderness, periorbital edema.

LATE OR TERTIARY MANIFESTATIONS   *Arthritis* Occurs in 60 % of untreated cases, 4 to 6 weeks after the tick bite (range 1 week to 22 months), sudden in onset, involves one or a few joints. Knee (89 %), shoulder (9 %), hip (9 %), ankle (7 %), and elbow (2 %) are commonly affected.

Neurologic Involvement Occurs in 10 % to 20 % of untreated LB cases, 1 to 6 weeks (or longer) following the tick bite. Manifested by meningitis (excruciating headache, neck pain), encephalitis (sleep disturbances, difficulty concentrating, poor memory, irritability, emotional lability, dementia); cranial neuropathies [unilateral or bilateral; optic neuropathy, sixth nerve palsy, facial (Bell's) palsy, eighth nerve deafness]; sensory and motor radiculopathies (severe radicular pain, dysesthesias, subtle sensory loss, focal weakness, loss of reflexes). Referred to as *Bannwarth's syndrome* or *tick-borne meningopolyneuritis of Garin-Bujadoux-Bannwarth.*

Cardiac Abnormalities Occur in 6 % to 10 % of untreated cases, usually within 4 weeks. Manifested by fluctuating degrees of atrioventricular block, myopericarditis, and left ventricular dysfunction. Usually transient and not associated with long-term sequelae.

Variants LB occurring in Europe usually milder than in United States, with more secondary EM-like skin lesions and fewer arthritic complications, probably due to strain differences in *B. burgdorferi.*

Differential Diagnosis

EM   Tinea corporis, herald patch of pityriasis rosea, insect (e.g., brown recluse spider) bite, cellulitis, urticaria, erythema multiforme, fixed drug eruption. Secondary lesions: secondary syphilis, pityriasis rosea, erythema multiforme, urticaria.

LC   Insect bite reaction, pseudolymphoma, cutaneous lymphoma

ACA   Arterial insufficiency of the lower leg, venous insufficiency with stasis dermatitis, and venous thrombosis/thrombophlebitis

FIBROTIC NODULES   Rheumatic nodules, gouty tophi, and erythema nodosum

Laboratory and Special Examinations

Skin Biopsy

EM   Deep and superficial perivascular and interstitial lymphohistiocytic infiltrate containing plasma cells. Spirochetes can be demonstrated in up to 40 % of EM biopsy specimens.

ACA   Early, perivascular inflammatory infiltrate and dermal edema. Subsequently, infiltrate broadens to a dense middermal band-like infiltrate. Ultimately, epidermal and dermal atrophy, dilated dermal blood vessels, plasma cell infiltrate, elastin and collagen defects.

Serology   A two-test approach for active disease and for previous infection using a sensitive enzyme immunoassay (EIA) or immunofluorescent assay (IFA) followed by a Western immunoblot (WIB) is recommended. All specimens positive or equivocal by a sensitive EIA or IFA should be tested by a standardized WIB. When WIB is used during the first 4 weeks of disease onset, both IgM and IgG procedures

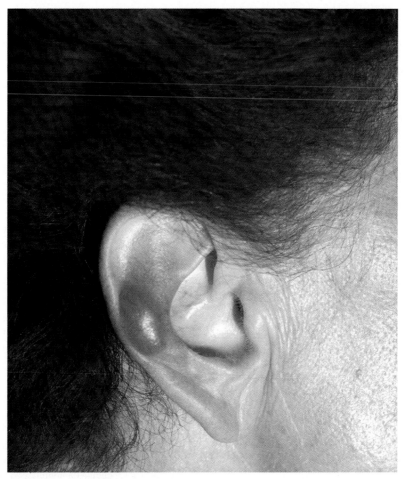

Figure 24-35 Lyme borreliosis: lymphocytoma cutis *Solitary, red-purple nodule occurring on the characteristic site of the ear.*

should be performed. A positive IgM test result alone is not recommended for use in determining active disease in persons with illness of >1 months' duration. If a patient with suspected early LD has a negative serology, serologic evidence of infection is best obtained by testing paired acute- and convalescent-phase serum samples. Serum samples from persons with disseminated or late-stage LB almost always have a strong IgG response to *B. burgdorferi* antigens. It is recommended that an IgM immunoblot be considered positive if 2 of 3 bands are present and that an IgG immunoblot be considered positive if 5 of 10 bands are positive.

Culture *B. burgdorferi* can be isolated from lesional skin biopsy specimen on Kelly's medium.

PCR Detects *B. burgdorferi* DNA in lesional skin biopsy specimen, blood, or joint fluid. May be the preferred confirmatory laboratory test.

Diagnosis

Acute Made on characteristic clinical findings in a person living in or having visited an endemic area

Late Confirmed by specific serologic tests. CDC case definition: physician-diagnosed EM in a person who acquired infection in a county with endemic LB, or for persons who acquired infection in a county without endemic LB, laboratory evidence of infection in addition to the presence of EM.

ACA Made on clinical findings confirmed by lesional biopsy

Pathophysiology

LB in many ways parallels the course of syphilis. EM, as with a syphilitic chancre, occurs at the site of entry of the spirochete soon after inoculation. Secondary lesions occur following hematogenous dissemination to the skin. The late joint manifestations appear to be mediated by immune-complex formation. Menin-

gitis results from direct invasion of the cerebrospinal fluid. The pathogenesis of cranial and peripheral neuropathies in LB is unknown but also might result from immune mechanisms.

Course and Prognosis

Untreated EM and secondary lesions fade in a median time of 28 days, but this ranges from 1 day to 14 months. Both EM and secondary lesions can fade and recur during this time. However, following adequate treatment, early lesions resolve within several days, and late manifestations are prevented. Late manifestations identified early usually clear following adequate antibiotic therapy; however, delay in diagnosis may result in permanent joint or neurologic disabilities.

ACA shows little response to adequate antibiotic therapy once atrophy has supervened. Adequately treated patients show declining titers of anti-*B. burgdorferi* antibody within 6 to 12 months.

Management

Prophylaxis Avoid known tick habitats. Other preventive measures include wearing long pants and long-sleeved shirts, tucking pants into socks, applying tick repellents containing *N,N*-diethyl-*m*-toluamide ("DEET") to clothing and/or exposed skin, checking regularly for ticks, and promptly removing any attached ticks. Acaracides containing permethrin kill ticks on contact and can provide further protection when applied to clothing.

Antimicrobial Treatment

EARLY LYME BORRELIOSIS Without neurologic, cardiac, or joint involvement

- Amoxicillin 500 mg PO t.i.d. for 21 days (if only EM, 10 days sufficient)
- Cefuroxime axetil 500 mg PO q.d. for 7 days
- Doxycycline 100 mg PO b.i.d. for 21 days (if only EM, 10 days sufficient)
- Azithromycin 500 mg PO q.d. for 7 days (*less effective*)

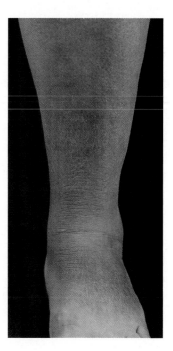

Figure 24-36 Lyme borreliosis: acrodermatitis chronica atrophicans, early *Ill-defined, violaceous erythema and edema of the leg and foot. Onset is usually several months after primary infection and often accompanied by symptoms of peripheral sensory neuropathy.*

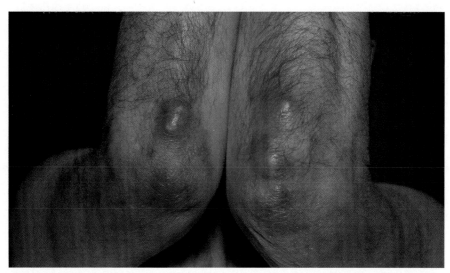

Figure 24-37 Lyme borreliosis: acrodermatitis chronica atrophicans, fibrotic nodules *Multiple, large, subcutaneous, fibrotic, violaceous nodules with surrounding erythema on the elbows.*

Neurologic Manifestations

- Bell's palsy (no other neurologic abnormalities). Oral regimens for early disease suffice.

  Meningitis (With or without radiculoneuropathy or encephalitis)

- Ceftriaxone 2 g IM q.d. for 14 to 28 days
- Doxycycline 100 mg PO or IV b.i.d. for 14 to 28 days
- Penicillin G 20 million units (divided doses) IV q.d. for 14 to 28 days

Arthritis

- Amoxicillin and probenecid 500 mg each PO t.i.d. for 30 days
- Ceftriaxone 2 g IM q.d. for 14 to 28 days
- Doxycycline 100 mg PO b.i.d. for 30 days
- Penicillin G 20 million units (divided doses) IV q.d. for 14 to 28 days

Carditis

- Amoxicillin 500 mg PO t.i.d. for 21 days
- Ceftriaxone 2 g IM q.d. for 14 days
- Doxycycline 100 mg PO b.i.d. for 21 days
- Penicillin G 20 million units (divided doses) IV q.d. for 14 days

Pregnancy

Localized early disease

- Amoxicillin 500 mg PO t.i.d. for 21 days

  Any manifestation of disseminated disease
- Penicillin G 20 million units (divided doses) IV q.d. for 14 to 28 days

Asymptomatic seropositivity

- No treatment necessary

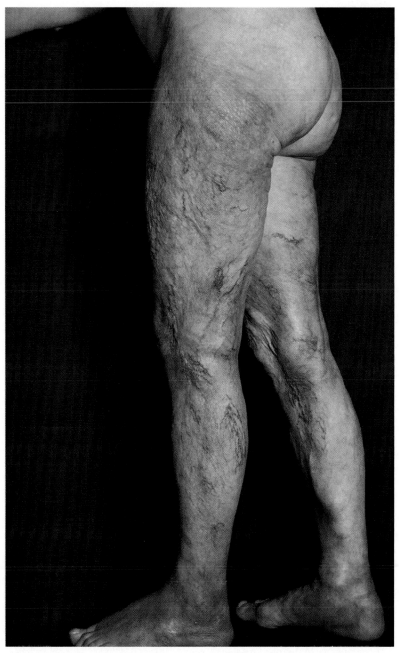

Figure 24-38 Lyme borreliosis: acrodermatitis chronica atrophicans, endstage *Advanced atrophy of the epidermis and dermis with associated violaceous erythema of legs and feet; the visibility of the superficial veins is striking.*

Section 25

CUTANEOUS FUNGAL INFECTIONS

DERMATOPHYTOSES

Dermatophytes are a unique group of fungi that are capable of infecting nonviable keratinized cutaneous tissues including stratum corneum, nails, and hair. Dermatophytic genera include *Trichophyton, Microsporum,* and *Epidermophyton.* The term dermatophytosis thus denotes a condition caused by dermatophytes. It can be further specified according to the tissue mainly involved: epidermomycosis, trichomycosis, or onychomycosis. The term *tinea* should be reserved for dermatophytoses and is modified according to the anatomic site of infection, e.g., tinea pedis.

Epidemiology and Etiology

Age Children have scalp infections (*Microsporum* and *Trichophyton*), and young adults have intertriginous infections.

Sex No profound differences

Race Adult blacks are said to have a lower incidence of dermatophytosis.

Etiology Three genera of dermatophytes: *Trichophyton, Microsporum,* and *Epidermophyton.* More than 40 species are currently recognized; approximately 10 species are common causes of human infection.

Geography Some species have a worldwide distribution; others are restricted to particular continents or regions. However, *T. concentricum,* the cause of tinea imbricata, is endemic to the South Pacific and parts of South America. The etiology of tinea capitis varies geographically. In North America and Europe, *T. tonsurans* is the most common cause, having replaced *M. audouinii.* In Europe, Asia, and Africa, *T. violaceum.*

Transmission Dermatophyte infections can be acquired from three sources: most commonly acquired from another person by fomites, from animals such as puppies or kittens, and least commonly from soil. Based on their ecology, dermatophytes are also classified as follows:

ANTHROPOPHILIC Person-to-person transmission by fomites

   Trichophyton species: *T. rubrum, T. mentagrophytes* (var. *interdigitale*), *T. schoenleinii, T. tonsurans, T. violaceum*
   Microsporum audouinii
   Epidermophyton floccosum

ZOOPHILIC Animal-to-human, direct contact, or by fomites

   Trichophyton species: *T. equinum, T. mentagrophytes* (var. *mentagrophytes*), *T. verrucosum*

   M. canis

GEOPHILIC Environmental

   Microsporum species: *M. gypseum, M. nanum*

Classification of Dermatophytoses Dermatophytes grow only on or within keratinized structures and, as such, involve

DERMATOPHYTOSES OF KERATINIZED EPIDERMIS (EPIDERMOMYCOSIS) (Figure 25-1)

   Tinea facialis
   Tinea corporis
   Tinea cruris
   Tinea manus
   Tinea pedis

DERMATOPHYTOSES OF NAILS (ONYCHOMYCHOSIS)

Tinea unguium (toenails, fingernails)
Onychomycosis (here it is a more inclusive term including nail infections caused by dermatophytes, yeasts, and molds)

DERMATOPHYTOSES OF HAIR (TRICHOMYCOSIS)

Dermatophytic folliculitis
Majocchi's (trichophytic) granuloma
Tinea capitis
Tinea barbae

Other Predisposing Factors *Immunosuppressed patients* have a higher incidence and more intractable dermatophytoses. With topical immunosuppression (i.e., with prolonged application of topical corticosteroids), there can be marked modification in the usual banal character of dermatophytosis; this is especially true of the face, groin, and hands. In immunocompromised patients, abscesses and granulomas may occur.

Laboratory and Special Examinations

Direct Microscopy (Figure 25-2)

SAMPLING

Skin: Collect scale using a no. 15 scalpel blade or edge of a glass microscope slide; scales are placed on center of microscope slide, sweeping them into a small pile and covered with a coverslip.

Nail: Keratinaceous debride is collected with a no. 15 scalpel blade or 1-mm curette:

Distal lateral subungual onychomycosis: distal lateral nail bed or undersurface of nail plate
Superficial white onychomycosis: superficial nail plate
Proximal subungual onychomycosis: undersurface of nail plate.

Hair: Remove hairs by epilation of broken hairs with a needle holder or forceps. Place on microscope slide and cover with glass coverslip.

Potassium Hydroxide (KOH) 5 % to 20 % solution is then placed at the edge of the cov-

erslip. Capillary action draws solution under coverslip. The preparation is gently heated with a match or lighter until bubbles begin to expand, clarifying the preparation. Excess KOH solution is blotted out with bibulous or lens paper. Condenser should be "racked down."

Examination Dermatophytes are recognized as septated, tubelike structures (hyphae or mycelia).

Wood's Lamp Hairs infected with *Microsporum* species fluoresce. Greenish. Darken room and illuminate affected site with Wood's lamp.

Fungal Cultures

• Specimens collected from scaling skin lesions, hair, nails. Scale and hair from the scalp are best harvested with a shampoo massage brush; the involved scalp is brushed vigorously with the brush, which is then pressed into a fungal culture plate. A toothbrush also can be used to harvest scale and infected hairs. Culture on Sabouraud's glucose medium.
• Repeat cultures recommended monthly

Dermatopathology Fungi are best demonstrated with periodic acid–Schiff (PAS) or methenamine silver stains.

Pathogenesis

Dermatophytes synthesize keratinases that digest keratin and sustain existence of fungi in keratinized structures. Cell-mediated immunity and antimicrobial activity of polymorphonuclear leukocytes restrict dermatophyte pathogenicity.

• *Host factors that facilitate dermatophyte infections:* atopy, topical and systemic corticosteroids, ichthyosis, collagen vascular disease
• *Local factors favoring dermatophyte infection:* sweating, occlusion, occupational exposure, geographic location, high humidity (tropical or semitropical climates)

The clinical presentation of dermatophytoses depends on several factors: site of infection, immunologic response of the host, species of fungus. Dermatophytes (e.g., *T. rubrum*) that initiate little inflammatory response are better able to establish chronic infection. Organisms such as *M. canis* cause an acute infection associated with a brisk inflammatory response and spontaneous resolution. In some individuals, infection can involve the dermis, as in kerion and Majocchi's granuloma.

Management

Prevention Apply powder containing miconazole or tolnaftate to areas prone to fungal infection after bathing.

Antifungal Therapy

TOPICAL AGENTS (Table 25-A)

These preparations are effective for treatment of dermatophytoses of skin but not for those of hair or nails. Topical agents should be continued for at least 1 week after lesions have cleared. Apply at least 3 cm beyond advancing margin of lesion.

These agents are comparable. Differentiated by cost, base, vehicle, and antifungal activity. Preparation is applied b.i.d. to involved area optimally for 4 weeks.

SYSTEMIC AGENTS

For infections of keratinized skin: use if lesions are extensive or if infection has failed to respond to topical preparations.
Usually required for treatment of tinea capitis and tinea unguium. Also may be required for inflammatory tineas and hyperkeratotic moccasin-type tinea pedis.

Griseofulvin: active only against dermatophytes; less effective than triazoles. Adverse effects include headache, nausea/vomiting, photosensitivity, lowers effect of crystalline warfarin sodium. *T. rubrum* and *T. tonsurans* infection may respond poorly. Should be taken with fatty meal to maximize absorption. In children, CBC and LFTs recommended if risk factors for hepatitis exist or treatment lasts longer than 3 months. *Micronized:* 250- or 500-mg tablets; 125 mg/teaspoon suspension. *Ultramicronized:* 165- or 330-mg tablets

Ketoconazole: 200-mg tablets. Imidazole. Needs acid gastric pH for dissolution of tablet. Take with food or cola beverage; antacids and H_2 blockers reduce absorption. The most hepatotoxic of azole drugs. Rarely: ventricular arrhythmia when coadministered with terfenadine/astemizole. Not approved for use in dermatophyte infections in the United States.

Itraconazole: 100-mg capsules. Triazole. Needs acid gastric pH for dissolution of tablet. Rarely: ventricular arrhythmia when coadministered with terfenadine/astemizole. Raises levels of digoxin and cyclosporine. Approved for onychomycosis in the United States.

Terbinafine: 250 mg/day. Allylamine. Rarely: nausea, dyspepsia, abdominal pain, loss of sense of taste, aplastic anemia. Most effective oral anti-dermophyte antifungal. Oral preparation not yet approved for use in the United States.

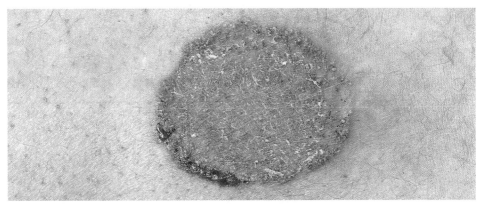

Figure 25-1 Epidermal dermatophytosis (Epidermomycosis) *Well-demarcated, red, scaling plaque with a raised border (note tiny vesicles) and a tendency toward central clearing is the essential lesion of epidermal dermatophytosis, i.e., "ring worm."*

TABLE 25-A TOPICAL ANTIFUNGAL AGENTS EFFECTIVE FOR TREATMENT OF EPIDERMAL DERMATOPHYTOSES

	Agents	Trade Names
Imidazoles	Clotrimazole	Lotrimin, Mycelex
	Miconazole	Micatin
	Ketoconazole	Nizoral
	Econazole	Spectazole
	Oxiconizole	Oxistat
	Sulconizole	Exelderm
Allylamines	Naftifine	Naftin
	Terbinafine	Lamisil
Naphthiomates	Tolnaftate	Tinactin
Substituted pyridone	Ciclopiroxalamine	Loprox

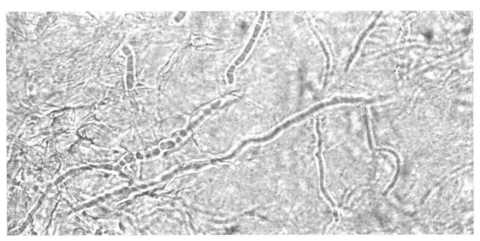

Figure 25-2 Potassium hydroxide (KOH) preparation *Multiple, septated, tubelike structures (hyphae or mycelia) and spore formation in scales obtained from an individual with epidermal dermatophytosis. In contrast, KOH preparation in candidiasis shows elongated yeast forms (pseudohyphae) without true septations.*

DERMATOPHYTOSES OF EPIDERMIS

Tinea Pedis

Tinea pedis is a dermatophytic infection of the feet, characterized by erythema, chronic diffuse desquamation, and/or bulla formation.
Synonym: Athlete's foot, moccasin-type tinea.

Classification

Interdigital Type (Acute and Chronic) Most common type; frequently overlooked.

Moccasin Type (Chronic Hyperkeratotic or Dry Type) Most often caused by *T. rubrum*. More common in atopic individuals.

Inflammatory or Bullous (Vesicular) Type Least common type; usually caused by *T. mentagrophytes*. Resembles an allergic contact dermatitis to a dermatophyte antigen.

Ulcerative Type An extension of interdigital type into dermis due to maceration and secondary (bacterial) infection.

Dermatophytid Presents as a vesicular eruption of the fingers and/or palmar aspects of the hands secondary to inflammatory tinea pedis; more commonly associated with *T. mentagrophytes* but also *T. rubrum* infection of feet. A combined clinical presentation also occurs. *Candida* and bacteria (*Staphylococcus aureus*, group A *Streptococcus, Pseudomonas aeruginosa*) may cause superinfection.

Etiology and Pathogenesis

Etiology *T. rubrum* is the most common cause of chronic tinea pedis; *T. mentagrophytes* causes more inflammatory lesions.

INTERDIGITAL TYPE *T. mentagrophytes* var. *interdigitale* (downy), *T. rubrum, E. floccosum*. Nondermatophytes: *Candida albicans, Scytalidium hyalinum, Hendersonula toruloidea*.

MOCCASIN TYPE Most often caused by *T. rubrum*, especially in atopic individuals; also *E. floccosum*.

INFLAMMATORY OR BULLOUS TYPE Least common type; usually caused by *T. mentagrophytes* var. *mentagrophytes* (granular). Resembles an allergic contact dermatitis; hapten is a dermatophyte antigen.

ULCERATIVE TYPE *T. rubrum, E. floccosum, T. mentagrophytes, C. albicans*.

Age Onset, late childhood or young adult life. Most common 20 to 50 years.

Sex Males > females

Predisposing Factors Hot, humid weather; occlusive footwear; excessive sweating

Transmission Walking barefoot on contaminated floors. Arthrospores can survive in human skin scales >12 months.

History

Duration Months to years

History Often, prior history of tinea pedis, ±tinea unguium of toenails

Skin Symptoms Asymptomatic frequently. Pruritus. Pain with secondary bacterial infection.

Physical Examination

Skin Lesions

TYPES
Interdigital Type Maceration, peeling, fissuring of toe webs (Figure 25-3). Underlying skin red, ±weeping.
Moccasin Type Well-demarcated erythema with minute papules on margin, fine white scaling, and hyperkeratosis (Figure 25-4)

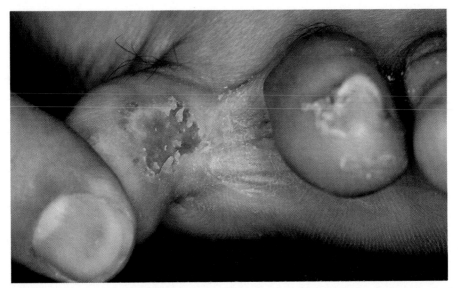

Figure 25-3 Tinea pedis: interdigital type *Scaling, maceration, erythema, and erosion in the webspace between the fourth and fifth toes; tinea unguium of the toenail of the fourth toe is also present.*

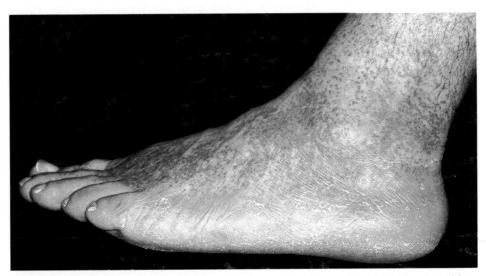

Figure 25-4 Tinea pedis: mocassin type *Erythema, fine white scaling of the plantar and lateral foot, and keratoderma (thickening of the keratin layer); the arciform pattern of scaling is characteristic. The multiple brown macules are incidental findings and represent progressive pigmentary purpura (Schamberg's disease).*

(confined to heels, soles, lateral borders of feet)

Inflammatory/Bullous Type Vesicles or bullae filled with clear fluid (Figure 25-5). Pus usually indicates secondary *S. aureus* infection. After rupturing, erosions with ragged ringlike border. May be associated with dermatophytid.

Ulcerative Type Extension of interdigital tinea pedis onto dorsal and plantar foot. Usually complicated by bacterial infection.

COLOR Red; opaque white scales

DISTRIBUTION One or both feet may be involved with any pattern; bilateral involvement more common.

Interdigital Type Most common site: between fourth and fifth toes. Infection may spread to adjacent areas of feet.

Moccasin Type The sole, involving area covered by a ballet slipper

Bullous Type Sole, instep, webspaces

Differential Diagnosis

Interdigital Type Erythrasma, impetigo, pitted keratolysis, *Candida* intertrigo, *P. aeruginosa* webspace infection

Moccasin Type Psoriasis vulgaris, eczematous dermatitis (dyshidrotic, atopic, allergic contact), pitted keratolysis, various keratodermas

Inflammatory/Bullous Type Bullous impetigo, allergic contact dermatitis, dyshidrotic eczema, bullous disease

Laboratory and Special Examinations

Direct Microscopy See page 691 (see Figure 25-2). In bullous type, examine scraping from the inner aspect of bulla roof for detection of hyphae.

Wood's Lamp Examination Negative fluorescence usually rules out erythrasma in inter-

digital infection. Erythrasma and interdigital tinea pedis may coexist.

Fungal Culture Dermatophytes can be isolated in 11 % of normal-appearing interspaces and 31 % of macerated toe webs. *Candida* species may be copathogens.

Bacterial Culture In individuals with macerated interdigital space, *S. aureus, P. aeruginosa,* and diphtheroids are commonly isolated.

Diagnosis

Demonstration of hyphae on direct microscopy, ±isolation of dermatophyte on culture

Course and Prognosis

Tends to be chronic, with exacerbations in hot weather. May provide portal of entry for lymphangitis or cellulitis, especially in patients whose leg veins have been used for coronary artery bypass surgery and have chronic low-grade edema of leg.

Management

Prevention Use of shower shoes while bathing at home or in public facility. Washing feet with benzoyl peroxide bar directly after shower. Diabetics and those who have undergone coronary artery bypass with harvesting of leg veins are especially subject to secondary bacterial infection (impetiginization, lymphangitis, cellulitis).

Special Considerations by Type of Infection

INTERDIGITAL TYPE Acutely: Burow's wet dressings; Castellani's paint. Chronically: aluminum chloride hexahydrate 20 % b.i.d. to reduce sweating.

MOCCASIN TYPE Most difficult to eradicate: many patients have a minor defect in cell-mediated immune response; stratum corneum thick, making it difficult for topical antifungal agents to penetrate; often associated with tinea unguium, a source of re-

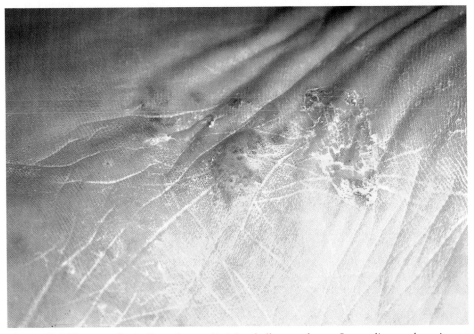

Figure 25-5 Tinea pedis: bullous type *Vesicles, bullae, erythema, fine scaling, and erosion on the plantar foot. Hyphae were detected on KOH preparation obtained from the roof of the inner aspect of the large bulla.*

infection of skin. Keratolytic agent (salicylic acid, lactic acid, hydroxy acid) with plastic occlusion useful in reducing hyperkeratosis. Nail reservoir must be eradicated to cure moccasin-type infection.

INFLAMMATORY/BULLOUS TYPE   Acutely, use cool compresses. If severe, systemic corticosteroids are indicated.

Antifungal Agents

TOPICAL AGENTS   See Dermatophytoses, page 691 (Table 25-A). Apply to all affected sites twice daily. Treat for 2 to 4 weeks.

SYSTEMIC AGENTS   Indicated for extensive infection or for failures of topical treatment or for those with tinea unguium and moccasin-type tinea.
Griseofulvin   660 to 750 mg/day for 21 days.
Itraconazole   200 mg b.i.d. for 7 days.
Terbinafine   250 mg/day for 14 days.

Secondary Prophylaxis   Important in preventing recurrence of interdigital and moccasin types of tinea pedis. Daily washing of feet while bathing with benzoyl peroxide bar is effective and inexpensive. Antifungal powders. Antifungal creams.

Tinea Manuum

Tinea manuum is a chronic dermatophytosis of the hand(s), often unilateral, most commonly on the dominant hand, and usually associated with tinea pedis.

Epidemiology and Etiology

Etiology   Most often *T. rubrum, T. mentagrophytes,* and *E. floccosum,* the same fungi that cause tinea pedis and tinea cruris

Pathogenesis

Usually associated with tinea pedis and, often, tinea cruris

History

Duration   Months to years

Skin Symptoms   Frequently symptomatic. Pruritus. Pain if secondarily infected or fissured. Dyshidrotic type: episodic symptoms of pruritus.

Physical Examination

Skin Lesions

TYPE   **Dyshidrotic Type**   Papules, vesicles, bullae (uncommon on the margin of lesion)
   Hyperkeratotic Type   Well-demarcated scaling patches, hyperkeratosis and scaling confined to palmar creases, fissures on palmar hand (Figure 25-6). Borders well demarcated; central clearing. Often extends onto dorsum of hand with follicular papules, nodules, pustules with dermatophytic folliculitis.
   Secondary Changes   Lichen simplex chronicus, prurigo nodules, impetiginization

COLOR   Erythematous

SHAPE   Annular, polycyclic, especially on the dorsum

DISTRIBUTION   Diffuse hyperkeratosis of the palms with pronounced involvement of palmar creases or patchy scaling on the dorsa and sides of fingers; 50 % of patients have *unilateral* involvement (Figure 25-6). Usually associated with tinea pedis, ±tinea cruris. If chronic, often associated with tinea unguium of fingernails.

Differential Diagnosis

Erythema/Scaling Hands   Atopic dermatitis, lichen simplex chronicus, allergic contact dermatitis, irritant contact dermatitis, psoriasis vulgaris, pityriasis rubra pilaris, *in situ* squamous cell carcinoma, tinea nigra

Laboratory and Special Examinations

Direct Microscopy   See page 689. Hyphae in scales.

Fungal Culture   Dermatophytes. Rule out *Scytalidium hyalinum, Hendersonula toruloidea, Candida albicans.*

Diagnosis

Clinical findings confirmed by direct microscopy or isolation of dermatophyte on culture

Course

Chronic, does not resolve spontaneously. After treatment, recurs unless dermatophytosis of fingernails, feet, and toenails is eradicated. Fissures and erosions provide portal of entry for bacterial infections.

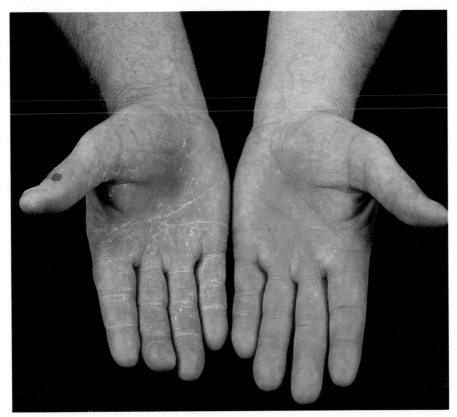

Figure 25-6 Tinea manuum *Erythema and scaling (seen best in the skin folds) of the right hand, which was associated with bilateral tinea pedum; the "one hand, two feet" distribution is typical of epidermal dermatophytosis of the hands and feet.*

Management

Prevention Must eradicate tinea unguium of fingernails as well as toenails, tinea pedis ±tinea cruris as well; otherwise, tinea manuum will recur.

Antifungal Agents

TOPICAL AGENTS See Dermatophytoses, page 691. Failure common.

SYSTEMIC AGENTS Because of thickness of palmar stratum corneum, and especially if associated with tinea unguium of fingernails, tinea manuum is impossible to cure by topical agents. Oral agents eradicate dermatophytoses of hands, feet, and nails.
Terbinafine 250 mg/day for 14 days.
Itraconazole 200 mg q.d. for 7 days.
Griseofulvin 500 mg micronized per day for 21 days.

NOTE: Eradication of dermatophytosis of nails requires longer use (see page 717)

Tinea Cruris

Tinea cruris is a subacute or chronic dermatophytosis of the groin, pubic regions, and thighs. *Synonym:* "Jock itch."

Epidemiology and Etiology

Age Adult

Sex Males > females

Etiology *Trichophyton* species (*T. rubrum, T. mentagrophytes*), *E. floccosum*

Predisposing Factors Warm, humid environment; tight clothing worn by men; obesity. Chronic topical corticosteroid application

Pathogenesis

Most individuals with tinea cruris have tinea pedis. Dermatophyte is transferred from feet to crural region by hands.

History

Duration Months to years

History Often, history of long-standing tinea pedis. Often prior history of tinea cruris.

Skin Symptoms Usually none. In some persons, pruritus causes patient to seek treatment.

Physical Examination

Skin Lesions *Usually associated with tinea pedis, ±tinea unguium of toenails*

TYPE Large, scaling, well-demarcated plaques (Figure 25-7). ±Central clearing. Papules, pustules may be present at margins. Treated lesions: lack scale; postinflammatory hyperpigmentation in darker-skinned persons. In atopics, chronic scratching may produce secondary changes of lichen simplex chronicus.

COLOR Dull red, tan, brown

ARRANGEMENT Arciform, polycyclic

DISTRIBUTION Groins and thighs (Figure 25-7). May extend to buttocks. Scrotum and penis are rarely involved.

Differential Diagnosis

Erythema/Scaling in Groins Erythrasma, intertrigo, *Candida* intertrigo, inverse-pattern psoriasis, pityriasis versicolor, Langerhans cell histiocytosis

Laboratory and Special Examinations

Direct Microscopy Visualize hyphae

Wood's Lamp Examination Negative for coral-red fluorescence rules out erythrasma

Diagnosis

Clinical findings, confirmed by direct microscopy

Course

Recurrence is common (20 % to 25 %) unless concomitant tinea pedis is eradicated.

Management

Prevention After eradication of tinea cruris, ±tinea pedis, ±tinea unguium, reinfection can be minimized by wearing shower shoes when using a public or home (if family members are infected) bathing facility; using antifungal powders; benzoyl peroxide wash.

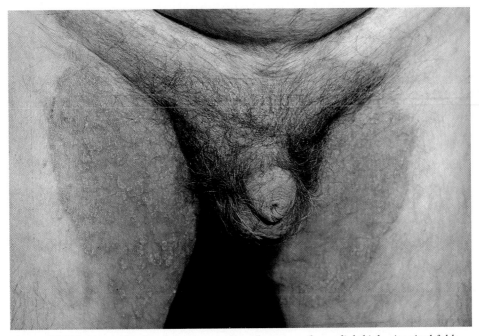

Figure 25-7 Tinea cruris *Erythematous, scaling plaques on the medial thighs, inguinal folds, and pubic area; areas of clearing are seen within the large plaques. The margins are raised and sharply marginated.*

Antifungal Agents

TOPICAL TREATMENT   See Table 25-A.

SYSTEMIC TREATMENT   If recurrent, if dermatophytic folliculitis is present, or if it has failed to respond to adequate topical therapy. See Dermatophytoses, page 688.

Griseofulvin   660 to 750 mg/day for 14 days.

Itraconazole   200 mg q.d. for 7 days.

Terbinafine   250 mg/day for 14 days.

Tinea Corporis

Tinea corporis refers to dermatophyte infections of the trunk, legs, and arms, excluding the feet, hands, and groin.
Synonym: "Ringworm."

Epidemiology and Etiology

Age All ages

Occupation Animal (large and small) workers

Etiology *E. floccosum, T. rubrum* most commonly; *M. canis*

Transmission Autoinoculation from other parts of the body, i.e., from tinea pedis and tinea capitis. Contact with animals or contaminated soil.

Geography More common in tropical and subtropical regions

Predisposing Factors Most commonly infection is spread from dermatophytic infection of the feet (*T. rubrum, T. mentagrophytes*). Infection also can be acquired from an active lesion of an animal (*T. verrucosum, M. canis*) or, rarely, from soil (*M. gypseum*).

History

Incubation Period Days to months

Duration Weeks to months to years

Symptoms Often asymptomatic. Mild pruritus.

Physical Examination

Skin Lesions

TYPES Small (Figures 25-1 and 25-8) to large (Figure 25-9), scaling, sharply marginated plaques with or without pustules or vesicles, usually at margins. Bullae. Granulomatous lesions (Majocchi's granuloma). Psoriasiform plaques (Figure 25-9). Verrucous lesions. Zoophilic infection (contracted from animals) lesions are more inflammatory (Figure 25-8) with marked vesiculation and crusting at margins, bullae

SHAPE AND ARRANGEMENT Peripheral enlargement and central clearing (Figure 25-8), producing an annular configuration with concentric rings. Arcuate. Fusion of lesions produces gyrate patterns.

DISTRIBUTION Single and occasionally scattered multiple lesions

SITES OF PREDILECTION Anywhere on the trunk and extremities.

Differential Diagnosis

Well-Demarcated Scaling Plaque(s) Allergic contact dermatitis, atopic dermatitis, annular erythemas, psoriasis, seborrheic dermatitis, pityriasis rosea, pityriasis alba, pityriasis versicolor, erythema migrans, subacute LE

Laboratory and Special Examinations

See Dermatophytoses, page 694.

Management

Antifungal Agents See Dermatophytoses, page 690.

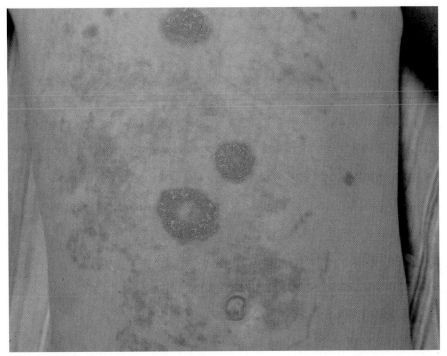

Figure 25-8 Tinea corporis *Multiple, bright red, sharply marginated lesions with only minimal scaling of several weeks duration on the trunk of a child. Three lesions are more inflammatory and thicker.* Microsporum canis *was isolated on fungal culture, which had been contracted from a pet guinea pig.*

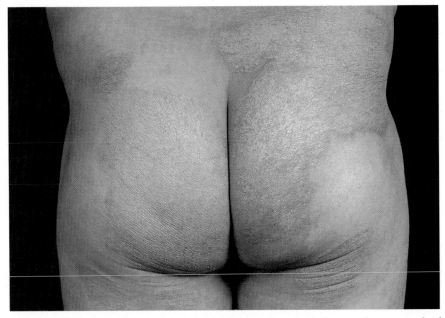

Figure 25-9 Tinea corporis *Sharply marginated, hyperpigmented plaques of many months duration on the back, buttocks, and thighs; scaling that gives the lesion the appearance of psoriasis. Associated tinea cruris and tinea pedis are usually present.*

Tinea Facialis

Tinea facialis is dermatophytosis of the glabrous facial skin, characterized by a well-circumscribed erythematous patch, and is more commonly misdiagnosed than any other dermatophytosis. *Synonyms:* Tinea faciei, ringworm of the face.

Epidemiology and Etiology

Age   More common in children

Etiology   *T. mentagrophytes, T. rubrum* most commonly; also *M. audouinii, M. canis*

Predisposing Factors   Animal exposure, chronic topical application of corticosteroids

History

Skin Symptoms   Most commonly asymptomatic. At times, pruritus and photosensitivity.

Physical Examination

Skin Lesions

TYPE   Well-circumscribed macule to plaque of variable size; elevated border and central regression (Figures 25-10 and 25-11). Scaling often is minimal but can be pronounced.

COLOR   Pink to red. In black patients, hyperpigmentation.

DISTRIBUTION   Any area of face but usually not symmetric

Differential Diagnosis

Scaling Facial Patches   Seborrheic dermatitis, contact dermatitis, erythema migrans, lupus erythematosus, polymorphic light eruption, phototoxic drug eruption, lymphocytic infiltrate

Laboratory and Special Examinations

Direct microscopic examination of scraping shows hyphae. Scrapings from patients who have used topical corticosteroid show massive numbers of hyphae.

Management

Topical antifungal preparations (see Table 25-A, page 691)
Eradicate dermatophyte infection at other sites such as feet and hands.

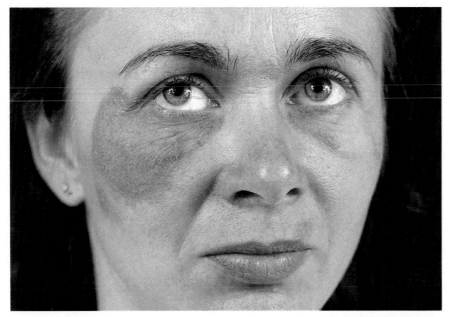

Figure 25-10 Tinea facialis *Sharply marginated, erythematous plaque with some central clearing and peripheral scaling on the lower eyelid and cheek of a young woman. Clinically, the lesion can be mistaken for chronic cutaneous (discoid) lupus erythematosus.*

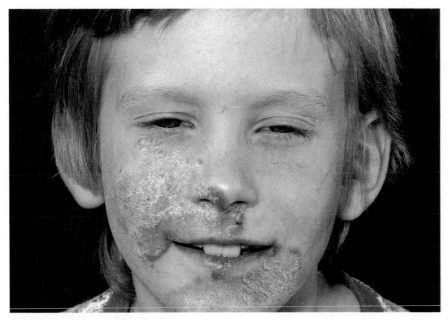

Figure 25-11 Tinea facialis *Sharply marginated, erythematous, scaling, and crusted plaques on the face of a child. Note asymmetry.*

DERMATOPHYTOSES OF HAIR

Dermatophytes are capable of hair invasion causing dermatophytic trichomycosis, with resultant tinea capitis, tinea barbae, and dermatophytic folliculitis.

Tinea Capitis

Tinea capitis is a dermatophytic trichomycosis of the scalp, the acute infection being characterized by follicular inflammation with painful, boggy nodules that drain pus and result in scarring alopecia, and the subacute to chronic infection, by scaling patches.

Epidemiology and Etiology

Etiology

UNITED STATES AND WESTERN EUROPE 90 % of cases of tinea capitis caused by *Trichophyton tonsurans;* less commonly *Microsporum canis.* Formerly, most cases were caused by *M. audouinii.* Less commonly, *M. gypseum, T. mentagrophytes, T. rubrum.*

EASTERN AND SOUTHERN EUROPE, NORTH AFRICA *T. violaceum*

Age Toddlers and school-aged children. Most common 6 to 10 years of age. Less common after age 16; in adults it occurs most commonly in a rural setting.

Race Much more common in blacks than in whites.

Transmission Person-to-person, animal-to-person, via fomites. Spores are present on asymptomatic carriers, animals, or inanimate objects.

Risk Factors For favus, debilitation, malnutrition, chronic disease

Pathogenesis Noninflammatory lesions: invasion of hair shaft by the dermatophytes, principally *M. audouinii* (child-to-child, via barber, hats, theater seats), *M. canis* (young pets-to-child and then child-to-child) or *T. tonsurans.* Inflammatory lesions: *T. tonsurans, M. canis, T. verrucosum,* and others. Spores enter through breaks in hair shaft or scalp to cause clinical infection.

Epidemiology Infections can become epidemic in schools and institutions, especially with overcrowding. Random fungal cultures in urban study revealed 4 % positive rate and a 12.7 % positive rate among black children.

Classification

ECTOTHRIX INFECTION Invasion occurs outside hair shaft. Hyphae fragment into arthroconidia, leading to cuticle destruction. Caused by *Microsporum* species (*M. audouinii* and *M. canis*) (Figure 25-12).

ENDOTHRIX INFECTION Infection occurs within hair shaft without cuticle destruction. Arthroconidia found within hair shaft. Caused by *Trichophyton* species (*T. tonsurans* in North America; *T. violaceum* in Europe, Asia, parts of Africa).
  "Black Dot" Tinea Capitis Variant of endothrix resembling seborrheic dermatitis (Figure 25-13)
  Kerion Variant of endothrix with boggy inflammatory plaques (Figure 25-14)
  Favus Variant of endothrix with arthroconidia and airspaces within hair shaft. Very uncommon in western Europe and North America. In some parts of the world (Middle East, South Africa), however, it is still endemic. (Figure 25-15)

History

Duration of Lesions Weeks to months

Skin Symptoms Loss of hair, pain and tenderness in inflammatory type

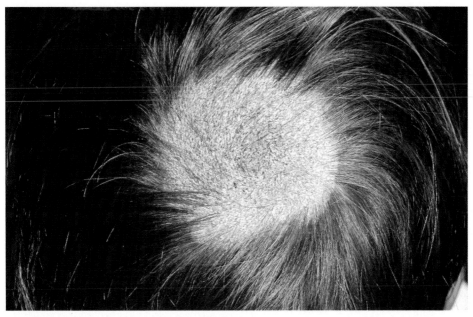

Figure 25-12 Tinea capitis: "gray patch" type *A large, round, hyperkeratotic plaque of alopecia due to breaking off of hair shafts close to the surface, giving the appearance of a mowed wheat field on the scalp of a child. Remaining hair shafts and scales exhibit a green fluorescence when examined with a Wood's lamp.* Microsporum canis *was isolated on culture.*

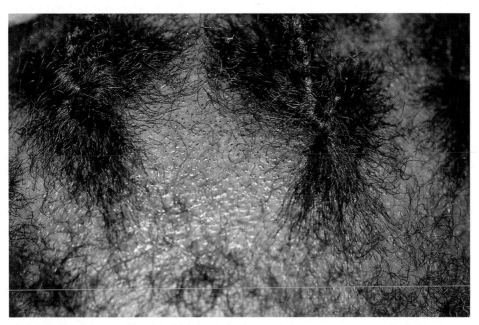

Figure 25-13 Tinea capitis: "black dot" variant *A subtle, asymptomatic patch of alopecia due to breaking off of hairs on the frontal scalp in a 4-year-old black child. The lesion was detected because her infant sister presented with tinea corporis.* Trichophyton tonsurans *was isolated on culture.*

Physical Examination

Skin Lesions and Hair Changes

CLASSIFICATION

> *Ectothrix Tinea Capitis* Presents as patches of scalp alopecia with scale (Figure 25-12), i.e., "gray patch" tinea capitis. Hair shaft becomes brittle, breaking off at or slightly above scalp. Small patches coalesce, forming larger patches. Inflammatory response minimal but massive scaling.

> *Endothrix Tinea Capitis* Clinical presentations include

- *"Black dot" tinea capitis* Broken-off hairs near surface give appearance of "dots" in dark-haired patients (Figure 25-13). Tends to be diffuse and poorly circumscribed. Resembles seborrheic dermatitis.
- *Kerion* Characterized by boggy, purulent, inflamed nodules and plaques (see Figure 25-14). Usually extremely painful; drains pus from multiple openings, like honeycomb. Hairs do not break off but fall out and can be pulled without pain. Heals with scarring alopecia.
- *Favus* Thick yellow adherent crusts (scutula) composed of skin debris and hyphae that are pierced by remaining hair shafts (Figure 25-15). Fetid odor. Untreated results in cutaneous atrophy, scar formation, and scarring alopecia.

Other Presentations Inflammatory pustules, cervical and occipital nodes, posterior and occipital lymphadenitis with minimal scalp changes.

Differential Diagnosis

"Gray Patch" Tinea Capitis Seborrheic dermatitis, psoriasis, atopic dermatitis, lichen simplex chronicus, alopecia areata

"Black Dot" Tinea Capitis Seborrheic dermatitis, psoriasis, seborrhiasis, atopic dermatitis, lichen simplex chronicus, chronic cutaneous lupus erythematosus, alopecia areata

Kerion Cellulitis, furuncle, carbuncle

Favus Impetigo, ecthyma, crusted scabies

Laboratory and Special Examinations

Wood's Lamp Examination Should be performed in any patient with scaling scalp lesions or hair loss of undetermined origin. *T. tonsurans,* the most common cause of tinea capitis in the United States, does not fluoresce. Formerly, *M. canis* and *M. audouinii,* which previously were the most common causes of tinea capitis, could be diagnosed by Wood's lamp examination, by bright green hair shafts with ectothrix infection.

Direct Microscopy Specimens should include hair roots and skin scales. Pluck hairs and use toothbrush to gather specimens. Skin scales contain hyphae and arthrospores. *Ectothrix:* arthrospores can be seen surrounding the hair shaft in cuticle. *Endothrix:* spores within hair shaft. *Favus:* loose chains of arthrospores and airspaces in hair shaft.

Fungal Culture With brush-culture technique, a dry toothbrush is rubbed over area of scale or alopecia; bristles are then inoculated into fungal media. A wet cotton swab also can be rubbed in affected area, which is then implanted into media. Growth of dermatophytes usually seen in 10 to 14 days.

ECTOTHRIX *Microsporum* species, *T. mentagrophytes, T. verrucosum*

ENDOTHRIX *T. tonsurans, T. violaceum, T. soudanense,* and *T. schoenleinii*

FAVUS *T. schoenleinii,* most commonly; also *T. violaceum, M. gypseum*

Bacterial Culture Rule out secondary bacterial infection, usually *Staphylococcus aureus* or group A streptococcus.

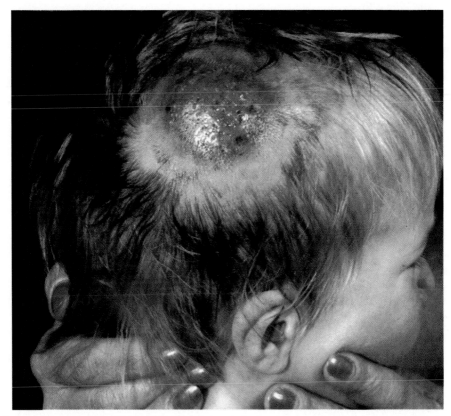

Figure 25-14 Tinea capitis: kerion type *Large, very painful, inflammatory tumor with hair loss, studded with multiple pustules on the scalp of a young child. Pressure on the lesion cause pus to discharge from multiple openings in a honeycomb pattern (*kerion *is the Greek term for honeycomb).*

Course

Chronic untreated kerion and favus, especially if secondarily infected with *S. aureus,* result in scarring alopecia. Regrowth of hair is the rule if treated with systemic antifungal agents. Favus may persist until adulthood.

Management

Prevention   Important to examine home and school contacts of affected children for asymptomatic carriers and mild cases of tinea capitis. Ketoconazole or selenium sulfide shampoo may be helpful in eradicating the asymptomatic carrier state.

Antifungal Agents   Topical agents are ineffective in management of tinea capitis. Duration of treatment should be extended until symptoms have resolved and fungal cultures negative.

NOTE: Of the systemic antifungals available, terbinafine and itraconazole are superior to ketoconazole and all three to griseofulvin. Side effects in increasing order: terbinafine, itraconazole < ketoconazole < griseofulvin

GRISEOFULVIN (ULTRAMICROSIZED)
  Pediatric Dose   Treatment duration: at least 6 weeks to several months; better absorption with fatty meal.

• Microsized: 15 mg/kg/day maximum 500 mg/day

• Ultramicrosized: 10 mg/kg/day

  Adult Dose

• "Gray patch" ringworm: 250 mg b.i.d. for 1 or 2 months
• "Black dot" ringworm: longer treatment and higher doses continued until KOH and cultures are negative
  Kerion   250 mg b.i.d. for 4 to 8 weeks, hot compresses; antibiotics for accompanying staphylococcal infection

KETOCONAZOLE   200-mg tablets. Treatment duration: 4 to 6 weeks.
  Pediatric Dose   5 mg/kg/day
  Adult Dose   200 to 400 mg/day

ITRACONAZOLE   100-mg capsules. Treatment duration: 4 to 6 weeks.
  Pediatric Dose   5 mg/kg/day
  Adult Dose   200 mg/day

TERBINAFINE   250-mg tablets. Treatment duration: 4 to 6 weeks.
  Pediatric Dose   10 mg/kg/day
  Adult Dose   250 mg/day

Adjunctive Therapy

PREDNISONE   1 mg/kg/day for 14 days for children with severe, painful kerion

SYSTEMIC ANTIBIOTICS   For secondary *S. aureus* or group A streptococcus infection, erythromycin, dicloxacillin, or cephalexin

Surgery   Drain pus from kerion lesions.

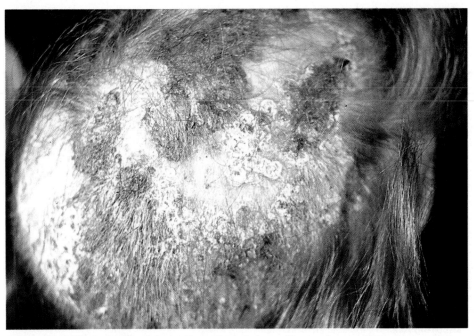

Figure 25-15 Tinea capitis: favus *Extensive hair loss with atrophy, scarring, and so-called scutula, i.e., yellowish adherent crusts present on the scalp; remaining hairs pierce scutula.* Trichophyton schoenleinii *was isolated on culture.*

Tinea Barbae

Tinea barbae is a dermatophytic trichomycosis involving the beard and moustache areas, closely resembling tinea capitis, with invasion of the hair shaft.
Synonym: Ringworm of the beard.

Epidemiology and Etiology

Age   Adult

Sex   Males only

Etiology   *T. verrucosum, T. mentagrophytes* most commonly. May be acquired through animal exposure.

Predisposing Factors   More common in farmers

History

Skin Symptoms   Pruritus, tenderness, pain

Physical Examination

Skin Lesions

TYPES   Pustular folliculitis (Figure 25-16), i.e., hair follicles surrounded by red inflammatory papules or pustules, often with exudation and crusting. Involved hairs are loose and easily removed. With less follicular involvement, there are scaling, circular, reddish patches in which hair is broken off at the surface. Papules may coalesce to inflammatory plaques topped by pustules. Kerion: boggy purulent nodules and plaques as with tinea capitis (Figure 25-17).

COLOR   Red

DISTRIBUTION   Beard and moustache areas, rarely eyelashes, eyebrows

Systemic Findings   Regional lymphadenopathy, especially if of long duration and if superinfected

Differential Diagnosis

Beard Folliculitis   *Staphylococcus aureus* folliculitis, furuncle, carbuncle, acne vulgaris, rosacea, pseudofolliculitis

Laboratory and Special Examinations

See Tinea Capitis, page 704.

Management

Topical Agents   Ineffective

Systemic Agents   See Tinea Capitis, page 704.

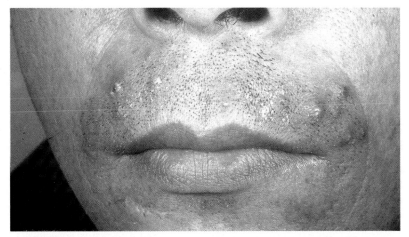

Figure 25-16 Tinea barbae *Scattered, discrete follicular pustules and papules in the moustache area, easily mistaken for* S. aureus *folliculitis.*

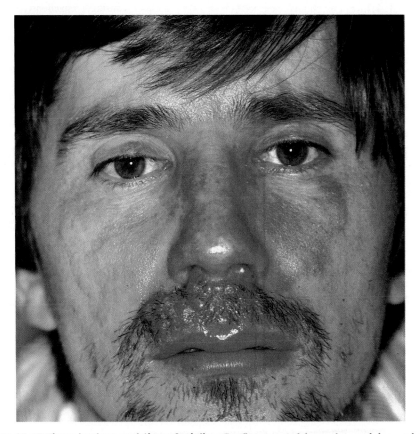

Figure 25-17 Tinea barbae and tinea facialis *Confluent, painful papules, nodules, and pustules on the upper lip. Epidermal dermatophytosis (tinea facialis) with sharply marginated erythema and scaling is present on the cheeks, eyelids, eyebrows, and forehead. Trichophyton mentagrophytes was isolated on culture. In this case, the organism caused two distinct clinical patterns (epidermal involvement, tinea facialis versus follicular inflammation, tinea barbae) depending on whether glabrous skin or hairy skin is infected.*

ONYCHOMYCOSIS AND TINEA UNGUIUM

Onychomycosis is an infection of the finger- or toenail caused by a wide variety of fungi, yeasts, and molds. *Tinea unguium* is a subtype of onychomycosis caused by the dermatophyte group of fungi.

Classification of the Anatomic Patterns of Onychomycosis

Distal and Lateral Subungual Onychomycosis (DLSO) (Figures 25-18 and 25-19)   Infection begins at the distal or lateral subungual margins and progressively involves the nail centripetally. May be either primary, i.e., involving a healthy nail, or secondary, i.e., involving a nail with established disease.

Superficial White Onychomycosis (SWO) The pathogen invades the nail plate on its surface.

Proximal Subungual Onychomycosis (PSO) (Figure 25-20)   The pathogen enters by way of the posterior nail fold–cuticle area and then migrates along the proximal nail groove to involve the underlying matrix, proximal to the nail bed, and finally the underlying nail plate.

Total Dystrophic Onychomycosis (TDO) (Figure 25-21)   May be either primary, i.e., involving a healthy nail, or secondary, i.e., involving a nail with established disease, and is often associated with chronic mucocutaneous candidiasis.

Etiology and Epidemiology

Etiology

ETIOLOGIC FACTORS   Toenail onychomycosis: The most important factor is wearing of occlusive footwear; others include overcrowding, communal bathing areas; disturbance of arterial circulation.

ETIOLOGIC AGENTS

Dermatophytes   Anthropophilic species: *Trichophyton rubrum, T. mentagrophytes* var. *interdigitale, T. violaceum, T. schoenleinii, Epidermophyton floccosum.* Zoo-

philic species: *T. verrucosum,* which usually infects only fingernails.

Yeasts   *Candida albicans, C. tropicalis, C. parapsilosis*

Molds   More than 40 mold species have been reported to cause onychomycosis. *Scopulariopsis brevicaulis,* the ubiquitous soil fungus, is the most commonly implicated pathogen in nondermatophyte nail infection and is capable of infecting normal as well as damaged nails. Other molds causing onychomycosis include: *Aspergillus* species, *Alternaria* species, *Acremonium* species, *Fusarium* species, *Scytalidium dimidiatum (Hendersonula toruloidea), S. hyalinum.* Most cases occur on the feet, which are more commonly exposed to soil. Onychomycosis caused by molds cannot be distinguished on clinical findings and may account for treatment failures.

ETIOLOGY OF ANATOMIC TYPES OF ONYCHOMY-
COSIS   *DLSO*   Most commonly, *T. rubrum*
PSO   Most commonly, *T. rubrum;* also
T. megnenii, T. schoenleinii, E. floccosum
SWO   Most commonly, *T. mentagrophytes*

Geographic Distribution   Worldwide. The etiologic agent varies in different geographic areas. More common in urban than in rural areas.

Age   Onset most common from 20 to 50 years. In one study, 1.3 % in 16- to 34-year-olds had onychomycosis, 2.4 % in 35- to 50-year-olds, and 4.7 % in those ≥55 years.

Prevalence   The incidence varies in different geographic regions. In the United States, an 8.1 % prevalence of tinea pedis and 2.2 % for onychomycosis has been reported (1979). In a report from Britain, the prevalence of onychomycosis was 2.8 % in men and 2.6 % in women. Currently in the United States, incidence reported to be 20 % of adults

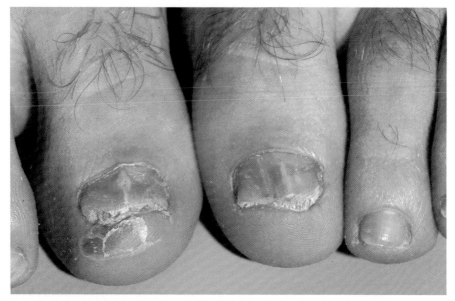

Figure 25-18 Onychomycosis of toenails: distal and lateral subungual type *Distal subungual hyperkeratosis and onycholysis involving most of the nail bed of the great toenails; these findings are usually associated with tinea pedis.*

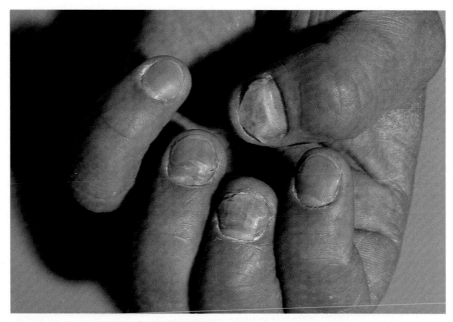

Figure 25-19 Onychomycosis of fingernails: distal and lateral subungual type *Distal onycholysis with subungual hyperkeratosis on two fingernails; the nail plates are relatively preserved. Associated tinea manuum with scaling and erythema is also present.*

Sex

TINEA UNGUIUM Somewhat more common in men

CANDIDA ONYCHOMYCOSIS More common in women

Transmission

DERMATOPHYTES Anthropophilic dermatophyte infections are transmitted from one individual to another, by fomite or direct contact, occurring commonly within family members. Some spore forms (arthroconidia) remain viable and infective in the environment for up to 5 years.

CANDIDA Part of the normal flora, which usually causes infection if the local ecology is changed in favor of the yeast or associated with altered immune status

MOLDS These organisms are ubiquitous in the environment and are not transmitted between humans.

History

PSO Previously a rare pattern, it occurs commonly on toenails in persons with HIV disease. May occur on the fingernails secondary to chronic paronychia.

Candidal Onychia and Paronychia History of frequent immersion in water is common. Occurs more commonly on the dominant hand, especially on the first and third fingers; infection of toenails uncommon. In comparison with other types of onychomycosis, *Candida* paronychia is painful and tender. Candidal onychia and paronychia are common in children with HIV disease and are usually associated with mucosal candidiasis.

Chronic Mucocutaneous Candidiasis (CMC) In patients with CMC with multiple endocrine gland failure, candidiasis at mucosal sites and paronychia occur in childhood followed by endocrinopathies, with hypoparathyroidism presenting first. CMC is associated with thymomas, myasthenia gravis, myositis, aplastic anemia, neutropenia, and hypogammaglobulinemia; onset is usually in adulthood.

Clinical Findings

Skin Findings Approximately 80 % of onychomycosis occurs on the feet, especially on the big toes; simultaneous occurrence on toe- and fingernails is not common.

DLSO A white patch is noted on the distal or lateral undersurface of the nail and nail bed, usually with sharply demarcated borders. In time, the whitish color can become discolored to a brown or black hue. Progressive involvement of the nail can occur in a matter of weeks, as in HIV disease, or more slowly over a period of months or years. With progressive infection, the nail becomes opaque, thickened, cracked, friable, raised by underlying hyperkeratotic debris in the nail bed (Figures 25-18 and 25-19). Sharply marginated white streaks beginning at the distal nail margin and extending proximate are filled with keratinaceous debris and air. DLSO caused by dermatophytes or mold is indistinguishable on clinical findings.

Toenails are involved much more commonly than fingernails. The first and fifth toenails are infected most frequently. Involvement of the fingernails is usually unilateral. When fingernails are involved, pattern is usually two feet and one hand.

SWO A white chalky plaque is seen on the proximal nail plate, which may become eroded with loss of the nail plate. Diagnostically, the involved nail can be removed easily with a curette in comparison with a traumatized nail, which has white, air-containing areas. In some cases, the entire superficial nail plate may become involved. SWO may coexist with DLSO. Occurs almost exclusively on the toenails, rarely on the fingernails.

PSO A white spot appears from beneath the proximal nail fold (Figure 25-20). In time the white spot fills the lunula, eventually moving distally to involve much of the undersurface of the nail plate. Patients treated with

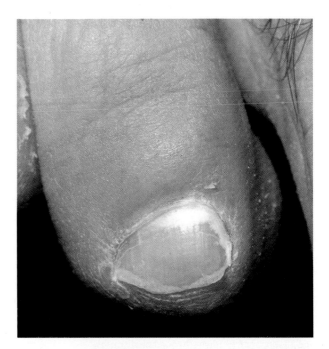

Figure 25-20 Tinea unguium: proximal subungual onychomycosis type *The proximal nail plate is a chalky white color due to invasion from the undersurface of the nail matrix. The patient had advanced HIV disease.*

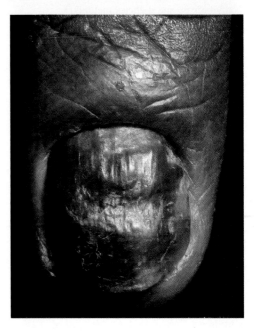

Figure 25-21 Onychomycosis: total dystrophic type *The entire fingernail plate is thickened and dystrophic and is associated with a paronychial infection; both findings were caused* Candida albicans *in an individual with advanced HIV disease.*

oral azoles show interruption of the involved nail. Occurs more commonly on the toenails.

CANDIDAL ONYCHOMYCOSIS (See also page 720) Begins with a proximal and later lateral paronychia, which appears clinically as edema, erythema, and pain of the nail fold; at times pus can be expressed (Figure 25-28). Secondary to paronychial infection, nail plate becomes dystrophic with areas of opacification, white, yellow, green, or black discoloration, with transverse furrowing (Figure 25-21). *Pressure on the nail is often painful.* About 70 % of cases occur on the fingernails, most commonly the middle finger. Uncommon presentation: subungual abscess

General Findings In patients with CMC, oropharyngeal and vulvovaginal candidiasis is often present. In those with CMC and endocrinopathy, vitiligo and alopecia areata also may be present, as well as polyglandular failure (hypoparathyroidism, hypoadrenalism, hypothyroidism, and diabetes mellitus).

Differential Diagnosis

Paronychial Disease *Candida* paronychia, herpetic whitlow, eczematous dermatitis, allergic contact dermatitis, lichen planus

DLSO Psoriatic involvement of the nails ("oil drop" staining of the distal nail bed and nail pits are seen in psoriasis but not onychomycosis), paronychial involvement of eczema, Reiter's syndrome and keratoderma blennorrhagicum, onychogryphosis, pincer nails, congenital nail dystrophies, pseudomonal nail infection (black-green discoloration)

SWO Traumatic injury to nail

Laboratory Studies

Obtaining Nail Samples All clinical diagnoses of onychomycosis should be confirmed by laboratory findings. Samples are best obtained from the distal edge of the involved nail, after the nail has been trimmed back, using a

1-mm curette or scalpel to scrape the undersurface of the nail and/or nail bed in DLSO. In SWO, the sample is obtained from the dorsal nail plate; in PSO, after removing the dorsal nail plate.

Direct Microscopy Direct microscopic examination of nail samples is used to confirm the clinical diagnosis. Keratinaceous material from the involved nail is placed on a glass slide, covered with a glass coverslip, suspended in a solution of potassium hydroxide (KOH), and gently heated. Addition of dimethyl sulfoxide and/or Parker Quink ink to the KOH solution may facilitate identification of fungal elements. Specific identification of the pathogen is usually not possible by microscopy but, in most cases, yeasts can be differentiated from dermatophytes.

Fungal Culture Isolation of the pathogen permits better use of oral antifungal agents. Samples of the infected nail are inoculated onto Sabouraud's agar with or without cyclohex-imide.

Histology of Nail Clipping Indicated if clinical findings suggest onychomycosis even after three KOH wet mounts and three cultures performed at weekly intervals have not detected pathogen. PAS stain is used to detect fungal elements in the nail. Probably the most reliable technique for diagnosing onychomycosis.

Diagnosis

Clinical findings confirmed by finding fungal forms in KOH preparation and/or isolation of pathogenic fungus on culture

Pathogenesis

Primary Onychomycosis Invasion of the nail occurs in an otherwise healthy nail. The probability of nail invasion by fungi increases with defective vascular supply (i.e., with increasing age, CVI, peripheral arterial disease), in post-traumatic states (lower leg fractures), or disturbance of innervation (e.g., injury to brachial plexus, trauma of spine).

Secondary Onychomycosis Infection occurs in an already altered nail, such as psoriatic or traumatized nail.

Toenail tinea unguium usually occurs after tinea pedis; fingernail involvement is usually secondary to tinea manuum, tinea corporis, or tinea capitis. Infection of the first and fifth toenails probably occurs secondary to damage to these nails by footwear.

DLSO The nail bed produces soft keratin stimulated by fungal infection that accumulates under the nail plate, thereby raising it, a change that clinically gives the involved nail an altered cream color rather than the normal transparent appearance. The dense keratin of the nail plate is not involved primarily. The accumulated subungual keratin promotes further fungal growth and keratin production. The nail matrix is not invaded and production of normal nail plate remains unimpaired despite fungal infection. In time, dermatophytes create air-containing tunnels within the nail plate; where the network is sufficiently dense, the nail is opaque. Often the invasion follows the longitudinal ridges of the nail bed. The subungual location of the infection could block effective topical antifungal agents.

Candida **Infection** In candidal infection of the nail, infection begins in the proximal nail fold, spreading around the nail. With subacute or chronic candidal paronychia, the nail plate becomes dystrophic.

Course and Prognosis

Without effective therapy, onychomycosis does not resolve spontaneously; progressive involvement of multiple toenails is the rule. Relapse occurs in the majority of persons (80 % to 90 %) with tinea unguium treated with griseofulvin. Long-term relapse rate with newer oral agents such as itraconazole or terbinafine is less than with griseofulvin but is yet to be determined with long-term follow-up studies. In persons with HIV disease, PSO, DLSO, and SWO may occur in the same nail, leading to rapid destruction of the nail.

Management (in Adults)

Topical Agents See Table 25-A. Available as lotions and lacquer. Usually not effective except for early DLSO and SWO after prolonged use (months). Amorolfine nail lacquer reported to be effective when applied >12 months. Needs confirmation.

Systemic Agents

GRISEOFULVIN (see page 690) Has to be administered over many months and at least as long as nail has completely regrown. High recurrence rate. Not in use in the United States and Europe anymore.

Azoles Drugs in this category are usually effective in treatment of nail infections caused by dermatophytes, yeasts, and molds.

ITRACONAZOLE (see page 690) 200 mg b.i.d. for first 7 days of each month for 2 months (fingernails) or 4 months (toenails); or 200 mg daily for 6 weeks (fingernails), 12 weeks (toenails). Effective in dermatophytes and candida

KETOCONAZOLE (see page 690) Effective at 200 mg daily; more effective for Candida than dermatophytes; however, infrequently hepatotoxicity and antiandrogen effect have limited its long-term use for onychomycosis.

FLUCONAZOLE Reported effective at dosing of 150 to 400 mg 1 day per week or 100 to 200 mg daily for 24 weeks. Needs confirmation. Effective in yeasts and less so in dermatophytes

Allylamines Most effective against dermatophyte infections

TERBINAFINE 250 mg/day for 6 weeks (fingernails); 250 mg/day for 12 weeks (toenails). Cure rate: 80 %

NOTE: In systemic treatment of onychomycosis the nail may not appear normal after the treatment times indicated because of slow growth of nail. If culture and KOH prep are negative after these time periods medication can nonetheless be stopped and nail will regrow normally.

CANDIDIASIS

CUTANEOUS CANDIDIASIS

Cutaneous candidiasis is a superficial infection occurring on moist cutaneous sites; many patients have predisposing factors such as increased moisture at the site of infection, diabetes, or alteration in systemic immunity.

Synonyms: Candidosis, moniliasis.

Epidemiology and Etiology

Age Any age. Infants (diaper area, mouth).

Sex Both. Women (vulvovaginitis), men (balanitis)

Etiology *Candida albicans.* Uncommonly, other *Candida* species.

Ecology *C. albicans* is seldom recovered from skin of normal individuals. Usually endogenous infection. *Candida* is a normal inhabitant of mucosal surfaces of oropharynx and GI tract. In males with balanitis, *Candida* may be transmitted from female sexual partner.

Occupation Persons who immerse their hands in water: housewives, mothers of young children, health care workers, bartenders, florists

Other Predisposing Factors Diabetes, obesity, hyperhidrosis, heat, maceration, polyendocrinopathies, systemic and topical corticosteroids, chronic debilitation

Classification

CANDIDA IN OCCLUDED SKIN Occurs where occlusion and maceration create warm, moist microecology.

Intertrigo

- Body folds: axillae, inframammary, groins, intergluteal
- Webspaces: fingers (erosio interdigitalis blastomycetica); associated with frequent wetting of hands. Toes.

Genital

- Balanoposthitis or balanitis
- Vulvitis

Occluded Skin Under occlusive dressing, under cast, back in hospitalized patient

Folliculitis Usually at sites of occlusion

Diaper Dermatitis May be primary or secondary infection

CANDIDA PARONYCHIA AND ONYCHIA Associated with frequent wetting of hands

CHRONIC MUCOCUTANEOUS CANDIDIASIS A group of uncommon conditions in which individuals with congenital immunologic (T-cell defects) or endocrinologic disorders (hypoparathyroidism, hypoadrenalism, hypothyroidism, diabetes mellitus) develop persistent or recurrent mucosal, cutaneous, or nail infections with *C. albicans*. Onset: within first 3 years of life. Mouth may be first site involved. Scalp, trunk, hands, feet also involved. Nail and fingertips affected.

History

Candida in Occluded Skin

- Intertrigo
  Axillae, inframammary, groins, intergluteal
  Webspaces: fingers (erosio interdigitalis blastomycetica), toes
- Balanoposthitis or balanitis: soreness, irritation of glans penis; subpreputial discharge
- Vulvitis: soreness, burning, dysuria, itching
- Occluded skin: under occlusive dressing, under cast, back in hospitalized patient
- Folliculitis: itching
- Diaper dermatitis: irritability, discomfort with urination, defecation, changing diapers

Candida Paronychia and Onychia Associ-

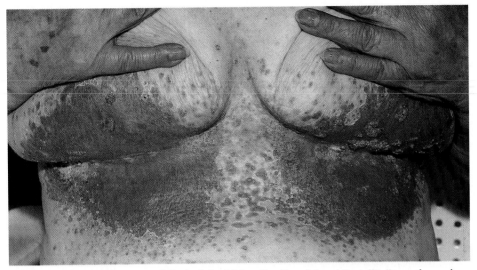

Figure 25-22 Cutaneous candidiasis: intertrigo *Small peripheral "satellite" papules and pustules that have become confluent centrally creating large eroded area in the inframammary area.*

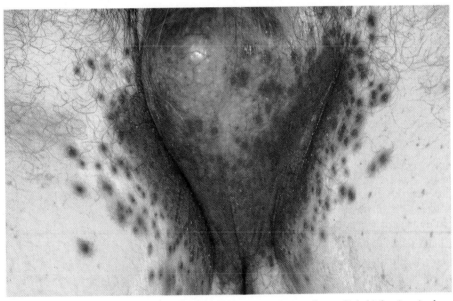

Figure 25-23 Cutaneous candidiasis: intertrigo *Erosions on the medial thighs, inguinal folds, and scrotum with "satellite" pustules and papules of an obese male.*

ated with frequent wetting of hands. History of intermittent painful swelling of lateral nail folds.

Physical Examination

Intertrigo Initial pustules on erythematous base become eroded and confluent. Subsequently, fairly sharply demarcated, polycyclic, erythematous, eroded patches with small pustular lesions at the periphery (satellite pustulosis). Distribution: inframammary (Figure 25-22), axillae, groins (Figure 25-23), perineal, intergluteal cleft.

Interdigital Erosio interdigitalis blastomycetica: Initial pustule becomes eroded, with formation of superficial erosion or fissure, ±surrounded by thickened white skin (Figure 25-24). May be associated with *Candida* onychia or paronychia. Distribution: on hands, usually between third and fourth fingers (Figure 25-24); on feet, similar presentation as interdigital tinea pedis.

Balanoposthitis, Balanitis Preputial sac: pustules, erosions (Figure 25-25). Maculopapular lesions with diffuse erythema. Edema, ulcerations, and fissuring of prepuce, usually in diabetic men; white plaques under foreskin.

Vulvitis Erosions, pustules, erythema (Figure 25-26), swelling, removable curdlike material

Diaper Dermatitis Erythema, edema with papular and pustular lesions; erosions, oozing, collarette-like scaling at the margins of lesions involving perigenital and perianal skin, inner aspects of thighs and buttocks (Figure 25-27)

Candida **Paronychia and Onychia** Initially, redness and swelling of proximal (also lateral) nail folds. Swelling lifts wall from underlying nail plate. Subsequently, infection becomes purulent, pressure releases creamy pus from nail fold (Figure 25-28). Painful. Nails may show onychodystrophy, onycholysis, discoloration (yellow, green, or black on lateral nail), and ridging (Figure 25-29). *Staphylococcus aureus* may cause superinfection. Subungual abscess

Follicular Candidiasis Small, discrete pustules in ostia of hair follicles

Differential Diagnosis

Intertrigo Nonspecific intertrigo, inverse pattern psoriasis, erythrasma

Interdigital Scabies

Balanoposthitis Psoriasis, eczema

Diaper Dermatitis Atopic dermatitis, psoriasis, irritant dermatitis, seborrheic dermatitis

Candida **Paronychia and Onychia** Dermatophytosis, *S. aureus* paronychia, herpetic whitlow

Folliculitis Bacterial *(S. aureus, Pseudomonas aeruginosa)* folliculitis, *Pityrosporum* folliculitis, acne

Laboratory and Special Examinations

Direct Microscopy Examination of scraping using Gram's stain or 10 % to 30 % KOH preparation visualizes pseudohyphae and yeast forms.

Fungal Culture Identification of *Candida* species.

Bacterial Culture Rule out bacterial superinfection.

Diagnosis

Clinical findings confirmed by direct microscopy or culture

Management

Prevention Keeping intertriginous areas dry is often difficult. Washing with benzoyl peroxide bar may reduce *Candida* colonization. Powder with miconazole applied daily.

Topical Treatment of Acute Episodes Castellani's paint brings almost immediate relief of symptoms. Short-term use of topical corticosteroid preparation speeds resolution of symptoms.

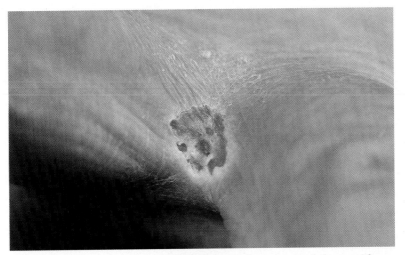

Figure 25-24 Cutaneous candidiasis: interdigital *Erythematous eroded area with surrounding maceration in a webspace of the hand occurring in a health care worker is a type of intertrigo.*

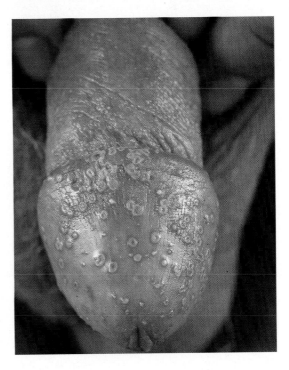

Figure 25-25 Candidiasis: balanoposthitis *Multiple, discrete pustules on the glans penis and inner aspect of the foreskin (the preputial sac). The "umbilicated" lesions can be mistaken for genital herpes, mollusca contagiosa, or condylomata acuminata.*

INTERTRIGO Castellani's paint. Nystatin or imidazole creams applied b.i.d.

BALANITIS/BALANOPOSTHITIS, VULVITIS Castellani's paint. Keep foreskin retracted if possi-

ble. Nystatin or imidazole creams applied b.i.d.

VULVITIS Castellani's paint, nystatin, azole, or imidazole creams applied b.i.d. Frequently

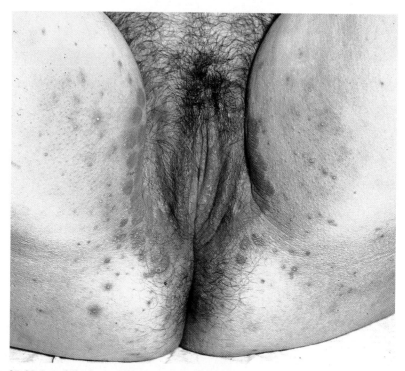

Figure 25-26 Candidiasis: vulvitis *Psoriasiform, erythematous lesions becoming confluent on the vulva with erosions and satellite pustules on the thighs.*

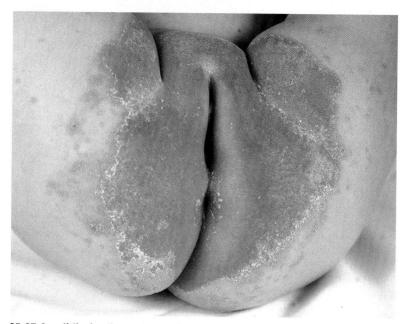

Figure 25-27 Candidiasis: diaper dermatitis *Confluent erosions, marginal scaling, and "satellite pustules" in the area covered by a diaper in an infant.*

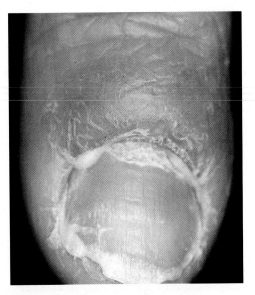

Figure 25-28 Candida paronychia *Painful, paronychial erythema and edema with pus exuding from under the proximal nail fold. Transverse grooves on the nail plate chronical prior episodes of infection.* Candida *parony-chia, which is an infection of the space between the undersurface of the cuticle and the proximal dorsal nail plate, is often mistaken for* S. aureus *paronychia, an infection of the paronychial tissue itself.*

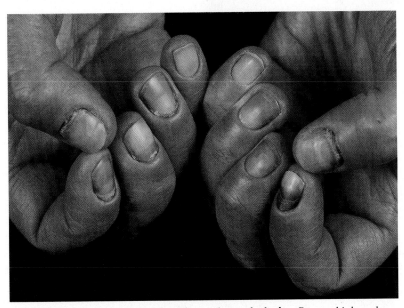

Figure 25-29 Candida paronychia, onychia, and onycholysis *Paronychial erythema and edema with proximal, as well as distal, onycholysis and onychodystrophy. The green-brown color was caused by* Pseudomonas aeruginosa *superinfection of the diseased nails. The patient was immunosuppressed following organ transplantation.*

associated with candidal vaginitis (vaginal candidiasis).

DIAPER CANDIDIASIS Dilute Castellani's paint. Nystatin or imidazole creams applied b.i.d. Oral nystatin (which is not absorbed from the gut) eliminates bowel candidal colonization, thus reducing frequent recurrences.

PARONYCHIA Castellani's paint. Eliminate immersion in water if possible. Nystatin or imidazole creams applied b.i.d. If topical therapy fails, systemic treatment is effective: fluconazole 200 mg weekly *or* itraconazole 200 mg/day until space between nail fold and nail plate has been eliminated.

MUCOSAL CANDIDIASIS

Mucosal candidiasis is a *Candida* infection occurring on the mucosa of the upper aerodigestive tract and vulvovagina; the course may be acute or chronic. Superficial mucosal candidiasis occurs in the oropharynx and vulvovagina in individuals with mild to moderate immunocompromise; deep mucosal candidiasis occurs in the esophagus and tracheobronchial tree in those with advanced immunocompromise. *Candida* can invade through eroded mucosa with resultant fungemia and invasive candidiasis.

Synonyms: Moniliasis; for oropharyngeal candidiasis, thrush, mycotic stomatitis, *Candida* leukoplakia.

Epidemiology and Etiology

Age   All ages

Sex   Equal

Etiology   *C. albicans,* most commonly, but also *C. tropicalis, C. (Torula) glabrata, C. Parapsilosis, C. krusei, C. lusitaniae, C. rugosa.* In some individuals, two or more species can be isolated. Increasingly, fluconazole-resistant strains of *C. albicans*. In HIV disease, >90 % of *Candida* infections are caused by *C. albicans,* serotype B.

Ecology   *Candida* species can be isolated from mouth and intestinal tract of a large portion of the normal population (30 % to 50 %) and from the genital tract in >20 % of normal women. *C. albicans* accounts for 60 % to 80 % of oropharyngeal isolates and 80 % to 90 % of genital isolates.

Incidence   Although a number of risk factors exist (see below) and almost obligatory involvement occurs in immunocompromised patients, it must be emphasized that the vast majority of mucosal candidiasis, in particular vaginal candidiasis, occurs in the *normal* population.

VAGINAL CANDIDIASIS (VC)   75 % of women experience at least one episode of VC during their lifetime, and 40 % to 45 % will experience two or more episodes. Often associated with vulvar candidiasis, i.e., vulvovaginal candidiasis (VVC). A small percentage of women (probably <5 %) experience recurrent VVC (RVVC).

HIV DISEASE   Oropharyngeal candidiasis (OPC) occurs in 50 % of those infected and 80 % to 95 % of those with AIDS; 60 % relapse within 3 months after treatment. Esophageal candidiasis occurs in 10 % to 15 % of individuals with AIDS.

BONE MARROW TRANSPLANT (BMT) RECIPIENTS   30 % to 40 % develop superficial mucosal candidiasis.

Transmission   Normal inhabitant of mucosal surfaces of the oropharynx and gastrointestinal tract; overgrowth associated with local or systemic suppression of immunity or antibiotic therapy. VC can be acquired sexually. In neonatal OPC, *C. albicans* is acquired from the genital tract of mother. Nosocomially transmission does occur.

Risk Factors   In addition to HIV-induced immunodeficiency, other risk factors include: general debilitation, diabetes mellitus, therapy with broad-spectrum antibiotics, topical or parenteral corticosteroids, parenteral hyperalimentation.

CDC Surveillance Case Definition for AIDS
Candidiasis of the esophagus, trachea, bronchi, or lungs is an AIDS-defining condition if the patient has no other cause of immunodeficiency and is without knowledge of HIV antibody status.

Classification

SUPERFICIAL MUCOSAL CANDIDIASIS   (May be associated with mild to moderate impairment of cell-mediated immunity.)
Vaginal and Vulvovaginal Candidiasis
Oropharyngeal Candidiasis

- Erythematous (atrophic) candidiasis
- Pseudomembranous candidiasis (thrush)
- Candidal leukoplakia (hyperplastic candidiasis)
- Angular cheilosis

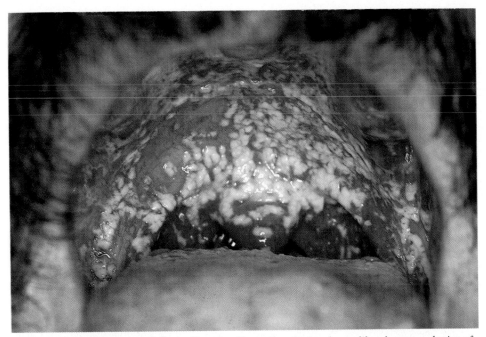

Figure 25-30 Mucosal candidiasis: thrush *Extensive cottage cheese-like plaques, colonies of* Candida *that can be removed by rubbing with gauze, on the palate and uvula of an individual with advanced HIV disease. Patches of erythema between the white plaques represent erythematous (atrophic) candidiasis. Involvement may extend into the esophagus and be associated with dysphagia.*

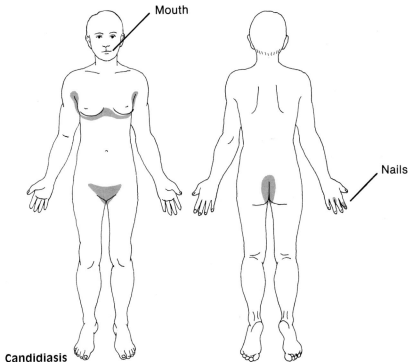

Mouth

Nails

Figure X Candidiasis

DEEP MUCOSAL CANDIDIASIS Occurs in states of advanced immunocompromise: esophageal candidiasis (EC), tracheobronchial candidiasis (TBC), both of which are AIDS-defining conditions. Bladder.

History

Incubation Period

HIV DISEASE *Candida* overgrowth occurs many years after primary HIV infection, with increasing immunodeficiency.

History

VC AND VVC Onset often abrupt, usually the week prior to menstruation; symptoms may recur prior to each menstruation. Pruritus, vaginal discharge, vaginal soreness, vulvar burning, dyspareunia, external dysuria.

OPC Most patients are asymptomatic. At times, burning sensation, diminished taste sensation. Cosmetic concern about white curds on tongue. Odynophagia. In HIV disease, OPC is a clinical marker for disease progression, first noted when CD4+ cell counts is 390/μl.

EC Occurs when CD4+ cell count is low (<200/μl) and is an AIDS-defining condition. Dysphagia. Odynophagia, resulting in difficulty eating and malnutrition.

Physical Examination

Mucosal Lesions

TYPES

VC/VVC Vaginitis with white discharge; vaginal erythema and edema; white plaques that can be wiped off on vaginal and/or cervical mucosa. Often associated with vulvar candidiasis and candidal intertrigo of inguinal folds and perineum.

OPC

- Pseudomembranous candidiasis (thrush) (Figure 25-30): removable white plaques on any mucosal surface; vary in size from 1 to 2 mm to extensive and widespread; removal with a dry gauze pad leaves an erythematous or bleeding mucosal surface.

- Erythematous (atrophic) smooth, red, atrophic patches
- Candidal leukoplakia: white plaques that cannot be wiped off but regress with prolonged anticandidal therapy
- Angular cheilitis: erythema, fissuring, i.e., intertrigo at the corner of mouth (Figure 25-31)

COLOR Thrush: white to creamy

PALPATION Thrush: removable with dry gauze

DISTRIBUTION *Thrush:* dorsum of tongue, buccal mucosa, hard/soft palate, pharynx extending down into esophagus and tracheobronchial tree. *Erythematous (atrophic) candidiasis:* hard/soft palate, buccal mucosa, dorsal surface of tongue. *Leukoplakia:* buccal mucosa, tongue, hard palate.

General Findings

INVASIVE CANDIDIASIS In individuals with severe prolonged neutropenia, *Candida* can invade into submucosa and blood vessels with subsequent hematogenous dissemination to skin and viscera. Candidemia also occurs in the setting of prolonged catheterization.

Differential Diagnosis

VC/VVC Trichomoniasis (caused by *Trichomonas vaginalis*), bacterial vaginosis (caused by replacement of normal vaginal flora by an overgrowth of anaerobic microorganisms and *Gardnerella vaginalis*), lichen planus, lichen sclerosus et atrophicus

OPC

PSEUDOMEMBRANOUS CANDIDIASIS (THRUSH) Oral hairy leukoplakia, condyloma acuminatum, geographic tongue, hairy tongue, lichen planus, bite irritation

ATROPHIC (ERYTHEMATOUS) CANDIDIASIS Lichen planus

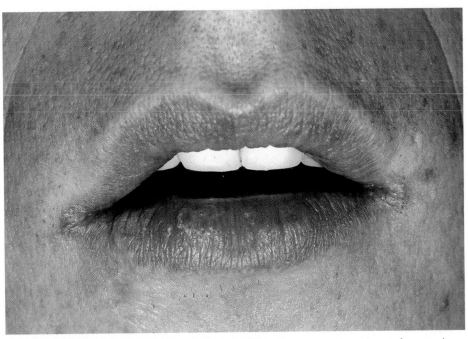

Figure 25-31 Mucosal candidiasis: angular cheilitis *Erythema and erosion at the commissures of the lips were associated with oropharyngeal candidiasis in an HIV-infected individual.*

Laboratory and Special Examinations

KOH Preparation   Scraping of an area suspected as candidiasis shows *Candida* pseudohyphae as well as budding yeast forms.

Culture   Identifies species of *Candida;* however, the presence of culture of *C. albicans* does not make the diagnosis of candidiasis because candidiasis is a normal inhabitant of the GI tract. Identifying *Candida* in the absence of symptoms should not lead to treatment, because 10 % to 20 % of normal women harbor *Candida* spp. and other yeasts in the vagina. Sensitivities to antifungal agents can be performed on isolate in cases of recurrent infection.

Endoscopy   Documents esophageal and/or tracheobronchial candidiasis.

Diagnosis

Clinical suspicion confirmed by KOH preparation of scraping from mucosal surface

Pathophysiology

C. albicans is part of the normal oral flora. Overgrowth with resultant oral candidiasis occurs when immunity is suppressed locally, as with use of corticosteroid inhalers or with the profound immunodeficiency that occurs with advancing HIV disease. Onset of candidiasis correlates with moderate degree of immunodeficiency in HIV-infected patients and portends that AIDS is imminent.

Course and Prognosis

RVVC   Defined as three or more episodes of symptomatic VVC annually. Affects a small proportion of women (<5 %). The natural history and pathogenesis of RVVC are poorly understood. The majority of women with RVVC have no apparent predisposing conditions.

Failure to Respond to Antifungal Agents
Clinical resistance to antifungal agents may be related to patient noncompliance, severe immunocompromise, drug-drug interaction (rifampin-fluconazole).

Bone Marrow Transplant (BMT) Recipients
Between 30 % and 40 % develop superficial mucosal candidiasis; 10 % to 25 % develop deep invasive candidiasis, of whom a quarter die from the infection and others go on to develop chronic visceral candidiasis.

HIV Disease   Oropharyngeal and esophageal candidiasis have been reported with primary HIV infection. In later HIV disease, OPC is nearly universal; vaginal infection extremely common, and esophageal infection occurs in 10 % to 20 % of patients. Relapse after topical or systemic treatment is expected. Virtually all HIV-infected individuals with CD4+ cell counts of ≤100/μl harbor oral *Candida;* chronic suppressive therapy is associated with changes in mouth flora rather than eradication.

Management

VC/VVC

TOPICAL THERAPY   Azoles/imidazoles are more effective than nystatin and result in relief of symptoms and negative cultures among 80 % to 90 % of patients after therapy is completed.

RECOMMENDED REGIMENS   Single-dose regimens probably should be reserved for cases of uncomplicated mild to moderate VVC. Multiday regimens (3- to 7-day) are the preferred treatment for severe or complicated VVC.

Butoconazole: 2 % cream 5 g intravaginally for 3 days *or*
Clotrimazole: 1 % cream 5 g intravaginally for 7 to 14 days *or*
   100-mg vaginal tablet for 7 days *or*
   100-mg vaginal tablet, two tablets for 3 days *or*
   500-mg vaginal tablet, one tablet in a single application *or*
Miconazole: 2 % cream 5g intravaginally for 7 days *or*

200-mg vaginal suppository, one suppository for 3 days *or*

100-mg vaginal suppository, one suppository for 7 days *or*

Tioconazole: 6.5 % ointment 5 g intravaginally in a single application *or*

Terconazole: 0.4 % cream 5 g intravaginally for 7 days *or*

0.8 % cream 5 g intravaginally for 3 days *or*

80-mg suppository, one suppository for 3 days

Fluconazole: 150 mg PO as a single dose

RVVC   Weekly dosing of the following may be effective:

Clotrimazole: 500-mg vaginal tablet, one tablet in a single application *or*

Fluconazole: 150 mg PO as a single dose

Intraconazole: 100 mg b.i.d.

OPC

TOPICAL THERAPY   These preparations are effective in the immunocompetent individual but relatively ineffective with decreasing cell-mediated immunity.

Nystatin: For OPC, vaginal tablets, 100,000 units q.i.d. dissolved slowly in the mouth, are the most effective preparation. The oral suspension, 1 to 2 teaspoons, held in mouth for 5 minutes and then swallowed may be effective.

Clotrimazole: For OPC, oral tablets (troche), 10 mg, one tablet 5 times daily may be effective.

MUCOSAL CANDIDIASIS IN HIV DISEASE   Responds to topical and/or systemic therapy; however, recurrence is the rule. May become refractory to intermittent therapy, requiring daily chemoprophylaxis, with either topical or systemic treatment.

Fluconazole: 200 mg PO once followed by 100 mg daily for 2 to 3 weeks, then discontinue. Increase the dose to 400 to 800 mg in resistant infection. Also available in IV form.

Alternative: Ketoconazole, 200 mg PO q.d. for 1 to 2 weeks; or itraconazole, 100 mg PO b.i.d. for 2 weeks. Increase dose with resistant disease.

NOTE: Itraconazole, ketoconazole need to be absorbed in an acidic environment but not fluconazole.

FLUCONAZOLE-RESISTANT CANDIDIASIS   Defined as clinical persistence of infection following treatment with fluconazole 100 mg/day PO for 7 days. Occurs most commonly in HIV-infected individuals with CD4+ cell counts $<50/\mu$l who have had prolonged fluconazole exposure. Chronic low-dose fluconazole treatment (50 mg/day) facilitates emergence of resistant strains; 50 % of resistant strains sensitive to itraconazole. Amphotericin B for severe resistant disease. New liposomal preparations are effective and less toxic. Recurrence is the rule; maintenance therapy is often required.

PITYRIASIS VERSICOLOR

Pityriasis versicolor (PV) is a chronic asymptomatic scaling dermatosis associated with the overgrowth of the hyphal form of *Pityrosporum* ovale, characterized by well-demarcated scaling patches with variable pigmentation, occurring most commonly on the trunk.
Synonym: Tinea versicolor.

Epidemiology and Etiology

Age   Young adults. Less common when sebum production is reduced or absent; tapers off during fifth and sixth decades.

Etiology   *P. ovale* (also known as *P. orbiculare* and *Malassezia furfur*), a lipophilic yeast that normally resides in the keratin of skin and hair follicles of individuals 15 years of age or older. It is an opportunistic organism, causing pityriasis versicolor, *Pityrosporum* folliculitis, and implicated in the pathogenesis of seborrheic dermatitis. *Pityrosporum* infections are not contagious, but an overgrowth of resident cutaneous flora occurs under certain favorable conditions.

Predisposing Factors   High humidity at the skin surface. High rate of sebum production. Application of grease such as cocoa butter predisposes young children to PV. High levels of cortisol appear to increase susceptibility—both in Cushing's syndrome and with prolonged administration of corticosteroids (topical as well as systemic).

Incidence   In temperate zones: 2 %. In subtropical and tropical zones: 40 %.

Season   In temperate zones, appears in summertime; fades during cooler months. In physically active individuals, may persist year round.

History

Duration of Lesions   Months to years

Skin Symptoms   Usually none. Occasionally, mild pruritus. Individuals with PV usually present because of cosmetic concerns about the blotchy pigmentation.

Physical Examination

Skin Lesions

TYPE   Macule, sharply marginated (Figures 25-32 through 25-34). Fine scaling is best appreciated by gently abrading lesions with a no. 15 scalpel blade or the edge of a microscope slide. Treated or burned-out lesions lack scale. Some patients have findings of *Pityrosporum* folliculitis and seborrheic dermatitis.

COLOR   In untanned skin, light brown. On tanned skin, white. In dark-skinned individuals, dark brown macules. Brown of varying intensities and hues (Figure 25-34); off-white macules (Figures 25-32 and 25-33).

SIZE AND SHAPE   Round or oval macules varying in size. In time, individual lesions may enlarge, merge, forming extensive geographic areas.

DISTRIBUTION   Upper trunk, upper arms, neck, abdomen, axillae, groins, thighs, genitalia. Uncommonly on the face.

Differential Diagnosis

Hypopigmented PV   Vitiligo, pityriasis alba, postinflammatory hypopigmentation, tuberculoid leprosy

Scaling Lesions   Tinea corporis, seborrheic dermatitis, pityriasis rosea, guttate psoriasis, nummular eczema

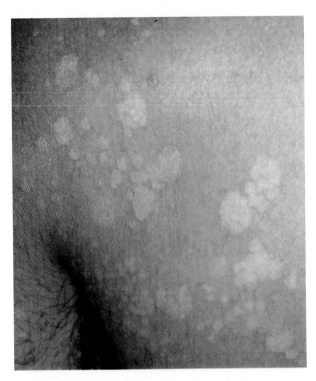

**Figure 25-32 Pityriasis versi-
color** *Hypopigmented, sharply
marginated, scaling macules on
the shoulder area of an individual with brown skin. Gentle
abrasion of the surface accentu-
ates the scaling.*

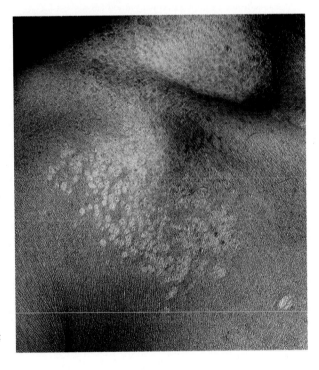

**Figure 25-33 Pityriasis versi-
color** *Follicular, hypopigmented macules on the upper
chest of an individual with black
skin.*

Laboratory and Special Examinations

Direct Microscopic Examination of Scales Prepared with KOH   Scale is best obtained using two microscope slides, using one to raise scale and move it onto the other. The harvested scale is moved into a small pile in the center of the slide and covered with a coverslip. KOH solution (15 % to 20 %) is added at the edge of the coverslip, the slide gently heated, and then examined. Filamentous hyphae and globose yeast forms, termed "spaghetti and meatballs," are seen.

Wood's Lamp Examination   Blue-green fluorescence of scales; may be negative in individuals who have showered recently in that the fluorescent chemical is water soluble. Vitiligo appears as depigmented, white, and has no scale.

Dermatopathology   Budding yeast and hyphal forms are seen in the most superficial layers of the stratum corneum, seen best with PAS stain. Variable hyperkeratosis, psoriasiform hyperplasia, chronic inflammation with blood vessel dilatation.

Diagnosis

Clinical findings, confirmed by positive KOH preparation findings

Pathophysiology

Dicarboxylic acids formed by enzymatic oxidation of fatty acids in skin surface lipids inhibit tyrosinase in epidermal melanocytes and thereby lead to hypomelanosis. The enzyme is present in the organism.

Management

Topical Agents

Selenium sulfide (2.5 %) lotion or shampoo: Apply daily to affected areas for 10 to 15 minutes, followed by shower, for 1 week.

Propylene glycol 50 % solution (in water): Apply b.i.d. for 2 weeks.

Ketoconazole shampoo applied as selenium sulfide shampoo.

Azole creams (ketoconazole, econazole, miconazole, clotrimazole): Apply q.d. or b.i.d. for 2 weeks.

Systemic Therapy   *None of these agents are approved for use in PV in the United States.*

Ketoconazole: 200 mg orally daily for 7 to 14 days

Ketoconazole (400 mg) or fluconazole (400 mg once); repeated after 1 week

Itraconazole: 200 mg b.i.d. on one day; 200 mg for 5 days

Secondary Prophylaxis   Ketoconazole shampoo once or twice a week. Selenium sulfide (2.5 %) lotion or shampoo. Salicylic acid/sulfur bar. Pyrithione zinc (bar or shampoo). Propylene glycol 50 % solution once a month.

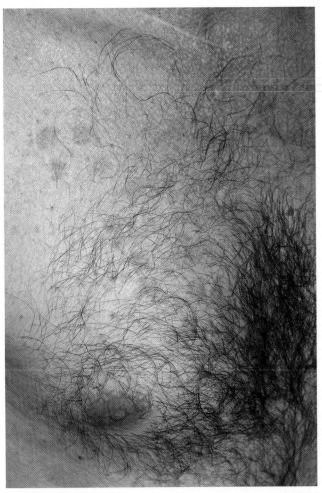

Figure 25-34 Pityriasis versicolor *Pink-tan macules on the chest of an individual with white skin are difficult to visualize and are often overlooked during physical examination.*

Section 26

SYSTEMIC FUNGAL INFECTIONS

MYCETOMA

Mycetoma is a local, chronic, slowly progressive infection of skin, subcutaneous tissues, fascia, bone, and muscle, most commonly of the foot or hand, characterized by swelling or tumorfaction, draining sinuses, and granules; the exudate contains grains that may be yellow, white, red, brown, or black depending on the causative microorganisms.
Synonyms: Madura foot, maduromycetoma.

Epidemiology and Etiology

Sex 90 % of patients are males.

Age 20 to 50 years

Etiology and Classification of Mycetoma-Like Clinical Presentation with Grain Formation

BOTRYOMYCOSES Caused by true bacteria. Not a true mycetoma.
Most Common *Staphylococcus aureus*
Also *S. epidermidis, Pseudomonas aeruginosa, Escherichia coli, Bacteroides* species, *Proteus* species, *Streptococcus* species

ACTINOMYCOTIC MYCETOMA Caused by Actinomycetales organisms
Actinomyces Cause mycetoma and actinomycosis (cervical, thoracic, abdominal)
Nocardia Cause mycetoma, lymphocutaneous infection (sporotrichoid pattern), superficial skin infections, disseminated infection with skin involvement
Actinomadura
Streptomyces

EUMYCOTIC MYCETOMA Caused by true fungi
Most Common *Pseudallescheria boydii, Madurella grisea, M. mycetomatis*

Also *Phialophora jeanselmei, Pyrenochaeta romeroi, Leptosphaeria senegaliensis, Curvularia lunata, Neotestudina rosatti, Aspergillus nidulans* or *flavus, Acremonium* species, *Fusarium* species, *Cylindrocarpon* species, *Microsporum audouinii*

Occupation Agricultural workers and laborers exposed to soil in tropical and subtropical regions

Transmission Cutaneous inoculation (thorn prick, wood splinter, stone cut) of organism, commonly with soil or plant debris, into foot or hand

Geography Fungi isolated from soil except *Actinomyces israelii.* Tropical and subtropical climate supports growth of organisms. In Central/South America, 90 % of cases caused by *Nocardia brasiliensis.* In Africa, *M. mycetomatis* common cause. Most commonly seen in India, Mexico, Nigeria, Saudi Arabia, Senegal, Somalia, Sudan, Venezuela, Yemen, Zaire.

Risk Factors Poor hygiene, walking barefoot, necrotic injured tissue, diminished nutrition

History

Incubation Period Lesion occurs at inoculation site weeks to years after trauma.

Duration of Lesion Lesions may continue to expand for decades.

Symptoms Relatively few, with little pain, tenderness or fever

Physical Examination

Skin Lesions

TYPES Primary lesion: papule/nodule at inoculation site. Swelling increases slowly. Epidermis ulcerates and pus-containing granules (grains) drain. Granules are microbial colonies, small <1 to ≥5 mm. Skin surrounding portals of fistula drainage is heaped up (Figure 26-1). Infection spreads to deeper tissues, into fascia, muscle, bone. Tissue becomes greatly distorted. Old mycetoma characterized by healed scars and draining sinuses.

PALPATION Usually not tender. Pus drains on pressure.

ARRANGEMENT Central clearing gives older lesions an annular shape.

DISTRIBUTION Unilateral on the leg, foot, hand. Uncommonly on torso, arm, head, thigh, buttock, head.

General Findings Fever with secondary bacterial infection. Regional lymphadenopathy occasionally.

Differential Diagnosis

Subcutaneous Inflammatory Mass(es) Chromoblastomycosis, blastomycosis, bacterial pyoderma, foreign-body granuloma, inflammatory dermatophytoses, leishmaniasis, pyoderma gangrenosum

Laboratory and Special Examinations

Smear of Pus from Lesion Granules (Medlar bodies) (see Table 26-A) visualized on KOH preparation as microbial colonies (see below).

Dermatopathology Pseudoepitheliomatous hyperplasia of epidermis. Suppurative acute and chronic inflammation with granules within. Surrounded by dense fibrous tissue.

Culture Isolate organism. Secondary bacterial infection common.

Imaging X-ray of bone shows multiple osteolytic lesions (cavities), periosteal new bone formation.

Diagnosis

Clinical suspicion confirmed by visualization of Medlar bodies on smear of pus or lesional biopsy specimen, and/or isolation of organism on culture. Medlar bodies (granules, grains) are white, black to gray, pinpoint globular grains that can be seen and felt in pus. Can be crushed on slide. They represent globular colonies of organism (see Table 26-A).

Pathophysiology

Only organism that can survive at body temperature can produce mycetoma. Infection begins in skin and subcutaneous tissues, extending into fascial planes, destroying contiguous tissues.

Course and Prognosis

Actinomycotic mycetoma usually enlarges more rapidly than eumycotic mycetoma. Secondary bacterial infections are common. Infection does not spread hematogenously. Relapse after antifungal or antibiotic therapy common.

Management

Individuals are advised to seek medical attention early.

Surgery Smaller lesions can be cured by surgical excision. More extensive lesions often recur after incomplete excision.

Medicosurgical Approach Bulk reduction surgery is performed; amputation/disarticulation avoided. Causative agent identified, and effective antimicrobial agent given.

Systemic Antimicrobial Therapy Usually continue for ≥10 months

BOTRYOMYCOSES Antimicrobial agents according to sensitivities of isolated organism

ACTINOMYCOTIC MYCETOMA Streptomycin sulfate combined with either dapsone or trimethoprim-sulfamethoxazole

EUMYCOTIC MYCETOMA Ketoconazole and itraconazole have been reported to be effective.

TABLE 26-A **COLOR GRAINS IN MYCETOMA AND ASSOCIATED ORGANISMS**

Color of Grain	Organism
Black	*Madurella mycetomatis*
	M. grisea
	Leptosphaeria senegalensis
White	*Pseudallescheria boydii*
	Acremonium species
	Nocardia brasiliensis
	Nocardia asteroides
White to yellow	*Nocardia caviae*
	Actinomyces israelii
Pink, white, to cream	*Actinomadura madurae*
Red	*Actinomadura pelletieri*

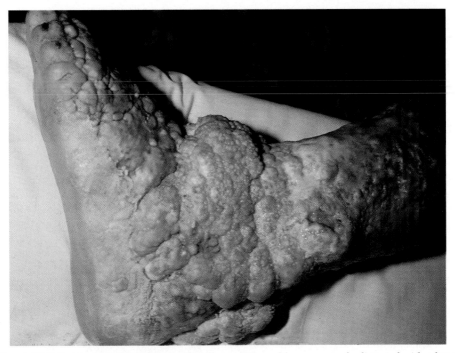

Figure 26-1 Eumycotic mycetoma *The foot, ankle, and leg are grossly distorted with edema and confluent subcutaneous nodules, cauliflower-like tumors, and ulcerations.*

CHROMOBLASTOMYCOSIS

Chromoblastomycosis is a localized chronic mycosis of skin and subcutaneous tissues characterized by verrucous plaques on the leg or foot, caused by dematiaceous (dark-colored) fungi. *Synonym:* Chromomycosis.

Epidemiology and Etiology

Sex Males > females

Age 20 to 60 years

Etiology Dematiaceous fungi: *Fonsecaea pedrosoi* (most commonly); also *F. compacta, Phialophora verrucosa, Cladosporium carrionii, Rhinocladiella aquaspersa, Botryomyces caespitosus*

Occupation Agricultural workers, mine workers, those exposed to soil while barefoot in tropical and subtropical regions

Transmission Cutaneous inoculation. Autoinoculation to other sites may occur. Transmission to other individuals does not occur.

Geography Fungi isolated from soil and vegetation, preferring regions with >100 in of rainfall per year and mean temperatures from 12° to 24°C.

History

Duration of Lesion Lesions may continue to expand for decades.

Symptoms Relatively few, with little pain, tenderness, or fever. Patients usually present with secondary infection, cosmetic disfigurement, lymphedema.

Physical Examination

Skin Lesions

TYPES Initial lesion: single scaling nodule at site of traumatic implantation (Figure 26-2). Later (months to years), new crops of nodules appear. Subsequently, expanding verrucous plaques with central clearing and islands of normal skin between verrucous macules. Large cauliflower-like lesions often form, which, in some cases, may become pedunculated. Surface of verrucous lesion: pustules, small ulcerations, "black dots" of hemopurulent material, ±friable granulation tissue that bleeds easily is common. Extension occurs via lymphatic spread or via autoinoculation. Chronic lesions may be 10 to 20 cm in diameter, enveloping calf or foot. In areas of long-standing, lymphedema of involved extremity (elephantiasis).

ARRANGEMENT Smaller lesions coalesce to form large verrucous masses. Central clearing gives older lesions an annular shape.

DISTRIBUTION Unilateral on the leg, foot. Rarely, hand, thorax.

Differential Diagnosis

Large Verrucous Plaques Blastomycosis, phaeohyphomycosis, lobomycosis, yaws, tertiary syphilis, tuberculosis verrucosa cutis, mycetoma, sporotrichosis, *Mycobacterium marinum* infection, lepromatous leprosy, botryomycosis, foreign-body granuloma, inflammatory dermatophytoses, leishmaniasis, pyoderma gangrenosum, squamous cell carcinoma

Laboratory and Special Examinations

Smear of Pus from Lesion Medlar bodies or "copper pennies" (see below) visualized on 10 % to 20 % KOH preparation as black dots. Hyphal forms can be seen in crusts, pus, exudate.

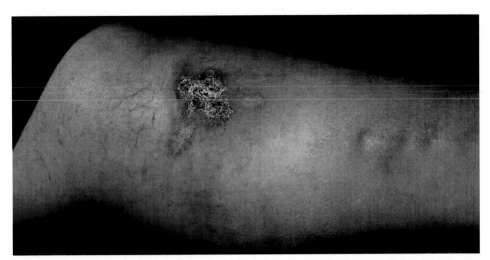

Figure 26-2 Chromoblastomycosis *Hyperkeratotic and crusted plaque with old scars on the leg had been present for several decades.*

Dermatopathology Warty granuloma: pseudoepitheliomatous hyperplasia, hyperkeratosis, intraepidermal abscesses containing inflammatory cells and Medlar bodies. Dense suppurative and granulomatous dermal response with histiocytes, giant cells, plasma cells, eosinophils, abscess formation. Medlar bodies (also known as sclerotic bodies, "copper pennies") are small brown fungal forms, which are round with thick bilaminate walls, 4 to 6 μm in diameter; occur singly or in clusters; all etiologic agents appear identical in tissue. Older lesions show dense fibrosis in and around granulomas.

Culture Organism in Sabouraud's glucose agar shows velvety green to black, restricted, slow-growing colonies. Agents grow very slowly, requiring 4 to 6 weeks for identification.

Diagnosis

Clinical suspicion confirmed by visualization of Medlar bodies on smear of pus or lesional biopsy specimen and/or isolation of organism on culture.

Course and Prognosis

Secondary bacterial infections are common. Recurrence after oral triazole therapy is common. Late complication is squamous cell carcinoma arising within verrucous area.

Management

Adjunctive Therapy Application of heat may be helpful in that lesions arise at cooler acral sites.

Surgery Smaller lesions can be cured by surgical excision.

Systemic Antifungal Therapy Amphotericin B usually is not effective at usual dosing.

ORAL ANTIFUNGAL AGENTS Treatment is usually continued for at least 1 year.

Itraconazole: 200 to 600 mg/day may be effective.
Ketoconazole: 400 to 800 mg/day may be effective.

SPOROTRICHOSIS

Sporotrichosis is a mycosis that most commonly follows accidental inoculation of the skin and is characterized by ulceronodule formation at the inoculation site, chronic nodular lymphangitis, and regional lymphadenitis. In the immunocompromised host, disseminated infection can occur from the skin involvement or from primary pulmonary infection.

Epidemiology and Etiology

Sex Males > females, especially disseminated disease

Etiology *Sporothrix schenckii,* a dimorphic fungus commonly found in soil. The tissue form is an oval, cigar-shaped yeast.

Occupation Occupation exposure important: gardeners, farmers, florists, lawn laborers, agricultural workers, forestry workers, paper manufacturers, gold miners, laboratory workers. In Uruguay, 80 % of cases occur following a scratch by an armadillo.

Transmission Commonly, subcutaneous inoculation by a contaminated thorn, barb, splinter, or other sharp object (laboratory). Rarely, inhalation, aspiration, or ingestion causes systemic infection. Most cases isolated. Epidemics do occur. Cutaneous sporotrichosis in cats has been transmitted to humans.

Geography Ubiquitous, worldwide. More common in temperate, tropical zones. Present on rose and barberry thorns, wood splinters, sphagnum moss, straw, marsh hay, soils.

Predisposing Factors For localized disease: diabetes mellitus, alcoholism. For disseminated disease: HIV infection, carcinoma, hematologic and lymphoproliferative disease, diabetes mellitus, alcoholism, immunosuppressive therapy.

History

Incubation Period 3 weeks (range 3 days to 12 weeks) after trauma or injury to site of lesion. Lesions are relatively asymptomatic, painless. Afebrile.

Physical Examination

Skin Lesions

TYPES *Local Cutaneous Type (Chancriform)* *(40 %)* Subcutaneous papule, pustule, or nodule appears at inoculation site several weeks after puncture wound. Surrounding skin is pink to purplish. In time, skin becomes fixed to deeper tissues. Painless indurated ulcer (Figure 26-3) may occur, resulting in sporotrichoid chancre. Border ragged and undermined. Draining lymph nodes become swollen and suppurative.
Chronic Lymphangitic Type (Sporotrichoid) *(60 %)* Follows lymphatic extension of local cutaneous type (Figure 26-4). Proximal to local cutaneous lesion, intervening lymphatics become indurated, nodular, thickened.
Fixed Cutaneous Sporotrichosis Crusted ulcers, ecthymatous, verrucous plaques, pyoderma gangrenosum-like, infiltrated papules and plaques.
Disseminated Sporotrichosis (Fungus disseminates hematogenously to skin, as well as joints, eyes, and meninges.) Crusted nodules, ulcers. Widespread.

ARRANGEMENT Primary chancre, nodular linear lymphatic spread (Figure 26-4) with enlarged regional lymph nodes described as "sporotrichoid"

DISTRIBUTION Primary lesion most common on dorsum of hand or finger with chronic nodular lymphangitis up arm. Fixed cutaneous—face in children, upper extremities in adults. Disseminated sporotrichosis: widespread lesions, usually sparing palms, soles.

General Examination

LUNGS Primary pulmonary infection does oc-

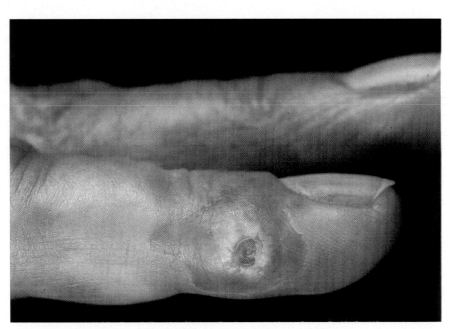

Figure 26-3 Sporotrichosis: chancriform type *An ulcerated nodule at the site of inoculation on the finger was associated with regional axillary lymphadenopathy.*

cur and has a worse prognosis than cutaneous infection.

JOINTS Swelling, painful joint(s) (hand, elbow, ankle, knee), often in the absence of skin lesion.

Hematogenous dissemination results in bone, muscle, joint, visceral, CNS lesions.

Differential Diagnosis

Chancriform Sporotrichosis Cutaneous tuberculosis, atypical mycobacterial infection, tularemia, cat-scratch disease, primary syphilis

Chronic Nodular Lymphangitic Sporotrichosis

"COMMON" INFECTING AGENTS *M. marinum, Nocardia brasiliensis, Leishmania brasiliensis, Francisella tularensis*

UNUSUAL INFECTING AGENTS *N. asteroides, M. chelonei, L. major.* Rare: *M. kansasii, Blastomyces dermatitidis, Coccidioides immitis, Cryptococcus neoformans, Histoplasma capsulatum, Streptococcus pyogenes, Staphylococcus aureus, Pseudomonas pseudomallei* (melioidosis), *Bacillus anthracis* (anthrax).

Fixed Cutaneous Sporotrichosis Bacterial pyoderma, foreign-body granuloma, inflammatory dermatophytoses, blastomycosis, chromoblastomycosis, leishmaniasis

Disseminated Sporotrichosis Acanthamebiasis, cryptococcosis

Laboratory and Special Examinations

Touch Preparation In disseminated sporotrichosis (usually with advanced HIV disease), KOH solution added to smear from back of lesional skin biopsy specimen helps visualize multiple yeast forms.

Gram's Stain In disseminated sporotrichosis (usually with advanced HIV disease), smear from crusted lesion shows multiple yeast forms.

Dermatopathology Granulomatous, Langhans-type giant cells, pyogenic microabscesses. Organisms rare, difficult to visualize in all except infection in immunocompromised host. Yeast appear as 1- to 3-μm by 3- to 10-μm cigar-shaped forms.

Culture Organism usually isolated within a few days from lesional biopsy specimen.

Serology Not helpful

Diagnosis

Clinical suspicion and isolation of organism on culture

Pathophysiology

Following subcutaneous inoculation, *S. schenckii* grows locally and slowly spreads along the draining lymphatics. Secondary skin lesions develop along the lymphatic chain. Rarely, following inhalation, the fungus causes a granulomatous pneumonitis, which resembles tuberculosis. The fungus can disseminate hematogenously from skin or pulmonary sites of infection.

Course and Prognosis

Shows little tendency to resolve spontaneously. Responds well to therapy, but a significant percentage relapse after completion of therapy. Disseminated infection in HIV-infected individuals responds poorly to all forms of therapy.

Management

Systemic Antifungal Therapy Saturated solution of potassium iodide (SSKI): 3 to 4 g three times a day is effective for lymphocutaneous infection. Less effective than oral antifungal agents.

ORAL ANTIFUNGAL AGENTS Itraconazole: 200 to 600 mg q.d. Very effective for lymphocutaneous infection. Not as effective for bone/

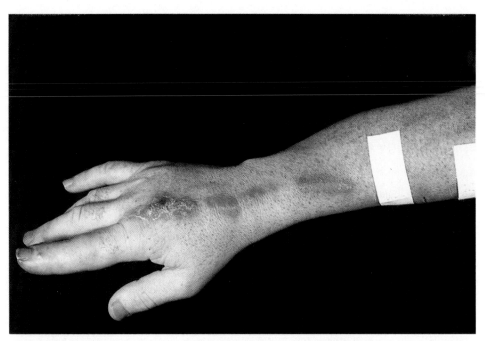

Figure 26-4 Sporotrichosis: chronic lymphangitic (sporotrichoid) type *An erythematous papule at the site of inoculation on the index finger with a linear arrangement of erythematous dermal and subcutaneous nodules extending proximally in lymphatic vessels of the dorsum of the hand and arm.*

joint and pulmonary infection.

Alternative

Fluconazole: 200 to 400 mg/day reported to be effective

Ketoconazole: 400 to 800 mg/day reported to be effective

INTRAVENOUS AMPHOTERICIN B For those with pulmonary or disseminated infection or who are unable to tolerate oral therapy for lymphocutaneous disease

DISSEMINATED CRYPTOCOCCOSIS

Systemic cryptococcosis is a systemic mycosis acquired by the respiratory route, with the primary focus of infection in the lungs, and with occasional hematogenous dissemination, characteristically to the meninges, and on occasion to skin.
Synonyms: Torulosis, European blastomycosis.

Epidemiology and Etiology

Age   More common over the age of 40 years

Sex   Males > females 3:1

Etiology   *Cryptococcus neoformans,* a yeast, serotypes A, B, C, D causing infection in humans. In tissue, encapsulated yeastlike globus fungi (3.5 to 7.0 μm in diameter). Bud connected to parent cell by narrow pore. Capsule thickness variable.

Incidence   Globally, cryptococcosis (usually meningitis) is the most common invasive mycosis in HIV disease, occurring in 6 % to 9 % of HIV-infected individuals in the United States and 20 % to 30 % in Africa. Incidence also high in Europe and South America. Currently, in the United States, the incidence is much less, presumably because of use of oral imidazoles for treatment of mucosal candidiasis. Cutaneous dissemination occurs in 10 % to 15 % of HIV-infected patients with cryptococcosis.

Transmission   Inhalation of aerosolized yeast, spread by air currents. Associated with avian feces worldwide (parakeets, budgerigars, canaries, and especially pigeons).

Risk Factors   Diabetes mellitus, lymphoma, Hodgkin's disease, sarcoidosis, transplant recipients. Currently, HIV infection is the major risk factor for disseminated cryptococcosis.

Geography   Worldwide, ubiquitous. Distribution of serotype varies in geographic areas.

History

Occurs in the setting of advanced HIV disease. Cutaneous lesions: usually asymptomatic. CNS: headache most common symptom (80 %), mental confusion, impaired vision for 2 to 3 months. Lungs: pulmonary symptoms uncommon.

Physical Examination

Skin Lesions

TYPES   ***Papules or Nodules***   With surrounding erythema that occasionally break down and exude a liquid, mucinous material. Molluscum contagiosum–like lesions commonly occur in HIV-infected patients (Figure 26-5).
Acneform
Herpetiform   Vesicular lesions.
Cryptococcal Cellulitis   Mimics bacterial cellulitis. Red, hot, tender, edematous plaque on extremity. Possibly multiple noncontiguous sites (Figure 26-6)

NOTE   *All types of lesions may ulcerate.*

DISTRIBUTION   In HIV disease, lesions occur most commonly on face and scalp.
Oral Mucosa   Occur in <5 % of patients, presenting as nodules or ulcers

General Findings   Meningitis. In HIV disease, cryptococcosis tends to be widespread with fungemia and infection of meninges, lungs, bone marrow, genitourinary tract including prostate, and skin. In HIV disease, hepatomegaly and splenomegaly.

Differential Diagnosis

Pyoderma, other bacterial or fungal skin lesions, blastomycosis, histoplasmosis. On the face of HIV-infected individuals, resembles molluscum contagiosum.

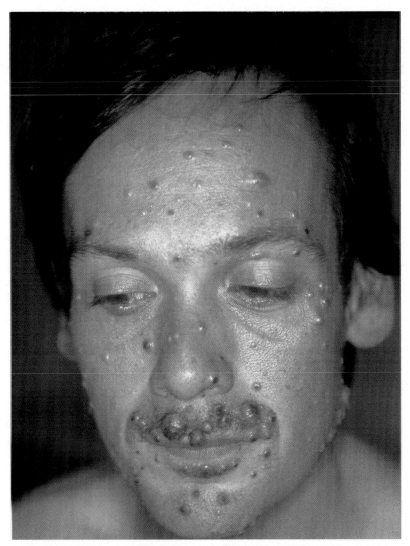

Figure 26-5 Cryptococcosis: disseminated *Multiple, skin-colored papules and nodules on the face in an HIV-infected individual represent dissemination of pulmonary cryptococcosis hematogenously to skin; meninges are also a common site of infection following fungemia. The lesions are easily mistaken for molluscum contagiosum, which occurs commonly in HIV disease. (Courtesy of Loïc Vallant, M.D.)*

Laboratory and Special Examinations

Dermatopathology Two patterns of histologic reactions are seen: gelatinous and granulomatous. Gelatinous reactions show numerous organisms in aggregates with little inflammatory response. Granulomatous reactions show tissue reaction with histiocytes, giant cells, lymphoid cells, and fibroblasts, ±areas of necrosis; organisms are present in smaller numbers. Capsules stain with mucicarmine stain, differentiating *C. neoformans* from *B. dermatitidis.*

Touch Preparation Lesional skin biopsy specimen or scrapings from skin lesion smear on microscope slide. Can be examined using KOH to identify *C. neoformans.*

CSF With meningitis, encapsulated budding yeast is seen with India ink preparations in 40% to 60 % of cases, lymphocytic pleocytosis, elevated protein, decreased glucose. Intracranial pressure may be moderately to extremely elevated.

Imaging X-ray findings of chest variable

Culture CSF. Lesional skin biopsy specimen. In HIV disease, cryptococcosis tends to be widespread, with cultures positive in blood, sputum, bone marrow, and urine. If *C. neoformans* isolated from lesional skin biopsy specimen, extent of disease should be determined by examination of CSF, bone marrow, sputum, urine, and prostate fluid.

Cryptococcal Antigens Sensitive and specific. Detect in CSF, serum, urine. Useful in following response to therapy and in determining prognosis.

Anticryptococcal Antibody Not useful

Diagnosis

Confirmed by skin biopsy and fungal cultures

Pathophysiology

C. neoformans is inhaled in dust and causes a primary pulmonary focus of infection with subsequent hematogenous dissemination to meninges, kidneys, and skin. Between 10 % and 15 % of patients have skin lesions. Cell-mediated immune deficiency is an important factor in pathogenesis in many patients.

Course and Prognosis

Acute pulmonary cryptococcosis is usually mild. Chronic cavitary forms lead to respiratory impairment. In HIV disease, cryptococcal meningitis relapses in 30 % of cases after amphotericin B plus 5-flucytosine therapy; lifelong secondary prophylaxis with fluconazole reduces relapse rate to 4 % to 8 %. Prostate is a site of extrameningeal disease and also a source of relapse after treatment.

Management

Primary Prophylaxis In some centers, fluconazole is given to HIV-infected individuals with low CD4+ cell counts; the incidence of disseminated infection is reduced, but there is no effect on the mortality.

Therapy of Meningitis

> *Amphotericin B* ± 5-flucytosine for 2 to 4 weeks in uncomplicated case; 6 weeks in complicated case
> *Alternative: fluconazole*

For high intracranial pressure, do repeated lumbar puncture aspirations using a large-bore needle to reduce the pressure.

Infection Limited to Skin

> *Fluconazole:* 400 to 600 mg/day
> *Itraconazole:* 400 mg/day

Secondary Prophylaxis In HIV disease, lifelong secondary prophylaxis is given.

> *Fluconazole:* 200 to 400 mg/day
> *Alternate: itraconazole* 200 to 400 mg/day

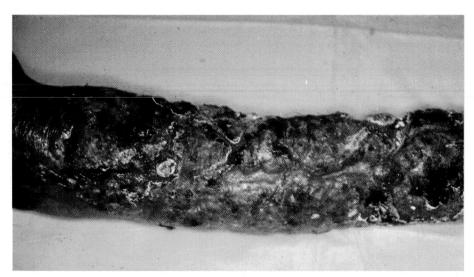

Figure 26-6 Cryptococcal cellulitis *Massive distortion of the forearm with ulceration, crusting, and scarring in an organ transplant recipient.*

HISTOPLASMOSIS

Histoplasmosis is a common systemic mycosis with a primary pulmonary infection but with uncommon hematogenous dissemination, characterized by chronic infection of mucous membranes, skin, and reticuloendothelial organs (liver, bone marrow, and spleen).
Synonyms: Darling's disease, cave disease, Ohio Valley disease.

Epidemiology and Etiology

Age   For disseminated infection, very old and very young

Etiology   *Histoplasma capsulatum,* a dimorphic fungus. In Africa, *H. capsulatum* var. *duboisii.* The fungus grows well in soil enriched with bird or bat guano.

Epidemiology   Farmers, construction workers, children, others involved in outdoor activities (cave exploration). Acute pulmonary histoplasmosis may occur in outbreaks in individuals with occupational or recreational exposure. In southern Kentucky, middle Tennessee, and surrounding areas, histoplasmin skin test positive in 95 % of population.

Transmission   Inhalation of spores in soil contaminated with bird or bat droppings

Risk Factors   For dissemination: immunosuppressed host (HIV infection, post-organ transplant, lymphoma, leukemia, chemotherapy), very old. Occurs in advanced HIV disease when CD4+ cell count is very low.

Incidence   Common opportunistic infection in HIV-infected individuals in highly endemic regions such as Indianapolis, Indiana. Early in the HIV epidemic, first cases of histoplasmosis were in immigrants from the endemic foci in the Caribbean Islands who developed AIDS while living in New York or California; disease presented as reactivation of latent foci of infection. In U.S. cities such as Indianapolis and Kansas City, 20 % to 25 % of patients with HIV disease have primary histoplasmosis. Incidence also increased in HIV disease in South America.

Geography   North America: eastern and central United States, especially Ohio/Mississippi River valleys (Kentucky, Illinois, Indiana, Missouri, Ohio, Tennessee, and western New York); in some areas, 80 % of residents are histoplasmin-positive. Caribbean Islands. Equatorial Africa.

Classification

Pulmonary histoplasmosis
 Acute pulmonary histoplasmosis (most cases are asymptomatic)
 Chronic cavitary pulmonary histoplasmosis
 Other pulmonary syndromes
Disseminated histoplasmosis infection
 Acute disseminated histoplasmosis
 Chronic progressive disseminated histoplasmosis

History

Incubation Period   For acute pulmonary infection, 5 to 18 days. For disseminated infection, ≥2 months. In severe forms of infection, presentation may be acute, resembling septicemia with associated disseminated intravascular coagulopathy.

ACUTE PRIMARY INFECTION   90 % of patients asymptomatic; if large numbers of spores inhaled, influenza-like syndrome may occur (fever ≥38.3°C, chills, night sweats, cough, headache, fatigue, myalgia).

DISSEMINATED INFECTION   Chronic disease syndrome. In HIV disease, can present as widely disseminated infection with symptoms of sepsis, adrenal insufficiency, diarrheal illness, or colonic mass.

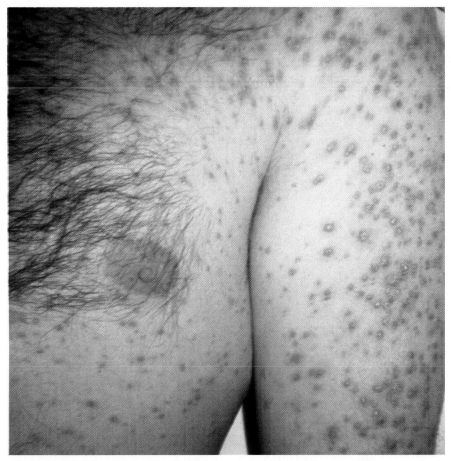

Figure 26-7 Histoplasmosis, disseminated *Multiple, erythematous, scaling papules on the trunk and upper arm occurred during a 2-week period and mimicked acute guttate psoriasis in an individual with HIV disease. The cutaneous lesions occurred following reactivation of pulmonary infection and fungemia. Multiple yeast-like* H. capsulatum *were demonstrated within macrophages in a lesional skin biopsy specimen. (Courtesy of J. D. Fallon, M.D.)*

Physical Examination

Skin Lesions

Acute pulmonary histoplasmosis: Cutaneous lesions represent hypersensitivity reactions to *Histoplasma* antigen(s).

Disseminated histoplasmosis to skin: Lesions caused by tissue infection. Historically, lesions of mucous membranes much more common than those on skin. However, in HIV infection, 10 % of patients with disseminated histoplasmosis have cutaneous lesions; in renal transplant patients, 4 % to 6 %.

TYPES **With Acute Pulmonary Infection** Erythema nodosum (see page 336), erythema multiforme (see page 332)

With Disseminated Infection Erythematous necrotic or hyperkeratotic papules and nodules (Figure 26-7); erythematous macules; folliculitis, ±pustules, ±acneform ulcers; vegetative plaques; panniculitis; erythroderma. Diffuse hyperpigmentation with Addison's disease secondary to adrenal infection.

DISTRIBUTION Face, extremities, trunk

MUCOUS MEMBRANES *Most common site of involvement;* nodules, vegetations, painful ulcerations of soft palate, oropharynx, epiglottis, nasal vestibule

General Examination Disseminated disease: hepatosplenomegaly, lymphadenopathy, meningitis

Differential Diagnosis

Disseminated Disease Miliary tuberculosis, coccidioidomycosis, cryptococcosis, leishmaniasis, lymphoma

Laboratory and Special Examinations

Dermatopathology Identify *H. capsulatum* in tissue by size and staining. Differentiate from

Coccidioides immitis, Blastomyces dermatitidis, Leishmania donovani, Toxoplasma gondii.

Smear *H. capsulatum* can be identified by smears obtained from touching lesional skin biopsy specimen to microscope slide (touch preparation), sputum, or bone marrow aspirate, stained with Giemsa's stain.

Culture Identify *H. capsulatum* from biopsy specimens of skin, oral lesions, bone marrow, sputum, lung biopsy specimen, blood, urine, lymph node, liver.

Antigen Detection Determination of *H. capsulatum* polysaccharide antigen titers in serum can be used for diagnosis and assessing response to treatment and in predicting later relapse. (Histoplasmosis Reference Laboratory, 1001 W. 10th St., OPW441, Indianapolis, IN 46202-2897; Tel: 317-630-6262, Fax: 317-630-7522.)

Antibody Detection Immunodiffusion and complement-fixation tests detect antibodies to *H. capsulatum.* Positive serologic test defined as presence of M or H band on immunodiffusion or 1:32 or higher titer by complement fixation.

Bone Marrow Aspiration *H. capsulatum* can be visualized in those with disseminated infection.

Imaging Chest x-ray: interstitial infiltrates and/or hilar adenopathy (acute)

Diagnosis

Clinical suspicion, confirmed by culture of organism

Pathogenesis

In HIV disease, can present as either primary histoplasmosis or reactivation of latent infection.

Course and Prognosis

Primary infection resolves spontaneously in most cases. Untreated chronic cavitary pulmonary infection or progressive disseminated form has a very high mortality rate, 80 % of patients dying within 1 year. Prognosis linked to underlying condition. Chronic maintenance often required. With itraconazole therapy, cure rate 80 %.

Management

Prevention When any material contaminated with bird or bat guano is to be disturbed in an area of endemic histoplasmosis, personal protective equipment (respirators, eye protection, gloves, or protective clothing) should be used during potential recreational or occupational exposure. Information regarding prevention and control of histoplasmosis can be obtained from the CDC's Division of Bacterial and Mycotic Diseases, National Center for Infectious Diseases (Mailstop A-13, 1600 Clifton Rd., N.E., Atlanta, GA 30333; Tel: 404-639-3158).

Systemic Antimycotic Therapy

FOR NON-LIFE-THREATENING INFECTIONS AND FOR THOSE UNABLE TO TOLERATE AMPHOTERICIN B Itraconazole 400 mg b.i.d. PO for 12 weeks, or fluconazole 800 mg q.d. PO for 12 weeks

FOR LIFE-THREATENING AND MENINGEAL INFECTION Amphotericin B given IV

Secondary Prophylaxis In HIV disease, itraconazole 200 mg/day or fluconazole 400 mg/day for life

NORTH AMERICAN BLASTOMYCOSIS

Blastomycosis is a chronic systemic mycosis characterized by primary pulmonary infection, which in some cases is followed by hematogenous dissemination to skin and other organs.
Synonyms: Gilchrist's disease, Chicago disease.

Epidemiology and Etiology

Age   Young, middle-aged

Sex   10 times more common in males than in females

Etiology   *Blastomyces dermatitidis,* a dimorphic fungus. In tissue, a yeast 10 μm in diameter with 1-μm-thick cell wall; pore of bud is wide.

Occupation   Outdoor vocation or avocation: farm workers, manual laborers. However, currently, many individuals infected during leisure activities: fishing, hunting, camping, hiking in areas of high endemicity.

Transmission   Commonly, inhalation of spores with primary pneumonitis. Uncommonly, accidental cutaneous inoculation. Most cases isolated; epidemics rare.

Geography   North America except Florida panhandle and New England; endemic in basins of Great Lakes and great rivers; southeastern United States. Africa.

Risk Factors for Dissemination   T-cell dysfunction. HIV-infected individuals with CD4+ cell counts <200/μl can experience widely disseminated infection.

History

Incubation Period   Estimated median 45 days. Depends on size of inoculum and immune status.

Symptoms   Primary pulmonary infection: usually asymptomatic; flulike or resembles bacterial pneumonitis. Chronic pulmonary infection: fever, cough, night sweats, weight loss. Cutaneous ulcers often painless.

Physical Examination

Skin Lesions

TYPES   ***Primary Infection***   Accompanied or followed by erythema nodosum or erythema multiforme
Disseminated Infection to Skin   Initial lesion, inflammatory nodule that enlarges and ulcerates (Figure 26-8); subcutaneous nodule, ±many small pustules on surface. Subsequently, verrucous/crusted plaque with sharply demarcated serpiginous borders. Peripheral border extends on one side, resembling a one-half to three-quarter moon. Pus exudes when crust lifted. Central healing with thin geographic atrophic scar.

SHAPE   May be serpiginous

DISTRIBUTION   Usually symmetrically on trunk but also face, hands, arms. Multiple lesions in half of patients. Primary cutaneous blastomycosis occurs at site of inoculation.

MUCOUS MEMBRANES   25 % of patients have oral or nasal lesions, half of whom have contiguous skin lesions. Laryngeal infection.

General Examination

LUNGS   Infiltrates, miliary, cavitary lesions

BONES   50 % involvement. Osteomyelitis in thoracolumbar vertebrae, pelvis, sacrum, skull, ribs, long bones. May extend to form large subcutaneous abscess. May occur in conjunction with cutaneous ulcer. Septic arthritis. Sinus tracts to skin can develop.

LYMPH NODES   Regional, enlarged only with primary cutaneous (inoculation) blastomycosis

GENITOURINARY TRACT   Prostate, epididymis

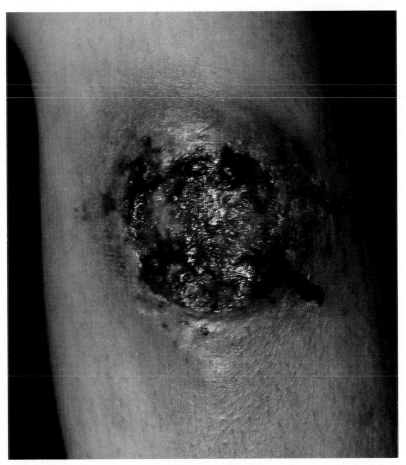

Figure 26-8 North American blastomycosis: disseminated   *Ulcerated, inflammatory plaque with surrounding erythema, edema, and fibrosis on the leg results from dissemination from pulmonary blastomycosis via blood to skin. The lesion must be differentiated from pyoderma gangrenosum. (Courtesy of Elizabeth M. Spiers, M.D.)*

Differential Diagnosis

Verrucous Skin Lesion   Squamous cell carcinoma, pyoderma gangrenosum tumor stage of mycosis fungoides, ecthyma, tuberculosis verrucosa cutis, actinomycosis, nocardiosis, mycetoma, syphilitic gumma, granuloma inguinale, leprosy, bromoderma

Laboratory and Special Examinations

Direct Examination   KOH preparation of pus or respiratory tract secretions shows large (8- to 15-μm), single, budding cells with a thick "double-contoured" wall and a wide pore of attachment. Specific diagnosis can be made using antibodies to *B. dermatitidis* antigens.

Culture   Of sputum, pus from skin lesion or biopsy, prostatic secretions

Dermatopathology   Pseudoepitheliomatous hyperplasia. Budding yeast with thick walls and broad-based buds in microabscess in dermis visualized by silver stain or periodic acid–Schiff stain. Mucicarmine stain differentiates *B. dermatitides* from *Cryptococcus neoformans.*

***B. dermatitidis* Antigens**   Can be detected in blood of infected individuals

Skin Tests   None available

Imaging   Acute (primary) infection shows pneumonitis, ±hilar lymphadenopathy. With chronic pulmonary infection, x-ray findings highly variable.

Diagnosis

Clinical suspicion, confirmed by culture of organism from skin biopsy, sputum, pus, urine

Pathophysiology

B. dermatitidis inhaled in dust; asymptomatic primary pulmonary infection most commonly resolves spontaneously. Hematogenous dissemination may occur to skin, skeletal system, genitalia, lungs. Reactivation may occur within lung or in sites of dissemination. Accidental inoculation into skin after trauma (autopsy prosectors and laboratory workers).

Course and Prognosis

Greater majority of primary pulmonary blastomycosis cases are asymptomatic, self-limited. Cutaneous infection can occur with primary pulmonary blastomycosis or months or years afterward. Skin most common site of extrapulmonary infection, followed by bones, prostate, and meninges; rarely, adrenals and liver. Prior to amphotericin B, mortality rate in individuals with disseminated infection was 80 % to 90 %. Cure rate with itraconazole 95 %.

Management

Prevention   Because of the widespread extent of *B. dermatitidis* in endemic regions, avoidance is not possible.

General Care   Patients with mild to moderate acute pulmonary blastomycosis often can be followed without antifungal therapy, especially if the patient is improving at time of diagnosis. Patients with meningitis or acute respiratory distress syndrome are best treated in hospital with IV amphotericin B.

Oral Antifungal Therapy   In those whose infection is non-life-threatening and those unable to tolerate amphotericin B;

> *Itraconazole:* 200 to 400 mg/day for >2 months
> *Ketoconazole (alternative):* 800 mg/day

Intravenous Amphotericin B   In life-threatening infections:

> *Amphotericin B:* 120 to 150 mg/week with a total dose of 2 g in adults. New liposomal preparations are less toxic. After initial improvement, therapy can be continued on an outpatient basis, three times weekly.

DISSEMINATED COCCIDIOIDOMYCOSIS

Coccidioidomycosis is a systemic mycosis characterized by primary pulmonary infection that usually resolves spontaneously but which can subsequently disseminate hematogenously and result in chronic, progressive, granulomatous infection in skin, lungs, bone, meninges.
Synonyms: San Joaquin Valley fever, valley fever, desert fever.

Epidemiology and Etiology

Race   Blacks, Filipinos

Sex   Risk of dissemination greater in males, pregnant females

Incidence   Greatly increased in southern California during the past few years. Approximately 100,000 cases in the United States per year; most asymptomatic. In endemic areas, infection rates, measured by skin test reactivity, may be 16 % to 42 % or higher by early adulthood. Occurs in up to 25 % of HIV-infected individuals in highly endemic regions such as Arizona or Bakersfield, CA.

Etiology   *Coccidioides immitis,* a dimorphic fungus. This mold grows in soil in arid areas of the western hemisphere.

Season   Late spring through fall, i.e., dry season

Acquisition   Inhalation of arthoconidia is followed by primary pulmonary infection. Rarely, percutaneous.

Risk Factors   Nonwhite, pregnancy, immunosuppression, HIV infection with low CD4+ cell counts

Geography   Regions endemic for *C. immitis* include: southern California (San Joaquin Valley), southern Arizona, Utah, New Mexico, Nevada, southwestern Texas; adjacent areas of Mexico; Central and South America. Primary pulmonary coccidioidomycosis occurs in individuals living in these regions (endemic) or in visitors to the regions (nonendemic).

Classification   Asymptomatic infection, febrile illness (valley fever) acute self-limited pulmonary coccidioidomycosis, disseminated coccidioidomycosis (cutaneous, osteoarticular, meningeal)

History

Incubation Period   1 to 4 weeks

History   About 40 % of persons infected with *C. immitis* will become symptomatic. With primary pulmonary infection, influenza- or grippelike illness with fever, chills, malaise, anorexia, myalgia, pleuritic chest pain. With disseminated infection, headache, bone pain. In HIV disease, clinical presentation is quite variable: focal pulmonary lesions, meningitis, focal disseminated lesions, or widespread disease. In HIV disease, usually presents when CD4+ cell count is $<200/\mu$l; the lower the CD4+ cell count, the more diffuse and widespread the mycosis.

Travel History   Living in or visit to endemic area. Disseminated coccidoidomycosis in individuals living in an endemic area is usually diagnosed more readily than in those with remote history of travel to an endemic region.

Physical Examination

Skin Lesions

TYPES   *Primary Infection* Toxic erythema (diffuse erythema, morbilliform, urticaria); erythema nodosum; erythema multiforme
Hematogenous Dissemination to Skin Initially, papule evolving with formation of pustules, plaques, nodules (Figure 26-9); abscess formation, multiple draining sinus tracts, ulcers; subcutaneous cellulitis; verrucous plaques; granulomatous nodules; scars
Primary Cutaneous Inoculation Site (Rare) Nodule eroding to ulcer. May have sporotrichoid lymphangitis, regional lymphadenitis.

Central face (Figure 26-9), especially nasolabial fold preferential site; extremities

MUCOUS MEMBRANES   Enanthem with primary infection

General Examination

BONE   Osteomyelitis. Psoas area produces draining abscess.

CNS   Signs of meningitis

Differential Diagnosis

Of skin lesions: warts, furuncles, ecthyma, bromoderma, rosacea, lichen simplex chronicus, prurigo nodularis, keratoacanthoma, blastomycosis, cryptococcosis, tuberculosis, tertiary syphilis, bacterial infection. In HIV-infected patient: may resemble folliculitis, molluscum contagiosum.

Laboratory and Special Examinations

Dermatopathology   Granulomatous inflammation; spores in tissue

Culture   Pus, biopsy specimen grows organism on Sabouraud's medium.

Diagnosis

Detection of *C. immitis* sporangia containing typical sporangiospores in sputum/pus; culture; skin biopsy

Pathophysiology

Spores inhaled resulting in primary pulmonary infection, which is asymptomatic or accompanied by symptoms of coryza. Failure to develop cell-mediated immunity is associated with disseminated infection and relapse after therapy.

Course and Prognosis

About 40 % of persons infected with *C. immitis* will become symptomatic. Disseminated disease is rare in immunocompetent persons but occurs at a higher rate in the United States among blacks, Filipinos, pregnant women, and immunosuppressed persons, particularly those with HIV infection. Most infected residents of endemic areas heal spontaneously. Meningeal infection difficult to cure. The incidence of relapse of pulmonary or dissemiated infection is relatively high. In HIV-infected individuals with coccidioidomycosis, the mortality rate in a study of 77 patients was 43 %; 60 % mortality with diffuse pulmonary disease; relapse rate very high.

Management

Systemic Antifungal Therapy

>Non-life-threatening infection:
>>Fluconazole 200 to 400 mg/day *or*
>>Itraconazole
>Life-threatening infection:
>>Amphotericin B deoxycholate

Secondary Prophylaxis   Lifelong therapy for meningeal infection may be required and is required in HIV disease.

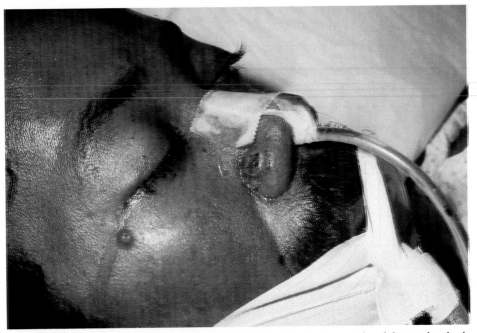

Figure 26-9 Coccidioidomycosis: disseminated *Ulcerated and crusted nodules on the cheek and nose in an individual with pulmonary coccidioidomycosis with dissemination to the skin. (Courtesy of Francis Renna, M.D.)*

Section 27

RICKETTSIAL INFECTIONS

SPOTTED FEVERS

The spotted fevers are Rocky Mountain spotted fever (RMSF), tick typhus, which is caused by several rickettsiae, and rickettsialpox. All except for rickettsialpox are transmitted to humans by the bite of ixodid ticks. Clinically, the spectrum of severity of clinical findings is broad, ranging from mild symptoms of general malaise and an exanthem to life-threatening illness.

Epidemiology and Etiology

Age More common in children and young adults, related to out-of-doors activities

Sex Males > females

Etiology, Geographic Distribution The rickettsiae causing the spotted fevers are collectively referred to as the *spotted fever group* (SFG) (Table 27-A).

Transmission All except rickettsialpox (transmitted by mite bite) are transmitted by tick bite.

Season Mediterranean spotted fever (MSF) occurs mainly in warm summer months (July, August, September).

History

Incubation Period Range 3 to 14 days (mean 7 days)

Prodrome Nonspecific

Travel History Residents of the United States have history of recent return from endemic region.

History of Tick Bite Often not elicited in that the *Rickettia* is transmitted by tiny immature larvae and nymphs

Symptoms Onset is sudden in 50% of patients. Most common: headache, fever. Also: chills, myalgias, arthralgias, malaise, anorexia.

Physical Examination

Skin Lesions

TYPES

   RMSF See Rocky Mountain Spotted Fever, page 762.

   Tache Noire Occurs in all except RMSF. A papule forms at the bite site; this evolves to a painless black crusted ulcer (eschar) (Figure 27-1) with a red areola in 3 to 7 days (looks like a cigarette burn).

   Tick Typhus About 3 to 4 days after appearance of the tache noire, an erythematous maculopapular eruption appears on the forearms and subsequently becomes generalized, involving the face, palms/soles. The density of the eruption heightens during the next few days. In severe cases, the lesions may become hemorrhagic.

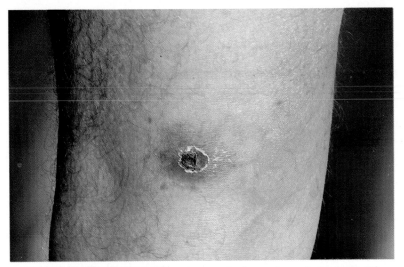

Figure 27-1 Rickettsialpox: tache noire *A crusted, ulcerated papule (eschar) with a red halo resembling a cigarette burn at the site of a tick bite.*

TABLE 27-A ETIOLOGY AND GEOGRAPHIC DISTRIBUTION OF SPOTTED FEVERS

Disease in Humans	Etiology	Distribution
Rocky Mountain spotted fever (RMSF)	*Rickettsia rickettsii*	Western hemisphere
Tick typhus		Primarily Mediterranean countries, Africa, India, Southeast Asia
Mediterranean spotted fever (MSF) (*fievre boutonneuse,* Marseilles fever, South African tick bite, Kenya tick typhus, Israeli spotted fever, Indian tick typhus)	*R. conorii*	Mediterranean Sea islands and surrounding lands; Africa
Siberian (North Asian) tick typhus	*R. sibirica*	Siberia, Mongolia, northern China
Australian (Queensland) tick typhus	*R. australis*	Australia
Oriental spotted fever	*R. japonica*	Japan
Rickettsialpox	*R. akari*	United States, Russia, South Africa, Korea, Europe

Rickettsialpox About 2 to 3 days after the onset of symptoms, a papulovesicular eruption appears. The initial lesions are erythematous papules (2 to 10 mm in diameter) (Figure 27-2). Papules evolve to vesicles and then heal after crust formation.

DISTRIBUTION Similar pattern of spread and distribution in all spotted fevers: trunk → extremities → face, except RMSF, which first appears at wrists and ankles and spreads centripetally

General Findings Conjunctivitis, pharyngitis, photophobia. CNS symptoms (confusion, stupor, delirium, seizures, coma) common in RMSF but not seen in other spotted fevers.

LYMPH NODES Nodes proximal to eschar are usually enlarged and nontender.

Differential Diagnosis

Tick Typhus Viral exanthems, drug eruption

Rickettsialpox Varicella, pityriasis lichenoides et varioliformis acuta (PLEVA), viral exanthems, disseminated gonococcal infection

Laboratory and Special Examinations

Skin Biopsy

ROUTINE HISTOLOGY *Rickettsialpox* Basal layer of epidermis shows vacuolar degeneration; vesiculation is subepidermal. Superficial and middermal neutrophilic and mononuclear cell infiltrate is present.

Direct Immunofluorescence Rickettsiae can be detected in lesional biopsy specimens from site of tick bite and cutaneous lesions; also in circulating endothelial cells and various tissues obtained postmortem.

PCR Detects rickettsial DNA in lesions and blood.

Serodiagnosis Various tests are available. Antirickettsial therapy usually blunts antibody responses. Demonstration of antibodies to SFG rickettsiae by microimmunofluorescence, latex agglutination, enzyme immunoassay, Western blot, or complement fixation. Enzyme-linked immunosorbent assay (ELISA) (IgM capture assays) among the most sensitive.

Culture Not available as a routine test. Rickettsiae can be cultured in the guinea pig and in a shell vial cell culture system.

Diagnosis

Clinical findings with identification of a tache noire confirmed by demonstration of rickettsiae by immunohistologic techniques in lesional skin biopsy specimens

Pathophysiology

Rickettsiae reproduce within endothelial cells at the bite site; the subsequent injury results in dermal and epidermal necrosis and perivascular edema, which presents clinically as a papule that evolves to a crusted ulcer at the bite site (tache noir or eschar). Rickettsiae then seed from this site into blood and systemically. In severe cases, disseminated vascular infection occurs with meningoencephalitis and vascular lesions in kidneys, lungs, GI tract, liver, pancreas, heart, spleen, and skin.

Course and Prognosis

In France and Spain, the mortality rate ranges from 1.4 % to 5.6 %, similar to that of RMSF. Spotted fevers are usually milder in children. Morbidity and mortality are higher in individuals with diabetes mellitus, cardiac insufficiency, alcoholism, old age, and G6PD deficiency.

Rickettsialpox Clinical symptoms usually mild. Morbidity and mortality uncommon. In untreated cases, symptoms resolve in 2 to 3 weeks.

Figure 27-2 Rickettsialpox *Multiple, erythematous papules and pustules, some with central hemorrhage and crusting, on the back following hematogenous dissemination of the* R. akari *from the tick bite site.*

Management

Prevention Control host animals and vectors.

Antirickettsial Therapy

Specific antirickettsial therapy abbreviates the length and severity of illness.

DRUG OF CHOICE Doxycycline (except for pregnant patients, history of allergy to doxycycline, or possibly a child <9 years of age): 200 mg/day PO or IV in two divided doses for adults. Tetracycline 25 to 50 mg/kg/day in four divided doses.

ALTERNATIVE Chloramphenicol 50 to 75 mg/kg/day in four divided doses or ciprofloxacin (1.5 g/day)

ROCKY MOUNTAIN SPOTTED FEVER

Rocky Mountain spotted fever (RMSF), the most severe of the rickettsial spotted fevers, is characterized by sudden onset of fever, severe headache, myalgia, and a characteristic acral exanthem; it is associated with significant morbidity and mortality.

Epidemiology and Etiology

Age and Sex Majority of cases in young adult males (55 %).

Etiology Caused by *Rickettsia rickettsii.*

Transmission Occurs through bite of an infected tick or inoculation through abrasions contaminated with tick feces or tissue juices. The reservoirs and vectors are the wood tick *Dermacentor andersoni* in the western United States, the dog tick *D. variabilis* in the eastern two-thirds and areas of the West Coast, *Rhipicephalus sanguineus* in Mexico, and *Amblyomma cajennense* in Mexico and Central and South America. Patient either lives in or has recently visited an endemic area, *but only 60 % have knowledge of a recent tick bite during the 2 weeks prior to onset of illness.*

Exposure to ticks occurs in tick-infested areas or in association with dogs who bring the dog tick into the patient's yard and home.

Season 95 % of patients become ill during the period April 1 to September 30. The longest season and greatest number of wintertime cases occur further south.

Geography Occurs only in the western hemisphere. Reported from each state except Hawaii and Vermont. In the United States during the period 1981 to 1991, the states with the highest incidence of RMSF were Oklahoma, North Carolina, Virginia, Maryland, Georgia, Missouri, Arkansas, Montana, and South Dakota; more recently, Tennessee and South Carolina have had a high incidence as well. Also reported from New York City. Although first recognized in the Rocky Mountains, currently rarely occurs in this region. Travelers to the western hemisphere may import RMSF to their homeland.

Incidence In the United States, ~600 cases of RMSF are reported to the CDC annually. The actual incidence is probably significantly higher. Four states (NC, OK, TN, SC) account for 48 % of U.S. cases.

History

Incubation Period Range, 3 to 14 days (mean, 7 days) after the tick bite

Prodrome Anorexia, irritability, malaise, chilliness, and feverish feeling

History of Tick Bite Given in only 60 % of cases

Symptoms Onset of symptoms is usually abrupt with fever (94 %), severe headache (86 %), generalized myalgia especially the back and leg muscles (83 %), a sudden shaking rigor, photophobia, prostration, nausea with occasional vomiting, all within the first 2 days. However, onset is at times less striking. Symptoms are similar to those of many acute infectious diseases, making specific diagnosis difficult during the first few days. On first day of illness, only 14 % of patients have characteristic rash; during first 3 days, 49 % of patients have rash. In 20 % of cases, rash appears only on day 6 or after. In 13 % of cases, no rash is detected (spotless RMSF).

Physical Examination

Skin Lesions The patient first seeking medical care may have no rash or a few small, pink macules that are identified only after a complete and careful examination of the skin. The temporal evolution of the rash is extremely helpful in the diagnosis. Extensive cutaneous necrosis due to DIC occurs in 4 % of cases and may be

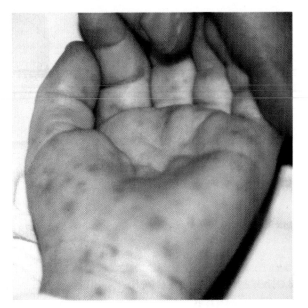

Figure 27-3 Rocky Mountain spotted fever *Erythematous and hemorrhagic macules and papules appeared initially on the wrists and later on the palms, soles, and trunk.*

associated with gangrene of extremities requiring amputation.

TYPES Early lesions 2 to 6 mm, pink, blanchable macules (Figure 27-3). In 1 to 3 days evolve to deep red papules (Figure 27-4). In 2 to 4 days become hemorrhagic, no longer blanchable. Rarely, an eschar (round crusted ulcer associated with an acute rickettsial infection) is present at the site of the tick bite. Necrosis of the skin and underlying structures. With DIC, skin infarcts (gangrene) occur.

COLOR Pink, evolving to deep red, evolving to violaceous

DISTRIBUTION Characteristically, rash begins on wrists, forearms, and ankles and somewhat later on palms and soles. Within 6 to 18 hours rash spreads centripetally to the arms, thighs, trunk, and face. The hemorrhagic rash involving the palms and soles occurs in 36 % to 82 % of cases and appears after day 5 of illness in 43 %. Necrosis occurs in acral extremities and scrotum.

General Findings Fever to 40°C. Hypotensive, shock later in course. Hepatomegaly, splenomegaly, GI hemorrhage, altered consciousness, transient deafness, incontinence, oliguria, and secondary bacterial infections of the lung, middle ear, and parotid gland may occur.

VARIANTS

Spotless fever: 13 % of cases. Associated with higher mortality because diagnosis is overlooked.

Abdominal syndrome: Can mimic acute abdomen, acute cholecystitis, acute appendicitis.

Thrombotic thrombocytopenic purpura

Differential Diagnosis

Usually of a tick-exposed patient who presents between May and September with a 1- to 3-day history of fever, headache, myalgia, malaise, and rash: meningococcemia, disseminated gonococcal infection, secondary syphilis, *Staphylococcus aureus* septicemia, toxic shock syndrome, typhoid fever, leptospirosis, other rickettsioses (ehrlichiosis, murine typhus, epidemic typhus, rickettsialpox), viral exanthem (measles, varicella, rubella, enterovirus), adverse cutaneous drug reaction, immune-complex vasculitis, idiopathic thrombocytopenic purpura, thrombotic thrombocytopenic purpura, Kawasaki's syndrome

Laboratory and Special Examinations

Skin Biopsy

H&E   Necrotizing vasculitis. *Rickettsia* can at times be demonstrated within the endothelial cells by immunofluorescence or immunoenzyme staining techniques.

DIRECT IMMUNOFLUORESCENCE   Specific *R. rickettsii* antigen within endothelial cells. False-negative rate approximately 30 %; treatment with antirickettsial drugs within 48 hours or less reduces sensitivity.

Serodiagnosis   Immunofluorescent antibody test (IFA) can be used to measure both IgG and IgM anti-*R. rickettsii* antibodies. Fourfold rise in titer between acute and convalescent stages is diagnostic, with a titer of ≥ 64 detectable between 7 and 10 days after onset of illness.

Diagnosis

Suspect in febrile children, adolescents, and men > 60 years old—particularly those who reside in or have traveled to the southern Atlantic states and South-Central states from May through September and participated in outdoor activity. Diagnosis must be made clinically and confirmed later. Only 3 % of cases with RMSF present with the triad of rash, fever, and history of a tick bite during the first 3 days of illness.

Pathophysiology

Following inoculation of rickettsiae into the pool of blood in the dermis while the tick feeds, initial local replication in endothelial cells is followed by hematogenous dissemination. Feeding usually takes place for ≥ 6 hours, after which rickettsiae are released from the salivary glands. Organisms spread hematogenously throughout the body and attach to the vascular endothelial cells, the principal target. Foci infected by *R. rickettsii* enlarge as rickettsiae spread from cell to cell, forming a network of contiguously infected endothelial cells in the microcirculation of the dermis, brain, lungs, heart, kidneys, stomach, large and small intestines, pancreas, liver, testes, skeletal muscle, and other organs and tissues. Focal infection of vascular smooth muscle causes a generalized vasculitis. Cases with severe infection of brain and lungs have a high mortality. Hypotension, local necrosis, gangrene, and DIC may follow. Rash results from extravasation of blood after vascular necrosis.

Course and Prognosis

Death is associated with older age, delay in diagnosis and delay in or no treatment, treatment with chloramphenicol (compared with tetracycline). Untreated (prior to the availability of effective antibiotics), the fatality rate was 23 %; treated, 3 % (6 % if age >40 years). Fatality rate 1.5 % with known tick bite but 6.6 % if no known tick exposure. Fulminant RMSF is defined as a fatal disease whose course is unusually rapid (i.e., ≤ 5 days from onset to death) and is usually characterized by early onset of neurologic signs and late or absent rash. In 1990, the case-fatality rate was 8 % for individuals <20 years and 6.8 % for those >20 years of age. In uncomplicated cases, defervescence usually occurs within 48 to 72 hours after initiation of therapy.

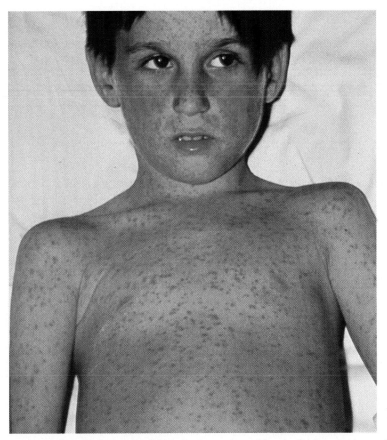

Figure 27-4 Rocky Mountain spotted fever *Disseminated hemorrhagic macules and papules on the face, neck, trunk, and arms on the fourth day of febrile illness; the initial lesions were noted on the wrists and ankles, subsequently extending centripetally.*

Long-term sequelae (complications that persist for 1 year or more after acute infection): neurologic (paraparesis; hearing loss; peripheral neuropathy; bladder and bowel incontinence; cerebellar, vestibular, and motor dysfunction; language disorders); nonneurologic (disability from limb amputation and scrotal pain following cutaneous necrosis)

Management

Specific antirickettsial therapy should be initiated as soon as the diagnosis is suspected clinically.

Antirickettsial Therapy

DRUG OF CHOICE Doxycycline (except for pregnant patients, history of allergy to doxycycline, or possibly a child <9 years of age): 200 mg/day PO or IV in two divided doses for adults. Tetracycline 25 to 50 mg/kg/day in four divided doses

ALTERNATIVE Chloramphenicol 50 to 75 mg/kg/day in four divided doses

Supportive Therapy For acute problems of shock, acute renal failure, respiratory failure, prolonged coma

Section 28

CUTANEOUS VIRAL INFECTIONS

HUMAN PAPILLOMAVIRUS INFECTIONS

Human papillomaviruses (HPV) are very widespread in human populations, causing subclinical infection or a wide variety of benign clinical lesions on skin and mucous membranes, and have a role in the oncogenesis of cutaneous and mucosal premalignancies and malignancies. More than 65 HPV types have been identified and are associated with certain clinical lesions (see Table 28-A).

Three clinical manifestations of cutaneous HPV infections occur with high incidence in the general population: common warts, plantar warts, and flat warts. Common warts represent approximately 70 % of all cutaneous warts, occurring in up to 20 % of all school-aged children. Plantar warts are common in older children and young adults, accounting for 30 % of cutaneous warts. Flat warts are also seen in children and adults, accounting for 4 % of cutaneous warts. Common in butchers, meat packers, and fish handlers are butcher's warts.

The most common presentation of mucosal HPV infection is condyloma acuminatum (genital wart), which is the most prevalent sexually transmitted disease in developed countries. Some HPV types have a major etiologic role in the pathogenesis of *in situ* as well as invasive squamous cell carcinoma of the anogenital epithelium. During delivery, maternal genital HPV infection can be transmitted to the neonate, resulting in anogenital warts or recurrent respiratory papillomatosis (RRP) following aspiration of the virus into the upper respiratory tract.

TABLE 28-A HPV TYPES AND ASSOCIATED CLINICAL LESIONS

	CUTANEOUS NONGENITAL HPV TYPES	
1	Deep plantar/palmar warts	Common warts
2, 4	Common warts	Plantar, palmar, mosaic, oral, anogenital warts
3, 10	Flat warts	
7	Butcher's warts	
5, 8, 9, 12, 14, 15, 17, 19–24	Macular warts in epidermodysplasia verruciformis (EDV)	
	MUCOSAL OROGENITAL HPV TYPES	
6, 11	Anogenital warts, cervical condylomata	Intraepithelial neoplasia, common warts
16, 18, 31, 33, 35	Intraepithelial neoplasia, cervical condylomata, anogenital warts	
13	Focal oral epithelial hyperplasia	

CUTANEOUS HUMAN PAPILLOMAVIRUS INFECTIONS

Certain human papillomavirus (HPV) types commonly infect keratinized skin. The common wart, a discrete benign epithelial hyperplasia, is manifested as papules and plaques.
Synonym: Myrmecia.

Epidemiology and Etiology

Etiology HPV, a double-stranded DNA virus of the papovavirus class (Table 28-A)

Transmission Skin-to-skin contact. Minor trauma with breaks in stratum corneum facilitates epidermal infection. Contagion occurs in groups—small (home) or large (school gymnasium). HPV in the plume from warts treated with laser or electrosurgery can cause nosocomial infection in medical workers.

Other Factors Immunocompromise such as occurs in HIV disease or following iatrogenic immunosuppression with organ transplantation is associated with an increased incidence of and more widespread cutaneous warts. Occupational risk associated with meat handling.

Inheritance Epidermodysplasia verruciformis (EDV): most commonly autosomal recessive

History

Duration of Lesions Warts often persist for several years if not treated.

Symptoms Cosmetic disfigurement. Plantar warts act as a foreign body and can be quite painful during normal daily activities such as walking. More aggressive therapies such as cryosurgery often result in much more pain than that caused by the wart itself. Bleeding, especially after shaving.

Physical Examination

Skin Lesions

VERRUCA VULGARIS (COMMON WARTS)
Type Firm papules, 1 to 10 mm or rarely larger (Figure 28-1), hyperkeratotic, clefted surface, with vegetations. Palmar lesions disrupt the normal line of fingerprints. Return of fingerprints is a sign of resolution of the wart.
Color Skin color. Characteristic "red dots" (thrombosing capillary loops) (Figure 28-2) are better seen with hand lens, are pathognomonic, representing thrombosed capillary loops.
Shape Round, polycyclic
Arrangement Isolated lesion, scattered discrete lesions. Annular at sites of prior therapy
Sites of Predilection Sites of trauma: hands, fingers, knees. Butcher's warts: hands.

VERRUCA PLANTARIS (PLANTAR WARTS) *Type* Early small, shiny, sharply marginated papule (Figure 28-3) → plaque with rough hyperkeratotic surface, studded with brown-black dots (thrombosed capillaries). As with palmar warts, normal dermatoglyphics are disrupted. Return of dermatoglyphics is a sign of resolution of the wart. Warts heal without scarring. Therapies such as cryosurgery and electrosurgery can result in lifelong scarring at treatment sites.
Color Skin-colored. To identify diagnostic red-brown dots, many plantar warts must be pared with a scalpel to remove the overlying hyperkeratosis.
Palpation Tenderness may be marked, especially in certain acute types and in lesions occurring over sites of pressure (metatarsal head).
Arrangement Confluence of many small warts results in a mosaic wart (Figure 28-3). "Kissing" lesion may occur on opposing surface of two toes.
Distribution Plantar foot, often solitary but may be three to six or more. Pressure points, heads of metatarsal, heels, toes.

VERRUCA PLANA (FLAT WARTS) *Type* Sharply defined, flat papules (1 to 5 mm); "flat" surface; the thickness of the lesion is 1 to 2 mm (Figure 28-4).

Color Skin-colored or light brown

Shape Round, oval, polygonal, linear lesions (inoculation of virus by scratching)

Arrangement Lesions that arise following trauma may have a linear arrangement.

Distribution Always numerous discrete lesions, closely set

Sites of Predilection Face, beard area, dorsa of hands, shins

EPIDERMODYSPLASIA VERRUCIFORMIS *Type* Flat wartlike lesions. Pityriasis versicolor-like lesions, particularly on the trunk. Lesions may be numerous, large, and confluent. Seborrheic keratosis-like lesions. Actinic keratosis-like lesions. Squamous cell carcinoma, *in situ* and invasive.

Color Skin-colored, light brown, pink, hypopigmented

Shape Round, oval

Arrangement Lesions often become confluent, forming large maplike areas. Linear arrangement following traumatic inoculation.

Distribution Face, trunk, extremities (flat wartlike lesions). Premalignant and malignant lesions arise most commonly on face.

Sites of Predilection Face, dorsa of hands, arms, legs, anterior trunk

Differential Diagnosis

Verruca Vulgaris Molluscum contagiosum, seborrheic keratosis

Verruca Plantaris Callus, corn (keratosis), exostosis

Verruca Plana Syringoma (facial), molluscum contagiosum

Epidermodysplasia Verruciformis Pityriasis versicolor, actinic keratoses, seborrheic keratoses, squamous cell carcinoma, basal cell carcinoma

Laboratory and Special Examinations

Dermatopathology Acanthosis, papillomatosis, hyperkeratosis. Characteristic feature is foci of vacuolated cells (koilocytosis), vertical tiers of parakeratotic cells, foci of clumped keratohyaline granules.

Diagnosis

Usually made on clinical findings

Course and Prognosis

In immunocompetent individuals, cutaneous HPV infections usually resolve spontaneously, without therapeutic intervention. In immunocompromised individuals, cutaneous HPV infections may be very resistant to all modalities of therapy.

Management

Aggressive therapies, which are often quite painful and may be followed by scarring, are usually to be avoided in that the natural history of cutaneous HPV infections is for spontaneous resolution in months or a few years. Plantar warts that are painful because of their location warrant more aggressive therapies.

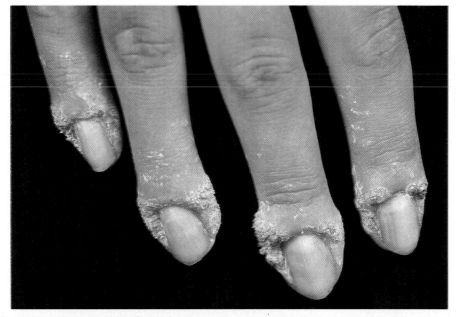

Figure 28-1 Verruca vulgaris: periungual *Hyperkeratotic papules becoming confluent around the periungual tissue of four fingers; the brown dots represent thrombosed capillaries and are pathognomonic for warts.*

Figure 28-2 Verruca plantaris
Deep-seated, painful, skin-colored, verrucous nodule disrupting the normal dermatoglyphics of the plantar foot. The thrombosed capillaries (brown dots) differentiate the lesion from a corn (an often painful, translucent, yellowish, keratotic granule) and a callus (a poorly demarcated, hyperkeratotic plaque with normal dermatoglyphics at pressure sites).

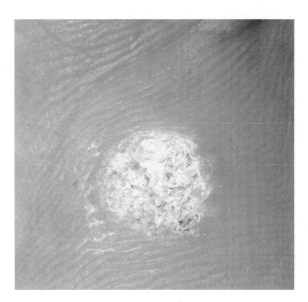

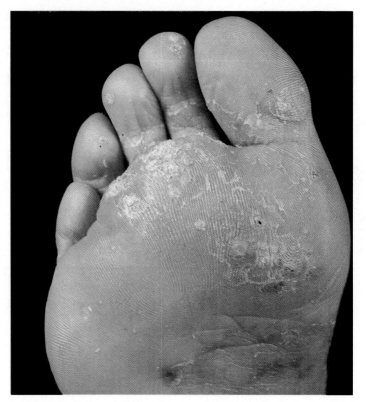

Figure 28-3 Verruca plantaris: mosaic type *Multiple, well-demarcated, skin-colored keratoses, discrete and confluent, forming a mosaic plaque on the distal volar foot. The warts are surrounded by nonwarty callus. Tinea pedis is also present in the webspaces and instep with sites of excoriation.*

Patient-Initiated Therapy

For small lesions: 10 %–20 % salicylic acid and lactic acid in collodion

For large lesions: 40 % salicylic acid plaster for 1 week, then application of salicylic acid–lactic acid in collodion

Cryosurgery If patients have tried home therapies and liquid nitrogen is available, light cryosurgery using a cotton-tipped applicator or cryospray, freezing the wart and 1 to 2 mm of surrounding normal tissue for approximately 30 seconds, is quite effective. Freezing kills the infected tissue but not HPV. Cryosurgery is usually repeated about every 4 weeks until the warts have disappeared. Painful

Electrosurgery More effective than cryosurgery, but also associated with a greater

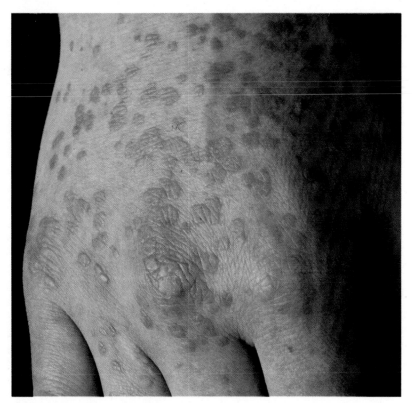

Figure 28-4 Verruca plana (flat warts) *Flat-topped, pink papules with sharp margination and minimal hyperkeratosis on the dorsum on the hands and fingers.*

chance of scarring. EMLA cream can be used for anesthesia for flat warts. Lidocaine injection is usually required for thicker warts, especially palmar/plantar lesions.

CO₂ Laser Surgery Effective for recalcitrant warts

Surgery Single, nonplantar verruca vulgaris: curettage after freon freezing; surgical excision of cutaneous HPV infections is not indicated in that these lesions are epidermal infections.

Hyperthermia for Verruca Plantaris Hyperthermia using hot water (113°F) immersion for 1/2 to 3/4 hour two or three times weekly for 16 treatments is effective in some patients.

MOLLUSCUM CONTAGIOSUM

Molluscum contagiosum is a self-limited epidermal viral infection, characterized clinically by skin-colored papules that are often umbilicated, occurring in children and sexually active adults. In HIV-infected individuals, however, numerous large mollusca often arise on the face, causing significant cosmetic disfigurement.

Epidemiology and Etiology

Etiology Molluscum contagiosum virus (MCV), a poxvirus. Types MCV-1 and MCV-2. The virus has not been cultivated. Not distinguishable from other poxviruses by electron microscopy.

Age Children. Sexually active adults.

Sex Males > females

Risk Factors HIV-infected individuals may have hundreds of small mollusca or giant mollusca on the face.

Transmission Skin-to-skin contact

Classification by Risk Groups

CHILDREN Commonly occur on exposed skin sites. Child-to-child transmission relatively low. Resolve spontaneously. Usually caused by MCV-1.

SEXUALLY ACTIVE ADULTS Occur in genital region. Virus transmitted during sexual activity. Resolve spontaneously.

HIV-INFECTED INDIVIDUALS Most commonly occur on the face, spread by shaving. Without aggressive therapy, mollusca enlarge. Spontaneous regression does not occur. Usually caused by MCV-2.

History

Duration of Lesions In the normal host, mollusca usually persist up to 6 months and then undergo spontaneous regression. In HIV-infected individuals, mollusca persist and proliferate even after aggressive therapy.

Skin Symptoms None; rarely pruritic if secondarily infected

Physical Examination

Skin Lesions

TYPE Papules (1 to 2 mm), nodules (5 to 10 mm) (rarely giant) (see Figure 28-5). Hundreds of lesions occur in HIV-infected patients. The majority of large mollusca have a central keratotic plug, which gives the lesion a central dimple or umbilication, best observed after light liquid nitrogen freeze. Gentle pressure on a molluscum causes the central plug to be extruded. Mollusca undergoing spontaneous regression have an erythematous halo.

COLOR Pearly white or skin-colored. In dark-skinned individuals, significant postinflammatory hyperpigmentation following treatment or spontaneous regression may occur.

SHAPE Round, oval, hemispherical, umbilicated (Figure 28-5)

ARRANGEMENT Isolated single lesion or multiple scattered discrete lesions. Autoinoculation is apparent in that mollusca are clustered at a site such as the axilla. In HIV-infected males who shave, mollusca can be confined to the beard area.

DISTRIBUTION Face, eyelids, neck; trunk, especially axilla; anogenital area. Multiple facial mollusca suggest HIV infection.

Differential Diagnosis

Multiple Small Mollusca Flat warts, condylomata acuminata, syringoma, sebaceous hyperplasia

Large Solitary Molluscum Keratoacanthoma, squamous cell carcinoma, basal cell carcinoma, epidermal inclusion cyst

Multiple Facial Mollusca in HIV-Infected Individual Disseminated invasive fungal infection, i.e., cryptococcosis, histoplasmosis, coccidioidomycosis, penicillinosis

Laboratory Examination

Smear of Keratotic Plug Direct microscopic examination of Giemsa-stained central semisolid core reveals "molluscum bodies" (inclusion bodies).

Dermatopathology Epidermal cells contain large intracytoplasmic inclusion bodies, so-called molluscum bodies, that appear as single, ovoid eosinophilic structures in lower cells of stratum malpighii. Epidermis grows down into dermis. Infection also occurs in epithelium and follicle.

Diagnosis

Usually made on clinical findings. Biopsy lesion in HIV-infected individual if disseminated invasive fungal infection is in the differential diagnosis.

Course and Prognosis

In healthy individuals, mollusca resolve spontaneously. In HIV-infected individuals, mollusca often progress even with aggressive therapies, creating significant cosmetic disfigurement, especially by facial lesions.

Management

In immunocompetent children and sexually active adults, mollusca regress spontaneously. Painful aggressive therapy is best avoided.

Prevention Avoid skin-to-skin contact with individual having mollusca. HIV-infected individuals with mollusca in the beard area should be advised to minimize shaving facial hair or grow a beard.

Therapy

CURETTAGE Small mollusca can be removed with a small curette with little discomfort or pain.

CRYOSURGERY Freezing lesions for 10 to 15 seconds is effective and minimally painful, using either a cotton-tipped applicator or cryospray.

ELECTRODESICCATION For mollusca refractory to cryosurgery, especially in HIV-infected individuals with numerous and/or large lesions, electrodesiccation or laser surgery is the treatment of choice. Patients to be treated can be anesthetized with EMLA for small papular lesions and injected lidocaine beneath large lesions. Giant mollusca may require several cycles of electrodesiccation and curettage to remove the large bulk of lesions; these lesions may extend through the dermis into the subcutaneous fat.

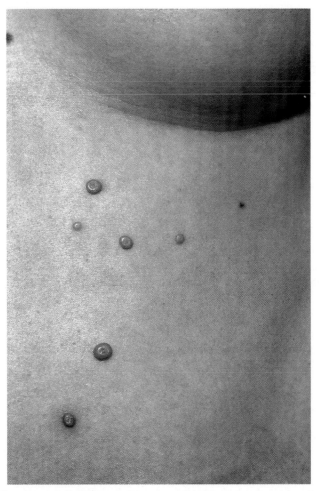

Figure 28-5 Molluscum contagiosum *Discrete, solid, skin-colored papules, 1 to 2 mm in diameter with central umbilication on the chest of an adolescent female. The lesion with an erythematous halo is undergoing spontaneous regression.*

Section 29

SYSTEMIC VIRAL INFECTIONS

INFECTIOUS EXANTHEMS

An infectious exanthem is a generalized cutaneous eruption associated with a primary systemic infection; it is often accompanied by oral mucosal lesions, i.e., an enanthem. Most often it is of viral nature but can be caused by *Rickettsia*, bacteria, and parasites.

Epidemiology and Etiology

Age   Usually younger than 20 years

Etiology   Adenoviruses, *Borrelia burgdorferi,* cytomegalovirus (CMV), Epstein-Barr virus (EBV), enteroviruses (e.g., coxsackie viruses, echo virus), flavivirus (dengue), hepatitis B virus, human herpesvirus 6 (exanthem subitum, roseola infantum), human immunodeficiency virus, *Legionella, Leptospira, Listeria,* meningococci, mycoplasma, orbivirus (Colorado tick fever), paramyxovirus (measles), parvovirus B19 (erythema infectiosum), reoviruses, respiratory syncytial virus, rhinovirus, *Rickettsia* (Rocky Mountain spotted fever, rickettsialpox, murine and epidemic typhus), rotaviruses, rubella virus, *Staphyloccus* (toxic shock syndrome), *Streptococcus* (scarlet fever). *Strongyloides, Toxoplasma, Treponema pallidum*

Transmission   Respiratory, food, sexual, blood

Season   Enterovirus infections, summer months

Geography   Worldwide

History

Incubation Period   Usually less than 3 weeks; hepatitis B virus several months

Prodrome   Fever, malaise, coryza, sore throat, nausea, vomiting, diarrhea, abdominal pain, headache

Physical Examination

Skin Lesions

TYPES   Erythematous macules and/or papules (Figure 29-1A and 29-1B); less frequently, vesicles, petechiae

COLOR   Pink to red

DISTRIBUTION   Usually central, i.e., head, neck, trunk, proximal extremities. Diffuse erythema of cheeks, i.e., "slapped cheek" with erythema infectiosum. Palms and soles usually spared except for hand-foot-and-mouth disease caused by coxsackie A16.

MUCOUS MEMBRANES   Koplik's spots in measles; microulcerative lesions in herpangina due to coxsackie virus A (Figure 29-2); palatal petechiae in mononucleosis syndrome of EBV or CMV; conjunctivitis

General Examination   Lymphadenopathy, hepatomegaly, splenomegaly

Differential Diagnosis

Exanthematous Eruption   Drug eruption, systemic lupus erythematosus, Kawasaki's syndrome

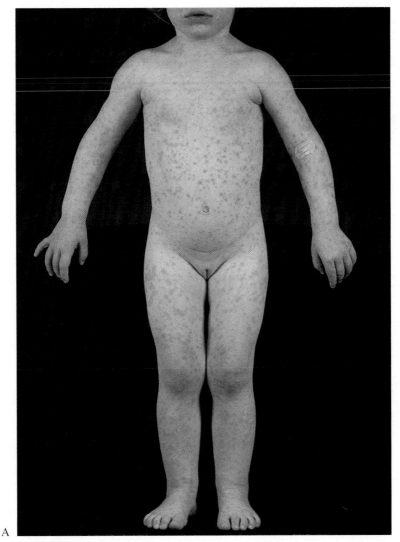

A

Figure 29-1 Infectious exanthem *Disseminated, erythematous macules and papules, typical of the cutaneous changes with many acute infections. The eruption must be differentiated from an exanthematous (morbilliform) drug eruption. A. Typical distribution of lesions on the trunk and extremities.*

Laboratory and Special Examinations

Cultures If practical

Serology Acute and convalescent titers most helpful in specific diagnosis

Diagnosis

Usually made on history and clinical findings

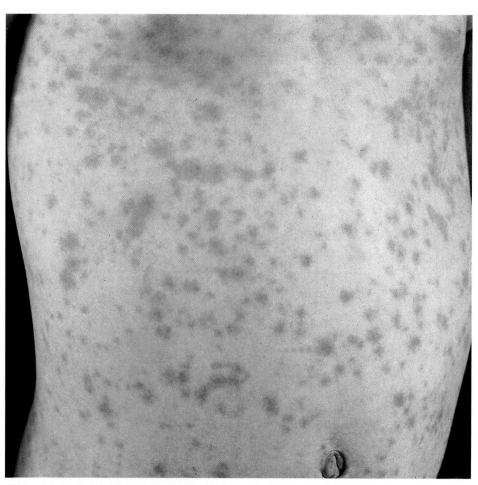

Figure 29-1 Infectious exanthem   B. *Close-up of pink macules and papules becoming confluent in some areas.*

Pathophysiology

Skin lesions may be produced by the direct effect of microbial replication in infected cells, the host response to the microbe, or the interaction of these two phenomena.

Course and Prognosis

Usually resolves in less than 10 days. Patient with primary EBV or CMV infection very often develops an exanthematous eruption if given ampicillin or amoxicillin.

Management

Symptomatic

Antimicrobial Therapy   Specific antimicrobial therapy when available

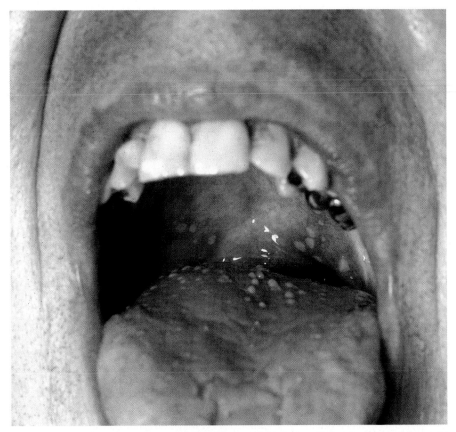

Figure 29-2 Infectious enanthem: herpangina *Multiple, small vesicles and erosions with erythematous halos on the soft palate; some taste buds on the posterior tongue are inflamed and prominent.*

RUBELLA

Rubella is a common benign childhood infection manifested by a characteristic exanthem and lymphadenopathy; however, occurring in pregnancy, it may result in the congenital rubella syndrome with serious chronic fetal infection and malformation.
Synonyms: German measles, "3-day measles."

Epidemiology and Etiology

Age Prior to widespread immunization, children <15 years. Currently, young adults.

Etiology Rubella virus

Occupation Young adults in hospitals, colleges, prisons, prenatal clinics

Transmission Inhalation of aerosolized respiratory droplets; moderately contagious; 10 % to 40 % of cases asymptomatic; period of infectivity from end of incubation period to disappearance of rash.

Risk Factors Lack of active immunization, lack of natural infection. Following immunization begun in 1969, incidence has decreased by 99 %.

Season Prior to 1969, epidemics in United States every 6 to 9 years, occurring in spring

Geography Worldwide. Marked reduction in incidence in developed countries following immunization.

History

Incubation Period 14 to 21 days

Prodrome Usually absent, especially in young children. In adolescents and young adults: anorexia, malaise, conjunctivitis, headache, low-grade fever, mild upper respiratory tract symptoms.

History Arthralgia, especially in adult women following immunization

Immune Status *In women, rubella-like illness frequently follows administration of attenuated live rubella virus.*

Physical Examination

Skin Lesions

TYPES Pink macules, papules (Figure 29-3A). Trunkal lesions may become confluent, creating a scarlatiniform eruption (Figure 29-3B).

DISTRIBUTION Initially on forehead, spreading inferiorly to face, trunk and extremities during first day. By second day, facial exanthem fades. By third day, exanthem fades completely without residual pigmentary change or scaling.

MUCOUS MEMBRANES Petechiae on soft palate (Forchheimer's sign) during prodrome (also seen in infectious mononucleosis)

General Examination

LYMPH NODES Enlargement noted during prodrome. Postauricular, suboccipital, and posterior cervical lymph nodes enlarged and possibly tender. Mild generalized lymphadenopathy may occur. Enlargement usually, persists for 1 week, but may last for months.

SPLEEN May be enlarged

JOINTS Arthritis occurs in adults. Possible effusion.

Differential Diagnosis

Exanthem Other viral exanthems, drug eruption, scarlet fever

Exanthem with Arthritis Acute rheumatic fever, rheumatoid arthritis

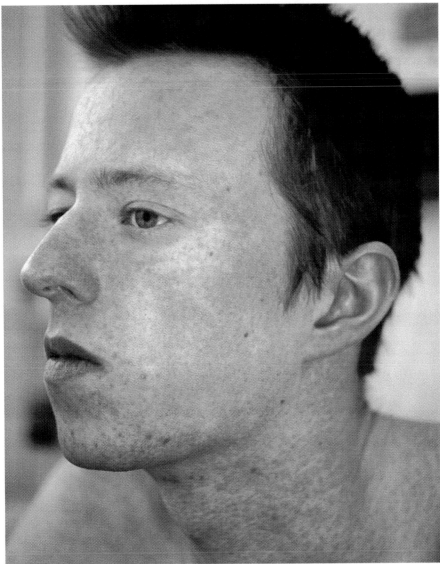

A

Figure 29-3 Rubella *Erythematous macules and papules appearing initially on the face and spreading inferiorly to the trunk and extremities usually within the first 24 hours. Postauricular and posterior cervical lymph nodes were enlarged. A. Lesions becoming confluent (scarlatiniform) on the cheeks while clear on the forehead.*

Laboratory and Special Examinations

Serology Acute and convalescent rubella antibody titers show fourfold or greater rise.

Culture Virus can be isolated from throat, joint fluid aspirate.

Diagnosis

Clinical diagnosis; can be confirmed by serology

Course and Prognosis

In most persons, rubella is a mild, inconsequential infection. However, when rubella occurs in a pregnant woman during the first trimester, the infection can be passed transplacentally to the developing fetus. Approximately half of infants who acquire rubella during the first trimester of intrauterine life will show clinical signs of damage from the virus. Manifestations of the congenital rubella syndrome are congenital heart defects, cataracts, microphthalmia, deafness, microcephaly, hydrocephaly.

Management

Prevention Rubella is preventable by immunization. Prior rubella should be documented in young women; if antirubella antibody titers are negative, rubella immunization should be given.

Acute Infection Symptomatic

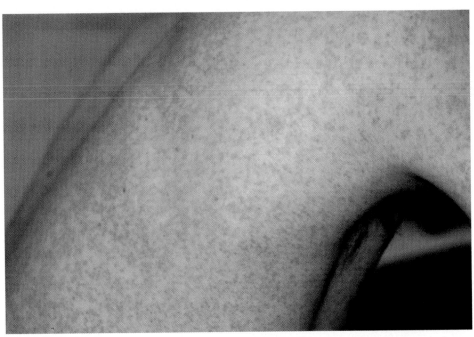

B

Figure 29-3 Rubella   B. *Truncal lesions appear 24 hours after onset of facial lesions.*

MEASLES

Measles is a highly contagious childhood viral infection characterized by fever, coryza, cough, conjunctivitis, pathognomonic enanthem (Koplik's spots), and an exanthem, it can be complicated, acutely and chronically, by significant morbidity and mortality.
Synonym: Rubeola, morbilli.

Epidemiology and Etiology

Age Prior to measles immunization: 5 to 9 years in the United States. In underdeveloped countries, up to 45 % of cases occur before the age of 9 months.

Etiology Measles virus, a paramyxovirus

Incidence

UNITED STATES   Greater than fourfold increase, 1988 to 1989. Since 1993, an historic low of 312 cases were reported. In 1994, 92 % of cases were indigenous and 8 % imported from other countries.

WORLDWIDE   Hyperendemic in many underdeveloped countries, resulting in >1.5 million deaths annually

Risk Factors Following immunization begun in 1963, incidence has decreased by 98 %. Current outbreaks in the United States occur in inner-city unimmunized preschool-aged children, school-aged persons immunized at early age, and imported cases. Most outbreaks are in primary or secondary schools, colleges or universities, day-care centers.

Transmission Spread by respiratory droplet aerosols produced by sneezing and coughing. Infected persons contagious from several days before onset of rash up to 5 days after lesions appear. Attack rate for susceptible contacts exceeds 90 % to 100 %. Asymptomatic infection rare.

Season Prior to widespread use of vaccine, epidemics occurred every 2 to 3 years, in late winter to early spring.

Geography Worldwide

History

Incubation Period   10 to 15 days

History Symptoms of upper respiratory infection with coryza and *hacking, barklike cough,* photophobia, malaise, fever. As exanthem progresses, systemic symptoms subside.

Physical Examination

Skin Lesions

TYPES   Exanthem: on the fourth febrile day, erythematous macules and papules. Initial discrete lesions may become confluent, especially on face (Figure 29-4), neck, and shoulders. Lesions gradually fade in order of appearance with subsequent residual yellow-tan stain or faint desquamation. Exanthem resolves in 4 to 6 days. Periorbital edema in prodrome.

COLOR   Initially erythematous, fading to yellow-tan

DISTRIBUTION   Appear on forehead at hairline, behind ears; spread centrifugally and inferiorly to involve the face, trunk (Figure 29-5), and extremities, reaching the feet by third day

MUCOUS MEMBRANES   Koplik's spots: cluster of tiny bluish white papules with an erythematous areola, appearing on or after second day of febrile illness, on buccal mucosa opposite premolar teeth. Bulbar conjunctivae: conjunctivitis.

General Examination Generalized lymphadenopathy common. Otherwise unremarkable.

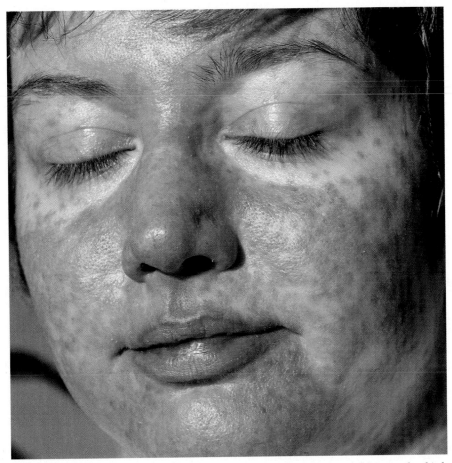

Figure 29-4 Measles *Confluent erythematous macules and papules on the face on the third day of febrile illness; conjunctivitis and Koplik's spot on the buccal mucosa were also present.*

Differential Diagnosis

Other viral exanthems (e.g., rubella), secondary syphilis, scarlet fever, drug eruption

Laboratory and Special Examinations

Cultures Isolate virus from blood, urine, pharyngeal secretions

Serology Demonstrates fourfold or greater rise in measles titer

PCR Detects genomic sequences of measles virus DNA in serum, throat swabs, and CSF

Diagnosis

Clinical diagnosis, at times, confirmed by serology (see Figure 29-5)

Pathophysiology

Virus enters cells of respiratory tract, replicates locally, spreads to local lymph nodes, and disseminates hematogenously to skin and mucous membranes. Viral replication also occurs on skin and mucosa.

Course and Prognosis

Self-limited infection in most patients. Complications more common in malnourished third-world children, the unimmunized, and those with congenital immunodeficiency and leukemia. Acute complications (9.8 % of cases): otitis media, pneumonia (bacterial or measles), diarrhea, measles encephalitis (1 in 800 to 1000 cases), thrombocytopenia. In unimmunized HIV-infected children, fatal measles pneumonia has occurred without rash. Chronic complication: subacute sclerosing panencephalitis.

Management

Prevention Prophylactic immunization. The goal of eliminating indigenous measles transmission in the United States is based on four components: (1) maintaining high coverage with a single dose of measles-mumps-rubella vaccine (MMR) among preschool-aged children, (2) achieving coverage with two doses of MMR for all school and college attendees, (3) enhancing surveillance and outbreak response, and (4) increasing efforts to develop and implement strategies for global measles elimination.

Acute Infection Symptomatic

Secondary Bacterial Infections Administration of appropriate antibiotics

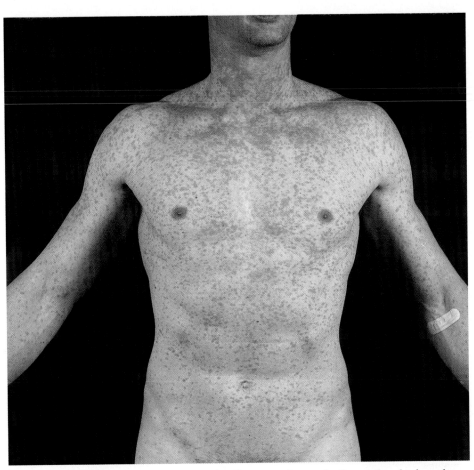

Figure 29-5 Measles *Erythematous papules, first appearing on the face and neck where they have become confluent, spreading to the trunk and arms in 2 to 3 days where they remain discrete. In contrast, rubella also first appears initially on the face but spreads to the trunk in one day.*

HAND-FOOT-AND-MOUTH DISEASE

Hand-foot-and-mouth disease (HFMD) is a systemic infection caused by coxsackie virus A16, characterized by ulcerative oral lesions and a vesicular exanthem on the distal extremities in association with mild constitutional symptoms.

Epidemiology and Etiology

Age Usually children <10 years old, but also young and middle-aged adults

Sex Equal

Season Epidemic outbreaks every 3 years. In temperate climates, outbreaks during warmer months.

Etiology Coxsackie virus A16. Sporadic cases have been reported with coxsackie virus A4-7, A9, A10, B2, and B5 and enterovirus 71.

Transmission Highly contagious, spread from person to person by oral-oral and fecal-oral routes

History

Incubation Period 3 to 6 days

Prodrome 12 to 24 hours of low-grade fever, malaise, and abdominal pain or respiratory symptoms

Symptoms Frequently 5 to 10 *painful* ulcerative oral lesions, leading to refusal to eat in children. Few to 100 cutaneous lesions appear together or shortly after the oral lesions and may be asymptomatic or *tender* and *painful.*

Physical Examination

Skin Lesions

TYPES Lesions begin as 2- to 8-mm *macules* or *papules* that quickly evolve to *vesicles* (Figure 29-6). Lesions on palms and soles usually do not rupture. At other cutaneous sites, vesicles can rupture, with formation of *erosions* and *crusts.* Lesions heal without scarring.

COLOR Early papules, pink to red. Vesicles have clear fluid with a watery appearance or yellowish hue.

SHAPE Cutaneous lesions have a characteristic "linear" shape on the palms and soles.

DISTRIBUTION Characteristically, lesions arise on palms and soles, especially on sides of fingers, toes, and buttocks.

Mucosal Lesions

TYPE 5- to 10-mm, small, punched out painful ulcers preceded by macules → grayish vesicles.

DISTRIBUTION Hard palate, tongue, buccal mucosa (Figure 29-7)

General Findings Typically, HFMD is accompanied by low-grade fever, malaise, and a sore mouth. In some patients, it may be associated with high fever, severe malaise, diarrhea, and joint pains.

Differential Diagnosis

A sudden outbreak of oral and distal extremity lesions is pathognomonic for HFMD; however, if only the oral lesions are present, the differential diagnosis would include: herpes simplex virus infection, aphthous stomatitis, herpangina, erythema multiforme major.

Laboratory and Special Examinations

Histopathology Epidermal reticular degeneration leads to an intraepidermal vesicle filled with neutrophils, mononuclear cells, and proteinaceous eosinophilic material. The dermis reveals a perivascular mixed cell infiltrate.

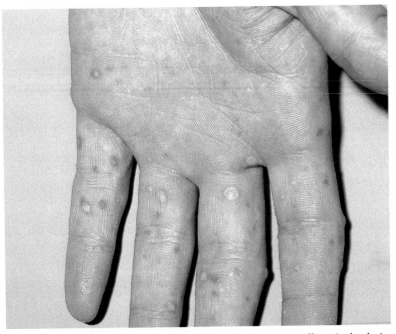

Figure 29-6 Hand-foot-and-mouth disease *Multiple, discrete, small, vesicular lesions on the fingers and palms; similar lesions were also present on the feet. Some vesicles are typically linear.*

Electron Microscopy Intracytoplasmic particles in crystalline array characteristic of coxsackie viral infections

Serology In acute serum, neutralizing antibodies may be detected but disappear rapidly. In convalescent serum, elevated titers of complement-fixing antibodies are found.

Tzanck Preparation Negative for both multinucleated giant cells and inclusion bodies

Viral Culture Virus may be isolated from vesicles, throat washings, and stool specimens.

Diagnosis

Usually made on clinical findings

Pathophysiology

Enteroviral implantation in the GI tract (buccal mucosa and ileum) leads to extension into regional lymph nodes, and 72 hours later a viremia occurs with seeding of the oral mucosa and skin of the hands and feet.

Course and Prognosis

Most commonly, HFMD is self-limited, and a rise in serum antibodies eliminates the viremia in 7 to 10 days. A few cases have been more prolonged or recurrent. Serious sequelae rarely occur; however, coxsackie virus has been implicated in cases of myocarditis, meningoencephalitis, aseptic meningitis, paralytic disease, and a systemic illness resembling rubeola. Infection acquired during the first trimester of pregnancy may result in spontaneous abortion.

Management

Symptomatic treatment, including topical application of dyclonine HCl solution or lidocaine, may reduce oral discomfort.

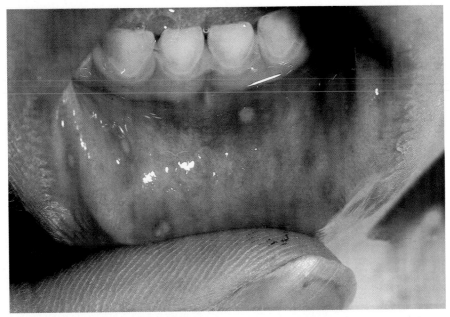

Figure 29-7 Hand-foot-and-mouth disease *Multiple, superficial erosions and small, vesicular lesions surrounded by an erythematous halo on the lower labial mucosa; the gingiva is normal. In primary herpetic gingivostomatitis, which presents with similar oral vesicular lesion, a painful gingivitis usually occurs as well.*

HERPES SIMPLEX VIRUS

NONGENITAL HERPES SIMPLEX VIRUS INFECTION

Nongenital herpes simplex virus (HSV) infection, whether primary or recurrent, is characterized clinically by grouped vesicles arising on an erythematous base on keratinized skin or mucous membrane. (For Genital Herpes Simplex Virus Infection, see page 910).
Synonyms: Herpes, herpes simplex, cold sore, fever blister, herpes febrilis, herpes labialis, herpes gladiatorum, scrum pox, herpetic whitlow.

Epidemiology and Etiology

Age Most commonly young adults; range, infancy to senescence

Etiology Labialis: HSV-1 (80 % to 90 %); HSV-2 (10 % to 20 %). Urogenital: HSV-2 (70 % to 90 %); HSV-1 (10 % to 30 %). Herpetic whitlow in patients <20 years usually HSV-1; >20 years, usually HSV-2. Neonatal: HSV-2 (70 %); HSV-1 (30 %).

Transmission Usually skin-skin, skin-mucosa, mucosa-skin contact. Herpes gladiatorum transmitted by skin-to-skin contact in wrestlers. Increased HSV-1 transmission associated with crowded living conditions and lower socioeconomic status.

Precipitating Factors for Recurrence Approximately one-third of persons who develop herpes labialis will experience a recurrence; of these, one-half will experience at least two recurrences annually. Usual factors for herpes labialis: skin/mucosal irritation (UV radiation), altered hormonal milieu (menstruation), fever, the common cold, altered immune states, site of infection (genital herpes recurs more frequently than labial).

Immunocompromising Factors Predisposing to HSV Reactivation HIV infection, malignancy (leukemia/lymphoma), transplantation (bone marrow, solid organ), chemotherapy, systemic corticosteroids, irradiation, immunosuppressive drugs

History

Incubation Period 2- to 20-day (average 6) incubation period for primary infection

Systems Review

PRIMARY HERPES Many individuals with primary HSV infection are either asymptomatic or have only trivial symptoms. Symptomatic primary herpes, which is uncommon, is characterized by vesicles at the site of inoculation associated with regional lymphadenopathy, at times accompanied by fever, headache, malaise, myalgia, peaking within the first 3 to 4 days after onset of lesions, resolving during the subsequent 3 to 4 days. Primary herpetic gingivostomatitis is the most common symptom complex accompanying primary HSV infection in children, in young women primary herpetic vulvivaginitis (see page 911).

RECURRENT HERPES Prodrome of tingling, itching, or burning sensation usually precedes any visible skin changes by 24 hours. Systemic symptoms are usually absent.

Physical Examination

Primary Herpes

SKIN FINDINGS Erythemas are often noted initially, followed soon by grouped, often umbilicated vesicles, which may evolve to pustules (Figure 29-9); these become eroded as the overlying epidermis sloughs. Erosions may enlarge to ulcerations, which may be crusted or moist. These epithelial defects

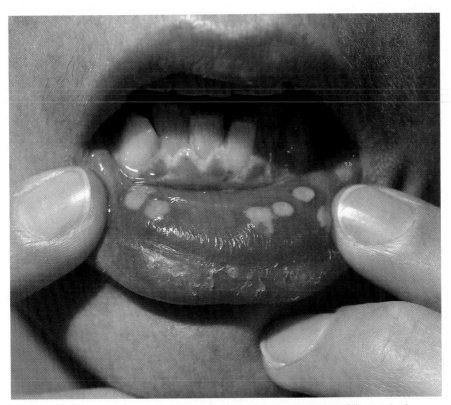

Figure 29-8 Herpes simplex virus infection: primary gingivostomatitis *Multiple, very painful erosions on the lower labial mucosa with erythema and edema of the gingiva; fibrin deposits on teeth and gingiva. Fever and tender submandibular lymphadenopathy were also present.*

heal in 2 to 4 weeks, often with resultant postinflammatory hypo- or hyperpigmentation, uncommonly with scarring. The area of involvement may be circumferential around the mouth.

MUCOUS MEMBRANES Oral mucosa usually involved only in primary HSV infection with vesicles that quickly slough to form erosions (Figure 29-8) at any site in oropharynx, scanty to numerous; gingivitis with gingival tenderness, edema, violaceous color. Sialorrhea. Documented recurrent intraoral HSV is uncommon.

GENERAL FINDINGS Fever is often present during symptomatic primary herpetic gingivostomatitis. Regional lymph nodes enlarged, firm, nonfluctuant, tender; usually unilateral. Signs of aseptic meningitis: headache, fever, nuchal rigidity, CSF pleocytosis with normal sugar content and positive HSV CSF culture.

Recurrent Herpes

TYPES OF LESIONS Lesions similar to primary infection but on a reduced scale. Often a 1- to 2-cm patch of erythema surmounted with vesicles. Heals in 1 to 2 weeks. May be associated with regional lymphadenitis

ARRANGEMENT Herpetiform, i.e., grouped vesicles (Figure 29-9A and 29-9B)

DISTRIBUTION May occur at any mucocutaneous site. Most common sites are perioral, cheek, nose tip, distal finger (herpetic whitlow) (Figure 29-10). Periocular localization requires examination of the cornea. Herpes gladiatorum occurs on the head, neck, or shoulder.

Widespread Cutaneous Infection in Underlying Dermatoses See page 806.

Chronic Herpetic Ulcer Relentlessly progressive ulcerative form of herpes in immunosuppressed individuals or patients with HIV infection (see Infections in the Immunocompromised Host, page 800)

Differential Diagnosis

Primary Intraoral HSV Infection Aphthous stomatitis, hand-foot-and-mouth disease, herpangina, erythema multiforme

Recurrent Lesion Fixed drug eruption

Laboratory and Special Examinations

Tzanck Smear (Figure 29-11). Optimally, fluid from intact vesicle is smeared thinly on a microscope slide, dried, and stained with either Wright's or Giemsa's stain. Positive if giant acantholytic keratinocytes or multinucleated giant keratinocytes are detected (Figure 29-11). Positive in 75 % of early cases, either primary or recurrent.

Antigen Detection Monoclonal antibodies, specific for HSV-1 and HSV-2 antigens, detect and differentiate HSV antigens on smear from lesion.

Dermatopathology Ballooning and reticular epidermal degeneration, acantholysis and intraepidermal vesicles; intranuclear inclusion bodies, multinucleate giant keratinocytes; multilocular vesicles. Immunoperoxidase techniques can be used to identify HSV-1 and HSV-2 antigens in formalin-fixed tissue samples.

Cultures Positive HSV cultures from involved mucocutaneous site or tissue biopsy specimens

Serology Primary HSV infection can be documented by demonstration of seroconversion. Recurring herpes can be ruled out if seronegative for HSV antibodies. Type-specific antibodies to HSV-1 and HSV-2 are presently used on a research basis but are not widely available.

Polymerase Chain Reaction (PCR) To determine HSV-DNA sequences in tissue

Diagnosis

Clinical suspicion confirmed by Tzanck smear, viral culture, or antigen detection

Pathophysiology

Transmission and primary infection of HSV occur through close contact with a person shedding virus at a peripheral site, mucosal surface, or secretion. HSV is inactivated promptly at room temperature; aerosol or fomitic spread unlikely. Infection occurs via inoculation onto susceptible mucosal surface or break in skin. Following exposure of skin sites to HSV, the virus replicates in parabasal and intermediate epithelial cells, causing lysis of infected cells, vesicle formation, and local inflammation. Subsequent to primary infection at inoculation site, HSV ascends peripheral sensory nerves and enters sensory (trigeminal or sacral) or autonomic nerve root ganglia (vagal), where latency is established. Latency can occur after both symptomatic and asymptomatic primary infection. Recurrences result from viral reactivation and synthesis and migration of virus through sensory nerves. Usually occur in the vicinity of the primary infection, may be clinically symptomatic or asymptomatic.

Course and Prognosis

Recurrences of HSV tend to become less frequent with the passage of time. Eczema herpeticum (see Widespread Cutaneous Infection

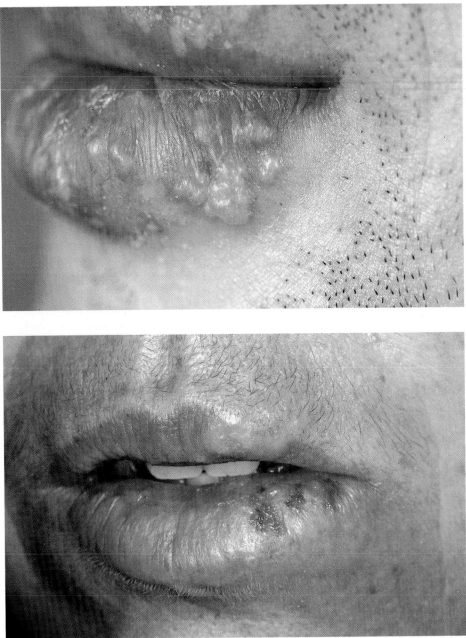

Figure 29-9 Herpes simplex virus infection: recurrent herpes labialis A. *Grouped and confluent vesicles with an erythematous rim on the lips.* B. *Edema with crusting of the lips which followed sun exposure; vesiculation is present but difficult to detect because of confluence of lesions. In some cases, crusting is the only finding.*

in Underlying Dermatoses, page 806) may complicate atopic dermatitis (eczema herpeticum), keratosis follicularis (Darier's disease), and second- and third-degree thermal burns. Patients with immunodeficiency may experience cutaneous and systemic dissemination of HSV and chronic herpetic ulcers (see Infections in the Immunocompromised Host, page 800). Erythema multiforme may complicate herpes, occurring 1 to 2 weeks after an outbreak.

Management

Prevention Skin-to-skin contact should be avoided during outbreak of cutaneous HSV infection.

Antiviral Therapy Currently, available drugs for HSV infections include acyclovir, valacyclovir, and famciclovir. Valacyclovir, the prodrug of acyclovir, has a better bioavailability and is nearly 85 % absorbed after oral administration; in the United States, it is currently approved for use in genital HSV infections. Famciclovir is equally effective for cutaneous HSV infections.

FOR PATIENTS WITH SEVERE DISEASE OR COMPLICATIONS NECESSITATING HOSPITALIZATION Acyclovir 5 mg/kg body weight IV every 8 hours for 5 to 7 days or until clinical resolution occurs. Oral valacyclovir or famciclovir may reduce the necessity for IV acyclovir therapy.

RECURRENT EPISODES Most episodes of recurrent herpes do not benefit from pulse apy with oral acyclovir. In severe recurrent disease, patients who start therapy at the beginning of the prodrome or within 2 days after onset of lesions may benefit from therapy by shortening and reducing severity of eruption; however, recurrences cannot be prevented.

Acyclovir 400 mg PO t.i.d. for 5 days *or*
Acyclovir 800 mg PO b.i.d. for 5 days
Valacyclovir 500 to 1000 mg b.i.d.
Famciclovir 125 mg b.i.d. for 5 days, both
   not yet approved in the United States

DAILY SUPPRESSIVE THERAPY Daily treatment reduces frequency of recurrences by at least 75 % among patients with frequent (>6 per year) recurrences. After 1 year of continuous daily suppressive therapy, acyclovir is discontinued so that the patient's recurrence rate may be reassessed.

Acyclovir 400 mg PO two times a day
Valacyclovir and famciclovir will probably
   also prove effective but studies are still
   ongoing.

Herpes Among HIV-Infected Patients Neither the need for nor the proper increased dosage of acyclovir has been established conclusively. Patients with herpes who do not respond to the recommended dose of acyclovir may require a higher oral dose of acyclovir, IV acyclovir, or be infected with an acyclovir-resistant HSV strain, requiring IV foscarnet. The role of valacyclovir and famciclovir are not yet established.

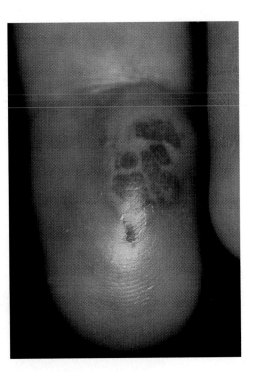

Figure 29-10 Herpes simplex virus infection: herpetic whitlow *Painful, grouped, confluent vesicles on the volar finger on an erythematous edematous base.*

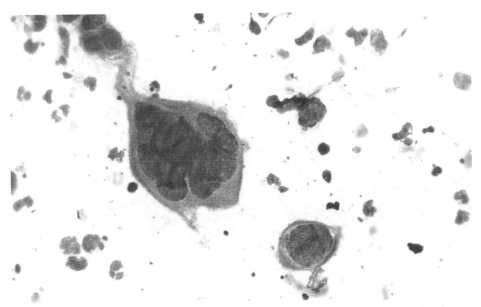

Figure 29-11 Herpes simplex virus infection: positive Tzanck smear *Giant and multinucleated keratinocytes on a Giemsa-stained smear obtained from a vesicle base. Compare size to that of neutrophils also seen in this smear.*

HERPES SIMPLEX VIRUS

NEONATAL HERPES SIMPLEX VIRUS INFECTION

Neonates may be infected during delivery or in the perinatal period. Eruption occurs on the mucous membranes or on the skin at innoculation sites. 70 % of infants with neonatal HSV infection are born to mothers with asymptomatic genital herpes; 73 % of cases occur in the first-born child. Difficulty in diagnosis of disseminated HSV infection in neonates is common in that up to 70 % of infants have no mucocutaneous lesions. IV acyclovir therapy is mandatory in these cases. For prophylaxis of neonatal HSV infection, see Section 32 (genital herpes infection, page 910).

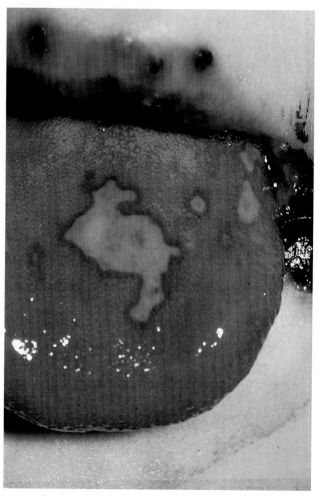

Figure 29-12 Herpes simplex virus infection: neonatal *Note necrotic lesions on the lips and large ulcers on the tongue.*

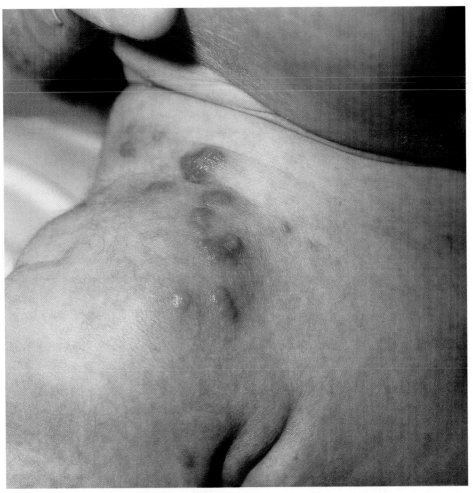

Figure 29-13 Herpes simplex virus infection: neonatal *Grouped and confluent vesicles with underlying erythema and edema on the shoulder of a newborn infant, arising at the inoculation site. Neonates become infected in the perinatal period, usually during vaginal delivery, 70 % of infants with neonatal HSV infection are born to mothers with asymptomatic genital herpes; 73 % of cases occur in the first-born child. Difficulty in diagnosis of disseminated HSV infection in neonates is common in that up to 70 % of infants have no mucocutaneous lesions.*

HERPES SIMPLEX VIRUS: INFECTIONS IN THE IMMUNOCOMPROMISED HOST

In the immunocompromised host, herpes simplex virus is capable of causing local infection, characterized by extensive local involvement (e.g., eczema herpeticum) or chronic herpetic ulcers, or widespread systemic infection, characterized by widespread mucocutaneous vesicles, pustules, erosions, and ulcerations, associated with signs of pneumonia, encephalitis, hepatitis, as well as involvement of other organ systems, usually occurring in an immunocompromised host. Also see Nongenital HSV Infections (page 792) and Genital Herpes (page 910).

Epidemiology and Etiology

Age   Any age

Etiology   Herpes simplex virus (HSV) type 1 and type 2

Incidence

- HSV-1: approximately 70 % of adults in the United States are seropositive. HSV-2: incidence of seropositivity has increased; highest in HIV-infected homosexual or bisexual men (68 % to 77 %).
- Incidence rising due to an increasing population of immunocompromised individuals: 80 % in bone marrow transplant recipients, 65 % in solid organ transplant recipients, 60 % of those with lymphoma and 55 % in leukemics, 25 % in individuals with HIV disease.
- Incidence of symptomatic outbreaks has decreased markedly because of the primary prophylaxis of HSV-seropositive individuals with acyclovir.

Risk Factors

IMMUNODEFICIENCY: HIV INFECTION   Frequency and duration increase sharply as CD4+ cell count falls below $50/\mu l$. In the majority of HIV-infected individuals, frequency, duration, and severity of HSV outbreaks similar to those in immunocompetent individuals. Disseminated cutaneous and visceral HSV infections are less common than in other immunocompromised states.

CDC Surveillance Case Definition for AIDS   HSV infection causing a mucocutaneous ulcer that persists longer than 1 month, or HSV infection causing bronchitis, pneumonitis, or esophagitis for any duration in a patient older than 1 month, is an AIDS-defining condition if the patient has no other cause of immunodeficiency and is without knowledge of HIV antibody status.

LEUKEMIA/LYMPHOMA   HSV reactivation typically occurs during induction or reinduction within 20 days in HSV-seropositive individuals.

BONE MARROW TRANSPLANTATION (BMT)   HSV reactivation occurs within the first 5 weeks after BMT (median, day 8 posttransplantation). Untreated, 3 % of patients die from disseminated HSV infection.

CHEMOTHERAPY for solid organ or bone marrow transplantation (BMT), congenital or acquired cellular immune defects. Cytotoxic cancer chemotherapy, corticosteroid therapy.

OTHER   Autoimmune diseases, malnutrition; rarely pregnancy. Radiotherapy. Instrumentation such as nasogastric tube in debilitated patient associated with HSV esophagitis.

History

History   Patients often hospitalized with underlying condition or disease

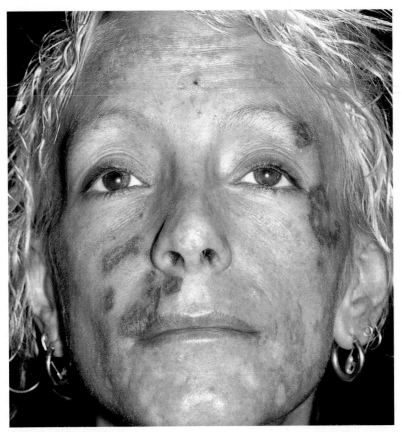

Figure 29-14 Herpes simplex virus infection: chronic ulcer in HIV disease *Shallow, well-demarcated ulcers and white depressed scars on the face of a 32-year-old HIV-infected female. The infecting HSV-1 strain was acyclovir-resistant; lesions resolved with intravenous foscarnet therapy.*

Skin Symptoms Tender and painful mucocutaneous ulcers

RECURRENT HERPETIC LESION Mild pain in ulcers

CHRONIC HERPETIC ULCERS (CHU) Mild to moderate pain

HERPETIC WHITLOW Severe pain

OROPHARYNGEAL ULCERS Oral pain on eating

ESOPHAGEAL ULCERS Retrosternal pain and/or painful swallowing (odynophagia) and/or dysphagia

ANORECTAL ULCERS Perianal/anal ulcers are usually quite painful. Anorectal ulcers are associated with pain, constipation, pain on defecation, discharge, tenesmus, and at times, sacral radiculopathy, impotence, neurogenic bladder.

MUCOCUTANEOUS DISSEMINATION Fever, deterioration of clinical status

Physical Examination

Skin Lesions

TYPES *Recurrent Herpetic Lesions* In the

majority of immunocompromised individuals, lesions appear as in the immunocompetent host. However, outbreaks may present with recurrent lesions (grouped crusts, erosions, ulcers) in a much larger area of involvement than usual. In HIV-infected individuals, large, necrotic, eroded lesions may appear over a period of a few days without apparent vesicle formation.

Chronic Herpetic Ulcers Recurrent lesions enlarge over weeks to months, forming large ulcers, 10 to 20 cm in diameter (Figures 29-14, 29-15, and 29-16). Margins may be slightly rolled, hyperplastic. Coalescence of ulcerations may result in linear ulcers in intergluteal cleft or inguinal fold. Base of ulcer may be crusted or moist. Painful on palpation. Perianal and/or rectal > genital > orofacial > digital. Uncommonly, ulcer on face and perineum simultaneously.

Oropharyngeal Ulcers Large ulcerations occur on the hard palate, often at the site of dental extraction. Linear ulcerations occur on the tongue.

Esophageal Ulcers Usually associated with oropharyngeal herpetic ulcer and swallowing HSV-infected saliva. Esophagoscopy: mucosal erosions/ulceration.

Anorectal Ulcers Anal ulcers usually occur via enlargement of perianal ulcers. Herpetic proctitis: Sigmoidoscopy shows friable mucosa and ulcerations.

Mucocutaneous Dissemination Disseminated (nongrouped) vesicles and pustules often hemorrhagic with inflammatory halo; quickly rupture, resulting in "punched-out" erosions. Lesions may be necrotic and then ulcerate (Figure 29-17). Ulcers may become confluent with polycyclic well-demarcated borders; edges may be slightly raised, rolled.

Infarctive Skin Lesions If complicated by purpura fulminans

DISTRIBUTION   Localized as described above; generalized, disseminated in mucocutaneous dissemination (Figure 29-15). Site of recurrent HSV infection, i.e., labial, oropharyngeal, esophageal, genital, perianal, may be apparent.

MUCOUS MEMBRANES   Oropharyngeal erosion: necrotizing gingivitis, palatal ulcers, glossitis.

General Examination   Oropharyngeal infection can occur in the absence of external facial lesions. HSV esophagitis, tracheobronchitis, and focal pneumonitis can be local infection associated with spread by aspirated or swallowed secretions. Diffuse interstitial pneumonitis can be a manifestation of hematogenous infection. HSV pneumonitis often results from endogenous reactivation. Widespread visceral involvement (liver, lungs, adrenals, GI tract, CNS) can occur in immunocompromised individual.

Variations with Specific States of Immunocompromise

LEUKEMIA/LYMPHOMA   HSV infection is often atypical, with extensive lesions on lips or nasolabial skin; oropharyngeal infection manifested as necrotic gingival papillae, intraoral ulcerations that mimic thrush, or mucositis from chemotherapy or radiotherapy.

HIV DISEASE   HSV reactivation is usually local, with chronic herpetic ulcers on the face or anogenital region. HSV esophagitis may coexist with candidal esophagitis. Persistent perianal herpes and herpetic proctitis. Disseminated visceral disease is uncommon.

Differential Diagnosis

Recurrent Herpetic Lesions   Mild pain in ulcers.

Chronic Herpetic Ulcers   Chronic VZV infection, impetigo, ecthyma, ecthyma gangrenosum, pressure ulcer, syphilitic chancre, deep mycotic (cryptococcal, histoplasmal, blastomycotic, coccidioidal) ulcer, fixed drug reaction.

Herpetic Whitlow   Paronychia, extragenital syphilitic chancre

Oropharyngeal Ulcers   Aphthous ulcers, lymphoma, histoplasmosis with oral ulcer.

Esophageal Ulcers   Cytomegalovirus ulcers, aphthous (idiopathic) ulcers, *Candida* esophagitis, histoplasmosis with esophageal ulcer.

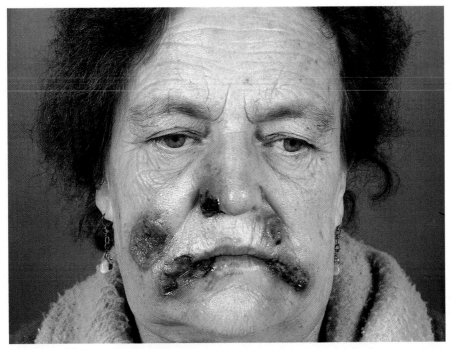

Figure 29-15 Herpes simplex virus infection: chronic ulcer in an immunocompromised host *Multiple, slowly spreading, deep ulcers with central necrosis and hemorrhagic crusts on the lips, cheeks, and nose in a female with leukemia.*

Anorectal Ulcers Carcinoma, Crohn's disease; amebiasis, chronic rectal abuse of ergot alkaloids.

Mucocutaneous Dissemination VZV infection (varicella, disseminated herpes zoster), eczema herpeticum, eczema vaccinatum, disseminated vaccinia in immunosuppressed patient (smallpox vaccination still given in U.S. military).

Laboratory and Special Examinations

Tzanck Preparation Multinucleated giant cells present in scraping of mucocutaneous erosions, tracheobronchial washing.

Antigen Detection Monoclonal antibodies, specific for HSV-1 and HSV-2 antigens, detect and differentiate HSV antigens on smear from lesion.

Lesional Skin Biopsy Typical multinucleate giant cells are seen but do not differentiate from VZV infection. Immunoperoxidase stains are specific for HSV-1 and HSV-2.

Cultures Positive HSV cultures from involved mucocutaneous site or tissue biopsy specimens

Serology Western blot (immunoblot) and enzyme immunoassay for antibody to HSV glycoprotein G differentiate antibodies to HSV-1 and HSV-2.

Urinalysis Hematuria due to HSV cystitis

Polymerase Chain Reaction (PCR) To detect HSV-DNA sequences

Diagnosis

Clinical suspicion confirmed by Tzanck smear, positive HSV antigen detection, or isolation of HSV on viral culture

Pathophysiology

During primary HSV infection, the virus spreads to involve sensory nerves at the primary cutaneous site. Monocyte/macrophage function and interferon production help determine whether HSV remains localized or disseminates. Subsequently, antibodies, natural killer cells, and sensitized T-lymphocytes help prevent spread. 60 % to 80 % of HSV-seropositive transplant recipients and patients undergoing chemotherapy for hematologic malignancies will experience reactivation of HSV. Following viremia, disseminated cutaneous or visceral HSV infection may follow. Factors determining whether severe localized disease, cutaneous dissemination, or visceral dissemination will occur are not well defined.

Course and Prognosis

In most immunocompromised individuals with reactivation of HSV, the infection differs little from infections in intact hosts. In renal transplant recipients, HSV is excreted in throat washings of 80 % of cases shortly after grafting; two-thirds of excreters will develop lesions shortly after excretion is detected. In some immunocompromised individuals, however, large ulcerations can persist for weeks to years. Herpetic ulcers provide a break in the epithelium, facilitating superinfection with bacteria or fungi.

When widespread, visceral dissemination of HSV may occur to liver, lungs, adrenals, GI tract, CNS. Visceral spread can be complicated by disseminated intravascular coagulation, which has a very high mortality rate. Factors determining whether severe localized disease, cutaneous involvement, or visceral dissemination will occur in an individual are not well defined. Disseminated HSV infection with visceral involvement in neonates has a 50 % to 80 % mortality rate if untreated.

CHUs that fail to respond to acyclovir should be evaluated promptly for the presence of resistant virus. Infection with acyclovir-resistant strains results in chronic, progressive ulcerations that persist and/or continue to enlarge despite oral and IV acyclovir treatment. These ulcers can enlarge to 20 to 30 cm in diameter and are associated with major morbidity and pain.

Management

Prevention *Acyclovir prophylaxis* for seropositive patients undergoing bone marrow transplantation, induction therapy for leukemia, or solid organ transplantation: acyclovir 5 mg/kg IV every 8 hours or 400 mg PO t.i.d., from the day of conditioning, induction, or transplantation for 4 to 6 weeks suppresses both HSV and VZV reactivation.

Systemic Antiviral Therapy

LOCALIZED HSV INFECTIONS   Acyclovir 200 mg PO five times daily or 400 mg t.i.d. for 10 days. If lesions fail to heal in 10 days, intravenous acyclovir should be given. Chronic herpetic ulcers superinfected with *Staphylococcus aureus* should be treated with appropriate antibiotics.

DISSEMINATED AND VISCERAL HSV INFECTIONS   Herpetic encephalitis, esophagitis, retinitis, pneumonitis, and disseminated disease should be treated as follows: acyclovir 10 mg/kg IV every 8 hours for 10 to 14 days or vidarabine 15 mg/kg IV daily for 10 to 14 days

NEW ANTIHERPES SIMPLEX VIRUS DRUGS   Famciclovir and valacyclovir are being evaluated.

ACYCLOVIR-RESISTANT HSV INFECTIONS   Acyclovir resistance results from loss of synthesis of the viral enzyme thymidine kinase (TK). In the absence of TK, acyclovir is not activated to its monophosphate form, and host cell enzymes cannot catalyze further phosphorylations that lead to acyclovir triphosphate. If herpetic lesion fails to heal after a 10-day course of intravenous acyclovir, and if HSV continues to be isolated from the lesion, acyclovir resistance is likely. Drug of choice: foscarnet 40 mg/kg IV every 8 hours; or vidarabine 15 mg/kg IV daily.

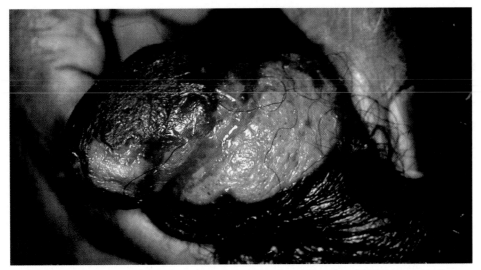

Figure 29-16 Herpes simplex virus infection: chronic penile ulcer in HIV disease *Large, shallow ulcer and a scar on the shaft and glans penis of a 26-year-old male with advanced HIV disease, who suffered from AIDS-dementia and was unaware of the lesion.*

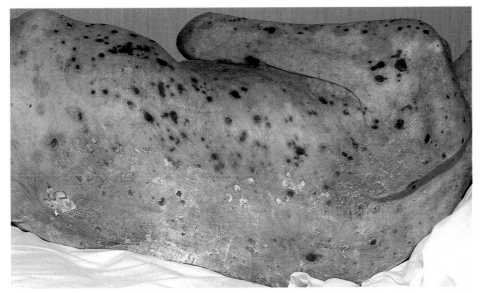

Figure 29-17 Herpes simplex virus infection: disseminated in an immunocompromised host *Disseminated erosion, ulcerations, vesicles with hemorrhagic crusts and necrotic bases in an individual with advanced lymphoma. Patients often have infection of lungs, liver, and brain.*

HERPES SIMPLEX VIRUS: WIDESPREAD CUTANEOUS INFECTION IN UNDERLYING DERMATOSES

Widespread herpes simplex virus (HSV) cutaneous infection in underlying dermatoses occurs most commonly in atopic dermatitis (eczema herpeticum) and is characterized by widespread vesicles and erosions; it may occur as a primary or recurrent infection.
Synonym: Kaposi's varicelliform eruption.

Epidemiology and Etiology

Age Children > adults

Etiology DNA virus *Herpesvirus hominis* (HSV) type 1, less commonly type 2

Transmission Commonly from parental herpes labialis

Risk Factors Most commonly, atopic dermatitis; more serious infections occur in erythrodermic atopic dermatitis. Also, Darier's disease, thermal burns, pemphigus vulgaris, bullous pemphigoid, ichthyosis vulgaris, mycosis fungoides, Wiscott-Aldrich syndrome.

History

Duration of Lesions Lesions begin in abnormal skin and may extend peripherally for several weeks during the primary infection or secondary eruption.

History Primary eczema herpeticum often associated with fever, malaise, irritability. When recurrent, prior history of similar lesions; systemic symptoms less severe.

Skin Symptoms Primary skin disease may be pruritic; onset of eczema herpeticum associated with pain and tenderness.

Physical Examination

Skin Lesions

TYPES Umbilicated vesicles evolving into "punched-out" erosions (Figures 29-18 and 29-19). Vesicles are first confined to eczematous skin and are, in contrast to primary or recurrent HSV eruptions, not grouped but disseminated (Figure 29-19). May later spread to normal-appearing skin. Erosions may become confluent, producing large denuded areas (Figure 29-19). Larger crusted lesions and follicular pustules occur with staphylococcal superinfection. Successive crops of new vesiculation may occur.

SHAPE Vesicle dome-shaped with umbilication

ARRANGEMENT Disseminated

DISTRIBUTION Common sites: face, neck, trunk

General Examination Primary infection often has fever and lymphadenopathy.

Differential Diagnosis

Widespread Vesiculopustules/Erosions Varicella zoster virus (VZV) infection with dissemination, disseminated (systemic) HSV infection, widespread bullous impetigo, staphylococcal folliculitis, pseudomonal ("hot tub") folliculitis, *Candida* folliculitis, Kaposi's varicelliform eruption caused by vaccinia virus

Laboratory and Special Examinations

Tzanck Preparation Multinucleated giant cells present in scraping of mucocutaneous erosions, tracheobronchial washing.

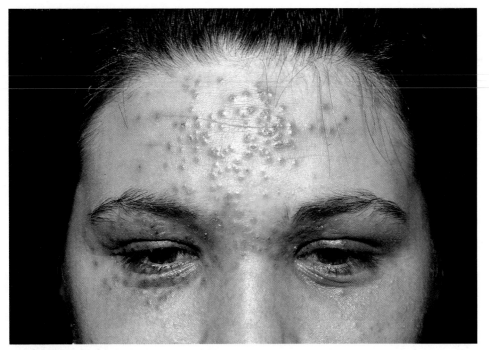

Figure 29-18 Herpes simplex virus infection: eczema herpeticum *Disseminated vesicles with punched out erosions and central crusting on the forehead and around the eyes in a patient with atopic dermatitis.*

Antigen Detection Monoclonal antibodies, specific for HSV-1 and HSV-2 antigens, detect and differentiate HSV antigens on smear from lesion.

Lesional Skin Biopsy Typical multinucleate giant cells are seen, but this does not differentiate from varicella-zoster virus infection. Immunoperoxidase stains are specific for HSV-1 and HSV-2.

Cultures Positive HSV cultures from involved mucocutaneous site or tissue biopsy specimens

Serology Western blot (immunoblot) and enzyme immunoassay for antibody to HSV glycoprotein G differentiate antibodies to HSV-1 and HSV-2.

Polymerase Chain Reaction (PCR) Detects viral DNA sequences.

Diagnosis

Clinical, confirmed by Tzanck test and HSV culture

Pathophysiology

See Nongenital Cutaneous Infections, page 792.

Course and Prognosis

Primary episode of eczema herpeticum runs course with resolution in 2 to 6 weeks. Recurrent episodes tend to be milder and not associated with systemic symptoms. Systemic dissemination can occur, especially in immunocompromised patients; reported mortality rates range from 10 % to 50 %. Widely distributed cutaneous HSV infection in burn patients can be difficult to detect clinically.

Management

Most cases are mild and localized and may not require specific therapy.

Antiviral Therapy

ACYCLOVIR For milder cases, acyclovir can be given orally for 7 days. In more severe cases (usually primary infection), acyclovir should be given IV 1.5 g/m^2/day.

VALACYCLOVIR To date, in the United States, approved only for use in treatment of herpes zoster and genital herpes; absorption is, however, four to six times that of acyclovir.

FAMCYCLOVIR To date, approved in the United States only for use in treatment of herpes zoster and genital herpes

Antibacterial Therapy Impetiginization with *Staphylococcus aureus* should be treated with erythromycin or dicloxacillin.

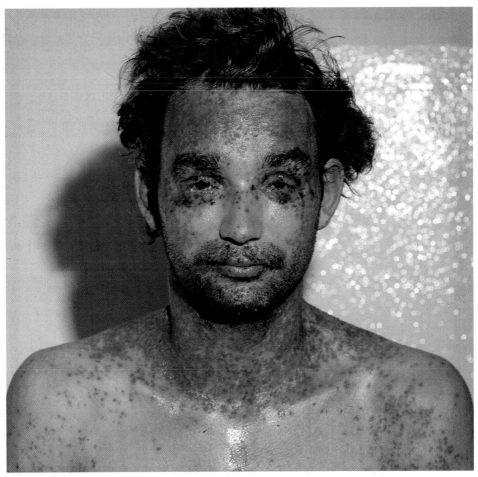

Figure 29-19 Herpes simplex virus infection: eczema herpeticum *Confluent, dissemi-nated, punched-out erosions with scattered, intact, peripheral vesicles on the face, eyelids, neck, upper trunk, and shoulders in a male with atopic dermatitis.*

VARICELLA ZOSTER VIRUS

VARICELLA

Varicella is the highly contagious primary infection caused by varicella zoster virus, characterized by successive crops of pruritic vesicles that evolve to pustules, crusts, and at times, scars, and is often accompanied by mild constitutional symptoms; primary infection occurring in adulthood may be complicated by pneumonia and encephalitis.
Synonym: Chickenpox.

Epidemiology and Etiology

Age 90% of cases occur in children <10 years, less than 5% in persons >15 years

Etiology Varicella zoster virus (VZV), a herpesvirus

Incidence 3 to 4 million cases in the United States annually

Transmission Airborne droplets as well as direct contact; indirect contact uncommon. Patients are contagious several days before exanthem appears and until last crop of vesicles. Crusts are not infectious. VZV also aerosolized from skin of individuals with herpes zoster and can cause varicella.

Season In metropolitan areas in temperate climates, varicella epidemics occur in winter and spring.

Geography Worldwide

History

Incubation Period 14 days (range 10 to 23 days)

Prodrome Characteristically absent or mild. Uncommon in children, more common in adults: headache, general aches and pains, severe backache, malaise. Exanthem appears within 2 to 3 days.

History Exposure at day care, school, to older sibling; relative with zoster

Skin Symptoms Exanthem usually quite pruritic

Physical Examination

Skin Lesions In most children, illness begins with appearance of exanthem, vesicular lesions evident in successive crops. Often single, discrete lesions or scanty in number in children, and much more dense in adults.

TYPES Initial lesions are *papules* (often not observed) that may appear as *wheals* and quickly evolve to *vesicles* and initially appear as small "drops of water" or "dewdrops on a rose petal" (Figure 29-20), superficial and thin-walled with surrounding erythema. Vesicles become umbilicated and rapidly evolve to *pustules* and *crusts* over an 8- to 12-hour period. With subsequent crops, all stages of evolution may be noted simultaneously, i.e., papules, vesicles, pustules, crusts. Crusts fall off in 1 to 3 weeks, leaving a pink, somewhat depressed base. Characteristic punched-out permanent scars may persist. Uncommonly, hemorrhage into pustular lesion occurs in otherwise healthy children, i.e., hemorrhagic varicella. Complicated by superinfection by staphylococci or streptococci; impetigo, furuncles, cellulitis, and gangrene may occur.

COLOR Vesicles, watery yellow; pustules, creamy white pus; crusts, brownish red

DISTRIBUTION First lesions begin on face and scalp, spreading inferiorly to trunk and extremities. Most profuse in areas least exposed to pressure, i.e., back between shoulder blades, flanks, axillae, popliteal and anticubital fossae. Density highest on trunk and face, less on extremities. Palms and soles usually spared.

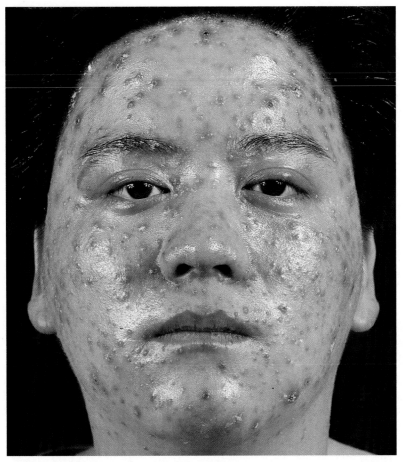

Figure 29-20 Varicella zoster virus infection: varicella *Multiple erythematous papules and vesicles on erythematous, edematous bases, so-called "dewdrops on a rose petal," of varying size on the face, neck, and shoulders of a young adult.*

MUCOUS MEMBRANES Vesicles (not often observed) and subsequent shallow erosions (2 to 3 mm) most common on palate but also occur on mucosa of nose, conjunctivae, pharynx, larynx, trachea, GI tract, urinary tract, vagina

Variants Varicella gangrenosa occurs in children with leukemia or other severe underlying disease, characterized by gangrenous ulceration of lesions. Hemorrhagic varicella with disseminated intravascular coagulation (purpura fulminans).

General Examination Low-grade fever. Vesicopustules may occur in respiratory, GU, and GI tracts.

Differential Diagnosis

Widespread Vesicles/Crusts Disseminated herpes simplex virus (HSV) infection, cutaneous dissemination of zoster, eczema herpeticum, eczema vaccinatum, disseminated vaccinia in immunosuppressed patient (smallpox vaccination still given in the U.S. military), rickettsialpox, enterovirus infections, bullous form of impetigo

Laboratory and Special Examinations

Tzanck Preparation Cytology of fluid or scraping from base of vesicle or pustule shows both giant and multinucleated epidermal cells (as does that of HSV infections).

Antigen Detection Fluorescent antibodies specific for VZV antigen identifies VZV on smears of vesicle fluid or base of vesicle.

Viral Cultures Isolation of virus on viral culture (human fibroblast monolayers) from vesicular skin lesions is possible, but more difficult than for HSV. Distinctive cytopathic effects usually appear in 3 to 10 days.

Bacterial Cultures Rule out superinfection with *Staphylococcus aureus* or group A *Streptococcus.*

Serology Seroconversion, i.e., fourfold or greater rise in VZV titers

Diagnosis

Usually made on clinical findings alone

Pathophysiology

Virus is thought to enter through mucosa of upper respiratory tract and oropharynx, followed by local replication and primary viremia; VZV then replicates in cells of reticuloendothelial system with subsequent secondary viremia and dissemination to skin and mucous membranes. Localization of VZV in the basal cell layer is followed by virus replication, vacuole formation, ballooning degeneration of epithelial cells, and accumulation of edema fluid. Second episodes of varicella have been documented but are rare. As with all herpesviruses, VZV enters a latent phase, residing in sensory ganglion; reactivation of VZV results in zoster.

Course and Prognosis

In healthy children, the course is self-limited; however, a mortality rate of 1 per 50,000 cases in the United States is reported (100 deaths annually in the 3 to 4 million cases). 6500 hospitalizations annually (U.S.) for varicella. The most common complication of varicella in young children (≤5 years) is bacterial (*S. aureus,* group A streptococcus) superinfection. In children 5 to 11 years, the most common complications are varicella encephalitis and Reye's syndrome.

In adults, prodromal symptoms are common and may be severe; exanthem may last for a week or more, with prolonged period of recovery. Primary varicella pneumonia, which presents 1 to 6 days after appearance of rash, is relatively common in adults, with 16 % of adults showing x-ray evidence of pneumonitis; however, only 4 % have clinical signs of pneumonitis. VZV encephalitis also may complicate varicella in adults. Less common complications of varicella include viral arthritis, uveitis, conjunctivitis, carditis, inappropriate antidiuretic hormone syndrome, nephritis, and orchitis. The mortality rate in adults is 15 per 50,000 cases; deaths in adults account for 25 % of varicella-associated mortality.

Maternal varicella during the first trimester of pregnancy may result in fetal varicella syndrome (limb hypoplasia, eye and brain damage, skin lesions) in 2 % of exposed fetuses. Neonatal varicella has higher incidence of pneumonitis and encephalitis than occurs in older children. Immunocompromised or corticosteroid-treated patients with varicella may manifest dissemination, hepatitis, encephalitis, and hemorrhagic complications. If varicella occurs at an early age when maternal antibody is still present, an individual can have a second episode of varicella. In HIV-infected patients, reactivation of VZV may result in chronic painful ecthymatous varicella.

In immunocompromised individuals, VZV hepatitis is relatively common and is associated with significant mortality.

Management

Prevention

IMMUNIZATION VZV immunization is now available (Varivax) and is 80 % effective in preventing symptomatic primary VZV infection. 5 % of newly immunized children develop rash. Those at high risk for varicella, who should be immunized, include: normal VZV-negative adults, children with leukemia, and immunocompromised individuals (treatment, HIV infection, cancer). VZV vaccine results in both cell-mediated immunity and antibody production against the virus.

Treatment of the Otherwise Healthy Patient

- Oral acyclovir: may reduce the severity of the infection and reduce secondary cases
- Oral valacyclovir: effective but not an approved use as yet
- Oral famciclovir: effective but not an approved use as yet
- Symptomatic treatment of pruritus: lotions and oral antihistamines
- Treatment of bacterial superinfection: Mupirocin ointment applied twice daily to lesions with secondary bacterial infection; oral erythromycin, dicloxacillin, cephalexin
- Antipyretic administration is of concern because of a possible link between aspirin and Reye's syndrome in children with varicella.

Treatment of Disseminated Varicella IV
acyclovir or vidarabine for severe varicella, varicella pneumonitis, varicella encephalitis, or varicella occurring in immunocompromised host

HERPES ZOSTER

Herpes zoster (HZ) is an acute dermatomal infection associated with reactivation of varicella-zoster virus (VZV) and is characterized by unilateral pain and a vesicular or bullous eruption limited to a dermatome(s) innervated by a corresponding sensory ganglion. The major morbidity is postzoster neuralgia.

Synonym: Shingles

Epidemiology and Etiology

Age   More than 66 % are over 50 years of age; 5 % of cases in children <15 years.

Sex and Race   No differences

Incidence

- In the United States, nearly 100 % of adults are seropositive for anti-VZV antibodies by the third decade of life and are thus at risk for reactivation of latent VZV. ~500,000 cases of HZ annually. Cumulative lifetime incidence: 10 % to 20 %. In one cohort, 5 % of individuals with HZ were HIV-infected and 5 % had cancer. Recurrent HZ <1 % of cases.
- Occurs in 25 % of HIV-infected individuals, an eight times higher incidence than the general population, aged 20 to 50 years; 7 % to 9 % of renal and cardiac transplant recipients. Recurrent HZ more common in immunocompromised individuals.

Risk Factors   Most common factor is diminishing immunity to VZV with advancing age, with majority of cases occurring in those ≥55 years old. Malignancy. Immunosuppression, especially from lymphoproliferative disorders and chemotherapy. Radiotherapy. HIV-infected individuals have an eightfold increased incidence of zoster.

Transmission   About one-third as contagious as varicella, and susceptible contacts can contract varicella by the airborne route.

Classification   HZ manifests in three distinct clinical phases: prodromal, active, and chronic stages.

History

Duration of Symptoms

PRODROMAL STAGE   Neuritic pain or paresthesia precedes cutaneous eruption by 3 to 5 days (range 1 to 14 days)

ACTIVE VESICULATION   3 to 5 days

CRUST FORMATION   Days to 2 to 3 weeks

POSTHERPETIC NEURALGIA (PHN)   Months to years

Skin Symptoms

PRODROMAL STAGE   Pain (stabbing, pricking, sharp, boring, penetrating, lancinating, shooting), tenderness, paresthesia (itching, tingling, burning, freeze-burning) in the involved dermatome precede the eruption. Allodynia: heightened sensitivity to mild stimuli.

ACTIVE VESICULATION   Neuritic pain. Pain in the involved skin.

ZOSTER *SINE* ZOSTER   Nerve involvement can occur without cutaneous zoster.

CHRONIC STAGES   PHN, described as "burning," "ice-burning," "shooting," or "lancinating," can persist for weeks, months, and years after the cutaneous involvement has resolved.

Constitutional Symptoms

PRODROMAL STAGE   Headache, malaise, fever occur in about 5 % of patients.

ACTIVE VESICULATION   Headache, malaise, fever

CHRONIC STAGES   Depression is very common in individuals with PHN.

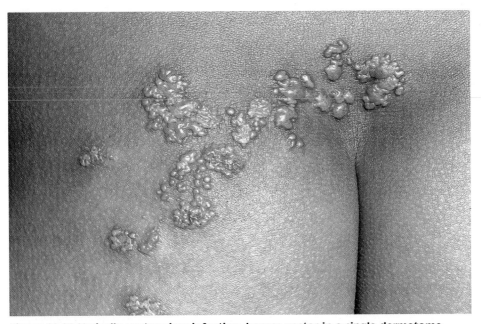

Figure 29-21 Varicella zoster virus infection: herpes zoster in a single dermatome
Dermatomal, grouped and confluent vesicles and pustules arising in the third sacral dermatome; note extension of lesions 1–2 cm across the midline.

Physical Examination

Skin Lesions

TYPE   Papules (24 hours) → vesicles-bullae (Figures 29-21 and 29-22) (48 hours) → pustules (96 hours) → crusts (7 to 10 days). New lesions continue to appear for up to 1 week. Necrotic and gangrenous lesions sometimes occur (Figure 29-23).

COLOR   Erythematous, edematous base with superimposed clear vesicles, sometimes, hemorrhagic

SHAPE   The vesicle-bulla is oval or round, may be umbilicated.

ARRANGEMENT   Herpetiform clusters (grouping) of lesions (see Figure 29-21)

DISTRIBUTION   Unilateral, dermatomal. Two or more contiguous dermatomes may be involved (Figure 29-22). Noncontiguous dermatomal zoster is rare. Hematogenous dis-

semination to other skin sites in 10 % of healthy individuals (Figure 29-23).

SITES OF PREDILECTION   Thoracic (>50 %), trigeminal (10 % to 20 %), lumbosacral and cervical (10 % to 20 %). In HIV-infected individuals, may be multidermatomal (contiguous or noncontiguous) and/or recurrent.

Mucous Membranes   Vesicles and erosions occur in mouth, vagina, and bladder depending on dermatome involved.

Lymphadenopathy   Regional nodes draining the area are often enlarged and tender.

Sensory or Motor Nerve Changes   Detectable by neurologic examination. Sensory defects (temperature, pain, touch) and (mild) motor paralysis, e.g., facial palsy

Eye   In ophthalmic zoster, nasociliary involvement of V1 (ophthalmic) branch of the trigeminal nerve occurs in about one-third of cases and is heralded by vesicles on the side and tip of the nose. Complications include uveitis, keratitis, conjunctivitis, retinitis, optic neuritis, glaucoma, proptosis, cicatricial lid retraction, and extraocular muscle palsies. *An ophthalmologist should always be consulted.*

Differential Diagnosis

Prodromal stage/localized pain: The prodromal pain of herpes zoster can mimic migraine, cardiac or pleural disease, an acute abdomen, or vertebral disease. *Dermatomal eruption:* zosteriform herpes simplex virus infection, phytoallergic (poison ivy, poison oak) contact dermatitis, erysipelas, bullous impetigo, necrotizing fasciitis

Laboratory and Special Examinations

Electrocardiogram Rule out ischemic heart disease in prodromal stage.

Imaging In prodromal stage, rule out organic, pleural, pulmonary, or abdominal disease.

Tzanck Preparation Smear of vesicle base (or fluid) shows giant and/or multinucleated epidermal cells.

VZV Antigen Detection Direct fluorescent antibody (DFA) detects VZV antigen in smear of vesicle base or fluid. Specific and very sensitive.

Viral Culture Isolation of VZV

Dermatopathology Lesional skin biopsy shows acantholysis, vesicle formation, and giant and/or multinucleated keratinocytes.

Diagnosis

Prodromal stage: headache, malaise, fever in about 5 % of patients. *Active vesiculation:* clinical findings confirmed by Tzanck test and possible DFA or viral culture to rule out HSV infection. *Chronic stages:* clinical findings confirmed by DFA, viral culture, or histologic findings.

Pathophysiology

VZV, during the course of varicella, passes from the skin lesions to the sensory nerves, travels to the sensory ganglia, and establishes latent infection. It is postulated that humoral and cellular immunity to VZV established with primary infection persists at low levels, and when this immunity ebbs, viral replication within the ganglia occurs. The virus then travels down the sensory nerve, resulting in initial dermatomal pain followed by painful skin lesions. Since the neuritis precedes the skin involvement, pain appears before the skin lesions are visible. The locations of pain are varied and relate directly to the ganglion where VZV has emerged from latency to active infection. Prodromal symptoms may appear initially in the trigeminal, cervical, thoracic, lumbar, or sacral dermatome. PHN probably occurs as damaged nerves continue to misfire in the absence of active viral infection.

Course and Prognosis

In immunocompetent host rash usually resolves in 2 to 3 weeks. Complications can be local: hemorrhage, gangrene; or general: meningoencephalitis, cerebral vascular syndromes, cranial nerve syndromes [trigeminal (ophthalmic) branch (herpes zoster ophthalmicus), facial and auditory nerves (Ramsay Hunt syndrome)], peripheral motor weakness, transverse myelitis, visceral involvement (pneumonitis, hepatitis, pericarditis/myocarditis, pancreatitis, esophagitis, enterocolitis, cystitis, synovitis), cutaneous dissemination, and superinfection of skin lesions. Pain with herpes zoster is associated with neural inflammation, nerve infection during the acute reactivation, and neural inflammation and scarring with PHN. The course in HIV-infected, renal and cardiac transplant recipients is usually uncomplicated without significant dissemination. Dissemination generally occurs 6 to 10 days after onset of localized lesions and is most often limited to cutaneous involvement. In immunosuppressed individuals, visceral dissemination can occur, involving CNS, lung, heart, and GI tract. The risk of PHN is > 40 % in patients over 60 years of age. In one large follow-

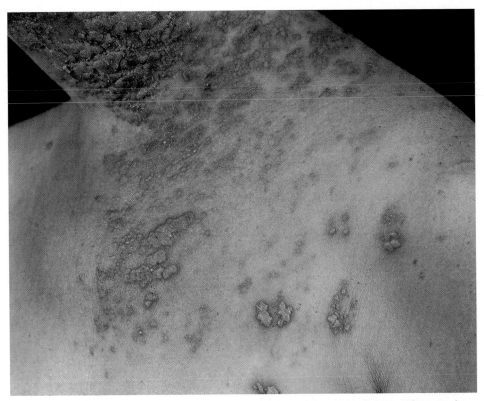

Figure 29-22 Varicella zoster virus infection: herpes zoster in multiple contiguous dermatomes *Grouped, hemorrhagic pustules on erythematous bases becoming confluent on the neck, upper trunk, and shoulder, involving multiple cervical and thoracic dermatomes; note the abrupt demarcation of lesions at presternal midline.*

up study, PHN was present 1 month after onset of the rash in 60 %, by 3 months there was some pain in 24 %, and by 6 months 13 % of the patients still had pain. The highest incidence of PHN is in ophthalmic zoster. Dissemination of zoster—20 or more lesions outside the affected or adjacent dermatomes —occurs in up to 10 % of patients, usually in immunosuppressed patients. Motor paralysis occurs in 5 % of patients, and especially when the virus involves the cranial nerves.

Management

Prevention

IMMUNIZATION   Immunization with VZV vaccine may boost humoral and cell-mediated immunity and decrease the incidence of zoster in populations with declining VZV-specific immunity.

ANTIVIRAL AGENTS   In individuals at high risk for reactivation of VZV infection, oral acyclovir can reduce the incidence of HZ.

Treatment of Acute Herpes Zoster The goals of management of HZ include: minimize pain; reduce viral shedding; speed crusting of lesions and healing; ease physical, psychological, emotional discomfort; prevent viral dissemination or other complications; prevent or minimize PHN.

PRODROMAL STAGE   Begin antiviral agent if diagnosis is considered likely. Analgesics.

ACTIVE VESICULATION   *Antiviral Agents* Antiviral treatment begun ≤72 hours accelerates healing of skin lesions, decreases the duration of acute pain, and may decrease the frequency of PHN.

Acyclovir: 800 mg PO q.i.d. for 7 to 10 days. The 50 % viral inhibitory concentration of acyclovir is three to six times higher for VZV than for HSV in vitro, and drug dose must be increased appropriately. The bioavailability of acyclovir is only 15 % to 30 % of the orally administered dose. For ophthalmic zoster and HZ in the immunocompromised host, acyclovir should be given intravenously. Acyclovir has been shown to hasten healing and lessen *acute* pain if given within 48 hours of the onset of the rash.

Valacyclovir: 1000 mg PO t.i.d. for 7 days 70 % to 80 % bioavailable.

Famciclovir: 500 mg PO t.i.d. for 7 days; 77 % bioavailable. Reduce dose in individuals with diminished renal function.

Foscarnet: Given IV for acyclovir-resistant strains of VZV infection

In immunosuppressed patients, IV acyclovir and recombinant interferon alpha-2a to prevent dissemination of herpes zoster is indicated.

Oral Corticosteroids Prednisone given early in the course of HZ is felt by some to reduce the likelihood and severity of PHN. Its benefit has not been demonstrated in controlled studies.

Dressings Application of moist dressings (water, saline, Burow's solution) to the involved dermatome is soothing and alleviates pain.

Pain Management Early control of pain with narcotic analgesics is indicated; failure to manage pain can result in failure to sleep, fatigue, and depression.

CHRONIC STAGES (**PHN**) ***Antiviral Agents*** Large controlled studies in patients >60 years of age have not demonstrated any effect on the incidence and severity of *chronic* PHN if high-dose oral acyclovir was given. A recent preliminary study of older patients (age 60 years) demonstrated a reduced frequency of persistent pain when IV acyclovir, 10 mg/kg every 8 hours for 5 days, was given within 4 days of the onset of the pain or within 48 hours after the onset of the rash. Studies are available indicating that a reduction of PHN can be achieved by oral valacyclovir or famciclovir treatment of early zoster in appropriate doses.

Pain Management Severe prodromal pain or severe pain on the first day of rash is predictive of severe PHN. Tricyclic antidepressants such as doxepin, 10 to 100 mg PO h.s. Capsaicin cream every 4 hours. Topical anesthetic such as EMLA or lidocaine gel or patch for allodynia. Nerve block to area of allodynia. Analgesics.

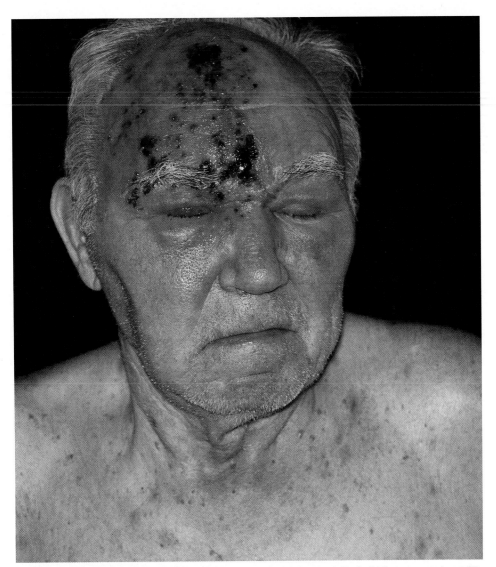

Figure 29-23 Varicella zoster virus infection: necrotizing ophthalmic herpes zoster with cutaneous dissemination *Hemorrhagic, crusted ulcerations and vesicles on the right forehead and periorbital area in the ophthalmic branch of the trigeminal nerve; note the bilateral facial edema and erythema. Hematogenous cutaneous dissemination has occurred with hundreds of vesicles and erythematous papules on the trunk. In spite of the extensive cutaneous infection, this immunocompetent patient was relatively painfree.*

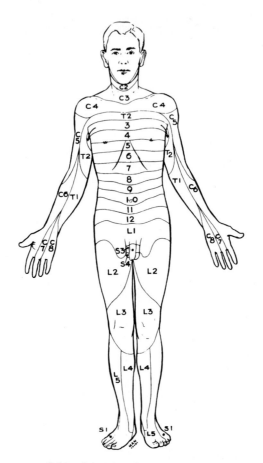

A

Dermatomes *The cutaneous fields of peripheral nerves. A. The segmental innervation of the skin from the anterior aspect. The uppermost dermatome adjoins the cutaneous field of the mandibular division of the trigeminal nerve. The arrows indicate the lateral extensions of dermatome T3. B. The dermatomes from the posterior view. Note the absence of cutaneous innervation by the first cervical segment. Arrows in the axillary regions indicate the lateral extent of dermatome T3; those in the region of the vertebral column point to the first thoracic, the first lumbar, and the first sacral spinous processes.* (After Foerster in Haymaker W, Woodhall B: Peripheral Nerve Injuries, 2d ed. Saunders, Philadelphia/London, 1953.) *C. Dermatomes of head.* (Modified from Steegmann AT: Examination of the Nervous System, 2d ed. Year Book Medical Publishers, Chicago, 1962.)

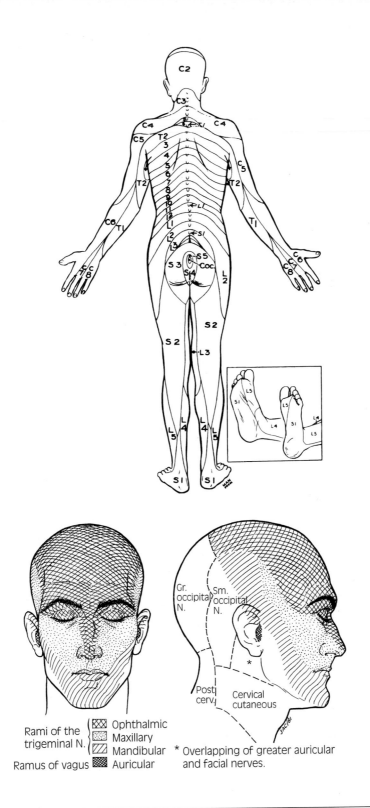

B

C

Rami of the trigeminal N. { ⊠ Ophthalmic / ▦ Maxillary / ▧ Mandibular

Ramus of vagus ▨ Auricular

Gr. occipital N. / Sm. occipital N.

Post. cerv. / Cervical cutaneous

* Overlapping of greater auricular and facial nerves.

VARICELLA ZOSTER VIRUS: INFECTIONS IN THE IMMUNOCOMPROMISED HOST

In immunocompromised individuals, varicella zoster virus infections can be disseminated hematogenously widely to mucocutaneous structures as well as to the viscera, often associated with high morbidity and mortality and chronic localized infections.

Epidemiology and Etiology

Incidence In the United States, >90 % of adults are seropositive for anti-VZV antibodies and are thus at risk for reactivation of latent virus. Population of immunocompromised individuals is increasing. Occurs in 25 % of HIV-infected individuals, a seven times higher incidence than in the general population aged 20 to 50 years. Most cases of recurrent herpes zoster occur in immunocompromised individuals.

Risk Factors

Associated with various causes of immunocompromise

FOR VISCERAL DISSEMINATION OF VARICELLA Children undergoing cancer chemotherapy; solid organ and bone marrow transplant recipients; HIV infection; certain cell-mediated immunodeficiency disorders of childhood.

FOR HERPES ZOSTER Often the first sign of HIV infection, preceding oral candidiasis and oral hairy leukoplakia by 1 year

FOR VISCERAL DISSEMINATION OF HERPES ZOSTER Hodgkin's disease (risk of developing zoster is 13 % to 15 % compared with 7 % to 9 % for non-Hodgkin's lymphoma patients and 1 % to 3 % for patients with solid tumors)

Other Factors Immunosuppression, especially from lymphoproliferative disorders, and cancer chemotherapy

Classification of VZV Infection in the Immunocompromised Host

Primary varicella with visceral dissemination
Herpes zoster with cutaneous dissemination
Herpes zoster with visceral and cutaneous dissemination
Herpes zoster with persistent dermatomal infection

Chronic cutaneous VZV infection following hematogenous dissemination

History

Skin Symptoms Symptoms of varicella and zoster. Chronic cutaneous VZV infections following hematogenous dissemination are often associated with significant lesional pain requiring narcotic analgesia for pain management.

Constitutional Symptoms Visceral dissemination usually accompanied by fever

Physical Examination

Skin Lesions
Varicella See Varicella, (page 810).
Herpes Zoster In HIV disease, involvement of several contiguous dermatomes is common (Figure 29-24).
Herpes Zoster with Cutaneous Dissemination A variable number of vesicle or bullae are seen at any mucocutaneous site, which evolve into crusted erosions (Figure 29-25). Lesions are disseminated and range from a few to hundreds. The condition thus appears clinically as zoster plus varicella.
Herpes Zoster with Persistent Dermatomal Infection Papules and nodules, which can become hyperkeratotic or verrucous, persist in a dermatomal pattern (single or multiple contiguous) after an outbreak of zoster. See also Section 33.
Chronic Cutaneous VZV Infection Following Hematogenous Dissemination Lesions on the palms or soles may present initially as bullae. Continual appearance of vesicles/bullae in a dermatomal or gen-

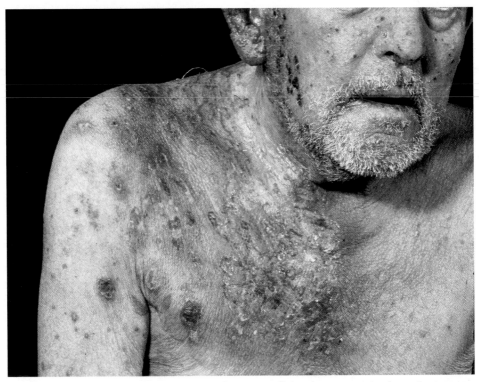

Figure 29-24 Varicella zoster virus infection: necrotizing herpes zoster in an immuno-compromised patient *Confluent, crusted ulcerations on an inflammatory base on the right face, ear, neck, and upper chest with vesicles, crusts, and ulcers at site of hematogenous, cutaneous dissemination in an elderly male with leukemia.*

eralized distribution. Chronic lesions present as nodules, ulcers, crusted nodules/ulcers (ecthymatous). ±Postinflammatory hyper- or hypopigmentation.

DISTRIBUTION Unilateral, hematogenous dissemination outside of the dermatome(s) is common with a few or hundreds of lesions on skin or mucosal sites.

Chronic Cutaneous VZV Infection Following Hematogenous Dissemination Can occur in a generalized distribution indicative of hematogenous dissemination or within a dermatome or contiguous dermatomes.

Systemic Findings

EYE In HIV disease, retinal VZV infection (acute retinal necrosis) can occur in the absence of apparent conjunctival or cutaneous involvement with subsequent loss of vision.

Bilateral involvement in one-third of cases with subsequent loss of vision. VZV optic neuritis rare.

CNS In HIV disease, VZV is the etiologic agent of up to 2 % of CNS disease (encephalitis, polyneuritis, myelitis, vasculitis).

Differential Diagnosis

Primary Varicella with Visceral Dissemination Pneumonia must be distinguished from *Pneumocystis carinii* pneumonia associated with varicella.

Herpes Zoster with Cutaneous Dissemination Zosteriform herpes simplex virus (HSV) with dissemination

Herpes Zoster with Visceral and Cutaneous

Dissemination Zosteriform herpes simplex with dissemination. Pneumonia must be distinguished from *P. carinii* pneumonia associated with varicella.

Herpes Zoster with Persistent Dermatomal Infection Chronic zosteriform HSV infection. Hypertrophic scars or keloids.

Chronic Cutaneous VZV Infection Following Hematogenous Dissemination Ecthyma, ecthyma gangrenosum, disseminated mycobacterial infection, deep fungal infection, syphilis

The prodromal pain of herpes zoster can mimic cardiac or pleural disease, an acute abdomen, or vertebral disease. The rash must be distinguished from zosteriform herpes simplex, which has a different course and prognosis, especially involving the eye, where herpes simplex is more pathogenic. These can be distinguished by viral culture. Contact dermatitis or localized bacterial infection also should be excluded.

Laboratory and Special Examinations

Tzanck Smear See Varicella, page 810

Viral Cultures Isolation of VZV from skin lesions or visceral tissue is possible but difficult. Vesicle fluid, biopsy specimens, corneal scraping, and CSF can be cultured.

Antiviral Sensitivities When isolated, VZV from cultured lesion can be tested for sensitivity to acyclovir and other antiviral agents.

VZV Antigen Detection Smear of vesicle fluid or scraping from ulcer base/margin is made on a glass microscope slide. Direct fluorescent antibody test (DFA) detects VZV-specific antigens. Sensitive and specific method for identifying VZV-infected lesions.

Bacterial Culture Rule out secondary bacterial infection, most commonly caused by *Staphylococcus aureus* or group A streptococcus.

Chemistries Abnormalities of liver function tests with VZV hepatitis

Histology Lesional skin or visceral biopsy specimen shows multinucleated giant epithelial cells indicating either HSV-1, HSV-2, or VZV infection. Immunoperoxidase stains specific for HSV-1, HSV-2, or VZV antigens can identify the specific herpes virus.

Pathophysiology

See Varicella (page 810) and Herpes Zoster (page 814).

Course and Prognosis

Approximately 2 % to 35 % of children with varicella who are undergoing cancer chemotherapy experience visceral dissemination; the associated mortality is 7 % to 30 %. Dissemination is more common in those with a peripheral blood lymphocyte count of $<500/\mu l$.

In children with varicella: Visceral involvement most commonly affects lungs, less often liver and brain. Varicella pneumonia occurs 3 to 7 days after onset of skin lesions; can progress rapidly over few days or remain indolent with gradual improvement over 2 to 4 weeks. Neurologic complications present 4 to 8 days after onset of rash; associated with poor prognosis.

In adults with herpes zoster: In HIV-infected adults, recurrent episodes occur in same or different dermatome(s); disseminated zoster infrequent. Between 15 % and 30 % of patients with Hodgkin's disease experience significant dissemination (most often cutaneous). Mortality rates for disseminated zoster much lower than for children with disseminated varicella. Postherpetic neuralgia does not appear to be more common in immunocompromised individuals than in the general population.

Management

Prevention

IMMUNIZATION VZV immunization is now available and is 80 % effective in preventing symptomatic primary VZV infection. About 5 % of newly immunized children develop rash. Those at high risk for varicella, who

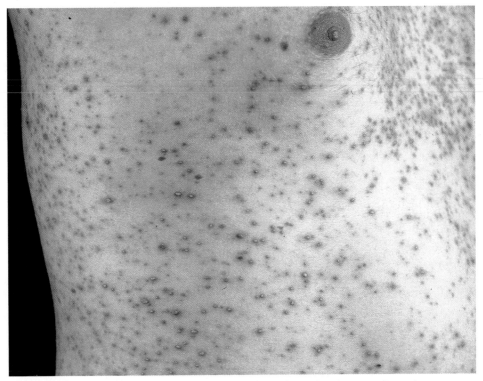

Figure 29-25 Varicella zoster virus infection: disseminated cutaneous in an immuno-compromised patient *Hundreds of vesicles and pustules on erythematous bases on the trunk of a patient with lymphoma: note the absence of grouping of lesions seen in herpes simplex or herpes zoster. The eruption is indistinguishable from varicella and must be differentiated from disseminated HSV infection.*

should be immunized, include: normal adults, children with leukemia, neonates, and immunocompromised individuals (treatment, HIV infection, cancer).

ANTIVIRAL AGENTS FOR VZV- AND HSV-SEROPOSITIVE INDIVIDUALS UNDERGOING BMT Acyclovir 400 mg PO b.i.d., from the day of conditioning, induction, or transplantation for 4 to 6 weeks, suppresses both HSV and VZV reactivation.

Systemic Antiviral Therapy

IN INDIVIDUALS WITH MILD TO MODERATE IMMUNOCOMPROMISE High-dose oral acyclovir, 800 mg five times daily for 7 days, has been shown to hasten healing and lessen *acute* pain if given within 48 hours of the on-

set of the rash. Large controlled studies in patients over 60 years of age have not, however, demonstrated any effect on the incidence and severity of *chronic* postherpetic neuralgia of high-dose oral acyclovir. A recent preliminary study of older patients (age 60) demonstrated a reduced frequency of persistent pain when IV acyclovir, 10 mg/kg every 8 hours for 5 days, was given within 4 days of the onset of the pain or within 48 hours after the onset of the rash.

IN INDIVIDUALS WITH ADVANCED IMMUNOCOMPROMISE OR SEVERE OR DISSEMINATED VZV INFECTION IV acyclovir or recombinant interferon alpha-2a to prevent dissemination of herpes zoster is indicated.

EXANTHEMA SUBITUM

Exanthema subitum (ES) (sudden rash) is a childhood exanthem associated with primary human herpesvirus type 6 (HHV-6) and HHV-7 infection, characterized by the sudden appearance of rash as high-fever lysis in a healthy-appearing infant.
Synonym: Roseola infantum.

Epidemiology and Etiology

Age 6 to 24 months

Sex Equal

Etiology HHV-6 and HHV-7, recently identified human herpesviruses

History

Incubation Period 5 to 15 days

Prodrome High fever ranging from 38.9° to 40.6°C. Remains consistently high, with morning remission, until the fourth day, when it falls precipitously to normal, coincident with the appearance of rash. Infant remarkably well despite high fever. Asymptomatic primary HHV-6 and HHV-7 infection is common.

Symptoms Usually absent

Physical Examination

Skin Lesions

TYPE Small blanchable macules and papules, 1 to 5 mm in diameter (Figure 29-26)

COLOR Pink, often with a white halo

PALPATION Only slightly elevated with side lighting

ARRANGEMENT Lesions may remain discrete or become confluent.

DISTRIBUTION Trunk and neck

General Findings Absent in presence of high fever. Febrile seizures are common.

Differential Diagnosis

Rubella, measles, scarlet fever, erythema infectiosum, other viral infections with exanthems (enterovirus, adenovirus, echovirus, coxsackievirus, rotavirus), adverse cutaneous drug reaction

Laboratory and Special Examinations

Serology Demonstration of IgM anti-HHV-6 or anti-HHV-7 antibodies or IgG seroconversion

Other Viral culture and isolation from peripheral blood mononuclear cells. Demonstration of HHV-6 of HHV-7 DNA by PCR.

Diagnosis

Usually made on clinical findings

Pathophysiology

Pathogenesis of ES rash is not known.

Course and Prognosis

Course self-limited with rare sequelae. In some cases, high fever may be associated with seizures. Intussusception association with hyperplasia of intestinal lymphoid tissue, and hepatitis has been reported. As with other human herpesvirus infections, HHV-6 and HHV-7 persist throughout the life of the patient; however, any clinical manifestations associated with HHV-6 and HHV-7 reactivation have not yet

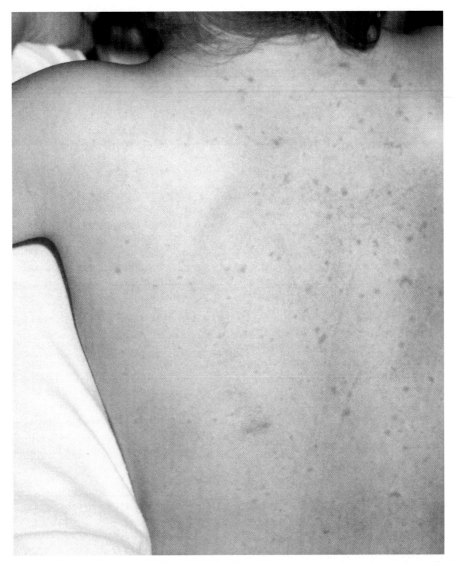

Figure 29-26 Exanthema subitum *Multiple, blanchable macules and papules on the back of a febrile child, which appeared as the temperature fell.* (Courtesy of Karen Wiss, M.D.)

been identified. An infant with HHV-6 ES may experience a second clinical syndrome, HHV-7 ES, and vice versa.

Management

Symptomatic

ERYTHEMA INFECTIOSUM

Erythema infectiosum (EI) is a childhood exanthem occurring with primary parvovirus B19 infection, characterized by edematous erythematous plaques on the cheeks ("slapped cheeks") and an erythematous lacy eruption on the trunk and extremities.
Synonym: Fifth disease.

Epidemiology and Etiology

Age All ages, but more common in young. Up to 60 % of adolescents and adults are seropositive for anti-HPV B19 IgG. Symptomatic rheumatic involvement is more common in adults.

Sex Symptomatic illness with arthralgias more common in adult women

Season Late winter, early spring

Etiology Human parvovirus B19 (HPV B19), a small single-stranded DNA virus

Transmission Virus present in respiratory tract during the viremic stage of HPV B19 infection and spread via droplet aerosol. Secondary attack rate among close contacts 50 %.

History

Incubation Period 4 to 14 days

Contacts Exposure to classmates or siblings with EI

Symptoms

IN CHILDREN Prodrome of fever, malaise, headache, coryza 2 days prior to rash. Headache, sore throat, fever, myalgias, nausea, diarrhea, conjunctivitis, cough may coincide with rash. Uncommonly arthralgias. Pruritus is variably present.

IN ADULTS May be asymptomatic. Constitutional symptoms more severe, with fever, adenopathy, arthritis/arthralgias involving small joints of hands, knees, wrists, ankles, feet. Numbness and tingling of fingers. Pruritus ±rash. Rash usually absent in adults.

Physical Examination

Skin Lesions

TYPES Edematous, confluent plaques on malar face ("slapped cheeks") (Figure 29-27). Nonfacial lesions: macules and papules that become confluent, giving a lacy or reticulated appearance (Figure 29-28). Less commonly, morbilliform, confluent, circinate, annular. Rarely, purpura, vesicles, pustules, palmoplantar desquamation.

COLOR Pink to red

SHAPE Round to oval

DISTRIBUTION "Slapped cheeks." Reticulated lesions on extensor surfaces of extremities, trunk, neck. Uncommonly, palmar and plantar. Uncommonly, enanthem with glossal and pharyngeal erythema; red macules on buccal and palatal mucosa. In adults with rash, "slapped cheeks" usually absent, reticulated macules on extremities.

Differential Diagnosis

Children with Erythema Infectiosum Childhood exanthems—rubella, measles, scarlet fever, erythema subitum, enteroviral infection, *Hemophilus influenzae* cellulitis, adverse cutaneous drug reaction

Adults with Arthritis Lyme arthritis, rheumatoid arthritis, rubella

Laboratory and Special Examinations

Serology Demonstration of IgM anti-HPV

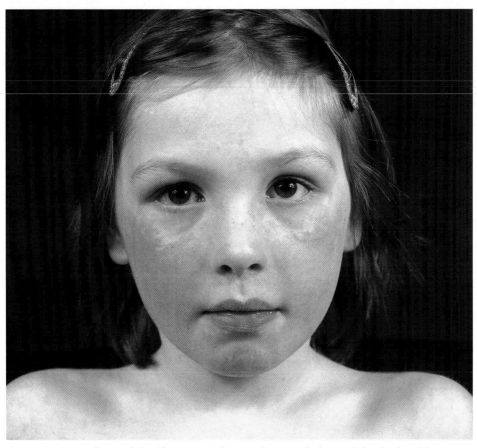

Figure 29-27 Erythema infectiosum *Diffuse erythema and edema of the cheeks with "slapped cheek" facies in a child.*

B19 antibodies or IgG seroconversion. Demonstration of HPV B19 in serum.

Electron Microscopy   Infected erythroid precursor cells show parvovirus-like particles.

Hematology   During aplastic crisis: absence of reticulocytes, falling hemoglobin, hypoplasia or aplasia of erythroid series in bone marrow

Diagnosis

Usually made on clinical findings

Pathophysiology

Pathogenesis of EI is not known but may be mediated by immune complexes.

Course and Prognosis

Erythema Infectiosum   "Slapped cheeks" are noted first. As these lesions fade over 1 to 4 days, reticulated rash appears on the trunk, neck, and extensor extremities. Eruption lasts 5 to 9 days but characteristically can recur for weeks or months, triggered by sunlight exposure, exercise, temperature change, bathing, emotional stress.

Arthralgias   Self-limited but may persist for several months

Aplastic Crisis   In patients with chronic hemolytic anemias (sickle cell anemia, hereditary spherocytosis, heterozygous beta-thalassemia, pyruvate kinase deficiency, autoimmune hemolytic anemia), transient aplastic crisis may occur, manifested by fatigue, pallor, worsening anemia.

Fetal HPV B19 Infection   Intrauterine infection may be complicated by nonimmune fetal hydrops secondary to infection of erythroid precursors, hemolysis, severe anemia, tissue anoxia, high-output heart failure. Risk less than 10% after maternal infection.

Management

Symptomatic

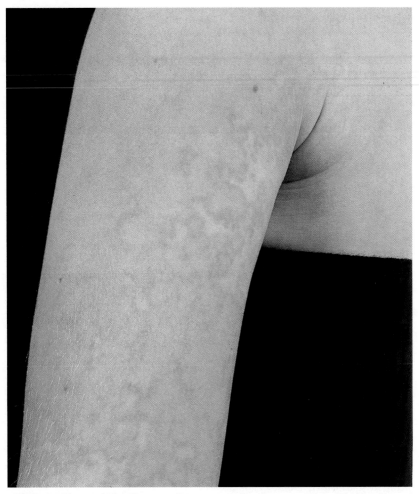

Figure 29-28 Erythema infectiosum *Discrete, erythematous macules with ring formation on the upper arm.*

KAWASAKI'S DISEASE

Kawasaki's disease (KD) is an acute febrile illness of infants and children, characterized by cutaneous and mucosal erythema and edema with subsequent desquamation, cervical lymphadenitis, and complicated by coronary artery aneurysms (20%).
Synonyms: Mucocutaneous lymph node syndrome, juvenile periarteritis nodosa.

Epidemiology and Etiology

Age   Peak incidence at 1 year, mean 2.6 years, uncommon after 8 years. Most cases of KD in adults probably represent toxic shock syndrome.

Sex   Male predominance, 1.5:1.

Race   United States: incidence>Japanese>Afro-Americans>white children

Etiology   Idiopathic, probably infectious

Season   Winter and spring

Geography   First reported in Japan, 1961; United States, 1971. Epidemics.

Clinical Phases of Kawasaki's Disease

PHASE I: ACUTE FEBRILE PERIOD   Abrupt onset of fever, lasting approximately 12 days, followed (usually within 1 to 3 days) by most of the other principal features

PHASE II: SUBACUTE PHASE   Lasts approximately until day 30 of illness; fever, thrombocytosis, desquamation, arthritis, arthralgia, carditis resolve; highest risk for sudden death

PHASE III: CONVALESCENT PERIOD   Begins within 8 to 10 weeks after onset of illness; begins when all signs of illness have disappeared and ends when ESR returns to normal; very low mortality rate during this period

History

Prodrome   Usually none

Symptoms   Fever, sudden onset. Constitutional symptoms of diarrhea, arthralgia, arthritis, meatitis, tympanitis, photophobia.

Physical Examination

Skin Lesions

PHASE I   Lesions appear 1 to 3 days after onset of fever. Duration 12 days average. Nearly all mucocutaneous abnormalities occur during this phase.

Exanthem   Erythema usually first noted on palms/soles, spreading to involve trunk and extremities within 2 days. First lesions erythematous macules; lesions enlarge and become more numerous (Figure 29-29). Type: urticaria-like lesions most common; morbilliform pattern second most common; scarlatiniform and erythema multiforme–like in <5 % of cases. Confluent macules to plaque-type erythema on perineum, which persist after other findings have resolved. Edema ofhands/feet: deeply erythematous to violaceous; brawny swelling with fusiform fingers. Palpation: lesions may be tender. Distribution: hands/feet, striking erythema, ±indurative edema; truncal erythema. Perineal.

Mucous Membranes   Bulbar conjunctivae: bilateral vascular dilatation (conjunctival injection); noted 2 days after onset of fever; duration, 1 to 3 weeks (throughout the febrile course). Lips: red, dry, fissured, hemorrhagic crusts; duration, 1 to 3 weeks. Oropharynx: diffuse erythema. Tongue: "strawberry" tongue (erythema and protuberance of papillae of tongue).

General Findings   Cervical lymphadenopathy (at least one lymph node >1.5 cm in diameter). Diarrhea, hepatic dysfunction, aseptic meningitis

PHASE II   *Exanthem*   Desquamation highly characteristic; follows resolution of exanthem (Figure 29-30). Begins on tips of fin-

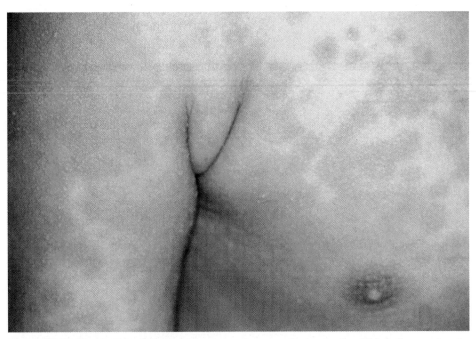

Figure 29-29 Kawasaki's disease *Blotchy erythema on the trunk of a child; bulbar conjunctival injection and strawberry tongue were also present.*

gers and toes at junction of nails and skin; desquamating sheets of palmar/plantar epidermis are progressively shed.

General Findings Meningeal irritation. Pneumonia. Lymphadenopathy, usually of a single cervical node, ≥1.5 cm, slightly tender, firm. Arthritis/arthralgias, knees, hips, elbows. Pericardial tamponade, dysrhythmias, rubs, congestive heart failure, left ventricular dysfunction.

PHASE III Beau's lines (transverse furrows on nail surface) may be seen. Possible telogen effluvium.

Differential Diagnosis

Juvenile rheumatoid arthritis, infectious mononucleosis, viral exanthems, leptospirosis, Rocky Mountain spotted fever, toxic shock syndrome, staphylococcal scalded-skin syndrome, erythema multiforme, serum sickness, systemic lupus erythematosus. Reiter's syndrome

Laboratoy and Special Examinations

Chemistry Abnormal liver functional tests

Hematology Leukocytosis ($>$18,000/μl)

PHASE II Thrombocytosis after the tenth day of illness. Elevated ESR.

PHASE III ESR returns to normal

Urinalysis Pyuria

Dermatopathology Arteritis involving small and medium-sized vessels with swelling of endothelial cells in postcapillary venules, dilatation of small blood vessels, lymphocytic/monocytic perivascular infiltrate in arteries/arterioles of dermis

Electrocardiography Prolongation of PR and QT intervals; ST-segment and T-wave changes

Echocardiography Coronary aneurysms

Cardiac Angiography Coronary aneurysms in 25 % of cases

Diagnosis

Diagnostic criteria: fever spiking to >39.4°C, lasting ≥5 days without other cause, associated with four of five criteria—(1) bilateral conjunctival injection, (2) at least one of following mucous membrane changes: injected/fissured lips, injected pharynx, "strawberry" tongue, (3) at least one of the following extremity changes: erythema of palms/soles, edema of hands/feet, generalized/periungual desquamation, (4) diffuse scarlatiniform erythroderma, diffuse centrally/sharply demarcated borders on extremities, deeply erythematous maculopapular rash, iris lesions, (5) cervical lymphadenopathy (at least one lymph node ≥1.5 cm in diameter)

Pathophysiology

Generalized vasculitis. Endarteritis of vasa vasorum involves adventitia/intima of proximal coronary arteries with ectasia, aneurysm formation, vessel obstruction, and distal embolization with subsequent myocardial infarction. Other vessels: brachiocephalic, celiac, renal, iliofemoral arteries.

Course and Prognosis

Clinical course triphasic. Uneventful recovery occurs in majority. CVS complications in 20 %. Coronary artery aneurysms occur within 2 to 8 weeks, associated with myocarditis, myocardial ischemia/infarction, pericarditis, peripheral vascular occlusion, small bowel obstruction, stroke. Mortality 1 %.

Management

Diagnosis should be made early and attention directed at prevention of the cardiovascular complications.

Hospitalization Recommended during the phase I illness, monitoring for cardiac and vascular complications

Aspirin 100 mg/kg/day until fever resolves or until day 14 of illness, followed by 5 to 10 mg/kg/day until ESR and platelet count have returned to normal

Intravenous Gamma Globulin High-dose (400 mg/kg/day in 2-hour infusions) IV gamma globulin for 4 days may reduce risk of coronary artery aneurysms and myocardial infarction.

Corticosteroids *Contraindicated.* Associated with a higher rate of coronary aneurysms.

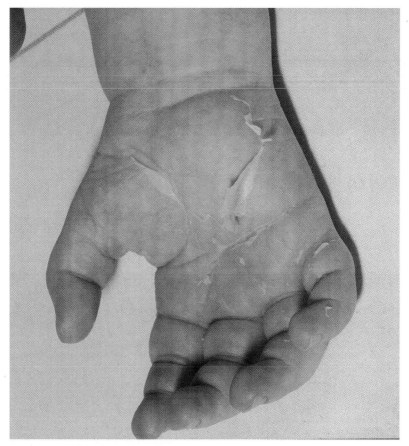

Figure 29-30 Kawasaki's disease *Shedding of the skin on the palm of this child 10 days after the acute illness.*

INSECT BITES AND INFESTATIONS

PEDICULOSIS CAPITIS

Pediculosis capitis is an infestation of the scalp by the head louse, which feeds on the scalp and neck and deposits its eggs on the hair; presence of head lice is associated with few symptoms but much consternation.

Epidemiology and Etiology

Age More common in children, but all ages

Sex Females > males

Etiology The subspecies of *Pediculus humanus capitis.* Unlike *P. humanus corporis,* the head louse is not a vector of infectious diseases.

Race More common in whites than in blacks in the United States. In Africa, pediculosis capitis is relatively common.

Transmission Shared hats, caps, brushes, combs; head-to-head contact. Epidemics in schools. Head lice can survive off the scalp for up to 55 hours.

Incidence Estimated that 6 to 10 million children in the United States are infested annually

History

Skin Symptoms Children said to be distracted, restless, and inattentive at school. Pruritus of the back and sides of scalp. Scratching and secondary infection associated with occipital and/or cervical lymphadenopathy.

Physical Examination

Skin Lesions

TYPES

Head lice are identified with eye or with hand lens but are difficult to find. The majority of patients have a population of <10 head lice.

Nits (Figure 30-1) or oval grayish-white egg capsules (1 mm long) firmly cemented to the hairs; vary in number from only a few to thousands. Nits are deposited by head lice on the hair shaft as it emerges from the follicle. With recent infestation, nits are near the scalp; with infestation of long standing, nits may be 10 to 15 cm from scalp. In that scalp hair grows 0.5 mm daily, the presence of nits 15 cm from the scalp indicates that the infestation is approximately 9 months old. New viable eggs have a creamy-yellow color; empty eggshells are white.

Eczema and lichen simplex chronicus occur on the occipital scalp and neck secondary to chronic scratching and rubbing.

Excoriations, crusts, and secondarily impetiginized lesions are seen commonly and mask the presence of lice and nits; may extend onto neck, forehead, face, ears. In the extreme, scalp becomes a con-

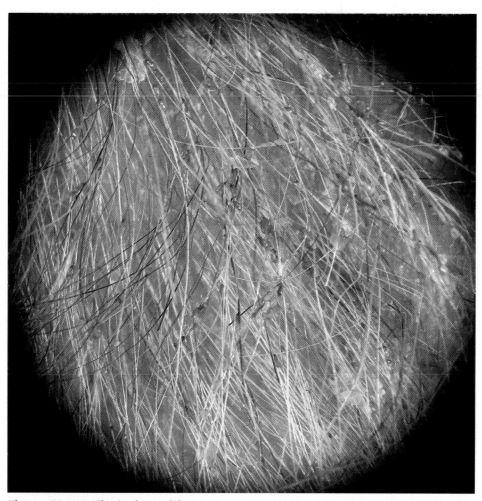

Figure 30-1 Pediculosis capitis *Myriads of nits (oval, grayish-white egg capsules) are firmly attached to the hair shafts. On close examination these have a bottle shape.*

fluent, purulent mass of matted hair, lice, nits, crusts, and purulent discharge

Papular urticaria, i.e., site of the lice bite, is sometimes apparent on the neck.

SITES OF PREDILECTION   Head lice nearly always confined to scalp, especially occipital and postauricular regions. Rare head lice infest beard or other hairy sites. Although more common with crab lice, head lice also can infest the eyelashes (pediculosis palpebrarum).

REGIONAL LYMPH NODES   Postoccipital lymphadenopathy secondary to impetiginization of excoriated sites

Differential Diagnosis

Small White Hair "Beads"   Hair casts, hair lacquer, hair gels, dandruff (epidermal scales)

Scalp Pruritus   Impetigo, lichen simplex chronicus

Laboratory and Special Examinations

Microscopy   The louse or a nit on a hair shaft can be examined to confirm the gross examination of the scalp and hair.

NITS   0.5-mm oval, whitish eggs. Nonviable nits show an absence of an embryo or operulum.

LOUSE   Insect with six legs, 1 to 4 mm in length, wingless, translucent grayish-white body that is red when engorged with blood

Wood's Lamp   Live nits fluoresce with a pearly fluorescence; dead nits do not.

Culture   If impetiginization is suspected, bacterial cultures should be obtained.

Diagnosis

Clinical findings, confirmed by detection of nits and/or lice

Management

Information   Available through the National Pediculosis Association, Box 149, Newton, MA 02161; Tel: 1-617-449-6487

Prevention   Avoid contact with possibly contaminated items such as hats, headsets, clothing, towels, combs, hair brushes, bedding, upholstery. The environment should be vacuumed. Bedding, clothing, and head gear should be washed and dried on the hot cycle of a dryer. Combs and brushes should be soaked in rubbing alcohol or Lysol 2 % solution for 1 hour.

Removal of Nits   Viability of residual nits cannot be ascertained; remaining nits should be removed with a fine-toothed nit comb. Application of white vinegar to the hair loosens the nits and facilitates removal.

Topically Applied Insecticides   Pyrethrins and lindane are not totally ovicidal and lack residual activity; in that the incubation period of louse eggs is 6 to 10 days, the agents should be reapplied in 7 to 14 days.

RECOMMENDED REGIMEN   Permethrin (over-the-counter preparation, Nix) or pyrethrins (over-the-counter preparations include RID, A-200 Pediculicide Shampoo or Gel Concentrate) applied to scalp and washed off after 10 minutes *or* 0.5% malathion (Ovide lotion) that is left on the scalp for 8 to 12 hours

ALTERNATIVE REGIMEN   Pyrethrins with piperonyl butoxide applied to scalp and washed off after 10 minutes *or* Lindane 1 % shampoo applied for 4 minutes and then thoroughly washed off. (Not recommended for pregnant or lactating women.) Patients should be reevaluated after 1 week if symptoms persist. Re-treatment may be necessary if lice are found or eggs are observed at the hair-skin junction.

Pediculosis Palpebrarum   Apply petrolatum to lashes twice daily for 8 days, followed by removal of nits, *or* physostigmine ophthalmic preparations applied twice daily for 1 or 2 days.

Secondary Bacterial Infection   Should be treated with appropriate doses of erythromycin *or* dicloxacillin.

PEDICULOSIS PUBIS (PHTHIRIASIS)

Pediculosis pubis is an infestation of hair-bearing regions, most commonly the pubic area but at times the hairy parts of the chest and axillae and the upper eyelashes; it is manifested clinically by mild to moderate pruritus.

Synonyms: Crabs, crab lice, pubic lice.

Epidemiology and Etiology

Age Most common in young adults; range from childhood to senescence

Sex More extensive infestation in males

Etiology *Phthirus pubis,* the crab or pubic louse. The life cycle from egg to adult is 22 to 27 days; the incubation period for the egg is 7 to 8 days; the rest of the life cycle is taken up with larval and nymphal development. The average life span is 17 days for the female and 22 days for the male. Lives exclusively on humans. Prefers a humid environment; does not tend to wander.

Transmission Close physical contact such as sexual intercourse; sleeping in same bed; possibly exchange of towels

History

Skin Symptoms May be asymptomatic. Mild to moderate pruritus for months. Patient may note a nodularity to hairs (nits or eggs) that is detected while scratching. With excoriation and secondary infection, lesions may become tender and be associated with enlarged regional, e.g., inguinal, lymph node.

Physical Examination

Skin Lesions

TYPES

> *Lice* appear as 1- to 2-mm, brownish-gray specks (see Figure 30-2) in the hairy areas involved. Remain stationary for days; mouth parts embedded in skin; claws grasping a hair on either side. Usually few in number.

> *Eggs (nits)* attached to hair appear as tiny white-gray specks (Figure 30-3). Few to numerous. Eggs found at hair-skin junction indicate active infestation.

> *Papular urticaria* (small erythematous papules) noted at sites of feeding, especially periumbilical (Figure 30-4); rarely feeding sites may become bullous.

> Secondary changes of lichenification, *excoriations,* and *impetiginized excoriations* detected in patients with significant pruritus. Serous crusts may be present along with lice and nits when eyelids are infested; occasionally, edema of eyelids with severe infestation.

> *Maculae caeruleae (taches bleues)* are slate-gray or bluish-gray macules 0.5 to 1.0 cm in diameter, irregular in shape, nonblanching. Pigment thought to be breakdown product of heme affected by louse saliva.

DISTRIBUTION Most commonly found in pubic and axillary areas; also, perineum, thighs, lower legs, trunk, especially periumbilical (Figure 30-4). In hairy males: nipple areas, upper arms, rarely wrists; rarely, beard and moustache area. In children, eyelashes and eyebrows may be infested without pubic involvement. Maculae caeruleae most common on lower abdominal wall, buttocks, upper thighs.

General Findings With secondary impetiginization, regional lymphadenopathy

Differential Diagnosis

Pruritic Dermatosis Eczema, seborrheic dermatitis, tinea cruris, folliculitis, molluscum contagiosum

Taches Bleues Ashy dermatosis

Laboratory and Special Examinations

Microscopy Lice and nits may be identified with hand lens or microscope.

Cultures Bacterial cultures if excoriation impetiginized

Serology Patients should be screened with blood tests for syphilis and HIV infection.

Diagnosis

Clinical diagnosis

Course and Prognosis

Patients should be evaluated after 1 week if symptoms persist. Re-treatment may be necessary if lice are found or if eggs are observed at hair-skin junction. Patients not responding to one regimen should be re-treated with an alternative.

Management

Lindane is the least expensive therapy; toxicity has not been reported when treatment is limited to a 4-minute period. Permethrin has less potential for toxicity in the event of inappropriate use.

Recommended Regimens

> Lindane 1 % shampoo applied for 4 minutes and then thoroughly washed off (not recommended for pregnant or lactating women or for children <2 years of age) *or*
>
> Permethrin 1 % cream rinse applied to affected areas and washed off after 10 minutes *or*
>
> Pyrethrins with piperonyl butoxide applied to affected area and washed off after 10 minutes

Infestation of Eyelids Recommended regimens should not be applied to eyelids. Apply occlusive ophthalmic ointment to eyelid margins two times a day for 10 days.

Decontamination of Environment Bedding and clothing should be decontaminated (machine washed or machine dried using heat cycle or dry-cleaned) or removed from body contact for at least 72 hours.

Management of Sex Partner(s) Sex partners within last month should be treated.

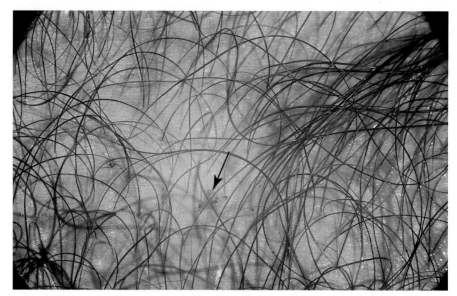

Figure 30-2 Pediculosis pubis: crab louse *A crab louse* (see arrow) *on the skin in the pubic region.*

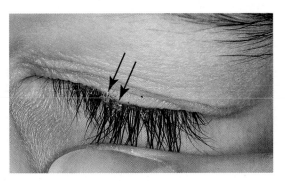

Figure 30-3 Pediculosis "pubis": crab lice and nits *Crab lice* (see arrow) *and nits on the upper eyelashes of a child; this was the only site of infestation.*

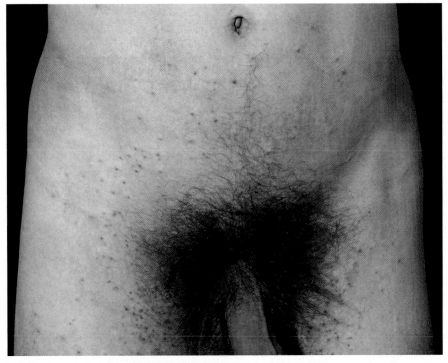

Figure 30-4 Pediculosis pubis: papular urticaria *At this magnification only inflammatory papules (sites of crab lice bites) which are extremely pruritic on the abdomen and the inner aspects of the thighs. Closer examination reveals nits on the pubic hairs.*

SCABIES

Scabies is an infestation by the mite *Sarcoptes scabiei,* usually spread by skin-to-skin contact, and characterized by generalized intractable pruritus often with minimal cutaneous findings. The diagnosis may be missed easily and should be considered in a patient of any age with persistent generalized severe pruritus.

Synonym: Chronic undiagnosed scabies is the basis for the colloquial expression, "the 7-year itch."

Epidemiology and Etiology

Age Young adults (usually acquired by sexual contact) or contact with mite-infested sheets in elderly and bedridden patients in the hospital; children (often 5 years or under). Nodular scabies more common in children.

Etiology *S. scabiei.* Thrive and multiply only on human skin. Burrow into skin shortly after contact. Burrow 2 to 3 mm daily. Usually burrow at night and lay eggs during day. Female lives 4 to 6 weeks, laying 40 to 50 eggs. Eggs hatch after 72 to 96 hours.

Other Factors Epidemics of scabies occur in cycles every 15 years; the latest epidemic began in the late 1960s but curiously has continued to the present.

Transmission Mite transmitted by skin-to-skin contact as with sex partner, children playing, or health care worker providing care. Mites can remain alive for over 2 days on clothing or in bedding, and therefore, scabies can be acquired without skin-to-skin contact. Patients with crusted scabies shed many mites into their environment daily and pose a high risk of infecting those around them.

Risk Factors Institutionalization in facilities such as nursing homes

Pathogenesis

For pruritus to occur, sensitization to *S. scabiei* must take place. Among persons with their first infection, sensitization takes several weeks to develop; after reinfestation, pruritus may occur within 24 hours. Various immunocompromised states or individuals with neurologic disease (see below) predisposed to crusted Norwegian scabies. Infestation is usually by only approximately 10 mites. In contrast, the number of infesting mites in crusted scabies may exceed a million.

History

History Patients are often aware of similar symptoms in family members or sexual partners. Patients with crusted scabies usually are immunocompromised (HIV disease, organ transplant recipient) or have neurologic disorders (Down's syndrome, dementia, strokes, spinal cord injury, neuropathy, leprosy).

Incubation Period With first episode of scabies, pruritus usually begins within 1 month after exposure and the generalized hypersensitivity eruption 1 or 2 weeks after. With reinfestation, pruritus begins immediately.

Duration of Lesions Weeks to months unless treated. Crusted scabies may be present for years.

Skin Symptoms

PRURITUS Intense, widespread, usually sparing head and neck. Itching often interferes with or prevents sleep. Half of patients with crusted scabies do not itch.

RASH Ranges from no rash to generalized erythroderma. Patients with atopic diathesis scratch, producing eczematous dermatitis. Other individuals experience pruritus for many months with no rash. Tenderness of lesions suggests secondary bacterial infection.

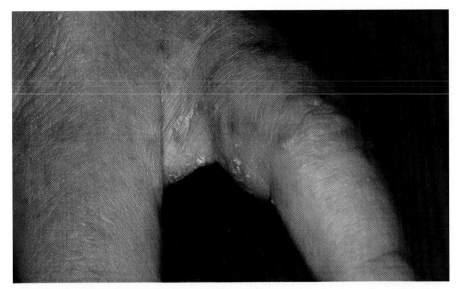

Figure 30-5 Scabies *Papules and burrows in typical location on the finger webs. Burrows are tan or skin-colored ridges with linear configuration with a minute vesicle or papule at the end of the burrow and are often difficult to locate.*

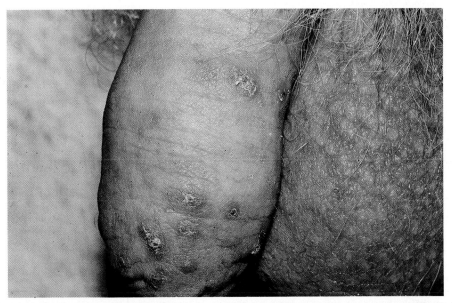

Figure 30-6 Scabies *Multiple, crusted, and excoriated papules and burrows on the penile shaft.*

Physical Examination

Skin Lesions Common cutaneous findings can be classified: lesions occurring at the sites of mite infestation, cutaneous manifestations of hypersensitivity to mite, lesions secondary to chronic rubbing and scratching, secondary infection, variants of scabies in special hosts.

LESIONS AT SITE OF INFESTATION

- Intraepidermal burrows: gray or skin-colored ridges, 0.5 to 1.0 cm in length (see Figures 30-5 and 30-6), either linear or wavy (serpiginous) with minute vesicle or papule at end of tunnel. Each infesting female mite produces one burrow. Mites are about 0.5 mm in length. Burrows average 5 mm in length but may be up to 10 cm. In light-skinned individuals, burrows have a whitish color with occasional dark specks (due to fecal scybala). Fountain-pen ink applied to infested skin concentrates in tunnels, highlighting and marking the burrow. Blind end of burrow where mite resides appears as a minute elevation with tiny halo of erythema or as a veiscle. *Distribution of burrows:* areas with few or no hair follicles, usually where stratum corneum is thin and soft, i.e., interdigital webs of hands > wrists > shaft of penis > elbows > feet > genitalia > buttocks > axillae > elsewhere (see Figure XI). In infants, infestation may occur on head and neck.
- A burrow is sometimes seen on the surface of a very early scabetic nodule.
- In areas of heavily infested crusted scabies, well-demarcated plaques covered by a very thick crust or scale

CUTANEOUS MANIFESTATIONS OF HYPERSENSITIVITY TO MITE

- Some individuals experience only pruritus without any cutaneous findings.
- "Id" or autosensitization-type reactions characterized by widespread small urticarial edematous papules mainly on anterior trunk, thighs, buttocks, and forearms
- Urticaria
- Eczematous dermatitis at sites of heaviest infestation: hands, axillae

LESIONS SECONDARY TO CHRONIC RUBBING AND SCRATCHING

- Excoriation, lichen simplex chronicus, prurigo nodules
- In individuals with atopic diathesis, atopic dermatitis occurs at sites of excoriation, most commonly on the hands, webspaces of hands, wrists, axillae, areolae, waist, buttocks, penis, scrotum. *Distribution:* In adults, the scalp, face, and upper back are usually spared, but in infants, the scalp, face, palms, and soles are involved.
- Postinflammatory hyperpigmentation
- Generalized eczematous dermatitis
- Erythroderma

SECONDARY INFECTION

- Impetiginized excoriations (crusted, tender, surrounding erythema), ecthyma
- *Staphylococcus aureus* folliculitis, abscess formation
- Lymphangitis, lymphadenitis
- Cellulitis
- Bacteremia
- Acute poststreptococcal glomerulonephritis

VARIANTS OF SCABIES IN SPECIAL HOSTS

Nodular Scabies Nodular lesions develop in 7 % to 10 % of patients with scabies. Nodules are 5 to 20 mm in diameter, red, pink, tan, or brown in color, smooth (Figure 30-7). A burrow may be seen on the surface of early nodule. *Distribution:* penis, scrotum, axillae, waist, buttocks, areolae. Resolve with postinflammatory hyperpigmentation. May be more apparent after treatment, as eczematous eruption resolves. Upper back, lateral edge of foot (infants). Nodules are usually countable.

Crusted or Norwegian Scabies May begin as ordinary scabies. In others, clinical appearance is of chronic eczema, psoriasiform dermatitis, seborrheic dermatitis, or erythroderma. Lesions often markedly hyperkeratotic and/or crusted. *Distribution:* generalized (even involving head and neck in adults) or localized. Scale/crusts found on dorsal surface of hands, wrists, fingers, metacarpophalangeal joints, palms, extensor aspect of elbows,

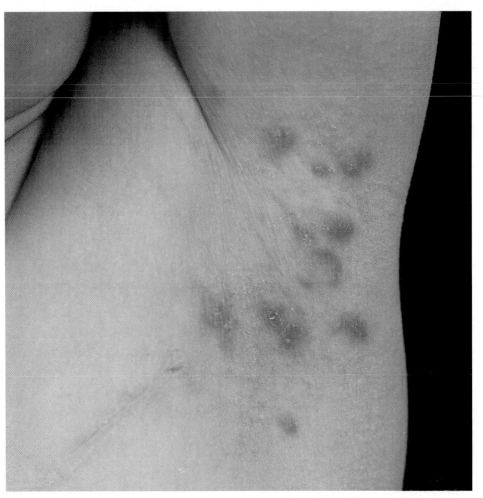

Figure 30-7 Scabetic nodules *Papules and nodules in the axillary fold in a child; these brownish-red, relatively deep-seated, pruritic lesions are pathognomonic for chronic scabies, particularly in children.*

scalp, ears, soles, and toes. In patients with neurologic deficit, crusted scabies may occur only in affected limb.

Differential Diagnosis

Pruritus, Localized or Generalized, ±Rash Adverse cutaneous drug reaction, atopic dermatitis, contact dermatitis, fiberglass dermatitis, dyshidrotic eczema, dermatographism, physical urticaria, pityriasis rosea, dermatitis herpetiformis, animal scabies, pediculosis corporis, pediculosis pubis, lichen planus, delusions of parasitosis, metabolic pruritus

Pyoderma Impetigo, ecthyma, furunculosis

Nodular Scabies Urticaria pigmentosa (in young child), papular urticaria (insect bites), Darier's disease, prurigo nodularis, secondary syphilis

Crusted Scabies Psoriasis, eczematous dermatitis, seborrheic dermatitis, erythroderma, Langerhans cell histiocytosis

Laboratory and Special Examinations

Finding the Mite A healthy adult with scabies has an average of 6 to 10 adult mites infesting the body. The highest yield in identifying a mite is in typical burrows on the finger webs, flexor aspects of wrists, and penis. A drop of mineral oil is placed over a burrow, and the burrow is scraped off with a no. 15 scalpel blade and placed on a microscope slide. A drop of immersion or mineral oil is placed on the scraping, which is then covered by a coverslip. Three findings are diagnostic of scabies: *S. scabiei* mites, their eggs, and their fecal pellets (scybala) (see Figure 30-8).

Hematology Eosinophilia in crusted scabies

Dermatopathology *Scabetic burrow:* located within stratum corneum; female mite situated in blind end of burrow. Body round, 400 μm in length. Spongiosis near mite with vesicle formation common. Eggs also seen. Dermis shows infiltrate with eosinophils. *Scabetic nodules:*

dense chronic inflammatory infiltrate with eosinophils. In some cases, persistent arthropod reaction resembling lymphoma with atypical mononuclear cells. *Crusted scabies:* thickened stratum corneum riddled with innumerable mites.

Cultures Scabetic lesions may become secondarily infected with *Staphylococcus aureus* or group A streptococcus.

Diagnosis

Clinical findings, confirmed, if possible, by microscopy. Assiduous search for burrows should be made in every patient with severe generalized pruritus. Sometimes when the mite cannot be demonstrated, a "therapeutic test" will clinch the diagnosis.

Course and Prognosis

Pruritus Often persists up to several weeks after successful eradication of mite infestation, understandable in that the pruritus is a hypersensitivity phenomenon to mite antigen(s). If reinfestation recurs, pruritus becomes symptomatic within a few days. Majority of cases resolve following recommended regimen of therapy. Glomerulonephritis has followed group A streptococcal secondary infection. Bacteremia and death have followed secondary *S. aureus* infection of crusted scabies in an HIV-infected patient.

Crusted Scabies May be impossible to irradicate in HIV-infected individuals.

Nodular Scabies In treated patient, 80 % resolve in 3 months, but may persist up to 1 year.

Management

Scabicides Permethrin is effective and safe but costs more than lindane. Lindane is effective in most areas of the world, but resistance has been reported. Seizures have occurred when lindane was applied after a bath or used by patients with extensive dermatitis. Aplastic anemia following lindane use was also reported.

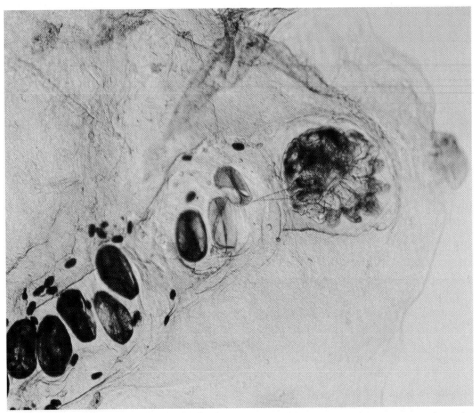

Figure 30-8 Burrow with Sarcoptes scabiei (female), eggs, and feces *A mite at the end of a burrow with 8 eggs and smaller fecal particles obtained from a papule on the webspace of the hand.*

Permethrin cream 5 % applied to all areas of the body from the neck down; wash off after 8 to 14 hours; *or*

Lindane (gamma-benzene hexachloride) 1 %, 1 oz of lotion or 30 g of cream, applied thinly to all areas of the body from the neck down; wash off thoroughly after 8 hours. Infants, young children, and pregnant and lactating women should not be treated with lindane. *Note:* Lindane should not be used following a bath or shower, and it should not be used by persons with extensive dermatitis, pregnant or lactating women, and children <2 years of age. Mite resistance to lindane has developed in some countries.

ALTERNATIVE REGIMEN

Crotamiton cream 10 % applied thinly to the entire body from the neck down, nightly for 2 consecutive nights; wash off 24 hours after second application.

Sulfur ointment 6 % to 10 % applied to skin for 2 to 3 days

Systemic Ivermectin *Ivermectin* 200 μg/kg PO; single dose reported to be very effective for common as well as crusted scabies.

Infants and Young Children Mites may infest the head and neck. Permethrin or crotamiton regimens or precipitated sulfur ointment should be used with application to all body areas.

Treatment of Eczematous Dermatitis

Antihistamines: systemic sedating antihistamine such as hydroxyzine hydrochloride or diphenhydramine 25 mg at bedtime.

Topical corticosteroid ointment applied to areas of extensive dermatitis associated with scabies

Systemic corticosteroids: A tapered course of prednisone (1 to 2 weeks) gives symptomatic relief of severe hypersensitivity reaction.

Postscabetic Itching Generalized itching that persists a week or more is probably caused by hypersensitivity to remaining dead mites and mite products. Nevertheless, a second treatment 7 days after the first is recommended by some physicians. For severe, persistent pruritus, especially in individuals with history of atopic disorders, a 14-day tapered course of prednisone (70 mg on day 1) is indicated.

Secondary Bacterial Infection Treat with mupirocin ointment or systemic antimicrobial agent.

Scabetic Nodules May persist associated with pruritus for up to a year after eradication of infestation. Intralesional triamcinolone 5 to 10 mg/ml into each lesion effective; repeat every 2 weeks if necessary.

Crusted Scabies Single application of a scabicide kills 90 % to 95 % of mites. Multiple applications are therefore required to all the skin. In HIV-infected individuals, eradication of infestation may be impossible. Treatment also should be directed at removing scale/crusts that protect mites from scabicide.

Decontamination of Environment Bedding and clothing should be decontaminated (machine washed or machine dried using heat cycle or dry-cleaned) or removed from body contact for at least 72 hours.

Management of Sex Partner(s) Sexual partners and close personal or household contacts within last month should be examined and treated.

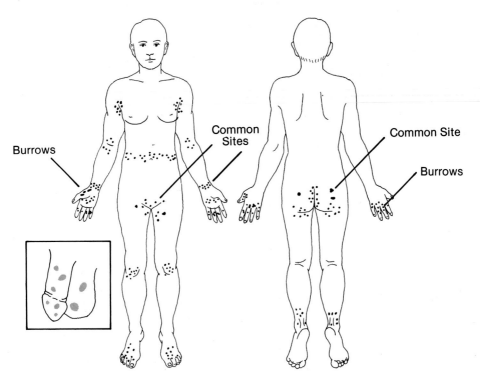

Burrows

Common
Sites

Common Site

Burrows

Figure XI Scabies

CUTANEOUS REACTIONS TO FLEA BITES

Cutaneous reaction to flea bites (CRFB) is an immunologic-mediated reaction, characterized by an intensely pruritic eruption occurring at the bite sites hours to days after the bite, manifested by grouped urticarial papules, papulovesicles, and/or bullae that persist for days to weeks; patients are unaware of being bitten.

Epidemiology and Etiology

Age   Any age, but more common in children

Season   Summer in temperate climates

Etiology   Cat fleas *Ctenocephalides felis,* dog fleas *C. canis,* human fleas *Pulex* species, *Xenopsylla* species, fowl fleas *Ceratophyllidae* species

History

Incubation Period   CRFB appears hours to days after the bite.

Duration of Lesions   Days, weeks

Skin Symptoms   Individuals are not aware of being bitten by fleas. Most patients who present with CRFB are incredulous when first given the diagnosis. Their association is with poor housekeeping practices or poor personal hygiene. Fleas commonly live in carpeting, emerging to hop onto and bite the lower legs. If dogs or cats are allowed onto furniture or bed, bites may occur on the trunk. Individuals holding the animal may have bites on the frontal chest. CRFB is associated with intermittent, mild to severe, intense pruritus. Several members of a household may have similar lesions.

Physical Examination

Skin Lesions

TYPES   *Erythematous Macules*   Occur at bite sites and are usually transient
Papular Urticaria   Persistent urticarial papules, often surmounted by a vesicle (Figure 30-9), usually <1.0 cm (lesions persist more than 48 hours). Excoriations and excoriated urticarial papules, vesicles. Crusted painful lesions, usually purulent, may represent impetigo, ecthyma, or cutaneous diphtheria. Excoriated or secondarily infected lesions may heal with hyper- or hypopigmentation, and/or raised or depressed scars, especially in more darkly pigmented individuals.
Bullous Lesions   Tense bullae with clear fluid on a slightly inflamed base. Excoriation results in large erosive lesions.

COLOR   Red. Bullae have clear amber fluid.

SHAPE   Round, domed

ARRANGEMENT   Usually in groups of three ("breakfast, lunch, and dinner"). Lesions may be clustered around areas where clothing is restricted.
DISTRIBUTION   *Extent*   Generalized groups or clusters
Pattern   The most common sites are the legs from ankles to knees. Thighs, forearms and arms, lower part of trunk, and waist, but sparing anogenital area and axillae.

Differential Diagnosis

Allergic contact dermatitis, especially to plants such as poison ivy or poison oak. Papular urticaria also follows bites of mites, bedbugs, mosquitoes.

Laboratory and Special Examinations

Cultures   Bacterial cultures are indicated if secondary infection is considered.

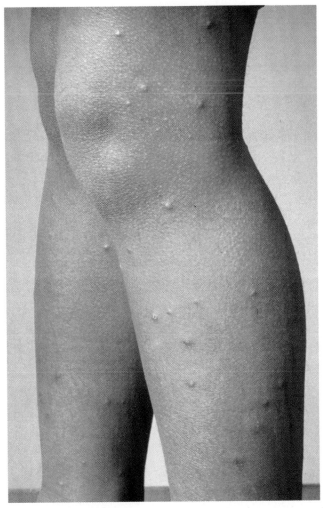

Figure 30-9 Papular urticaria to flea bites *Multiple, very pruritic, urticaria-like papules at the sites of flea bites on the knees and legs of a child; these persistent urticaria-like papules are usually < 1 cm in diameter and may have a vesicle on the top. When scratched, they exhibit erosions or crusts.*

Dermatopathology Epidermis: intercellular and intracellular edema and occasional spongiotic vesicle. Dermis: chronic deep inflammatory infiltrate with eosinophils predominantly around blood vessels.

Diagnosis

Clinical diagnosis, at times confirmed by lesional biopsy

Pathogenesis

The cutaneous lesion following an arthropod bite is caused by an immunologic tissue response to an injected anthropodal antigen.

The intensity of the reaction varies according to the geographic areas, as there are hundreds of species of fleas.

Course and Prognosis

Excoriation of CRFB commonly results in secondary infection of the eroded epidermis by group A beta-hemolytic *Streptococcus* and/or *Staphylococcus aureus* causing impetigo or ecthyma. This is especially common in humid tropical climates. Less common is secondary infection with *Corynebacterium diphtheriae,* with resultant cutaneous diphtheria. Streptococcal skin infections are, at times, complicated by glomerulonephritis.

At times, fleas are vectors for infectious agents causing the following flea-borne diseases: bubonic plague, tularemia, murine typhus, boutonneuse fever, Q fever, lymphocytic choriomeningitis, tick-borne encephalitis.

Management

Prevention Avoid contact with cats and dogs. Treat flea-infested cats and dogs. Spray household with insecticides (e.g., malathion 1 % to 4 % dust) with special attention to baseboards, rugs, floors, upholstered furniture, bed frames, mattresses, and cellar.

Corticosteroids Potent topical corticosteroids given for a short time are helpful for intensely pruritic lesions. In some cases, a short tapered course of oral corticosteroids can be given for extensive CRFBs that are persistent.

Antimicrobial Agents Antibiotic treatment with topical agents such as mupirocin ointment (Bactroban) or antistaphylococcal/antistreptococcal agents if secondary infection is present.

CUTANEOUS LARVA MIGRANS

Cutaneous larva migrans is a cutaneous lesion produced by percutaneous penetration and migration of larvae of various nematode parasites, characterized by erythematous, serpiginous, papular, or vesicular linear lesions corresponding to the movements of the larvae beneath the skin.
Synonym: Creeping eruption.

Etiology and Epidemiology

Etiology *Ancylostoma braziliense* in central and southeastern United States; *A. caninum, Uncinaria stenocephala* (hookworm of dogs), *Bunostomum phlebotomum* (hookworm of cattle); also *A. duodenale, Necator americanus*

Epidemiology Ova of hookworms are deposited in sand and soil in warm, shady areas, hatching into larvae that penetrate human skin. Persons at risk include gardeners, farmers, sea bathers.

Occupation Workers exposed to hookworm larvae include plumbers ("plumber's itch"), electricians, carpenters, pest exterminators while in contact with warm, moist sandy soil as in crawl spaces of dwellings, gardeners, and fishermen.

History

Skin Symptoms Local pruritus begins within hours after larval penetration.

Physical Examination

Skin Lesions

TYPE   Serpiginous, thin, linear, raised, tunnel-like lesion 2 to 3 mm wide containing serous fluid (Figure 30-10). Several or many lesions may be present depending on the number of penetrating larvae. Larvae move a few to many millimeters daily, confined to an area several centimeters in diameter. If multiple larvae are present, multiple tracts are seen (Figure 30-11).

COLOR   Erythematous

DISTRIBUTION   Exposed sites, most commonly the feet, lower legs, buttocks, hands

Variant

LARVA CURRENS   Caused by *Strongyloides stercoralis*. Papules, urticaria, papulovesicles at the site of larval penetration (Figure 30-11). Associated with intense pruritus. Occurs on skin around anus, buttocks, thighs, back, shoulders, abdomen. Pruritus and eruption disappear when larvae enter blood vessels and migrate to intestinal mucosa.

Systemic Findings Visceral larva migrans characterized by persistent hypereosinophilia, hepatomegaly, and frequently pneumonitis. Caused by *Toxocara canis, T. cati, A. lumbricoides.*

Differential Diagnosis

Curvilinear Inflammatory Lesion Phytoallergic contact dermatitis, phytophotodermatitis, erythema migrans of Lyme borreliosis, jelly fish sting, epidermal dermatophytosis, granuloma annulare

Diagnosis

Clinical findings

Course

Self-limited; humans are "dead-end" hosts. Most larvae die and the lesions resolve within 4 to 6 weeks.

Management

Symptomatic relief is provided by topical application of a corticosteroid preparation under occlusion.

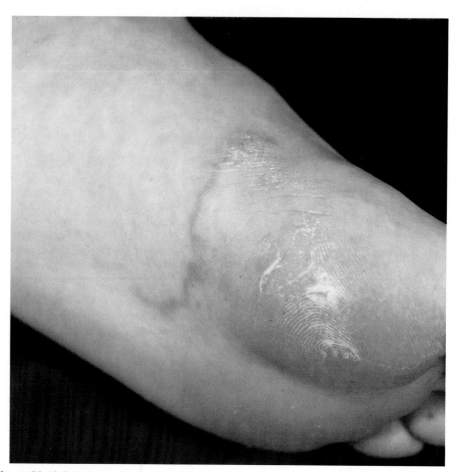

Figure 30-10 Cutaneous larva migrans *A thin, erythematous, serpiginous (snakelike), papular eruption that marks the burrow created by the parasite.*

Antihelminthic Agents

THIABENDAZOLE   Orally 50 mg/kg/day in two doses (maximum 3 g/day) for 2 to 5 days. Also effective when applied topically under occlusion.

ALBENDAZOLE   400 mg daily for 3 days, highly effective

Cryosurgery   Liquid nitrogen to progressing end of larval burrow

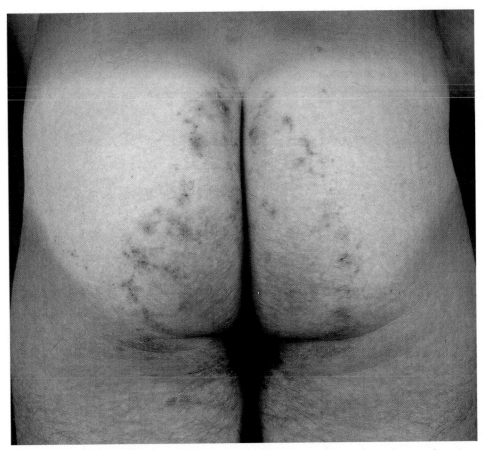

Figure 30-11 Cutaneous larva migrans: larva currens *A widespread eruption starting on the buttocks consisting of urticarial papules and serpiginous papular lesions with occasional vesiculation. Close inspection reveals the serpiginous configuration of the lesions and thus facilitates diagnosis of* Strongyloides stercoralis *infestation.*

TUNGIASIS

Tungiasis is an infestation by the flea *Tunga penetrans,* characterized by painful papules at the site of penetration, most often under the toenails or between the toes. Travelers to endemic areas may acquire the infestation while walking barefoot on beaches.
Synonyms: Nigua, bicho de pe. Flea called *chigoe* or *jigger.*

Epidemiology and Etiology

Etiology   *T. penetrans.* The larvae are free-living in earth floors of human dwellings, in sandy soil, or on beaches; require shade. The flea is red-brown in color, 1 mm in length; it is capable of invading the skin of humans, pigs, and other mammals. Only the female flea burrows into the skin until the last abdominal segment is parallel with the skin surface. Larvae emerge from eggs 3 to 4 days after being laid and thrive best in dry, sandy soil. Larvae feed on organic matter. Here the larvae develop into pupae and finally adult fleas within 3 weeks.

Geographic Distribution   Central and South America, the Caribbean Islands. Tropical Africa, the Seychelles, Pakistan, the west coast of India. The flea was probably transported from South America to the West Coast of Africa in the mid-1800s in sand ballast or in the feet of infested sailors. From there, the flea spread to Zanzibar and India.

History

History   For individuals residing in industrialized countries, there usually has been recent travel history to subtropical or tropical areas.

Incubation Period   8 to 12 days after penetration

Duration of Lesions   The flea usually lives 2 to 3 weeks in the skin, then lays eggs and dies.

Skin Symptoms   Infestation occurs most commonly on the feet and lower extremities but can occur at any site. Minor irritation can be noted at time of penetration. Pain and/or pruritus at infested sites; swelling. Subungual lesions are very painful.

Constitutional Symptoms   Only if lesions are secondarily infected

Physical Examination

Skin Lesions

TYPES   Papule or vesicle (6 to 8 mm in diameter) (Figure 30-12) with central black dot produced by the posterior part of the flea's abdominal segments. As eggs mature and abdomen swells, papule becomes a white, pea-sized nodule. With intralesional hemorrhage, it becomes black (Figure 30-12). With severe infestation, nodules and plaques with a honeycombed appearance. If lesions are squeezed, eggs, feces, and internal organs are extruded through pore.

COLOR   Red, bluish, white, black

ARRANGEMENT   Scattered, single or multiple

DISTRIBUTION   Feet, especially under toenails, between toes, plantar aspect of the feet, sparing weight-bearing areas. In sunbathers, any area of exposed skin.

Differential Diagnosis

Staphylococcus aureus paronychia, *Candida* paronychia, myiasis, cercarial dermatitis, scabies, fire ant bite, folliculitis

Laboratory Findings

Microscopic Examination   Material extruded by squeezing lesion shows eggs and body parts of *T. penetrans.*

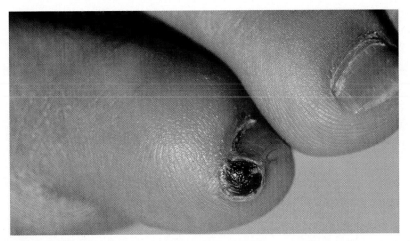

Figure 30-12 Tungiasis *A necrotic, periungual papule with surrounding erythema on the lateral margin of the fifth toe; the larva is visualized by removing the overlying crust.*

Gram's Stain Rule out secondary infection.

Culture Rule out secondary infection.

Dermatopathology Flea in epidermis except for the head, which penetrates into the dermis. Flea has thick cuticle, internal parts, ova, thick band of striated muscle extending from head to terminal abdominal orifice, minute head dwarfed and almost surrounded by engorged body. Lymphocytic, plasmacytic, eosinophilic dermal infiltrate.

Diagnosis

Clinical findings; morphology of flea

Pathogenesis

The recently impregnated female flea penetrates skin of a human host, burrows into epidermis to dermal-epidermal junction, where she feeds on blood drawn from host vessels in superficial dermis. Enlargement of the buried flea to 5 to 8 mm causes local pain in the infested skin. Mature eggs (150 to 200) are extruded singly from a terminal abdominal orifice during a period of 7 to 10 days. The female dies shortly after egg extrusion, and the infested tissues collapse around it; ulcerations can occur at the site. Inflammation and secondary infection can arise if parts of the flea are retained in the tissue.

T. penetrans jumps, most often biting the human host on the feet or, in the natives who frequently squat, the perineum or buttocks.

Course and Prognosis

Most infestations are mild and resolve without complication; they can, however, be complicated by *S. aureus* or streptococcal secondary infection (abscess formation, cellulitis), tetanus, gas gangrene, or autoamputation. Prior infestation does not protect against reinfestation.

Management

Prevention Wear closed-toe footwear and protective clothing; prevent direct contact of skin with soil. Spray heavily infested areas with insecticides.

Treatment Remove flea with needle, scalpel, or curette. Attempt should be made to remove all flea parts. Treat secondary infection. Tetanus prophylaxis. Oral thiabendazole 25 mg/kg/day, or albendazole 400 mg/day for 3 days, effective for heavy infestations.

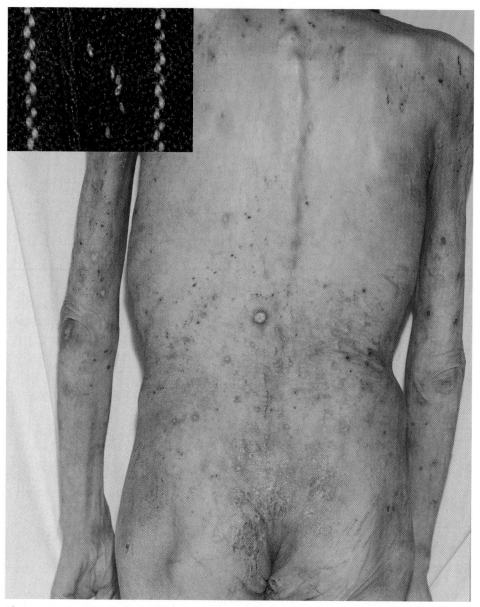

Figure 30-13 Pediculosis corporis   *Pediculosis corporis is caused by* Pediculus humanus corporis *(body louse), which resembles the head louse but is larger in size. The body louse lives in clothing or bedding (insert) and visits the human host only to feed. The host invariably has very poor hygiene. Clinically, nits are seen in the seams of clothing. Sites of feeding may present as red macules, papules, or papular urticaria with central hemorrhagic punctum. Because of the associated pruritus, primary lesions are commonly scratched, resulting in excoriations, eczematous dermatitis, and lichen simplex chronicus, which, in turn, can become secondarily infected.*

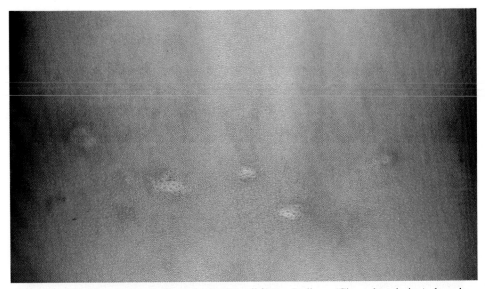

Figure 30-14 Cutaneous reactions to bedbug bites *Bedbugs (*Cimex lectularius*) share human domains, residing in crevices of floors and walls, in bedding, and in furniture. They usually feed only once a week, and less often in cold weather. Bedbugs can travel long distances in search of a human host and can survive for 6 to 12 months without feeding. Bite reactions occur on exposed sites such as the face, neck, arms, and hands, with two to three lesions in a row ("breakfast, lunch, dinner"). In previously unexposed individuals, bite sites appear as erythematous, pruritic macules. In sensitized individuals, intensely pruritic papules, papular urticaria, or vesicles/bullae may arise at the bite sites. Changes secondary to scratching include excoriations, eczematous dermatitis, and secondary infections.*

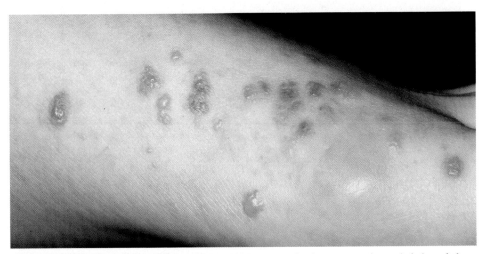

Figure 30-15 Cercarial dermatitis *Cercarial dermatitis, also known as* swimmer's itch *and* clam digger's itch, *is an acute pruritic papular eruption at the sites of cutaneous penetration by* Schistosoma cercariae. *Exposure can be to fresh, brackish, or salt water. In comparison with seabather's eruption, which occurs on areas of the body covered by swimsuits, cercarial dermatitis occurs on exposed sites. Papular urticaria occurs at each site of penetration in previously sensitized individuals. In highly sensitized persons, lesions may progress to eczematous plaques, urticarial wheals, and/or vesicles, reaching a peak 2 to 3 days after exposure. Lesions usually resolve within a week.*

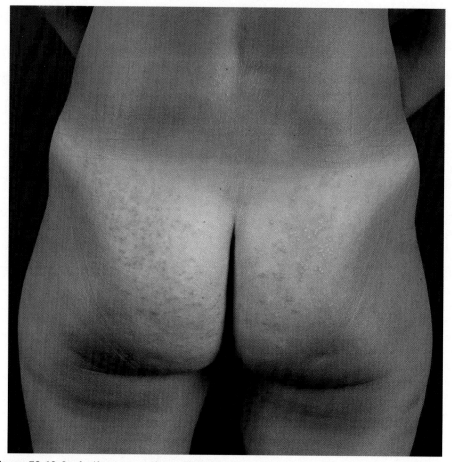

Figure 30-16 Seabather's eruption *Seabather's eruption is caused by exposure to the planula larvae of the sea anemone,* Edwardsiella lineata, *and presents clinically as inflammatory papules hours or days after exposure. In comparison with cercarial dermatitis, which occurs on exposed sites, seabather's eruption occurs at sites covered by bathing apparel while bathing in salt water. Some affected individuals recall a stinging or prickling sensation while in the water. A monomorphous eruption of erythematous papules or papulovesicles is seen most commonly: vesicles, pustules, and papular urticaria. On average, lesions persist for 1 to 2 weeks. In sensitized individuals, the eruption can become progressively more severe with repeated exposures. Topical or systemic corticosteroids provide symptomatic relief.*

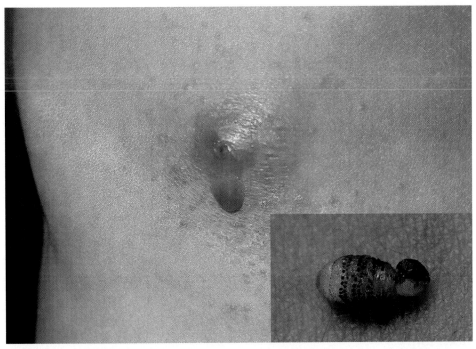

Figure 30-17 Myiasis *Myiasis is an infestation of tissues by the larval form of nonbiting dipterous insects (flies). Flies commonly feed on open wounds, exudates, and skin ulcers and may deposit eggs at these sites. Fly larvae can burrow into injured or normal skin, invading through the epidermis into the dermis. In some cases, larvae move about the subcutis (migratory myiasis), mimicking the pattern of cutaneous larva migrans. Myiasis can arise at any exposed skin site, including the ear, nose, paranasal sinuses, mouth, eye, anus, and vagina, or at any wound site (leg ulcers, ulcerated SCC and BCC, hematomas, umbilical stump).*

In wound myiasis, larvae initially consume necrotic debris but may proceed to feed on normal tissue. Furuncular myiasis occurs following penetration of normal skin by fly larvae; a pruritic papule develops at the site, slowly enlarging over several weeks into a domed nodule (resembles a furuncle). The lesion has a central pore through which the posterior end of the larve intermittently protrudes. The larva can be induced to exit the lesion by covering it with pork fat or petrolatum.

Section 31

SYSTEMIC INFESTATIONS

CUTANEOUS AND MUCOCUTANEOUS LEISHMANIASIS

Leishmaniasis is a parasitic infection caused by many species of the protozoa *Leishmania,* manifested clinically as four major syndromes—cutaneous leishmaniasis (CL) of Old and New World types, mucocutaneous leishmaniasis, diffuse cutaneous leishmaniasis, and visceral leishmaniasis. CL is characterized by development of single or multiple cutaneous papules at the site of a sandfly bite, often evolving into nodules and ulcers, which heal spontaneously with a depressed scar.

Synonyms: Old World leishmaniasis: Baghdad/Delhi boil or button, oriental/Aleppo sore, *bouton d'Orient.* Mucocutaneous leishmaniasis: Espundia. Visceral leishmaniasis: Kala-azar.

Taxonomy

1. Old world leishmaniasis (*a.* urban or dry, recidivans; *b.* rural or wet). 2. New World/American leishmaniasis [*a.* purely cutaneous (ACL); *b.* mucocutaneous (MCL); *c.* disseminated cutaneous (DCL)].

Epidemiology and Etiology

Incidence Estimated 12 million people infected worldwide; 400,000 new cases reported annually; 350 million individuals are at risk of infection

Etiology The clinical symptomatology, whether cutaneous, mucocutaneous, or visceral, depends on the infecting species.

OLD WORLD CUTANEOUS LEISHMANIASIS (OWCL)
  L. tropica major causes wet (rural). *L. t. minor* causes dry (urban).

AMERICAN CUTANEOUS LEISHMANIASIS (ACL)
  CL—*L. mexicana* (chiclero's ulcer, bay sore), *L. amazonensis, L. venezuelensis, L. lainsoni, L. peruviana* (uta), *L. colombiensis, L. guyanensis* (pian bois or forest yaws)

MUCOCUTANEOUS LEISHMANIASIS (MCL)
  L. brasiliensis complex *(L. b. brasiliensis, L. b. panamensis, L. b. guyanensis)*

DIFFUSE CUTANEOUS LEISHMANIASIS (DCL)
  L. m. pifanoi (Venezuela), *L. m. amazonensis* (Brazil), members of the *L. mexicana* complex (Dominican Republic), *L. aethiopica* (Africa)

VISCERAL LEISHMANIASIS (VL) (KALA-AZAR)
  Caused by *L. donovani* complex *(L. donovani, L. infantum, L. chagasi)*

Life Cycle *Leishmania* dimorphic. In mammalian host: amastigote (leishmanial) form—2 to 3 μm in length, oval/round, aflagellate; lives intracellularly in cells of reticuloendothelial system. In GI tract of sandfly/in culture: promastigote (leptomonad) form—10 to 15 μm in length, spindle-shaped, flagellated; extracellular. Speciation: isoenzyme patterns, kinetoplast DNA buoyant densities, specific phlebotomine vectors, monoclonal antibodies, DNA hybridization, DNA restriction endonuclease fragment analysis.

Reservoir Varies with geography and leishmanial species. Zoonosis involves rodents/canines. Mediterranean littoral—dogs. Southern Russia—gerbils.

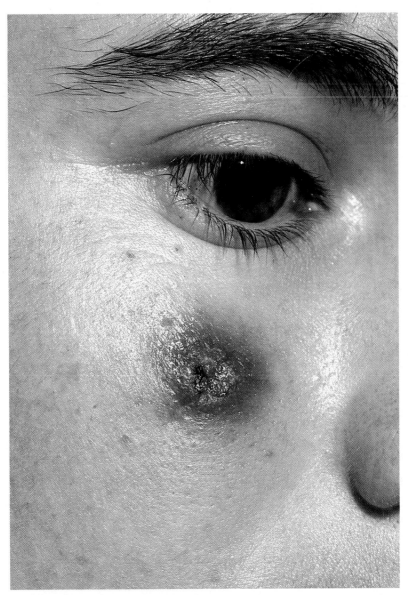

Figure 31-1 Old World cutaneous leishmaniasis *A solitary, inflamed nodule with central necrosis and ulceration on the cheek for one month arising at the site of a sandfly bite.*

Vector Female sandflies of genus *Phlebotomus* (Old World) and *Lutzomyia* and *Psychodopygus* (New World). Breed in cracks in buildings, rubbish, rubble; rodent burrows, termite hills, rotting vegetation. Weak fliers; remain close to ground near breeding site. Ingest amastigotes while feeding on infected mammals, converting to promastigotes in the gut of the sandfly; replicate in gut.

Transmission Promastigotes deposited on skin of host into a small pool of blood drawn by probing sandfly

Season OWCL *L. t. major*—summer through autumn epidemics; OWCL *L. t. minor*—year round; ACL—rainy season

Geography All inhabited continents except Australia

owcl Asia Minor, Middle East, southern Russia, China, the Mediterranean littoral, India, Africa (Sudan, Ethiopia, Congo Basin)

acl, mcl Forests of South and Central America. *L. mexicana* endemic in south-central Texas.

dcl South America, Dominican Republic, Africa

History

Incubation Period Inversely proportional to size of inoculum; shorter in visitors to endemic area. OWCL: *L. t. major,* 1 to 4 weeks; *L. t. minor,* 2 to 8 months; ACL: 2 to 8 weeks or more.

Symptoms Noduloulcerative lesions usually asymptomatic. With secondary bacterial infection, may become painful.

Physical Examination

Skin Findings

TYPES OF LESIONS Primary lesions occur at site of sandfly bite.

OWCL

L. t. minor—single dry ulcer. Papule on face; evolves slowly (Figure 31-1); healing in

>1 year with scar. After healing, peripheral papules may erupt and extend from scar (leishmaniasis recidivans).

L. t. major—multiple exudative ulcers (Figure 31-2). Erythematous papule. Numerous lesions may be present initially, some resolving, others evolving into CL. Persistent papule enlarges to nodule (Figures 31-2 and 31-3). Summit of nodule crusts, oozes; evolves to shallow ulcer with spongy base. *Volcano sign:* volcanic nodule with sloping sides, shallow apical crater covered with crust (Figure 31-2). *Iceberg nodules:* nodules with subcutaneous, endophytic component. Satellite papules: multiple inflammatory papules surrounding (up to 2 cm distant) primary nodule, 2 to 5 mm, lack punctum or crust, appear later in evolution. Lesion fixed for months. Healing begins centrally, spreading centrifugally with resultant scar formation. Scar atrophic, hyperpigmented, irregular (cribriform). Recurrent CL (RCL) occurs several months to several years after the original lesion has healed; small, firm papules to nodules appear on periphery or in scar; duration 60+ years.

ACL or New World CL *L. m. mexicana*—chiclero ulcer or bay sore. Small, erythematous, firm papule. Usually ulcerates, encrusted (Figure 31-4). Enlarges to 3 to 12 cm with raised border. Nonulcerating nodules may become verrucous. ±Lymphangitis, ±regional lymphadenopathy. Isolated lesions on hand or head usually do not ulcerate; heal spontaneously. Ear lesions may persist for years, destroying cartilage.

MCL *L. b. brasiliensis*—one or several lesions on lower extremities, ulcerate, heal spontaneously. After months to years, metastatic lesions may appear in nasopharynx and/or perineum. Associated with nasal obstruction, epistaxis, painful mutilating ulcers (Figure 31-5) (espundia).

DCL Resembles lepromatous leprosy

SHAPE OF INDIVIDUAL LESION May be elongated with long axis along skin crease (Figure 31-2)

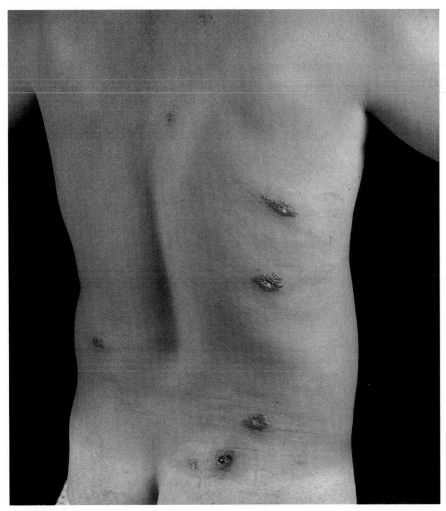

Figure 31-2 Old World cutaneous leishmaniasis *Multiple, crusted nodules on the exposed back, arising at sites of sandfly bites. Many of the lesions resemble a volcano with a central depressed center, i.e., volcano sign.*

DISTRIBUTION OF LESIONS *L. t. major*—exposed sites, especially ankles and legs; in children only, face

MUCOUS MEMBRANES MCL occurs 3 to 10 years after primary ACL in one-third of cases. Nasal mucosa—inflamed, edematous, ulcerative; associated with coryza, epistaxis. Perforation of septum. Ulceration with destruction of nasal fossa, mucosa, cartilage. Lips, pharynx, tonsils, floor of mouth, tongue may be affected; may extend to larynx, trachea, bronchi. Mucosa thickened, granulomatous, bleeds easily. Complicated by difficulty in breathing, feeding, swallowing; malnutrition.

General Examination OWCL: regional lymphadenopathy common. In visceral leishmaniasis VL (kala-azar), bone marrow, liver, spleen are involved.

Differential Diagnosis

Acute CL Insect bite reaction, impetigo, furuncle, carbuncle, ecthyma, anthrax, orf, milker's nodule, tularemia, swimming pool granuloma, tuberculosis cutis, syphilitic gumma, yaws, sporotrichosis, blastomycosis, kerion, myiasis, dracunculosis, molluscum, warts, pyogenic granuloma, tropical ulcer, foreign-body granuloma, keratoacanthoma, basal cell carcinoma, squamous cell carcinoma, metastases, lymphoma, leukemia

Chronic CL and Relapsing CL Lupus vulgaris, leprosy, sarcoidosis, granuloma faciale, Jessner's lymphocytic infiltrate, lymphocytoma cutis, discoid lupus erythematosus, psoriasis, acne, rosacea, cellulitis, erysipelas, keloids, Wegener's granulomatosis, syphilitic gumma

Laboratory and Special Examinations

Leishmanin (Montenegro) Skin Test Of no use in endemic areas. Negative in DCL.

Serology Lacks specificity

Dermatopathology Large macrophages filled with 2- to 4-μm amastigotes (Leishman-Donovan bodies); mixed lymphocytic, plasmacytic infiltrate. In Wright- and Giemsa-stained preparations, the amastigote cytoplasm appears blue, nucleus relatively large and red, distinctive kinetoplast rod-shaped and stains intensely red.

Culture Novy-MacNeal-Nicolle medium at 22° to 28°C for 21 days grows motile promastigotes.

Touch Preparation Macrophages containing organisms: dark, slightly flattened nucleus and rod-shaped kinetoplast observed

Needle Aspiration Visualize amastigote within macrophages

Diagnosis

Clinical suspicion, confirmed by demonstrating amastigotes on smear or in skin biopsy specimen or promastigotes on culture of aspirates or tissue

Pathophysiology

Course determined by host's cellular immunity and species of *Leishmania*. MCL: destructiveness of metastatic lesions due to hypersensitivity to parasite antigens. DCL: leishmanin reaction negative, i.e., selective anergy.

Course and Prognosis

CL Whether caused by *L. tropica* or *L. mexicana*, CL is self-limited. Scarring is increased by secondary bacterial infection.

MCL May extend to secondary sites. Secondary infection common. Mortality from pneumonia.

DCL Progressive; refractory to treatment; cures rare

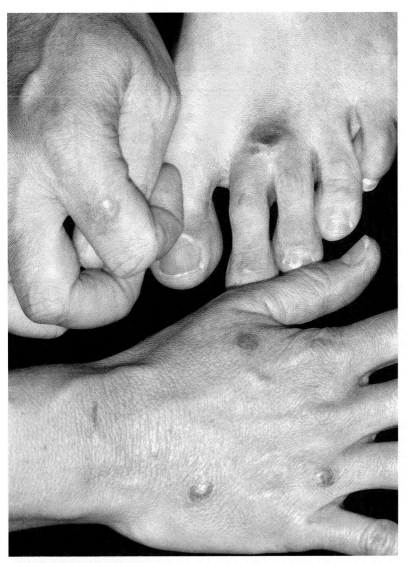

Figure 31-3 Old World cutaneous leishmaniasis *Multiple erythematous papules and nodules on the dorsum of hands and foot in a husband and wife who had been camping in Israel. A facial papule was present in the wife. All lesions resolved spontaneously within 2 to 3 months.*

Management

No chemoprophylaxis for travelers exists. OWCL: Delay specific treatment until ulceration occurs, allowing protective immunity to develop, unless lesions are disfiguring, disabling, persist >6 months.

Lesional Therapy   Local injection of antimonials with or without steroids, cryosurgery, ultrasound-induced hyperthermia, excision, electrosurgery. Topical 15 % paramomycin sulfate, 12 % methylbenzethonium chloride in white paraffin twice daily for 10 days.

Systemic Therapy   For selected CL, MCL, DCL. *Sodium antimony gluconate (Pentostam)* IV or IM in single daily dose of 10 mg/kg for adults and 20 mg/kg for patients <18 years of age for 10 days. *Meglumine antimoniate (Glucantime)* 20 mg/kg daily for 10 days. ECG control. *Amphotericin B* or *pentamidine* or *sodium antimony gluconate plus interferon gamma* for resistant cases. Ketoconazole.

Combined Immunotherapy   Leishmanial antigen in BCG

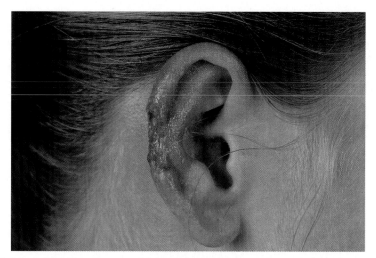

Figure 31-4 New World cutaneous leishmaniasis: chiclero ulcer *A deep ulcer on the helix at the site of a sandfly bite. This variant typically occurs in leishmaniasis acquired in Central and South America.*

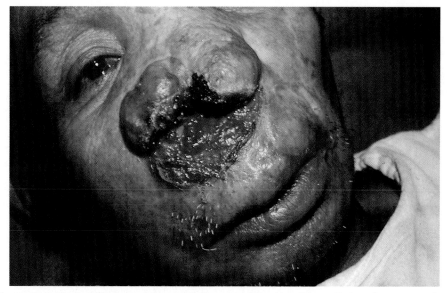

Figure 31-5 Mucocutaneous leishmaniasis: espundia *Painful, mutilating ulceration with destruction of portions of the nose. (Courtesy of Eric Kraus, M.D.)*

Section 32

SEXUALLY TRANSMITTED DISEASES

NEISSERIA GONORRHOEAE

LOCALIZED INFECTION (GONORRHEA)

Gonorrhea is an acute sexually transmitted infection of the mucocutaneous surfaces of the lower genitourinary tract, anorectum, and oropharynx characterized clinically in males by a purulent urethral discharge, but in females infection is often asymptomatic; if untreated, infection can spread to deeper structures with abscess formation and disseminated gonococcal infection (DGI).
Synonyms: Clap, blennorrhagia, blennorrhea.

Epidemiology and Etiology

Age   Young, sexually active; infection of conjunctiva in newborns

Sex   Symptomatic infection more common in males. Pharyngeal and anorectal in homosexual males.

Etiology   *Neisseria gonorrhoeae,* the gonococcus, a gram-negative diplococcus

Incidence   Current estimates are that slightly <1 million new infections with *N. gonorrhoeae* occur in the United States each year, half of which go unreported.

Transmission   Sexually, from partner who is either asymptomatic or who has minimal symptoms. Neonate exposed to infected secretions in birth canal.

Geography   Worldwide

History

Incubation Period

MALES   90 % of males develop urethritis within 5 days of exposure.

FEMALES   Usually >2 weeks when symptomatic; however, up to 75 % of women are asymptomatic.

Skin Symptoms   Urethral discharge, dysuria. Vaginal discharge; deep pelvic or lumbar pain. Copious purulent anal discharge; burning or stinging pain on defecation; tenesmus; blood in/on stool. Mild sore throat.

Physical Examination

Site of Infection

EXTERNAL GENITALIA

Males   Urethral discharge ranging from scanty and clear to purulent and copious

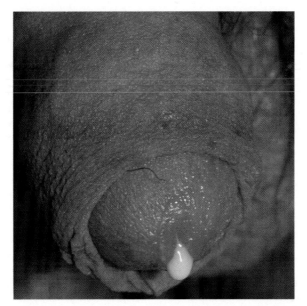

Figure 32-1 Gonorrhea *Purulent, creamy urethral discharge from the distal urethra of a male.*

(Figure 32-1); meatal edema; preputial or penile edema. Balanoposthitis with subpreputial discharge in uncircumcised men; balanitis in circumcised men. Folliculitis or cellulitis of thigh or abdomen. Rare complications of anterior urethritis include infection of: parafrenal sebaceous glands of Tyson, paraurethral ducts, Littré's glands, lacunae of Morgagni, subepithelial and periurethral tissue of the urethra, median raphe, Cowper's ducts, and glands.

Females Periurethral edema, urethritis. Purulent discharge from cervix but no vaginitis. In prepubescent females, vulvovaginitis. Bartholin's abscess.

GENITALIA

Males Prostatitis, epididymitis, vesiculitis, cystitis

Females Pelvic inflammatory disease with signs of peritonitis, endocervicitis, endosalpingitis, endometritis.

ANORECTUM

In females and homosexual males, proctitis with pain and purulent discharge

OROPHARYNX

In females and homosexual males, pharyngitis with erythema.

EYE

Conjunctivitis In newborn, organism is transmitted as newborn passes through birth canal. In adults, rare in industrialized nations but in epidemics in third world countries such as Ethiopia. Usually occurs in the absence of genital infection, copious purulent conjunctival discharge. Can be complicated by corneal ulceration and perforation.

General Examination
DGI Acral hemorrhagic pustules

Differential Diagnosis

Urethritis Genital herpes with urethritis, *Chlamydia trachomatis* urethritis, *Ureaplasma urealyticum* urethritis, *Trichomonas vaginalis* urethritis, Reiter's syndrome

Laboratory and Special Examinations

Gram's Stain Gram-negative diplococci intracellularly in PMNs in exudate (Figure 32-2)

Culture Isolation on gonococcal-selective media, i.e., chocolatized blood agar, Martin-Lewis medium, Thayer-Martin medium. Antimicrobial susceptibility testing important due to resistant strains. Specimen collection sites: heterosexual men—urethra, oropharynx; homosexual men—urethra, rectum, oropharynx; women—cervix, rectum, oropharynx.

Serologic Tests None available for gonorrhea. All patients should have a serologic test for syphilis and should be offered HIV testing.

Diagnosis

Clinical suspicion, confirmed by laboratory findings, i.e., presumptively by identifying gram-negative diplococci intracellularly in PMNs, confirmed by culture

Pathophysiology

Gonococcus has affinity for columnar epithelium, while stratified and squamous epithelia are more resistant to attack; epithelium is penetrated between epithelial cells, causing a submucosal inflammation with PMN reaction with resultant purulent discharge.

Course and Prognosis

Most infections among men produce symptoms that cause the person to seek curative treatment soon enough to prevent serious sequelae—but not soon enough to prevent transmission to others. If not treated, complications due to ascending infection occur: prostatitis—pain upon defecation; epididymitis—swelling of epididymis and pain in walking; cystititis. Many infections among women do not produce recognizable symptoms until complications such as pelvic inflammatory disease (PID) occur. PID, whether symptomatic or asymptomatic, can cause tubal scarring leading to infertility or ectopic pregnancy. Because gonococcal infections among women are often asymptomatic, a primary measure for controlling gonorrhea in the United States has been the screening of high-risk women. DGI more common in women with asymptomatic cervical, endometrial, or tubal infection and homosexual men with asymptomatic rectal or pharyngeal gonorrhea.

Management

Prevention Use of condoms should be encouraged.

Antimicrobial Regimens Most patients with incubating syphilis may be cured by any of the regimens containing ceftriaxone or doxycycline. There is a high frequency of chlamydial infections in persons with gonorrhea, and treatment regimens cover this possibility.

UNCOMPLICATED URETHRAL, ENDOCERVICAL, OR RECTAL INFECTIONS
Recommended Regimens

Ceftriaxone 250 mg IM in a single dose *or*
Cefixime 400 mg PO in a single dose *or*
Ciprofloxacin 500 mg PO in a single dose *or*
Oxofloxacin 400 mg PO in a single dose
  plus
A regimen effective against possible coinfection with *C. trachomatis*, such as doxycycline 100 mg PO b.i.d. for 7 days

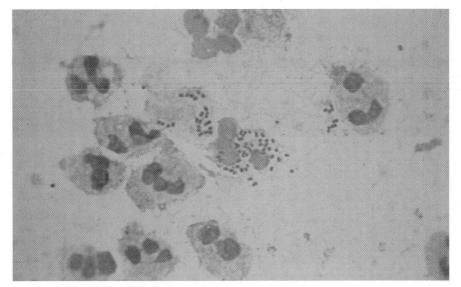

Figure 32-2 *Neisseria gonorrhoeae* *Multiple, gram-negative diplococci within polymorphonuclear leukocytes as well as in the extracellular areas of a smear from a urethral discharge.*

Alternative Regimen

Spectinomycin 2 g IM in a single dose *or*

An injectable cephalosporin (ceftizoxime 500 mg IM in a single dose, cefotaxime 500 mg IM in a single dose, cefotetan 1 g IM in a single dose, or cefoxitin 2 g IM in a single dose)

If gonococcus is known not to be penicillin-resistant, amoxicillin 3 g PO with 1 g probenecid

All of the preceding alternative regimens should be followed by doxycycline 100 mg PO b.i.d for 7 days.

PHARYNGEAL CONOCOCCAL INFECTION Ceftriaxone 250 mg IM once *or* ciprofloxacin 500 mg PO once

Follow-Up Persons with uncomplicated gonorrhea and who are cured with any of the preceding regimens need not return for test-of-cure. Persons with persisting symptoms after treatment should be evaluated by culture for *N. gonorrhoeae,* and any gonococci isolated should be evaluated for antimicrobial susceptibility. Infections detected after treatment with one of recommended regimens more commonly occur because of reinfection rather than treatment failure, indicating a need for improving sex partner referral and patient education. Persistent urethritis, cervicitis, or proctitis also may be caused by *C. trachomatis* and other organisms.

Management of Sex Partners Sex partners should be referred for evaluation and treatment.

DISSEMINATED GONOCOCCAL INFECTION

Disseminated gonococcal infection (DGI) is a systemic infection following the hematogenous dissemination of the gonococcus from infected mucosal sites to skin, tenosynovium, and joints and is characterized by fever, petechial or pustular acral lesions, asymmetric arthralgias, tenosynovitis, or septic arthritis. It is occasionally complicated by hepatitis and, rarely, endocarditis or meningitis. *Synonyms:* Gonococcemia, gonococcal arthritis-dermatitis syndrome.

Epidemiology and Etiology

Age   Young, sexually active

Sex   Young females, homosexual males

Race   Incidence higher in whites than in blacks

Etiology   Gonococcus, i.e., *Neisseria gonorrhoeae,* a gram-negative diplococcus

Incidence   Decreasing in United States

Geography   Worldwide. Incidence varies with local incidence of DGI strains of gonococcus.

Transmission   Sexual. About 1 % of patients with untreated mucosal gonococcal infection develop DGI.

History

Incubation Period   7 to 30 days of mucosal infection (range, from few days to 1 year). Varies with host factors such as menstruation, invasiveness of infecting organism.

Prodrome   Fever, anorexia, malaise, ± shaking chills

History   Recurring symptoms around menses, migratory polyarthralgias

Physical Examination

Skin Findings

TYPES OF LESIONS   1- to 5-mm erythematous macules evolving to hemorrhagic pustules (Figure 32-3) within 24 to 48 hours. Centers at times hemorrhagic/necrotic. Rarely, large hemorrhagic bullae, 3 to 20 in number.

DISTRIBUTION OF LESIONS   Acral, arms more often than legs, near small joints of hands or feet. Difficult to detect in black patients; look in web spaces. Face spared.

MUCOUS MEMBRANES   Usually asymptomatic colonization of oropharynx, urethra, anorectum, endometrium

General Examination

SPECTRUM OF DISEASE   Fever 38° to 39°C usual. Severity varies: DGI with skin lesions alone, classic DGI with skin lesions and tenosynovitis, DGI with septic arthritis, DGI with metastatic infection at other sites.

TENOSYNOVITIS   Common. Single or few sites, acrally. Extensor/flexor tendons and sheaths of hands/feet. Erythema, tenderness, swelling along tendon sheath aggravated by moving tendon.

SEPTIC ARTHRITIS   Joint—red, hot, tender with effusion; asymmetric. Most commonly involved: knee, elbow, ankle, metacarpophalangial/interphalangeal joints of hand, shoulder, hip. Usually only one to two joints involved.

OTHER   Hepatitis, perihepatitis (Fitz-Hugh-Curtis syndrome), myopericarditis, endocarditis, meningitis, perihepatitis. Rarely, pneumonitis, adult respiratory distress syndrome, osteomyelitis.

Differential Diagnosis

Scant, Acral, Hemorrhagic Pustules   Bacteremia: meningococcemia, other bacteremias, endocarditis. Tenosynovitis/arthritis: infectious

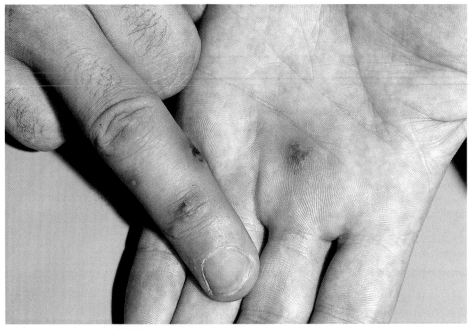

Figure 32-3 Disseminated gonococcal infection *Hemorrhagic, painful pustules on erythe-matous bases on the palm and the finger of the other hand. These lesions occur at acral sites and are few in number.*

arthritis, infectious tenosynovitis, Reiter's syndrome, psoriatic arthritis, SLE.

Laboratory and Special Examinations

Dermatopathology Immunofluorescence of skin lesion biopsy shows gonococcus in 60 %.

Gram's Stain From the male urethra or cervix, may show gonococci.

Culture Mucosal sites yield 80 % to 90 % positive cultures. Skin biopsy, joint fluid, blood have only a 10 % to 30 % chance of positive culture.

Diagnosis

Made on clinical criteria, confirmed by culture of gonococcus from mucosal sites

Pathophysiology

Strains of gonococcus that cause DGI tend to cause little genital inflammation and thereby escape detection. These strains have become uncommon in the United States during the past decade. Most signs and symptoms of DGI are manifestations of immune-complex formation and deposition. Multiple episodes of DGI may be associated with abnormality of terminal complement-component factors.

Course and Prognosis

Untreated, skin/joint lesions often gradually resolve; endocarditis usually fatal.

Management

Prevention Safe sex practices including condom use prevent infection.

Antimicrobial Therapy Hospitalization is recommended for initial therapy, especially for patients who cannot reliably comply with treatment, have uncertain diagnoses, or have purulent synovial effusions or other complications. Patients should be examined for clinical evidence of endocarditis or meningitis. Patients treated for DGI should be treated presumptively for concurrent *C. trachomatis* infection.

> *Recommended initial regimen:* Ceftriaxone 1 g IM or IV every 24 hours
> *Alternative initial regimen:*
> Cefotaxime 1 g IV every 8 hours *or*
> Ceftizoxime 1 g IV every 8 hours *or*
> *For persons allergic to beta-lactam drugs:*
> Spectinomycin 2 g IM every 12 hours
> All regimens should be continued for 24 to 48 hours after improvement begins; then therapy may be switched to one of the following regimens to complete a full week of antimicrobial therapy:
> Cefixime 400 mg PO b.i.d. *or*
> Ciprofloxacin 500 mg PO b.i.d.

NOTE: *Ciprofloxacin is contraindicated for children, adolescents ≤17 years of age, and pregnant and lactating women.*

Management of Sex Partners Gonococcal infection is often asymptomatic in sex partners of patients with DGI. As for uncomplicated infections, patients should be instructed to refer sex partner(s) for evaluation and treatment.

SYPHILIS

Syphilis is a sexually transmitted infection caused by *Treponema pallidum* and characterized by the appearance of a painless ulcer or chancre at the site of inoculation, often associated with regional lymphadenopathy; shortly after inoculation, syphilis becomes a systemic infection with characteristic secondary and tertiary stages. During the past few years, the incidence of syphilis has increased and the clinical course and response to standard therapy may be altered in HIV-infected patients. *Synonyms:* Lues, the great imitator.

Epidemiology

Age In decreasing order: 20 to 39 years, 15 to 19 years, 40 to 49 years

Race All races; in the United States, incidence increasing in African-Americans and Hispanics

Sex Males outnumber females 2:1 to 4:1

Other Factors Until recently, nearly half of all males with syphilis in the United States were homosexual, but this percentage has decreased due to safer sexual practices. The incidence of syphilis, however, has markedly increased in minorities and is associated with exchange of sex for drugs. Associated with the increase in sexually transmitted syphilis is a marked increase in the number of cases of congenital syphilis.

Etiology *T. pallidum*

Classification
Primary syphilis
Secondary syphilis
Early latent syphilis
Late latent syphilis
Syphilis of unknown duration
Late (tertiary) syphilis
Congenital syphilis

PRIMARY SYPHILIS

History

Incubation Period 21 days (average); range 10 to 90 days

Physical Examination

Skin Lesions

TYPE Chancre: button-like papule that develops into a painless erosion and then ulcer with raised border and scanty serous exudate (Figures 32-4 to 32-6). Surface may be crusted. Size: few millimeters to 1 or 2 cm in diameter. Border of lesion may be raised.

COLOR Red, "meaty colored"

PALPATION Most commonly, firm with *indurated* border. Painless. Extragenital chancres particularly on the fingers may be painful. Atypically, genital chancres painful, especially if secondarily infected with *Staphylococcus aureus.*

SHAPE Round or oval

ARRANGEMENT Single lesion. May be few or multiple; kissing lesions. Multiple chancres may occur in HIV-infected patients.

DISTRIBUTION *Sites of Predilection* Male: inner prepuce, coronal sulcus of the glans, shaft, base. Female: cervix, vagina, vulva, clitoris, breast; chancres observed less frequently in women because of their location within vagina or on cervix.
Extragenital Chancres (Figure 32-6) Anus or rectum, mouth, lips, tongue, tonsil, fingers (painful!), toes, breast, nipple

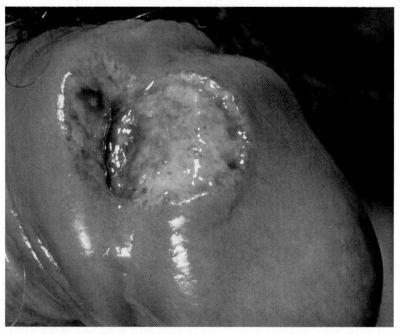

Figure 32-4 Primary syphilis: penile chancre *Large, painless ulcer on the proximal glans penis and adjacent foreskin with erythema and edema of the foreskin; the area surrounding the ulcer is indurated. The chancre arises at the site of inoculation of* T. pallidum.

General Findings Syphilis is a systemic infection; all patients should have a thorough clinical examination. Regional lymphadenopathy appears within 1 week. Nodes are discrete, firm, rubbery, nontender, more commonly unilateral.

Differential Diagnosis

In the differential diagnosis of any genital lesion, primary syphilis should be considered as suspect until ruled out clinically and by specific testing. Chancroid, genital herpes, fixed drug eruption, lymphogranuloma venereum, donovanosis, traumatic ulcer, furuncle, aphthous ulcer.

Diagnosis

Clinical suspicion, confirmed by dark-field examination or serologically

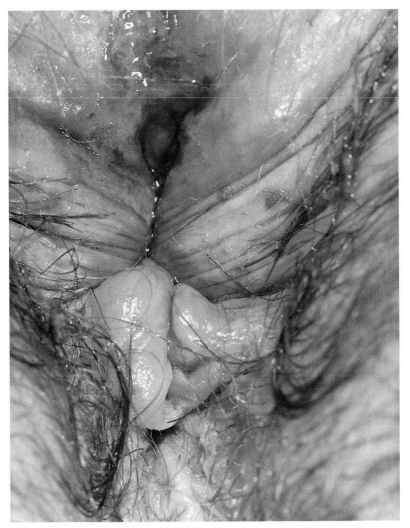

Figure 32-5 Primary syphilis: vulvar chancre *Large, painless ulcer with jagged margins on the posterior introitus.*

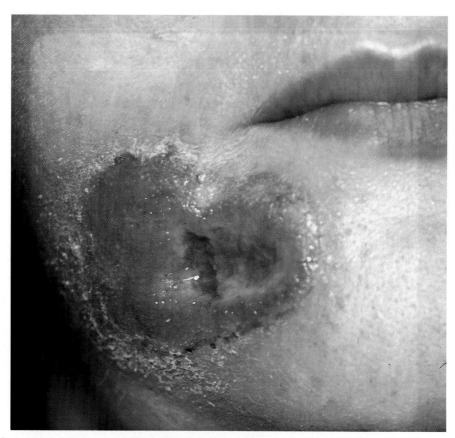

Figure 32-6 Primary syphilis: extragenital chancre *Large, painless ulcer with surrounding erosion on the chin at the site of inoculation of* T. pallidum.

SECONDARY SYPHILIS

History

Secondary syphilis appears 2 to 6 months after primary infection and 2 to 10 weeks after appearance of the primary chancre. Chancre may still be present when secondary lesions appear. Concomitant HIV infection may alter course of secondary syphilis. "Acute illness" syndrome: headache, chills, feverishness, arthralgia, myalgia, malaise, photophobia. Mucocutaneous lesions are asymptomatic.

Duration of Lesions   Weeks

Physical Examination

Skin Lesions

TYPES   Macules and papules 0.5 to 1.0 cm, round to oval (Figure 32-7). However, may be papulosquamous (Figures 32-7 and 32-8), pustular, or acneform. Vesiculobullous lesions occur only in neonatal congenital syphilis (palms and soles). Condylomata lata: soft, flat-topped, moist, red-to-pale papules, nodules, or plaques (Figure 32-9), which may become confluent. Uncommonly, lesions of secondary syphilis and chancre of primary syphilis occur concomitantly.

COLOR   Macules: Pink; papules: brownish red, pink

PALPATION   Papules—firm, Condylomata lata—soft.

SHAPE   Annular, polycyclic, especially on face in dark-skinned individuals. In relapsing secondary syphilis, arciform lesions. Always sharply defined except for macular exanthem.

ARRANGEMENT   Scattered, discrete lesions. Symmetry usual, Asymmetric lesions in relapsing eruption.

DISTRIBUTION   Generalized eruption on the trunk (Figure 32-7); localized eruptions most commonly are scaling and papular localizing, especially on the head (hairline, nasolabial, scalp), neck, *palms* (Figure 32-8), and *soles*. Condylomata lata (Figure 32-9): most commonly in anogenital region and mouth; can be seen on any body surface where moisture can accumulate between intertriginous surfaces, i.e., axillae or toe webs.

HAIR   Two types: diffuse hair loss, including temples and parietal scalp; or patchy, "moth-eaten" alopecia on the scalp and beard area. Loss of eyelashes, lateral third of eyebrows.

MUCOUS MEMBRANES   *Mucous patches,* i.e., small, asymptomatic, round or oval, slightly elevated, flat-topped macules and papules 0.5 to 1.0 cm in diameter, covered by hyperkeratotic white to gray membrane, occurring on the oral or genital mucosa; *split papules* at the angles of the mouth

General Examination   ±Fever. Generalized lymphadenopathy (cervical, suboccipital, inguinal, epitrochlear, axillary) and splenomegaly.

ASSOCIATED FINDINGS   *Diffuse pharyngitis. Acute bacterial iritis. Periostitis* of long bones, particularly tibia (nocturnal pain) and arthralgia or hydrarthrosis of knees or ankles without x-ray changes. *Meningovascular reaction* (CSF positive for inflammatory markers). Hepatosplenomegaly, cardiac arrhythmia, nephritis, cystitis, prostatitis, gastritis.

Course

In secondary syphilis there may be only one or several recurrent eruptions that appear after month-long asymptomatic intervals. The first secondary syphilis eruption is a relatively faint exanthem, always macular, pink, and lesions are ill-defined; later lesions of early syphilis are papular, brownish (Figure 32-7), and tend to be more localized (Figures 32-8 and 32-9).

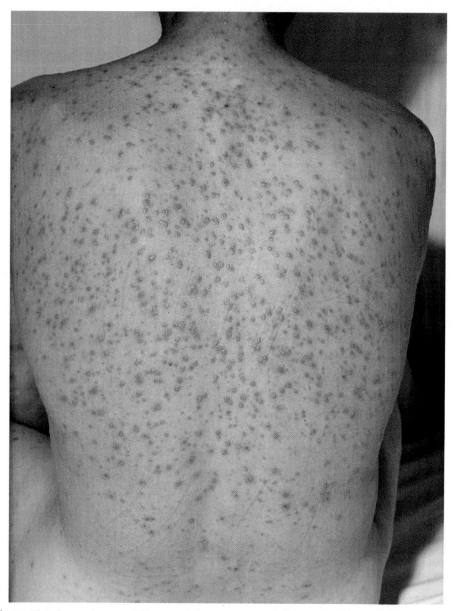

Figure 32-7 Secondary syphilis: papulosquamous eruption on trunk *Scaling, erythematous papules and macules on the back. The eruption must be differentiated from guttate psoriasis and pityriasis rosea.*

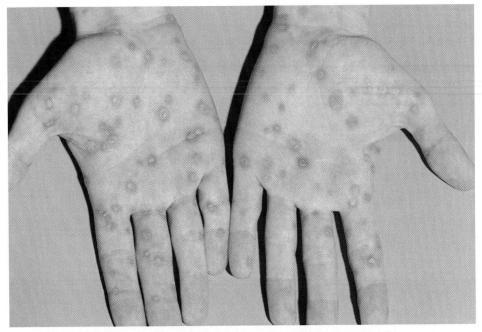

Figure 32-8 Secondary syphilis: papulosquamous eruption on palms *Discrete, copper-colored, keratotic papules on the palms and fingers.*

Differential Diagnosis

Drug eruption (e.g., captopril), pityriasis rosea, viral exanthem, infectious mononucleosis, tinea corporis, tinea versicolor, scabies, "id" reaction, condylomata acuminata, acute guttate psoriasis, lichen planus

Diagnosis

Clinical suspicion confirmed by dark-field examination and/or serology. Dark-field is positive in all secondary syphilis lesions except for macular exanthem.

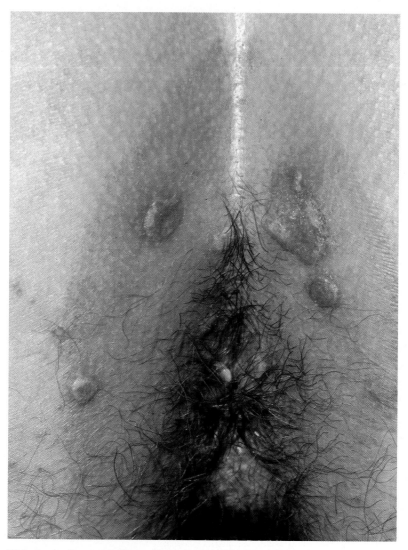

Figure 32-9 Secondary syphilis: condylomata lata *Soft, flat-topped, moist, pink-tan papules and nodules on the perineum and perianal area. The lesions are teeming with* T. pallidum.

LATENT SYPHILIS

Latent syphilis is that stage in which there are no clinical signs or symptoms of the infection. The diagnosis is made only after a careful history and physical examination have ruled out symptoms and signs of active infection. The serologic tests for syphilis (STS) are positive; CSF is normal. Early latent syphilis (<2 years) is distinguished from late latent disease (>2 years). All patients with syphilis have latent disease at some time during the course of the illness; some patients have only latent-stage syphilis and are diagnosed by a positive STS. Latent disease does not preclude infectiousness, nor development of gummatous skin lesions, cardiovascular lesions, or neurosyphilis. A pregnant woman with latent disease can infect her fetus, with congenital syphilis occurring in her baby.

TERTIARY SYPHILIS

History

Duration of Lesions In *untreated* syphilis, 15 % of patients developed late benign syphilis, mostly skin lesions; tertiary syphilis is now very rare. Previously, patients presenting with tertiary syphilis gave history of lesions of 3 to 7 years' duration (range 2 to 60 years); gumma develop by fifteenth year.

Skin Symptoms None

Physical Examination

Skin Lesions

NODULOULCERATIVE SYPHILIDES Simulate lupus vulgaris (cutaneous tuberculosis)
  Type Plaques and nodules with scars healed in the center with or without psoriasiform scales and with or without ulceration (Figure 32-10). Typically, and in contrast to lupus vulgaris, syphilides do not recur in scars but rather on their periphery.
  Color Brown
  Palpation Firm
  Arrangement Grouped, serpiginous (snake-like), annular, polycyclic, scalloped borders
  Distribution Solitary isolated lesions (Figure 32-10): arms (extensor aspects), back, or face

GUMMA The term *gumma* (Latin: "gum") describes the rubbery lump or deep granulomatous lesion found in the subcutaneous tissue, having a tendency for necrosis and ulceration.
  Type Nodule, with ulceration, "punched out"

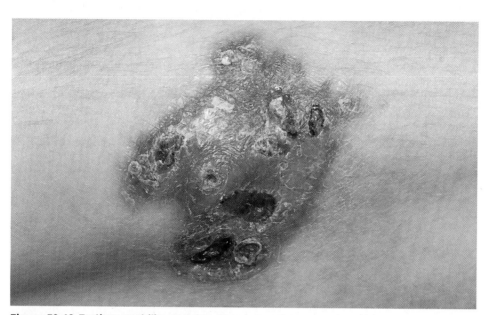

Figure 32-10 Tertiary syphilis: nodular ulcer type *Asymptomatic, red-brown, translucent, crusted, ulcerated plaque with serpiginous borders.*

Palpation   Hard

Arrangement   Isolated

Distribution   Anywhere, but especially on the scalp, face, chest (sternoclavicular), and calf

General Examination   25 % of patients have neurosyphilis or cardiovascular syphilis.

Differential Diagnosis

Cutaneous tuberculosis, cutaneous atypical mycobacterial infection, malignancy such as lymphoma, deep fungal infections, furuncle

Diagnosis

Clinical findings, confirmed by STS and lesional skin biopsy; dark-field examination always negative, silver impregnation of histologic sections for demonstration of spirochetes only very rarely positive.

SYPHILIS IN HIV DISEASE

HIV-infected individuals with neurosyphilis are more likely to present with uveitis or retinitis and have significantly higher serum RPR titers. Some, however, fail to respond to *T. pallidum* infection with antibody formation (i.e., negative STS).

Diagnosis

HIV testing is advised for all sexually active patients with syphilis. Neurosyphilis should be considered in the differential diagnosis of neurologic disease in HIV-infected persons. When clinical findings suggest syphilis but serologic tests are negative or confusing, alternative tests such as biopsy of lesions, dark-field examination, and direct fluorescent antibody staining of lesion material should be used.

LABORATORY AND SPECIAL EXAMINATIONS IN SYPHILIS

Dark-Field Examination Dark-field examination is a simple and reliable test to demonstrate the causative agent. The chancre is debrided from crusts and cleaned with saline swabs and, if not primarily eroded or ulcerated, scarified with a scalpel by gentle scraping, blotted until bleeding stops, and then squeezed between fingers (gloves!) until serous fluid emerges on surface or base of the ulcer. Serous exudate is removed by a glass capillary and pipetted onto microscopic slide, covered with a coverslip, and examined in a dark-field microscope. *Treponema pallidum* is recognized as a corkscrew-like organism, 5 to 20 μm in length, showing rotatory, pocket knife-like kinking and harmonica-like contractile movements. In contrast to saprophytic spirochetes, it does not, however, exhibit locomotion. Dark-field examination is positive in primary chancre and papular lesions of secondary syphilis, in particular condylomata lata. Unreliable in oral cavity because of the presence of saprophytic spirochetes, and negative in patients treated systematically or topically with antibiotics. In the latter case the regional lymph node is punctured and the aspirate is examined in the dark-field microscope.

Direct Fluorescent Antibody Test Fluorescent antibodies are used to detect *T. pallidum* in exudate from lesion, lymph node aspirate, or tissue. Identification of *T. pallidum* makes a definitive diagnosis.

Serologic Tests Presumptive diagnosis is possible with use of two types of serologic tests for syphilis (STS): (1) nontreponemal (cardiolipin-VDRL, RPR) and (2) treponemal (FTA-ABS, MHA-TP). The use of one type of test alone is not sufficient for diagnosis. Nontreponemal test antibody titers usually correlate with disease activity; results are reported quantitatively. A four-fold change in titer is necessary to demonstrate a substantial difference between two nontreponemal test results. A positive treponemal test usually remains so for a lifetime, regardless of treatment or disease activity (15 % to 25 % of patients treated during primary stage may revert to being serologically nonreactive after 2 to 3 years). Treponemal test antibody titers correlate poorly with disease activity and should not be used to assess response to treatment.

PRIMARY SYPHILIS Positive reactions develop in the third to fourth week after infection or concomitantly and up to 1 week after appearance of the chancre. Untreated primary syphilis has a positive FTA-ABS *T. pallidum* hemagglutination (TPHA)] test (91 %) at 6 weeks after infection, compared with VDRL (88 %). Cardiolipin tests become nonreactive 1 year after adequate treatment. Specific *Treponema* antigen tests (FTA-ABS, TPHA) usually remain positive at low titers.

SECONDARY SYPHILIS Nontreponemal serologic tests (e.g., VDRL) are always positive (>1:32). FTA-ABS is 99.2 % positive, as is TPHA. HIV-infected individuals with secondary syphilis rarely may have negative STS. Beware of false-negative STS resulting from *prozone phenomenon* (presence of excess antibody results in failure of the flocculation reaction and thus a false nonreactive test). Nontreponemal serologic tests become nonreactive 24 months after adequate treatment; treponemal serologic tests usually remain reactive.

TERTIARY SYPHILIS STS is usually highly reactive, but false-negative nontreponemal tests are possible.

NOTE *Testing for HIV infection is advised for all patients with syphilis.*

False-Positive Serologic Tests for Syphilis

FALSE-POSITIVE REACTIONS OCCUR WITH FTA-ABS FOR THE FOLLOWING REASONS Technical error, inefficient sorbents, genital herpes simplex, pregnancy, lupus erythematosus (systemic or skin only), alcoholic cirrhosis, scleroderma, mixed connective tissue disease

FALSE-POSITIVE REACTIONS OF NONTREPONEMAL TESTS ARE ASSOCIATED WITH THE FOLLOWING *Transient reactors:* technical error (low titer), *Mycoplasma* pneumonia, enterovirus infection, infectious mononucleosis, pregnancy, IVDU, and less common causes (advanced tuberculosis, scarlet fever, viral pneumonia, brucellosis, rat-bite fever, relapsing fever, leptospirosis, measles, mumps, lymphogranuloma venereum, malaria, trypanosomiasis, varicella. *Chronic*

reactors: malaria, leprosy, SLE, IDVU, other connective tissue disorders, elder population, Hashimoto's thyroiditis, rheumatoid arthritis, reticuloendothelial malignancy, familial false-positives, idiopathic.

NOTE *If no history of possible early lesions, or no evidence of congenital syphilis based on patient's history, or no sexual exposure except to individuals who are known to have a negative STS, then diagnosis of false-positive is probably correct. False positive reactions to* both *treponemal and nontreponemal tests are highly unlikely.*

Dermatopathology In primary and secondary syphilis, lesional skin biopsy shows central thinning or ulceration of epidermis. Lymphocytic and plasmacytic dermal infiltrate. Proliferation of capillaries and lymphatics with endarteritis; may have thrombosis and small areas of necrosis. Dieterle stain demonstrates spirochetes.

Pathophysiology

Treponeme invades through mucous membrane or skin and divides locally, with resulting host inflammatory response and chancre formation, either a single lesion or, at times, multiple lesions. Later syphilis is essentially a vascular disease, lesions occurring secondary to obliterative endarteritis of terminal arterioles and small arteries and by the resulting inflammatory and necrotic changes.

Course and Prognosis

Even without treatment, chancre will heal completely within a 4- to 6-week period, the infection either becoming latent or clinical manifestations of secondary syphilis appearing. Secondary syphilis usually manifests as macular exanthem initially; after weeks, lesions will resolve spontaneously and recur as maculopapular or papular eruptions. In 20 % of untreated cases, up to three to four such recurrences followed by periods of clinical remission may occur over a period of 1 year. The infection then enters a latent stage, in which there are no clinical signs or symptoms of the disease. After untreated syphilis has persisted for more than 4 years, it is rarely communicable, except in the case of the pregnant woman, who, if untreated, may transmit syphilis to the fetus, regardless of the duration of her disease. Gummas hardly ever heal spontaneously. Noduloulcerative syphilides undergo spontaneous partial healing, but new lesions appear at the periphery.

Management

Antimicrobial Therapy

PRIMARY AND SECONDARY SYPHILIS AND EARLY LATENT SYPHILIS OF LESS THAN 1 YEAR'S DURATION

Recommended Regimen   Benzathine penicillin G, 2.4 million units IM, in one dose

Alternative Regimen for Penicillin-Allergic Patients (Nonpregnant)

Doxycycline, 100 mg PO b.i.d. for 2 weeks, *or*

Tetracycline, 500 mg PO q.i.d. for 2 weeks, *or*

Erythromycin, 500 mg PO q.i.d. for 2 weeks, *or*

Ceftriaxone, 250 mg IM once a day for 10 days

Jarisch-Herxheimer Reaction   An acute febrile reaction, often accompanied by chills, fever, malaise, nausea, headache, myalgia, arthralgia, that may occur after any therapy for syphilis. May occur within hours after treatment, subsiding within 24 hours. More common in patients with early syphilis; developing lesions of secondary syphilis may first appear at this time. Treatment: reassurance, bed rest, aspirin. Pregnant patients should be warned that early labor may occur.

LATE LATENT SYPHILIS OF MORE THAN 1 YEAR'S DURATION, GUMMAS, AND CARDIOVASCULAR SYPHILIS

Recommended Regimen   Benzathine penicillin G, 7.2 million units total, administered as three doses of 2.4 million units IM, given 1 week apart for 3 consecutive weeks.

Alternative Regimen for Penicillin-Allergic Patients (Nonpregnant)

Doxycycline, 100 mg PO b.i.d. for 4 weeks, *or*

Tetracycline, 500 mg PO q.i.d. for 4 weeks

NEUROSYPHILIS

Recommended Regimen   Aqueous crystalline penicillin G, 12 to 24 million units administered 2 to 4 million units every 4 hours IV, for 10 to 14 days

Alternative Regimen (If Outpatient Compliance Can Be Ensured)   Procaine penicillin, 2 to 4 million units IM daily, *and* probenecid, 500 mg PO q.i.d., both for 10 to 14 days

SYPHILIS IN HIV-INFECTED PATIENTS   Penicillin regimens should be used whenever possible for all stages of syphilis in HIV-infected patients. Some authorities advise CSF examination and/or treatment with a regimen appropriate for neurosyphilis for all patients coinfected with syphilis and HIV, regardless of the clinical stage of syphilis. Patients should be followed clinically and with quantitative nontreponemal serologic tests (VDRL, RPR) at 1, 2, 3, 6, 9, and 12 months after treatment. Patients with early syphilis whose titers increase or fail to decrease fourfold within 6 months should undergo CSF examination and be re-treated. In such patients, CSF abnormalities could be due to HIV-related infection, neurosyphilis, or both.

Management of Sex Partners   Sex partners should be referred for evaluation and treatment.

CHANCROID

Chancroid is an acute, sexually transmitted infection characterized by a *painful* ulcer at the site of inoculation, usually on the external genitalia, and the development of suppurative regional lymphadenopathy.

Synonyms: Soft chancre, ulcus molle, sore sore, chancre mou.

Epidemiology and Etiology

Sex Young males. Lymphadenitis more common in males.

Etiology *Hemophilus ducreyi,* a gram-negative streptobacillus

Transmission Most likely during sexual intercourse with partner who has *H. ducreyi* genital ulcer

Incidence Underreported. In 1994, 773 cases reported to CDC in the United States.

Geography Uncommon in industrialized nations; microepidemics introduced sporadically from tropical countries. Endemic in tropical and subtropical third world countries, especially in poor, urban, and seaport populations.

History

Incubation Period 4 to 7 days

Prodrome None

Travel History Sexually active during visit to country where chancroid is endemic. Possible contact with prostitute.

Physical Examination

Skin Findings

TYPES OF LESIONS Primary lesion: tender papule with erythematous halo that evolves to pustule, erosion, and ulcer. Ulcer is usually quite *tender* or *painful.* Its borders are sharp, undermined, and *not* indurated (Figure 32-11). Its base is friable with granulation tissue and covered with gray to yellow exudate. Edema of prepuce common.

SHAPE OF INDIVIDUAL LESION Ulcer may be singular or multiple, merging to form large or giant ulcers (>2 cm) with a serpiginous shape.

DISTRIBUTION OF LESIONS Multiple ulcers (Figure 32-12) develop by autoinoculation. Male: prepuce, frenulum, coronal sulcus, glans, shaft. Female: fourchette, labia, vestibule, clitoris, vaginal wall by direct extension from introitus, cervix, perianal. Extragenital lesions: breast, fingers, thighs, oral mucosa.

General Examination Painful inguinal lymphadenitis (usually unilateral) occurs in 50 % of patients 1 to 2 weeks after primary lesion. Buboes occur with overlying erythema and may drain spontaneously.

Differential Diagnosis

Genital ulcer: genital herpes, primary syphilis, donovanosis, lymphogranuloma venereum, secondarily infected human bites or traumatic lesions. *Tender inguinal mass:* incarcerated hernia, plague, tularemia.

Laboratory and Special Examinations

Gram's Stain Of scrapings from ulcer base or pus from bubo, attempt to see small clusters or parallel chains of gram-negative rods. Interpretation difficult due to presence of contaminating organisms in ulcers.

Culture Special growth requirements; isolation difficult. Using special media, sensitivity is no higher than 80 %.

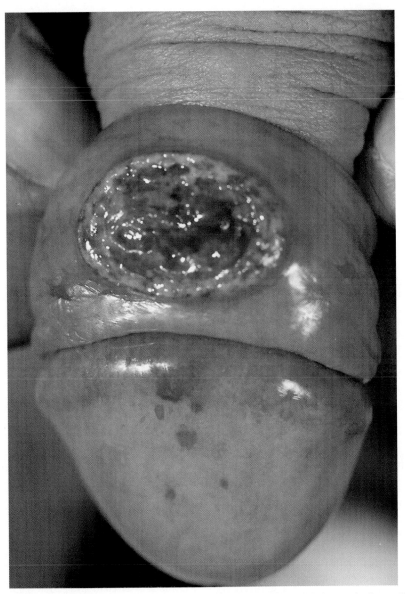

Figure 32-11 Chancroid *Painful ulcer with marked surrounding erythema and edema.* (Courtesy of Alfred Eichmann, M.D.)

Serologic Tests None available. Patients should be tested for HIV infection at time of diagnosis. Patients also should be tested 3 months later for both syphilis and HIV infection if initial results are negative.

Dermatopathology May be helpful. Organism rarely demonstrated.

PCR Detects *H. ducreyi* DNA sequences

Diagnosis

The combination of a painful ulcer with tender lymphadenopathy (which occurs in one-third of patients) is suggestive of chancroid and, when accompanied by suppurative inguinal lymphadenopathy, is almost pathognomonic.

Definitive Diagnosis Made by isolation of *H. ducreyi* on culture

Probable Diagnosis Made if a person has one or more painful genital ulcers and (1) no evidence of *T. pallidum* infection by dark-field examination of ulcer exudate or by STS performed at least 7 days after onset of ulcers and (2) either the clinical presentation of the ulcer(s) is not typical of disease caused by HSV or the HSV test results are negative.

Pathophysiology

Poorly studied. *H. ducreyi* is inoculated through small breaks in the epidermis or mucosa. Primary infection develops at the site of inoculation, followed by lymphadenitis. Bubo formation occurs with scant organisms and an exuberant acute inflammatory response. The role of the immune response is unknown. Cofactor for HIV transmission: Chancroid is the STD most strongly associated with increased risk for HIV transmission. About 10 % of patients with chancroid may be coinfected with *T. pallidum* or HSV.

Course and Prognosis

Patients should be reexamined 3 to 7 days after initiation of therapy. If treatment is successful, ulcers improve symptomatically within 3 days and improve objectively within 7 days after therapy. If no clinical improvement is evident, diagnosis may be incorrect, coinfection with another STD agent exists, the patient is HIV-infected, treatment was not taken as instructed, or the *H. ducreyi* strain causing infection is resistant to the prescribed antimicrobial. The time required for complete healing is related to the size of the ulcer; large ulcers may require ≥ 2 weeks. Complete resolution of fluctuant lymphadenopathy is slower than that of ulcers and may require needle aspiration through adjacent intact skin—even during successful therapy. In HIV-infected persons, healing may be slower, and treatment failures may occur; longer treatment regimens may be advisable.

Management

Prevention Condom use

Antimicrobial Therapy

RECOMMENDED REGIMEN

Azithromycin, 1 g PO in a single dose, *or*
Ceftriaxone, 250 mg IM in a single dose, *or*
Erythromycin, 500 mg PO q.i.d. for 10 days

ALTERNATIVE REGIMEN

Amoxicillin, 500 mg, plus clavulanic acid, 125 mg PO t.i.d. for 7 days, *or*
Ciprofloxacin, 500 mg PO b.i.d. for 3 days

Management of Sex Partners Sex partners should be referred for evaluation and treatment.

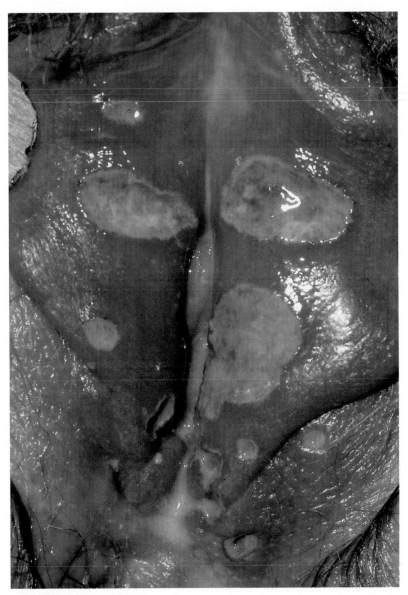

Figure 32-12 Chancroid *Multiple, painful, punched-out ulcers with undermined borders on the vulva occurring following autoinoculation.*

DONOVANOSIS

Donovanosis is a chronic, progressively destructive bacterial infection of the genital region, characterized by ulceration and epitheliomatous hyperplasia.
Synonyms: Granuloma inguinale, granuloma venereum.

Epidemiology and Etiology

Sex   Young males

Etiology   *Calymmatobacterium granulomatis,* an encapsulated gram-negative rod

Transmission   Poorly studied. Venereal but also nonvenereal transmission occurs.

Geography   Endemic foci in tropical and subtropical environments (India, Caribbean, Africa, aborigines in Australia). Rare in United States, Canada, Europe.

History

Incubation Period   8 to 80 days

Travel History   Sexual exposure in endemic area

History   Genital ulcers are relatively painless.

Physical Examination

Skin Lesions

TYPES   Primary lesion: button-like papule or subcutaneous nodule that ulcerates within a few days. Ulcers have beefy-red granulation tissue base with sharply defined edges. Fibrosis occurs concurrently with extension of ulcer. Lymphedema may follow with elephantiasis of penis, scrotum, vulva.

DISTRIBUTION   *Males*   Prepuce or glans, penile shaft, scrotum
Females   Labia minora, mons veneris, fourchette. Ulcerations then spread by direct extension or autoinoculation to inguinal and perineal skin. Extragenital lesions occur in mouth, lips, throat, face, GI tract, and bone.

VARIANTS   *Ulcerovegetative (Figure 32-13)*
Develops from the nodular variant; large, spreading, exuberant ulcers
Nodular   Soft, red nodules that eventually ulcerate with bright red granulating bases
Hypertrophic   Proliferative reaction; formation of large vegetating masses
Cicatricial   Spreading scar tissue formation associated with spread of infection

LATE SEQUELA   Squamous cell carcinoma of genital skin

General Examination   Regional lymph node enlargement is uncommon. Large subcutaneous nodule may mimic a lymph node, i.e., pseudobubo.

Differential Diagnosis

Genital ulcer(s): syphilitic chancre, chancroid, lymphogranuloma venereum, cutaneous tuberculosis, cutaneous amebiasis, filariasis, squamous cell carcinoma. *Perianal hypertrophic donovanosis:* condylomata acuminata, condylomata lata.

Laboratory and Special Examinations

Touch or Crush Preparation   Of punch biopsy stained with Wright's or Giemsa's stain shows Donovan bodies in cytoplasm of macrophages. Clinical variants differ in quantity of organisms.

Dermatopathology   Extensive acanthosis and dense dermal infiltrate, mainly plasma cells and histiocytes. Large mononuclear cells containing cytoplasmic inclusions (Donovan bodies), i.e., *C. granulomatis,* are pathognomonic.

Serology   STS to rule out syphilis

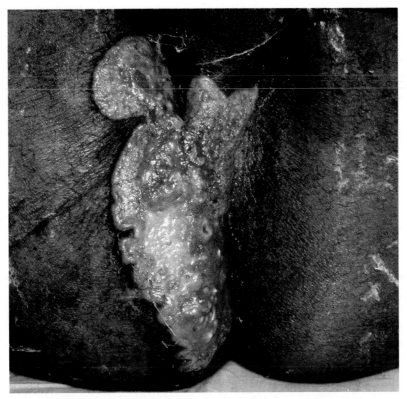

Figure 32-13 Donovanosis: ulcerovegetative type *Extensive granulation tissue formation, ulceration, and scarring of the perineum, scrotum, and penis.*

Diagnosis

Clinical diagnosis excluding other causes of genital ulcer(s) using touch preparation of biopsied tissue

Pathophysiology

Poorly understood. Mildly contagious. Repeated exposure necessary for clinical infection to occur. In most cases, lesions cannot be detected in sexual contacts.

Course and Prognosis

Little tendency toward spontaneous healing. Following antibiotic treatment, lesions often heal with depigmentation of reepithelialized skin.

Management

Prevention   Encourage use of condoms.

Most Effective

Chloramphenicol, 500 mg PO every 8 hours, *or*
Gentamycin, 1 mg/kg IV b.i.d., *or*
Tetracycline, 500 mg PO q.i.d. for 3 to 4 weeks (until ulcers have healed)

Alternatives

Streptomycin, 1 g IM b.i.d., *or*
Ampicillin, 500 mg PO q.i.d. for up to 12 weeks
Erythromycin, 500 mg PO q.i.d., *or*
Cotrimoxazole, 2 tablets PO every 12 hours for 10 days

Management of Sex Partners   Sex partners should be referred for evaluation and treatment.

LYMPHOGRANULOMA VENEREUM

Lymphogranuloma venereum (LGV) is a sexually transmitted infection manifested by an infrequent primary genital lesion, secondary lymphadenitis with bubo formation and/or proctitis, and late infrequent sequelae of fibrosis, edema, and fistula formation.
Synonym: Lymphogranuloma inguinale.

Epidemiology and Etiology

Age Third decade, while most sexually active

Race Most cases in nonwhites, but probably no true racial difference

Sex Acute infection much more common in males. Anorectal syndrome more common in women and homosexual men.

Etiology *Chlamydia trachomatis,* immunotypes or serovars L$_1$, L$_2$, L$_3$

Transmission *Chlamydia* in purulent exudate is inoculated onto the skin or mucosa of a sexual partner and gains entry through minute lacerations and abrasions.

Geography Sporadic in North America, Europe, Australia, and most of Asia and South America. Endemic in East and West Africa, India, parts of southeastern Asia, South America, and the Caribbean.

History

Incubation Period 3 to 12 days or longer for primary stage; 10 to 30 days (but up to 6 months) for secondary stage

Travel History In North America and Europe, most cases occur in patients who have traveled to endemic areas, where they were sexually active.

Symptoms

PRIMARY STAGE Painless herpetiform erosion or ulceration at the site of inoculation. The majority of patients do not present with this finding.

SECONDARY STAGE *Inguinal Syndrome* Constitutional symptoms (fever, malaise) associated with inguinal buboes. Severe local pain in buboes. Lower abdominal and back pain.
Anogenitorectal Syndrome Anal pruritus, rectal discharge, fever, rectal pain, tenesmus, constipation, "pencil" stools, weight loss

Physical Examination

Skin Lesions

PRIMARY STAGE *Types* Papule, shallow erosion or ulcer, grouped small erosions or ulcers (herpetiform), or nonspecific urethritis. In males, cordlike lymphangitis of dorsal penis may follow. Lymphangial nodule (bubonulus) may occur. Bubonuli may rupture, resulting in sinuses and fistulas of urethra and deforming scars of penis. In females, cervicitis, perimetritis, salpingitis may occur.
Distribution At the site of inoculation. Males: coronal sulcus, frenum, prepuce, penis, urethra, glans, scrotum. Females: posterior vaginal wall, fourchette, posterior lip of cervix, vulva. When primary lesion occurs intraurethrally, presentation is of a nonspecific urethritis with a thin, mucopurulent discharge.
Other Erythema nodosum in 10% of cases. Erythema multiforme, scarlatiniform eruptions, urticaria. Primary inoculation of mouth or pharynx results in lymphadenitis of submaxillary or cervical lymph nodes.

SECONDARY STAGE *Inguinal Syndrome* Unilateral bubo in two-thirds of cases (Figure 32-14). Marked edema and erythema of skin overlying node. One-third of inguinal buboes rupture; two-thirds slowly involute. "Groove" sign: inflammatory mass of fem-

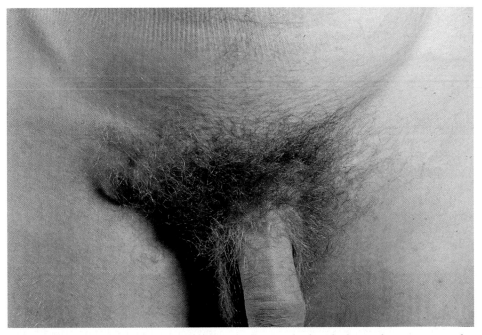

Figure 32-14 *Lymphogranuloma venereum* *Striking tender lymphadenopathy occurring at the femoral and inguinal lymph nodes separated by a groove made by Poupart's ligament (groove sign).*

oral and inguinal nodes separated by depression or groove made by Poupart's ligament. 75 % of cases have deep iliac node involvement with a pelvic mass which seldom suppurates.

Anogenitorectal Syndrome In individuals who practice receptive anal intercourse, proctocolitis, hyperplasia of intestinal and perirectal lymphatic tissue. Resultant perirectal abscesses, ischiorectal and rectovaginal fistulas, anal fistulas, rectal stricture. Overgrowth of lymphatic tissue results in lymphorrhoids (resembling hemorrhoids) or perianal condylomata.

Esthiomene Elephantiasis of genitalia, usually females, which may ulcerate, occurring 1 to 20 years after primary infection

General Examination

ANOGENITORECTAL SYNDROME Lower abdominal tenderness, pelvic colon thickened, enlarged perirectal nodes

Differential Diagnosis

Primary Stage Genital herpes, primary syphilis, chancroid

Inguinale Syndrome Incarcerated inguinal hernia, plague, tularemia, tuberculosis, genital herpes, syphilis, chancroid, Hodgkin's disease

Anogenitorectal Syndrome Rectal stricture caused by rectal cancer, trauma, actinomycosis, tuberculosis, schistosomiasis

Esthiomene Filariasis, mycosis

Laboratory and Special Examinations

Frei Skin Test Of historical interest only. Positive delayed hypersensitivity to standardized antigen Lygranum indicates past or present infection. Positive 2 to 8 weeks after infection begins. Frei antigen is common to all *Chlamydia*. Positive test is not diagnostic of LGV.

Serologic Tests Complement-fixation (CF) test more sensitive and reactive earlier than Frei test. Active LGV usually has titer ≥1:64. Microimmunofluorescence test most sensitive and specific test, identifying infecting serovar.

Culture *C. trachomatis* can be cultured on tissue-culture cell lines in up to 30 % of cases.

Dermatopathology Not pathognomonic. Primary stage: small stellate abscesses surrounded by histiocytes, arranged in palisade pattern. Late stage: epidermal acanthosis/papillomatosis; dermis edematous, lymphatics dilated with fibrosis and lymphoplasmocytic infiltrate.

Diagnosis

By serologic tests and by exclusion of other causes of inguinal lymphadenopathy or genital ulcers

Pathophysiology

Primarily an infection of lymphatics and lymph nodes. Lymphangitis and lymphadenitis occur in drainage field of the inoculation site with subsequent perilymphangitis and periadenitis. Necrosis occurs, and loculated abscesses, fistulas, and sinus tracts develop. As the infection subsides, fibrosis replaces acute inflammation with resulting obliteration of lymphatic drainage, chronic edema, and stricture. Inoculation site determines affected lymph nodes: penis, anterior urethra—superficial, deep inguinal; posterior urethra—deep iliac, perirectal; vulva—inguinal; vagina, cervix—deep iliac, perirectal, retrocrural, lumbosacral; anus—inguinal; rectum—perirectal, deep iliac.

Course and Prognosis

Natural history is highly variable. Spontaneous remission is common.

Management

Prevention Condom use

Antimicrobial Therapy Cures infection and prevents ongoing tissue damage, although tissue reaction can result in scarring. Buboes may require aspiration or incision and drainage through intact skin.

RECOMMENDED REGIMEN

Doxycycline, 100 mg PO b.i.d. for 21 days

ALTERNATIVE REGIMEN

Erythromycin, 500 mg PO q.i.d. for 21 days, *or*

Sulfisoxazole, 500 mg PO q.i.d. for 21 days, or equivalent sulfonamide course

Follow-Up Patients should be followed clinically until signs and symptoms have resolved.

Management of Sex Partners Sex partners should be referred for evaluation and treatment.

HUMAN PAPILLOMAVIRUS

MUCOSAL WARTS

Mucosal warts are soft, skin-colored, fleshy warts occurring on anogenital or oral mucosa or skin, caused by infection with a mucosal type of human papillomavirus (HPV).
Synonyms: Condylomata acuminata, anogenital warts, acuminate or venereal warts, verruca acuminata.

Epidemiology and Etiology

Age   Young, sexually active adults

Etiology   HPV, a DNA papovavirus that multiplies in the nuclei of infected epithelial cells: types 6, 11 most commonly; also types 16, 18, 31, 33. Types 16, 18, 31, and 33 are strongly associated with genital dysplasia and carcinoma.

Transmission   Contagious, nonsexually and sexually transmitted; 90 % to 100 % of male sex partners of infected females become HPV infected, most subclinically. HPV infection probably persists throughout a patient's lifetime in a dormant state and becomes infectious intermittently. Exophytic warts are probably more infectious than subclinical infection. In infants and children, HPV may be acquired during delivery.

Incidence   Increased manyfold during the past two decades. Prevalence of HPV infection in women ranges from 3 % to 28 %, depending on the population studied.

History

Incubation Period   Several weeks to months to years

Duration of Lesions   Months to years

Skin Symptoms   Usually asymptomatic, except for cosmetic appearance. In infants and children, genital warts may be a marker for sexual abuse, although much less commonly so than initially thought.

Physical Examination

Skin Lesions

TYPE   Pinhead papules to cauliflower-like masses (Figures 32-15 to 32-18). Subclinical on penis, vulva, or other genital skin; visible only following application of acetic acid, appearing as white patches.

COLOR   Skin-colored, pink, or red

PALPATION   Soft

SHAPE   Filiform, sessile (especially on penis)

DISTRIBUTION   Rarely, a few isolated lesions; usually clusters

ARRANGEMENT   May be solitary. Grouped into grapelike or cauliflower-like cluster. Perianal cauliflower lesions; may be size of walnut to apple (Figure 32-18).

SITES OF PREDILECTION *Male* Frenulum, corona, glans, prepuce, shaft, scrotum
Female Labia, clitoris, periurethral area, perineum, vagina, cervix (flat lesions) (Figure 32-17)
Both Sexes Perineal, perianal, anal canal, rectal; urethral meatus, urethra, bladder; oropharynx

Differential Diagnosis

Condylomata lata, intraepithelial neoplasia, bowenoid papulosis, squamous cell carcinoma, molluscum contagiosum, lichen nitidus, lichen planus, normal sebaceous glands, angiokeratoma, pearly penile papules, folliculitis, moles, seborrheic keratoses, skin tags, pilar cyst, scabetic nodules

Laboratory and Special Examinations

Acetowhitening Subclinical lesions can be visualized by wrapping the penis with gauze soaked with 5 % acetic acid for 5 minutes. Using a 10× hand lens or colposcope, warts appear as tiny white papules.

Serology Occurrence of genital warts is a marker of unsafe sexual practices. STS should be obtained on all patients to rule out coinfection with *Treponema pallidum,* and all patients offered HIV testing.

Dermatopathology Indicated in some cases to confirm diagnosis and/or rule out *in situ* or invasive squamous cell carcinoma

Pap Smear All women should be encouraged to have annual Pap smear, in that HPV is the major etiologic agent in pathogenesis for cancer of cervix.

Detection of HPV DNA Presence of HPV DNA and specific HPV types can be determined on smears and lesional biopsy specimens by *in situ* hybridization.

Diagnosis

Clinical diagnosis, occasionally confirmed by biopsy

Course and Prognosis

Condylomata recur even after appropriate therapy in a high percentage of patients, due to persistence of latent HPV in normal-appearing perilesional skin (see Transmission). Recurrences more commonly result from reactivation of subclinical infection than from reinfection by a sex partner. If left untreated, genital warts may resolve on their own, remain unchanged, or grow. In placebo-treated cases, genital warts clear spontaneously in 20 % to 30 % of patients within 3 months.

Dysplasia and Carcinoma The major significance of HPV infection is its oncogenicity. HPV types 16, 18, 31, and 33 are the major etiologic factors for cervical dysplasia and cervical squamous cell carcinoma; bowenoid papu-

losis, *in situ* and invasive carcinoma of both the vulva and penis; anal squamous cell carcinoma of homosexual/bisexual males. Treatment of external genital warts is not likely to influence the development of cervical cancer. The importance of the annual Pap test must be stressed to women with genital warts.

Children delivered vaginally of mothers with genital HPV infection are at risk for developing recurrent respiratory papillomatosis in later life.

Management

Prevention Use of condoms reduces transmission to uninfected sex partners. Goal of treatment is removal of exophytic warts and amelioration of signs and symptoms—not eradication of HPV. No therapy has been shown to eradicate HPV. Treatment is more successful if warts are small and have been present for <1 year. Risk of transmission might be reduced by "debulking" genital warts. Selection of treatment should be guided by preference of patient—expensive therapies, toxic therapies, and procedures that result in scarring avoided.

External Genital/Perianal Warts

CRYOSURGERY WITH LIQUID NITROGEN Apply with cotton swab or cryospray. Repeat weekly or biweekly. Relatively inexpensive, does not require anesthesia, and does not result in scarring.

PODOFILOX (CONDYLOX) 0.5 % solution and gel. A purified and stable preparation of the active agent in podophyllin. Patient-initiated therapy. Solution or gel applied with a cotton swab to condylomata and/or site involved (including normal-appearing skin between lesions) twice daily for 3 days, followed by 4 days of no therapy. This cycle may be repeated as necessary for a total of four cycles. Total area of treatment should not exceed 10 cm², and total volume should not exceed 0.5 ml/day. The health care provider should apply the initial treatment to demonstrate the proper application technique and identify lesions and sites to be treated. *Podofilox is contraindicated during pregnancy.*

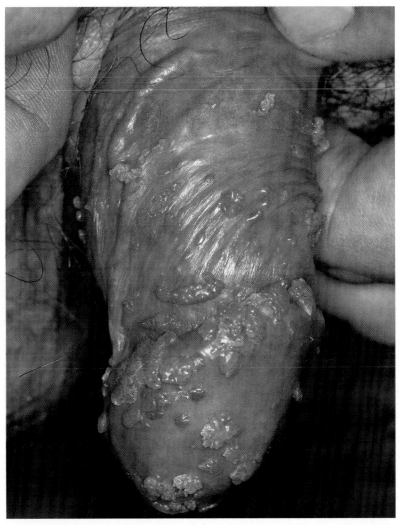

Figure 32-15 Condylomata acuminata of penis *Multiple, soft, filiform papules, discrete with some coalescing to raspberry-like lesions, on the glans penis and prepuce.*

PODOPHYLLIN 10 % to 25 % in compound tincture of benzoin. Limit the total volume of podophyllin solution applied to ≤0.5 ml or ≤10 cm² per session. Thoroughly wash off in 1 to 4 hours. Treat <10 cm² per session. Repeat weekly if necessary. If warts persist after 6 applications, other therapeutic methods should be considered. *Podophyllin contraindicated during pregnancy.*

TRICHLOROACETIC ACID 80 % to 90 %. Apply only to warts: powder with talc or sodium bicarbonate (baking soda) to remove unreacted acid. Repeat weekly if necessary. If warts persist after six applications, other therapeutic methods should be considered.

ELECTRODESICCATION/ELECTROCAUTERY

Highly effective in destruction of infected tissue and HPV. Should be attempted only by clinicians trained in the use of this modality. Electrodesiccation is contraindicated in patients with cardiac pacemakers.

INTRALESIONAL INTERFERON Is currently being used on an experimental basis. It is painful and requires repeated injections.

Urethral Meatus Warts

CRYOSURGERY WITH LIQUID NITROGEN

PODOPHYLLIN 10 % to 25 % in compound tincture of benzoin. Treatment area must be dry before contact with normal mucosa. Wash off in 1 to 2 hours. Repeat weekly if necessary. If warts persist after six applications, other therapeutic methods should be considered.

Perianal/Anal Warts

CRYOSURGERY WITH LIQUID NITROGEN

TRICHLOROACETIC ACID 80 % to 90 %. Apply only to warts; powder with talc or sodium bicarbonate (baking soda) to remove unreacted acid. Repeat weekly if necessary. If warts persist after six applications, other therapeutic methods should be considered.

PODOPHYLLIN 10 % to 25 % in compound tincture of benzoin.

Carbon Dioxide Laser and Electrodesiccation Useful in management of extensive warts, particularly for those patients who have not responded to other regimens; not appropriate for treatment of limited lesions.

Management of Sex Partners Examination of sex partners is not necessary because role of reinfection is probably minimal. Majority of partners are probably already subclinically infected with HPV, even if no warts are visible.

Subclinical Genital HPV Infection (Without Exophytic Warts) Subclinical genital HPV infection is much more common than exophytic warts among both men and women. Infection is often indirectly diagnosed on cervix by Pap smear, colposcopy, or biopsy and on the penis, vulva, and other genital skin by the appearance of white areas after application of acetic acid. Treatment is not indicated.

IMIQUIMOD (ALDARA) 5 % cream. Patient-initiated therapy. The mechanism of action is unknown but thought to be via local cytokine release (interferon, tumor necrosis factor, interleukin). Imiquimod has no direct antiviral activity. The cream, which is supplied in single dose packets, is applied to the involved site by the patient, three times per week, usually at bedtime. Some patients experience local irritation. Treatment duration 8–16 weeks.

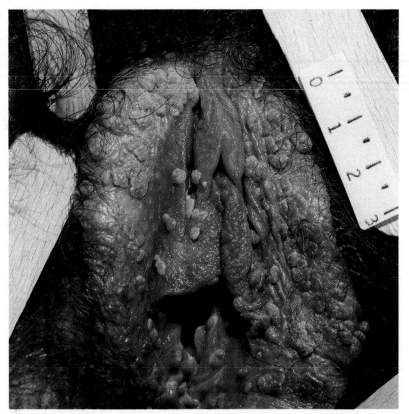

Figure 32-16 Condylomata acuminata of vulva *Multiple, pink-brown, soft papules on the labia.*

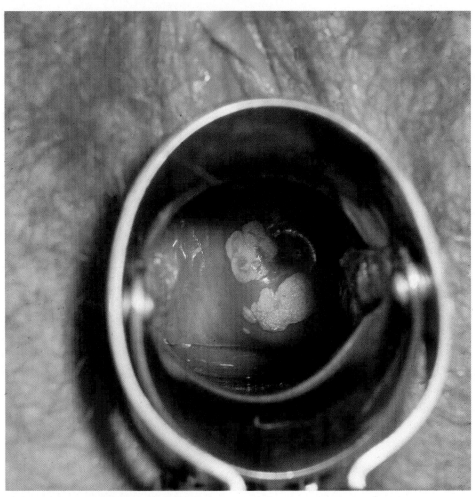

Figure 32-17 Condylomata acuminata on the cervix *Sharply demarcated, whitish, flat plaques becoming confluent around the os cervix.*

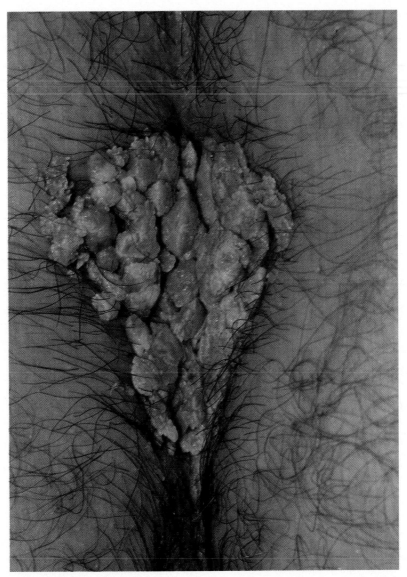

Figure 32-18 Condylomata acuminata, perianal *Fleshy papules becoming a confluent cauliflower-like mass on the perineum.*

INTRAEPITHELIAL NEOPLASIA OF THE ANOGENITAL SKIN

Intraepithelial neoplasia of the anogenital skin is characterized by multifocal benign-appearing maculopapular lesions occurring on the mucosa and anogenital and crural skin, exhibiting histologic changes of (bowenoid) squamous cell carcinoma *in situ,* but following a largely benign clinical course.

Synonyms: Bowenoid papulosis, vulvar intraepithelial neoplasia, penile intraepithelial neoplasm, squamous intraepithelial neoplasia.

Epidemiology and Etiology

Age Third and fourth decades

Etiology HPV types 16, 18, 31, and 33

Transmission HPV transmitted sexually. Autoinoculation. Rarely, HPV-16 transmitted from mother to newborn, with subsequent development of bowenoid papulosis (BP) on penis.

Incidence Marked increase during past two decades associated with increased sexual promiscuity

History

Duration of Lesions Weeks to months to years to decades

Incubation Period Months to years

Systems Review Prior history of condylomata acuminata. Female partners of males may have cervical intraepithelial neoplasia (CIN).

Skin Lesions

TYPES Erythematous macules. Lichenoid (flat-topped) or pigmented papules (several millimeters) (Figures 32-20 and 32-21); may show some confluence or form plaque(s) (Figure 32-19). Leukoplakia-like plaque. Surface usually smooth, velvety.

COLOR Tan, brown, pink, red, violaceous, white

ARRANGEMENT Characteristically clusters (multifocal), May be solitary.

DISTRIBUTION Males: glans penis, prepuce (75 %) (flat lichenoid papules or erythematous macules); penile shaft (25 %) (pigmented papules) (Figure 32-19). Females: labia majora and minora (Figure 32-20), clitoris. Both sexes: inguinal folds, perineal/perianal skin (Figure 32-21). Oropharyngeal mucosa.

ACETOWHITENING Application of 3 % to 5 % acetic acid to the area of involvement for 5 minutes may facilitate visualization of lesions.

OTHER May be associated with cervical dysplasia, cervical intraepithelial neoplasia, cervical squamous cell carcinoma. Rarely, BP of other sites, i.e., periungual, intraoral.

Differential Diagnosis

Psoriasis vulgaris; lichen planus; condylomata acuminata; angiokeratomas; Bowen's disease, i.e., squamous cell carcinoma *in situ* (occurs as single lesion in older individual rather than as multiple lesions in younger person)

Laboratory and Special Examinations

Dermatopathology Epidermal proliferation with numerous mitotic figures, abnormal mitoses, atypical pleomorphic cells with large hyperchromatic, often clumped nuclei, dyskeratotic cells; basal membrane intact. ±Koilocytosis. Recent application of podophyllin to condyloma acuminatum may cause changes similar to BP.

Southern Blot Analysis Identifies HPV type

Pap Smear Koilocytotic atypia

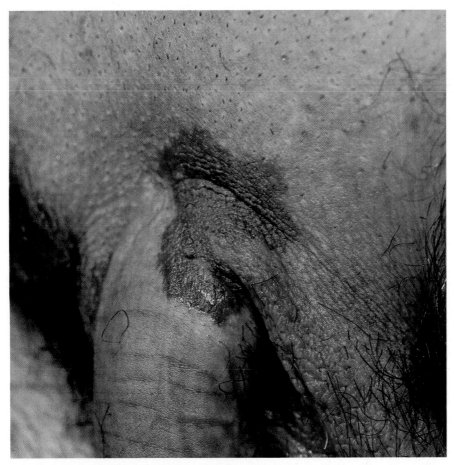

Figure 32-19 Intraepithelial neoplasia of penis *Sharply dark-brown, well-circumscribed plaque with microverrucous surface and irregular borders.*

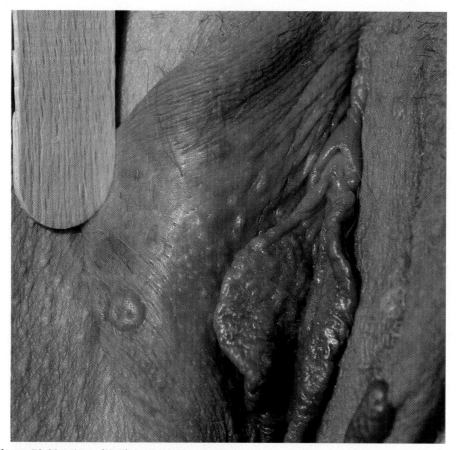

Figure 32-20 Intraepithelial neoplasia of vulva *Pink-to-dark-brown, well-demarcated, flat-topped papules on the labia majora; the lesions are clinically indistinguishable from condylomata acuminata. Lesions have the potential for undergoing malignant transformation to invasive squamous cell carcinoma.*

Diagnosis

Clinical suspicion, confirmed by lesional biopsy

Course and Prognosis

May resolve spontaneously. May persist for many years with the appearance of multiple new lesions. May rarely progress to invasive squamous cell carcinoma, ±metastasis.

Management

Current therapeutic options less than optimal: surgical excision, Mohs' surgery, electrosurgery, carbon dioxide laser vaporization, cryosurgery, topical 5-fluorouracil

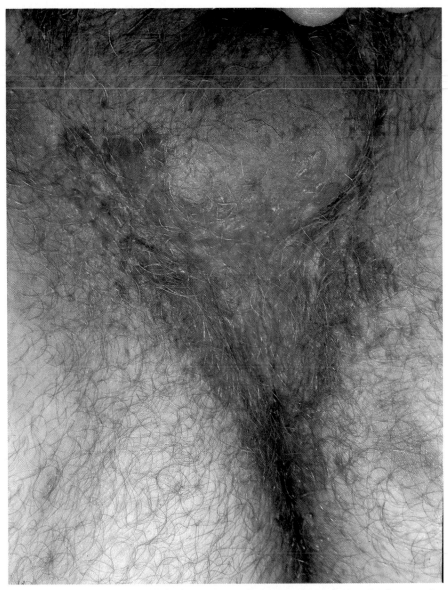

Figure 32-21 Intraepithelial neoplasia of the perineum and scrotum *Confluent, red-tan papules for a large plaque on the anogenital region in a male with advanced HIV disease. The lesions were successfully treated with 5-fluorouracil cream.*

HERPES SIMPLEX VIRUS: GENITAL INFECTION

Genital herpes is a sexually transmitted viral infection, characterized by primary infection with grouped vesicles at the site of inoculation and regional lymphadenopathy and a course of recurring outbreaks of vesicles at the same site. (See also HSV: Infections in the Immunocompromised Host, page 798).

Synonyms: Herpes progenitalis, herpes genitalis, genital herpes simplex.

Epidemiology and Etiology

Age Young, sexually active adults

Etiology Herpes simplex virus (HSV) type 2 > type 1. Currently in the United States, 30 % of new cases of genital herpes are caused by HSV-1.

Transmission Usually skin-to-skin contact. In most cases, transmission occurs during times of asymptomatic HSV shedding, which occurs during 1 % of days when no identifiable lesion is present. Transmission rate in discordant couples (one partner infected, the other not) approximately 10 % per year; 25 % of females become infected compared with only 4 % to 6 % of males. Prior HSV-1 infection is protective; in females with anti-HSV-1 antibodies, 15 % become HSV-2 infected, but in those without anti-HSV-1 antibodies, 30 % become infected.

Incidence >600,000 new infections in the United States annually; 30 million Americans are HSV-2 infected, i.e., approximately 1 in 5 adults. The presence of antibodies to HSV type 2 varies with the sexual history of the individual: nuns, 3 %; middle class, 25 %; heterosexuals at an STD clinic, 26 %; homosexuals, 46 %; lower classes, 46 % to 60 %; prostitutes, 70 % to 80 %.

Race and Sex By HSV-2 seropositivity studies in the United States, more common in blacks: 3 in 5 men, 4 in 5 women. Whites: 1 in 5 men, 1 in 4 women.

Diseases Characterized by Genital Ulcers In the United States, most patients with genital ulcers have genital herpes, syphilis, or chancroid. The relative frequency varies by geographic area and patient population, but in most areas of the United States genital herpes is the most common of these diseases. More than one of these diseases may be present among at least 3 % to 10 % of patients with genital ulcers. Each disease has been associated with an increased risk for HIV infection.

History

Incubation Period 2- to 20-day (average 6) incubation period

Symptoms 50 % to 70 % of HSV-2–infected individuals are asymptomatic or have only minor symptoms and are unaware of their infection.

PRIMARY GENITAL HERPES Frequently accompanied by fever, headache, malaise, myalgia, peaking within the first 3 to 4 days after onset of lesions, resolving during the subsequent 3 to 4 days. Depending on location, pain, itching, dysuria, vaginal or urethral discharge are common symptoms. Tender inguinal lymphadenopathy occurs during second and third weeks. Deep pelvic pain associated with pelvic lymphadenopathy. Some cases of first clinical episode of genital herpes are manifested by extensive disease that requires hospitalization.

RECURRENT GENITAL HERPES Prodrome of burning or itching sensation prior to eruption of vesicles. Dysuria, sciatica, rectal discomfort.

SYSTEMIC SYMPTOMS Symptoms of aseptic HSV-2 meningitis can occur with primary or recurrent genital herpes.

Physical Examination

Skin Lesions

TYPES *Primary Genital Herpes* An erythematous plaque is often noted initially, fol-

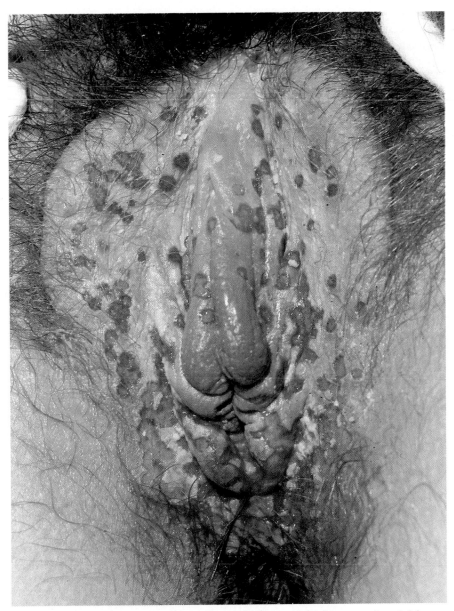

Figure 32-22 Genital herpes: primary vulvar infection *Multiple, extremely painful, punched-out, confluent, shallow ulcers on the vulva and perineum. Micturition is often very painful. Associated inguinal lymphadenopathy is common.*

lowed soon by grouped vesicles, which may evolve to pustules; these become eroded as the overlying epidermis sloughs Figure 32-22). Erosions are punched out and may enlarge to ulcerations, which may be crusted or moist. These epithelial defects heal in 2 to 4 weeks, often with resulting postinflammatory hypo- or hyperpigmentation, uncommonly with scarring. The area of involvement may be circumferential around the penis, or the entire vulva may be involved (Figure 32-22).

Recurrent Genital Herpes Lesions similar to primary infection but on a reduced scale (Figure 32-23). Often a 1- to 2-cm plaque of erythema surmounted with vesicles (Figure 32-24), which rupture with formation of erosions (Figure 32-23). Heals in 1 to 2 weeks.

ARRANGEMENT Herpetiform, i.e., grouped vesicles

DISTRIBUTION *Males* Primary infection: glans, prepuce, shaft, sulcus, scrotum, thigh, buttocks. Recurrences: penile shaft (Figure 32-24), glans, buttocks.

Females Primary infection: labia majora/minora, perineum, inner thighs. Recurrences: labia majora/minora, buttocks.

Anorectal Infection Occurs in male homosexuals (often HSV-1); characterized by tenesmus, anal pain, proctitis, discharge, and ulcerations (Figure 32-25) as far as 10 cm into anal canal.

General Findings

REGIONAL LYMPH NODES Inguinal/femoral lymph nodes enlarged, firm, nonfluctuant, tender; usually unilateral

SIGNS OF ASEPTIC MENINGITIS Fever, nuchal rigidity. Can occur in the absence of genital herpes. Pain along sciatic nerve.

Differential Diagnosis

Syphilitic chancre, fixed drug eruption, chancroid, gonococcal erosion, folliculitis, pemphigus, pemphigoid

---

Laboratory and Special Examinations

Evaluation of all persons with genital ulcers should include a serologic test for syphilis and possibly other tests. Although ideally all these tests should be conducted for each patient with a genital ulcer, use of such tests (other than STS) may be based on test availability and clinical or epidemiologic suspicion.

Tzanck Smear Optimally, fluid from intact vesicle and/or base is smeared thinly on a microscope slide, dried, and stained with either Wright's or Giemsa's stain. Positive if giant keratinocytes or multinucleated giant keratinocytes are detected (see Figure 29-11). Positive in 75 % of early cases, either primary or recurrent.

HSV Antigen Detection Sensitive and specific method [direct fluorescent antibody (DFA)] of identifying HSV-1 and HSV-2 on a smear from vesicle fluid or ulcer base

Dermatopathology Ballooning and reticular epidermal degeneration, acanthosis, acantholysis, and intraepidermal vesicles; intranuclear inclusion bodies, multinucleate giant keratinocytes; multilocular vesicles

Viral Culture Documents the presence of HSV in 1 to 10 days. Positive in 70 % of active lesions.

Serology

SYPHILIS STS to rule out syphilis

HSV Primary HSV infection documented by obtaining acute and convalescent sera that show seroconversion for HSV antibodies, as well as indicating whether HSV is type 1 or type 2. In a patient with recurrent genital lesions, genital herpes can be ruled out if HSV antibodies are absent. The most specific serologic tests are type-specific antibodies detected by Western blot technique.

HIV Rule out concomitant HIV infection.

CSF Pleocytosis with normal sugar content. HSV isolated on CSF viral culture. PCR detects HSV DNA.

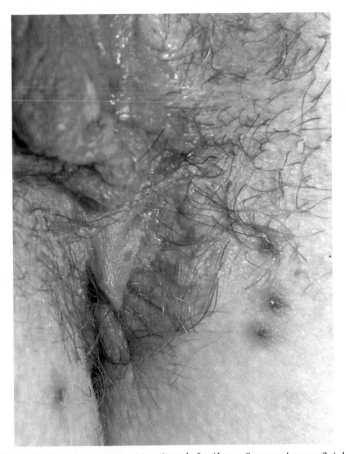

Figure 32-23 Genital herpes: recurrent vulvar infection *Scattered, superficial erosion with surrounding erythema on the posterior labia major and thighs. This episode was the first recognized recurrence; symptoms were minimal.*

Diagnosis

Clinical suspicion, confirmed by Tzanck smear, viral culture, or DFA

Pathophysiology

Transmission and infection of HSV occurs through close contact with a person shedding virus at a peripheral site, mucosal surface, or secretion. HSV is inactivated promptly at room temperature; aerosol or fomitic spread unlikely. Infection occurs via inoculation onto susceptible mucosal surface or break in skin. Subsequent to primary infection at inoculation site, HSV ascends peripheral sensory nerves and enters sensory or autonomic nerve root ganglia, where latency is established. Latency can occur after both symptomatic and asymptomatic primary infection. Recrudescences may be clinically symptomatic or asymptomatic.

Course and Prognosis

Genital herpes may be recurrent and has no cure. As many as 50 % to 70 % of HSV-2 infections are asymptomatic. From 50 % to 80 % of patients with HSV-2 infections experience recurrence(s) in 1 year; 2 % have monthly outbreaks, 13 % every 2 to 11 months, 24 % yearly or less often. Of individuals with initially symptomatic genital HSV-2 infection, almost all have symptomatic recurrences; recurrence rates are high in those with an extended first episode of infection, regardless of whether acyclovir therapy is given. The rate of recurrence is 20 % higher in men. Acyclovir does not completely suppress viral shedding but does reduce the quantity by 99 % to 99.9 % and thus may reduce transmission of the virus.

The incidence of primary infection with acyclovir-resistant HSV strains in individuals never exposed to acyclovir is 2.7 % in the United States.

Erythema multiforme may complicate genital herpes, occurring 1 to 2 weeks after an outbreak.

Management

Prevention

SEXUAL TRANSMISSION   Condom; chronic acyclovir prophylaxis

PERINATAL TRANSMISSION   Many experts recommend serotesting for HSV-1 and HSV-2 (Western blot) at the first prenatal visit. Infants born to women who asymptomatically shed HSV have reduced birth weight and increased prematurity.

Treatment   Systemic acyclovir provides partial control of symptoms and signs of herpes episodes when used to treat first clinical episode or when used as suppressive therapy. Acyclovir neither eradicates latent virus nor affects subsequent risk, frequency, or severity of recurrences after drug is discontinued. Even after laboratory testing, at least a quarter of patients with genital herpes have no laboratory-confirmed diagnosis. Many experts recommend treatment for chancroid and syphilis as well as genital herpes if the diagnosis is unclear or if the patient resides in a community in which chancroid is present.

First Clinical Episode of Genital Herpes Acyclovir 200 mg PO five times a day for 7 to 10 days or until clinical resolution occurs. *Note:* Only 10 % to 20 % of acyclovir is bioavailable following oral dosing. Valacyclovir, 500 mg b.i.d., famciclovir, 125 mg b.i.d.

First Clinical Episode of Herpes Proctitis Acyclovir 400 mg PO five times a day for 10 days or until clinical resolution occurs

Recurrent Episodes   When treatment is instituted during the prodrome or within 2 days of onset of lesions, patients with recurrent disease experience limited benefit from therapy in that the severity of the eruption is reduced. If early treatment cannot be administered, most immunocompetent patients with recurrent disease do not benefit from acyclovir treatment, and for these cases, it is not generally recommended.

> Acyclovir: 200 mg PO five times a day for 5 days, *or*
> 400 mg PO t.i.d. for 5 days, *or*
> 800 mg PO b.i.d. for 5 days
> Valacyclovir, 500 mg b.i.d.
> Famciclovir, 125 mg b.i.d.

Daily Suppressive Therapy   Daily treatment reduces frequency of recurrences by at least 75 % among patients with frequent (more than six per year) recurrences. Suppressive treatment with oral acyclovir does not totally eliminate symptomatic or asymptomatic viral shedding or the potential for transmission. Safety and efficacy have been documented among persons receiving daily therapy for as long as 5 years. Acyclovir-resistant strains of HSV have been isolated from some persons receiving suppressive therapy, but these strains have not been associated with treatment failure among immunocompetent patients. *After 1 year of continuous therapy, acyclovir should be discontinued to allow assessment of the patient's rate of recurrent episodes.*

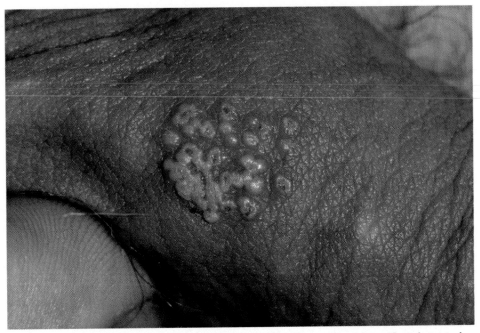

Figure 32-24 Genital herpes: recurrent of the penis *Group of vesicles with early central crusting on a red base arising on the shaft of the penis.*

RECOMMENDED REGIMEN   Acyclovir, 400 mg PO b.i.d.

ALTERNATIVE REGIMEN   Acyclovir, 200 mg PO three to five times a day. The goal of the alternative regimen is to identify for each patient the lowest dose that provides relief from frequently recurring symptoms. Valacyclovir, 500 mg b.i.d., famciclovir, 500 mg b.i.d.

Severe Disease   IV therapy should be provided for patients with severe disease or complications necessitating hospitalization (e.g., disseminated infection that includes encephalitis, pneumonitis, or hepatitis).

RECOMMENDED REGIMEN   Acyclovir, 5 mg/kg body weight IV every 8 hours for 5 to 7 days or until clinical resolution is attained

Other Management Considerations

- Patients should be advised to abstain from sexual activity while lesions are present.

- Patients with genital herpes should be told about the natural history of the disease, with emphasis on the potential of recurrent episodes, asymptomatic viral shedding, and sexual transmission. Sexual transmission of HSV has been documented to occur during periods without evidence of lesions. Many infections are transmitted during such asymptomatic periods.
- The use of condoms should be encouraged during all sexual exposures.
- The risk for neonatal infection should be explained to all patients—male and female—with genital herpes.

Special Considerations

HIV INFECTIONS   Lesions caused by HSV are relatively common among HIV-infected persons. Intermittent or suppressive therapy with oral acyclovir may be needed. Acyclovir, 400 mg PO three to five times per day, may be useful. Therapy should continue until clinical resolution is attained. For severe disease, IV acyclovir therapy may be required. If lesions persist among patients undergoing acyclovir treatment, resistance to acyclovir should be suspected. For severe disease caused by proven or suspected acyclovir-resistant strains, hospitalization should be considered. Forscarnet, 40 mg/kg body weight every 8 hours until clinical resolution is attained, appears to be the best available treatment.

PREGNANCY The safety of systemic acyclovir among pregnant women has not yet been established.

PERINATAL INFECTIONS Most mothers of infants who acquire neonatal herpes lack histories of clinically evident genital herpes. The risk for transmission to the neonate from an infected mother appears highest among women with first-episode genital herpes near the time of delivery and is low (<3%) among women with recurrent herpes. The results of viral cultures during pregnancy do not predict viral shedding at the time of delivery, and such cultures are not routinely indicated.

At the time of labor, all women should be questioned carefully about symptoms of genital herpes and should be examined. Women without symptoms or signs of genital herpes infection (or prodrome) may deliver babies vaginally. Among women who have a history of genital herpes or who have a sex partner with genital herpes, cultures of the birth canal at delivery may aid in decisions relating to neonatal management.

Infants delivered through an infected birth canal (proven by virus isolation or presumed by observation of lesions) should be followed carefully, including virus cultures obtained 24 to 48 hours after birth. Treatment should be reserved for infants who develop evidence of clinical disease and for those with positive postpartum cultures.

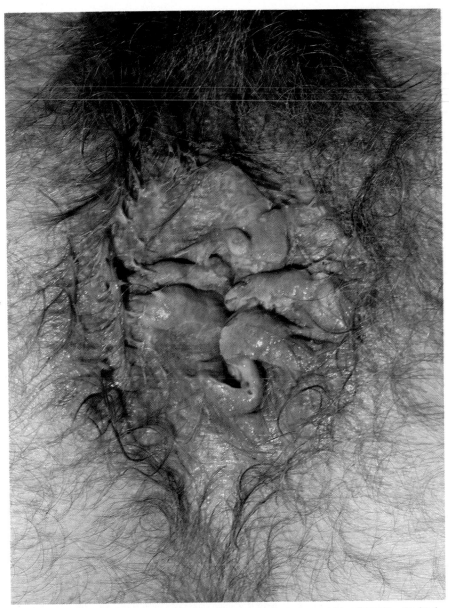

Figure 32-25 Genital herpes: recurrent of the rectum, anus, and perineum *Multiple, deep, sharply demarcated ulcers with purulent exudation in a male with advanced HIV disease. The lesions were very painful, and associated with very painful defecation.*

MUCOCUTANEOUS MANIFESTATIONS OF HUMAN IMMUNODEFICIENCY VIRUS DISEASE

MUCOCUTANEOUS FINDINGS IN HIV DISEASE

By year 2000, the human immunodeficiency virus (HIV)/acquired immunodeficiency syndrome (AIDS) pandemic will have been in place for 20 years. The dynamics of the pandemic are ever-changing. In the United States and other developed nations, a steady state has been reached, with the number of new infections equal to the number of those dying from HIV disease. As of the mid-1990s, estimates are that about 1 million individuals in the United States are HIV-infected, half of whom have advanced disease (AIDS); 40,000 to 50,000 individuals become newly infected and the same number die from complications of the disease each year. In western Europe, the epidemiology is similar to that in the United States, with the majority of infected individuals being men who have sex with men and injecting drug users. Of the 20 million HIV-infected individuals worldwide, two-thirds live in sub-Saharan Africa; in some western African countries, 20 % of the population is HIV-infected. The number of infected individuals is, however, increasing most rapidly in Southeast Asia, especially in India.

Nearly all HIV-infected individuals exhibit some dermatologic disorder attributable to progressive immunodeficiency during the course of the infection. Some disorders are highly associated with HIV infection, and their diagnosis often warrants HIV serotesting; they include: the exanthem of acute retroviral syndrome, Kaposi's sarcoma, oral hairy leukoplakia, proximal subungual ony-chomycosis, bacillary angiomatosis, eosinophilic folliculitis, chronic herpetic ulcers (>1 month du-ration), any sexually transmitted disease, multiple facial molluscum contagiosum in an adult, and skin findings of injecting drug use. Other findings are common in HIV disease and may be indica-tions for serotesting in some patients: herpes zoster, mucosal candidiasis (oropharyngeal, recurrent vulvovaginal), seborrheic dermatitis, and severe persistent aphthous ulcers.

Early diagnosis is critical in the management of HIV disease for several reasons. Given the knowl-edge of their HIV infection and its contagiousness, most patients will reduce or eliminate behav-iors associated with transmission of HIV. Early treatment with antiretroviral drugs retards progres-sion of HIV-induced immunodeficiency. Many of the opportunistic infections such as *Pneumocystis carinii* pneumonia (PCP) that plague HIV-infected patients are better treated by primary prophy-lactic regimens prior to development of clinical disease.

ACUTE RETROVIRAL SYNDROME

Acute retroviral syndrome (ARS) is characterized by an infectious mononucleosis-like syndrome or aseptic meningitis syndrome with fever, lymphadenopathy, meningitis, GI symptoms, and a characteristic infectious exanthem, an enanthem, and genital ulceration.
Synonym: Symptomatic primary HIV infection.

Epidemiology and Etiology

Age   Commonly young, but any age

Sex   Initially in the United States and Europe, much more common in males due to male-male sexual intercourse; currently, incidence in females increasing due to heterosexual transmission. In Africa, nearly equal incidence in sexes due to pattern of male-female sexual transmission.

Etiology   Nearly all cases in the United States and western Europe caused by HIV-1; some cases in western Africa caused by HIV-2. Both HIV-1 and HIV-2 can have a similar acute retroviral syndrome; clinical findings with HIV-2 infection are usually less severe.

Incidence   Current estimates are that by year 2000, 40 million individuals will have become HIV infected. In the United States, 1 million individuals are infected, with 40,000 to 50,000 new infections occurring annually. The incidence of symptomatic ARS is uncertain in that symptoms vary greatly, only those with significant illness seeking medical attention.

Transmission of HIV

SEXUAL EXPOSURE   Unprotected receptive intercourse (anal and vaginal) is the most efficient mode of transmission of HIV.

INJECTING DRUG USER (IDU)   Needle sharing transmits HIV.

BLOOD OR BLOOD PRODUCTS   Recipients of blood or blood products after 1978 but before 1985 were inadvertently infected with HIV. Currently, newly HIV-infected donors may be HIV-seronegative but are HIV-viremic.

HEALTH CARE WORKERS   HIV can be transmitted by needle sticks and cuts contaminated with HIV-infected blood during medical procedures.

ORGAN TRANSPLANT RECIPIENTS   Prior to HIV testing, HIV was transmitted during transplantation of solid organs, bone marrow, and corneae.

PERINATAL TRANSMISSION   Child born to mother with HIV infection, i.e., intrauterine, during birthing, or by breast feeding, may become infected.

Risk Factors   Genital ulcer disease, such as genital herpes, chancroid, or syphilis, increases the risk of HIV transmission. HIV-infected individuals with higher viral loads may transmit the virus more efficiently.

Geography   Worldwide epidemic with many cases in the United States, South America, Europe, Australia, and Africa. Presently, the greatest number of new HIV infections are occurring in Asia, especially in India.

History

Incubation Period   3 to 6 weeks (from presumed exposure to development of acute febrile illness); varies according to route and size of virus inoculation. Between 10 % and 20 % of recently infected individuals experience symptomatic primary infection.

History   Most patients are asymptomatic. Rash: usually appears 2 to 3 days after onset of fever; 5 to 8 days' duration. Exanthem asymptomatic. Ulcers: painful ulcers in mouth and/or anogenital region. Fever, rigors, malaise, lethargy, sore throat, arthralgias, myalgias, lasting 2 to 3 weeks. Also abdominal cramps, vomiting, diarrhea, headache, stiff neck, photophobia.

Physical Examination

Skin Lesions

TYPE   Morbilliform rash, i.e., infectious exanthem (Figure 33-1) with macules, papules up to 1 cm in diameter. Ulcers occur on penis and/or scrotum. Less commonly: urticaria. Also reported: vesicular and pustular exanthems, desquamation of palms/soles.

COLOR   Pink to red

ARRANGEMENT   Lesions remain discrete and do not become confluent.

DISTRIBUTION   Most common site of exanthem is upper thorax and collar region (100 %) > face (60 %) > arms (40 %) > scalp, thighs (20 %). Palms.

Mucous Membranes   Pharyngitis. Enanthem, spotty, on hard and soft palate. Ulcers: 5 to 10 mm in diameter, round to oval, shallow with white bases surrounded by a red halo, arising on the tonsils, palate, and/or buccal mucosa; esophageal ulcers. Uncommonly, oral candidiasis

ANOGENITALIA   Ulcers: prepuce of penis, scrotum, anal ulcers, anal canal

General Examination

LYMPH NODES   Lymphadenopathy

NEUROLOGIC FINDINGS   Acute meningitis; acute reversible encephalopathy with loss of memory, alteration of consciousness, and personality change

Differential Diagnosis

Fever, Exanthem, and Lymphadenopathy in Individuals at Risk for HIV Infection Primary Epstein-Barr virus (EBV) infection (infectious mononucleosis), primary cytomegalovirus (CMV) infection, rubella, toxoplasmosis, hepatitis, secondary syphilis, primary HSV infection

Fever, Exanthem, and Aseptic Meningitis in Individuals at Risk for HIV Infection   Lymphocytic (aseptic) meningitis, disseminated gonococcal infection

Laboratory and Special Examinations

Hematology   Leukopenia, elevated ESR

Viral Load Levels   (VLL) Usually extremely high initially. Subsequently reduced to low or undetectable levels. After a hiatus of years, the viral load eventually increases as immune function declines.

HIV Antigen   p24 antigen is detectable in serum during ARS prior to HIV seroconversion. Becomes undetectable following immune response. Recurs as immune function declines.

Viral Cultures   HIV isolation from blood or CSF during ARS. Virus is undetectable following immune response. Viremia recurs as immune function declines.

CD4+ T-Lymphocytes   Usually dip down by several hundred (normal in adults, approximately $1000/\mu l$), occasionally as low as $200/\mu l$ but return to normal levels within several weeks. After a latent period, CD4+ cells levels again fall.

Serology

ACUTE RETROVIRAL SYNDROME   Demonstrate seroconversion of anti-HIV-1 antibodies by ELISA confirmed by Western blot within 3 weeks of illness. HIV-2 infection is rare in industrialized countries.

ASYMPTOMATIC HIV INFECTION   HIV antibody is detectable in 95 % or more of individuals within 6 months of infection. Although a negative antibody test usually means an individual is not infected, antibody tests cannot rule out infection that occurred less than 6 months before the test.

CSF   Lymphocytic pleocytosis, p24 antigenemia

Dermatopathology   Sparse lymphohistiocytic infiltrate around blood vessels of the superficial dermal plexus and between collagen bundles in upper dermis

Diagnosis

Demonstrate seroconversion of HIV by ELISA or Western blot *or* isolation of HIV from blood or CSF *or* demonstration of p24 antigen

Pathophysiology

Following primary HIV infection, billions of

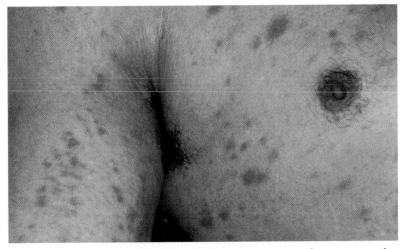

Figure 33-1 Acute retroviral syndrome: exanthem *Discrete, erythematous macules and papules on the trunk and arm; associated findings were fever, scrotal ulcers, erythematous macules on palate, and lymphadenopathy.*

virions are produced and destroyed each day; a concomitant daily turnover of actively infected CD4+ cells is also in the billions.

Course and Prognosis

The spectrum of symptoms associated with primary HIV infection is broad; the majority of individuals experience no or mild symptoms that do not prompt medical consultation. In those with symptomatic illness, the mean duration of illness in one study was 13 days (range 5 to 44 days). Long-term illness of greater than 2 weeks is associated with an eight times higher risk of developing AIDS within 3 years of seroconversion.

After an asymptomatic or symptomatic primary infection, HIV infection becomes latent with no clinical symptoms or findings. With disease progression and diminution of immune function, criteria for diagnosis of the acquired immunodeficiency syndrome occur. The pace of disease progression is variable. The median time between primary HIV infection (seroconversion) and the development of AIDS among young homosexual men is >10 years (in the United States), with a range from a few months to ≥12 years. Most adults and adolescents in-

fected with HIV remain symptom-free for long periods, but with viral replication occurring at a high rate. Factors that correlate with more rapid disease progression are HIV infection transmitted from someone with advanced HIV disease rather than an asymptomatic individual, older individuals (>30 years), and severe ARS. Essentially all HIV-infected individuals will eventually have symptoms related to the infection: 70 % to 85 % of infected adults develop symptoms and 55 % to 62 % develop AIDS within 12 years of seroconversion. Additional cases occur among those who have remained AIDS-free for >12 years.

Management

HIV Prevention Counseling

SEX EDUCATION The most common mode of HIV transmission is during sexual intercourse. Currently, in terms of numbers of new HIV infections, female-to-male and male-to-female transmission is much more common than male-to-male. Safer sexual practices must be taught at an early age.

TRANSFUSIONS AND TRANSPLANTATION Blood and blood by-products must be tested before administration. HIV infection must be ruled out in donors of any transplanted organ.

Treatment of ARS Symptomatic. Efficacy of antiretroviral therapy at this stage still controversial.

Treatment of Asymptomatic HIV Infection Early diagnosis offers the opportunity for counseling and for assistance in preventing the transmission of HIV infection to others.

Antiretroviral Therapy Combinations of zidovudine/didanosine and zidovudine/zalcitabine are preferred over zidovudine monotherapy. Protease inhibitors such as indinavir and ritonavir reduce viral load by 2 to 3 logs in some individuals. Triple combination is currently recommended.

Recent data on HIV pathogenesis, the development of methods for quantification of plasma HIV RNA, clinical trial data, and the availability of new drugs have resulted in profound changes of therapeutical approaches.

It is now evident that in all stages of the infection the virus replicates at high levels in the lymphoid tissue, as reflected by the amount of HIV RNA in the plasma. This large amount of virus turns over rapidly with a virion half-life of less then 6 hours and an estimated 10 billion (10^{10}) virus particle produced daily. Shortly after infection each individual establishes its individual quasi-steady-state levels of plasma HIV RNA that largely determines the rate of CD4 cell-destruction and ultimately the natural history of this infection. At any time point of the infection this set-point of plasma HIV RNA correlates inversely with prognosis and in fact can be used to predict the natural course of the disease.

It is well established that inhibition of viral replication with even potent antiretroviral agents at either suboptimal doses and/or as monotherapy by about 70–90% is gradually lost within a few months, coincident with the development of resistance. Nevertheless, when antiretroviral agents of different classes with nonoverlapping genetic patterns are used in combination, their genetic barrier to simultaneous resistance is significantly increased.

Antiretroviral agents approved for treatment of HIV in one or more countries of the world can be divided into three classes of drugs: nucleoside reverse transcriptase inhibitors (NRTI), nonnucleoside reverse transcriptase inhibitors (NNRTI), and protease inhibitors (PI). They are directed against two target-enzymes—HIV reverse transcriptase and HIV protease—thereby interfering with formation of proviral DNA and virus assembly, respectively.

Combination therapy can slow down or even prevent selection of drug-resistant strains and is associated with significant clinical benefit. Current treatment recommendations favor the combined usage of two NRTI and one PI (preferably IDV, NFV, or RTV) or two NRTI and one NNRTI.

Treatment is now recommended for all patients with HIV RNA levels above 5000–10000 copies/ml plasma but essentially be considered and provided for all HIV-infected patients with detectable HIV RNA in plasma. For patients at low risk of progression (low plasma HIV RNA level and high CD4 count), particularly those who are not committed to complex antiretroviral regimens, therapy might be safely deferred. These patients should be reevaluated every 3 to 6 months. (This text was provided by Armin Rieger, MD.)

Generic Name	Other Names	Principal Activities	Usual Adult Dose
NRTI: Didanosine	ddI	HIV-1, HIV-2	20 mg bid
Lamivudine	3TC	HIV-1, HIV-2, HBV	150 mg bid
Stavudine	d4T	HIV-1, HIV-2	40 mg bid
Zalcitabine	ddC	HIV-1, HIV-2	0.75 mg tid
Zidovudine	ZDV	HIV-1, HIV-2	300 mg bid
NNRTI: Delavirdine	DLV	HIV-1	400 mg tid
Nevirapine	NVP	HIV-1	200 mg bid
PI: Indinavir	IDV	HIV-1, HIV-2	800 mg tid
Nelfinavir	NFV	HIV-1, HIV-2	750 mg tid
Ritonavir	RTV	HIV-1, HIV-2	600 mg bid
Saquinavir	SQV	HIV-1, HIV-2	600 mg tid

EOSINOPHILIC FOLLICULITIS

Eosinophilic folliculitis (EF) is an idiopathic, extremely pruritic, papular follicular eruption of the upper trunk, face, neck, and proximal extremities occurring in advanced HIV disease, often associated with peripheral eosinophilia.

Etiology

Unknown

History

History Moderate to intense itching unrelieved by many therapies

Systems Review Occurs in HIV disease; all individuals have an AIDS-defining criterion.

Physical Examination

Skin Lesions

TYPES 3- to 5-mm, edematous, follicular papules and pustules (Figures 33-2A and 2B). Most patients have hundreds of lesions. Frequently, changes secondary to scratching/rubbing are seen: excoriations/crusting; atopic dermatitis, lichen simplex chronicus, prurigo nodularis. Secondary infections of excoriated sites include: impetiginization, deep infections such as furuncles, and/or cellulitis. Postinflammatory hyperpigmentation occurs in more darkly pigmented individuals.

COLOR Erythematous, new lesions. Postinflammatory hyperpigmentation of older excoriated sites.

DISTRIBUTION Trunk universally; head and neck; proximal extremities

Differential Diagnosis

Allergic contact dermatitis, adverse cutaneous drug reaction, atopic dermatitis, scabies, papular urticaria (insect bites), acne vulgaris, dermatophytic folliculitis, bacterial folliculitis (*Staphylococcus aureus*), fungal folliculitis (*Pityrosporum ovale*)

Laboratory and Special Examinations

Serology HIV ELISA and Western blot positive

Cultures Negative for pathogenic organisms

Dermatopathology Perifollicular and perivascular infiltrate with varying numbers of eosinophils. Epithelial spongiosis of follicular infundibulum and/or sebaceous glands associated with a mixed cellular infiltrate. Eosinophilic pustules occur uncommonly. Special stains for bacteria, fungi, and parasites are negative.

Hematology Many patients have either absolute or relative peripheral eosinophilia. CD4+ count usually <100 μl.

Diagnosis

Clinical diagnosis confirmed by skin biopsy, with cultures ruling out infectious causes

Pathophysiology

Unknown. May be similar to the rare dermatosis, eosinophilic pustular folliculitis (Ofuji's disease), which is reported mainly from Japan.

Course and Prognosis

Course tends to be chronic, characterized by spontaneous exacerbations and remissions.

Management

Pruritus is moderate to severe, significantly affecting quality of life. Changes secondary to chronic scratching such as secondary infections and lichen simplex chronicus also should be identified and treated.

Antihistamines Those causing sedation are more effective for symptomatic relief of pruritus.

Topical Agents

CORTICOSTEROIDS Class I (superpotent) corticosteroids applied to affected areas produce fair to moderate improvement in pruritus and lesions.

PERMETHRIN CREAM (ELIMITE) Reported to be effective

Systemic Agents Reported to Be Effective

PREDNISONE Initial dose of 70 mg, followed by a taper of 5 mg/day (14 days) provides rapid symptomatic improvement as well as resolution of EF. EF gradually recurs after completion of course.

ISOTRETINOIN (ACCUTANE) 1 to 2 mg/kg/day (about 80 mg) very effective in causing resolution of EF. Once symptoms and skin findings have resolved, dose is reduced to 40 mg/day for 2 to 4 weeks and then tapered to 40 mg q.o.d. Dosing may be discontinued in 1 to 2 months if symptoms do not recur.

ITRACONAZOLE 400 mg/day for 4 weeks reported to be effective

UVB Phototherapy or Natural Sunlight Treatments are usually given three times a week, tapering as symptoms of EF resolve. Moderately effective. Many individuals cannot, however, tolerate phototherapy because of treatment with photosensitizing drugs such as trimethoprimsulfamethoxazole (Bactrim).

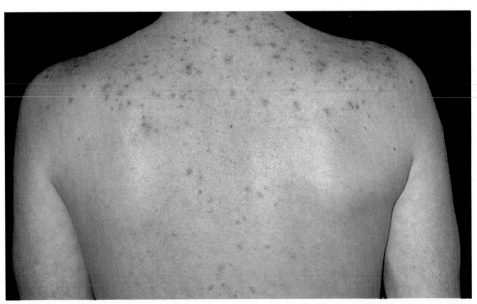

A

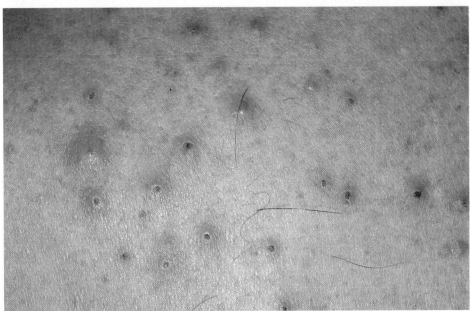

B

Figure 33-2 Eosinophilic folliculitits *Multiple, very pruritic, edematous papules and a few pustules of a male with advanced HIV disease (CD4+ cell count < 50/µL): A. Distribution on the upper trunk; lesions were also present on the face and neck. B. Close-up showing urticarial papules, pustules, and erosion secondary to rubbing; the primary lesions resemble papular urticaria (insect bites).*

KAPOSI'S SARCOMA

Kaposi's sarcoma (KS) is a multisystem vascular neoplasia characterized by mucocutaneous violaceous lesions and edema as well as involvement of nearly any organ. Many individuals with KS are in some degree immunocompromised, especially those with HIV disease.
Synonym: Multiple idiopathic hemorrhagic sarcoma.

Epidemiology and Etiology

Etiopathogenesis Recently, DNA of a new human herpesvirus, human herpesvirus type 8 (HHV-8), has been identified in tissue samples of several variants of KS.

Clinical Variants of KS

CLASSIC OR EUROPEAN KS Occurs in elderly males of eastern European heritage (Mediterranean and Ashkenazi Jewish). Predominantly arises on the legs; also occurs in lymph nodes and abdominal viscera (Figure 33-3).

AFRICAN-ENDEMIC KS (NON-HIV-ASSOCIATED) Four clinical patterns are recognized:
Nodular Type Runs a rather benign course with a mean duration of 5 to 8 years and resembles classic KS.
Florid or Vegetating Type Characterized by more aggressive biologic behavior. Is also nodular but may extend deeply into the dermis, subcutis, muscle, and bone.
Infiltrative Type Shows an even more aggressive course with florid mucocutaneous and visceral involvement.
Lymphadenopathic Type Predominantly affects children and young adults. Frequently confined to lymph nodes and viscera, but occasionally also involves the skin and mucous membrane.

IATROGENIC IMMUNOSUPPRESSIVE DRUG–ASSOCIATED KS Occurs in recipients of renal transplants and individuals with cancer treated with cytotoxic chemotherapy

HIV-ASSOCIATED KS

Sex Much more common in males in all variants. HIV-associated KS: Women who acquire HIV infection via heterosexual exposure are at risk of developing KS if sexual partner is a bisexual male.

Incidence

CLASSIC KS Increasing incidence in Sweden prior to onset of HIV pandemic

AFRICAN-ENDEMIC KS 9 % to 12.8 % of all malignancies in Zaire.

IMMUNOSUPPRESSIVE DRUG-ASSOCIATED KS In HIV-infected individuals, the risk for KS is 20,000 times that of the general population, 300 times that of other immunosuppressed individuals.

HIV-ASSOCIATED KS Early in the HIV epidemic in the United States and Europe, 50 % of homosexual men at the time of initial diagnosis of AIDS had KS; currently, the incidence is 18 % within this risk group.

Age

CLASSIC KS Peak incidence after the sixth decade

AFRICAN-ENDEMIC KS Two distinct age groups: young adults, mean age 35, and young children, mean age 3 years

Risk Factors

AFRICAN-ENDEMIC KS No evidence of underlying immunodeficiency

IMMUNOSUPPRESSIVE DRUG–ASSOCIATED KS Most commonly in solid-organ transplant recipients as well as a wide spectrum of indi-

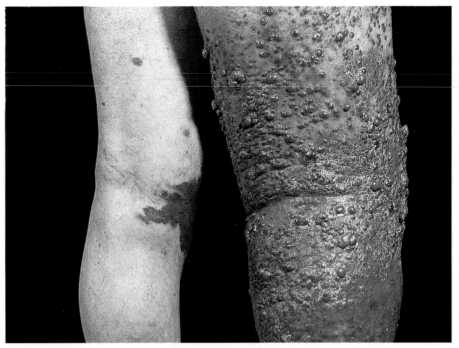

Figure 33-3 Kaposi's sarcoma, classic: confluent papules and nodules with edema
Massive infiltration of the right leg and thigh with confluent purple nodules with edema. Note the striking difference of involvement of the two legs.

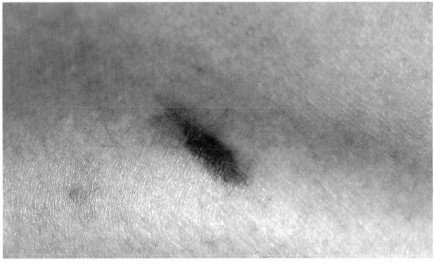

Figure 33-4 Kaposi's sarcoma, HIV-associated: very early macule *Oval, purple macule with a faint greenish halo overlying the clavicle.*

viduals treated chronically with immuno-suppressive drugs. Arises on average 16.5 months after transplantation.

HIV-ASSOCIATED KS At the time of initial presentation, less than one in six HIV-infected individuals with KS have CD4+ cell counts of ≥500/μl.

Geography

HIV-ASSOCIATED KS Homosexual men living in San Francisco, Los Angeles, and New York City are more likely to develop KS than are those living outside these areas.

CDC Surveillance Case Definition for AIDS

KS in a patient <60 years is an AIDS-defining condition if the patient has no other cause of immunodeficiency and is without knowledge of HIV antibody status.

History

History Cutaneous KS lesions most often begin as an ecchymotic-like macule. Mucocutaneous lesions are usually asymptomatic but are associated with significant cosmetic stigma. At times lesions may ulcerate and bleed easily. Large lesions on palms or soles may impede function. Lesions on the lower extremities that are tumorous, ulcerated, or associated with significant edema often give rise to moderate to severe pain. Urethral or anal canal lesions can be associated with obstruction. GI involvement rarely causes symptoms. Pulmonary KS can cause bronchospasm, intractable coughing, progressive respiratory failure, shortness of breath. Secondary malignancies occur in >35 % of individuals with classic KS.

Physical Examination

Skin Lesions

TYPES (FIGURES 33-4 THROUGH 33-9) Macules, papules, plaques, nodules (Figure 33-4), tumors located in dermis or hypodermis. In time, individual lesions may enlarge and become confluent, forming tumorous masses. Numerous small papules and nodules may arise in a large cluster (trunk, groin) in a follicular pattern, which in time can coalesce to very large tumor masses. Secondary changes to larger nodules and tumors include erosion, ulceration, crusting, and hyperkeratosis.

Lymphedema Confluent mass of lesions on an extremity may result in unilateral distal edema; deeper involvement of lymphatics and lymph nodes results in varying degrees of edema, usually symmetric, most pronounced on the lower legs, genitalia, and/or face. Areas of tense edema have a peau d'orange appearance.

Fibrosis Long-standing confluent lesions associated with edema of a limb can evolve to fibrosis, contracture, and atrophy with subsequent loss of function of the extremity.

COLOR Early dermal lesions violaceous, red, pink, or tan. Older lesions have purple-brownish hue with greenish hemosiderin halo.

PALPATION Small lesions that appear to be macules should be palpated with an ungloved finger. *Almost all KS lesions are palpable,* feeling firm to hard. Lesions that have the color of KS but are not palpable are probably ecchymoses. Lesions arising at the junction of the dermis and hypodermis (subcutaneous fat) are better defined by palpation than inspection.

SHAPE Often oval initially. On the trunk, oblong lesions are often parallel to skin tension lines.

ARRANGEMENT Truncal lesions have pityriasis rosea–like pattern. Lesions may occur at sites of trauma, koebnerization, or isomorphic phenomenon.

DISTRIBUTION Widespread: trunk; head, especially tip of nose, periorbital, ears, scalp; penis; legs; palms and soles

Mucous Membranes Oral lesions are the first manifestation of KS in 22 % of cases; often a marker for CD4+ cell counts of <200/μl.

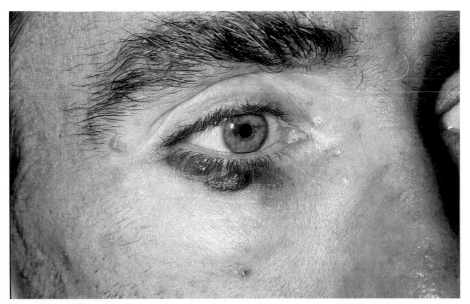

Figure 33-5 Kaposi's sarcoma, HIV-associated: nodules *A purple nodule on the lower eyelid with surrounding yellow-green halo. Mollusca contagiosa are also present on the cheek.*

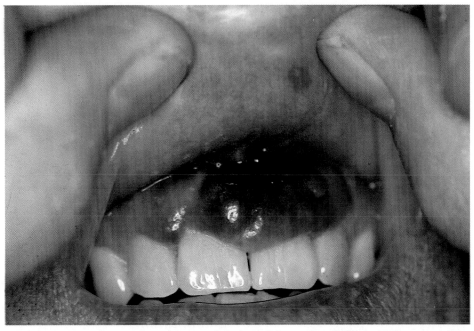

Figure 33-6 Kaposi's sarcoma, HIV-associated: nodule on the gingiva *Violaceous nodule on the upper gingiva, enlarging and covering the teeth.*

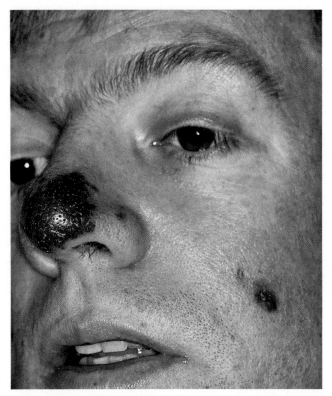

Figure 33-7 Kaposi's sarcoma, HIV-associated: plaque *A purple plaque on the nose with nodules on the cheek causing significant cosmetic disfigurement.*

Very common (50 % of individuals) on hard palate, appearing as a violaceous stain, which can become papules and nodules with a cobblestone appearance. Lesions also arise on soft palate, uvula, pharynx, gingiva, and tongue. Conjunctival lesions uncommon.

General Examination KS lesions of the viscera, though common, are often asymptomatic. At autopsy of HIV-infected individuals with mucocutaneous KS, 75 % have visceral involvement (bowel, liver, spleen lungs).

LYMPH NODES In HIV-associated KS, lymph nodes involved in half of cases

UROGENITAL TRACT Prostate, seminal vesicles, testes, bladder, penis, scrotum

LUNG Pulmonary infiltrates

GI TRACT GI hemorrhage, rectal obstruction, protein-losing enteropathy can occur.

OTHER Heart, brain, kidney, adrenal glands

Differential Diagnosis

Single Pigmented Lesion Dermatofibroma (sclerosing hemangioma), pyogenic granuloma, hemangioma, bacillary (epithelioid) angiomatosis, melanocytic nevus, ecchymosis, granuloma annulare, insect bite reactions, stasis dermatitis

Laboratory and Special Examinations

Skin Biopsy The diagnosis of KS should be confirmed histologically in all patients.

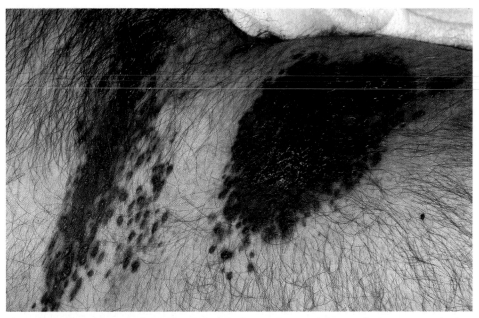

Figure 33-8 Kaposi's sarcoma, HIV-associated: papules, nodules, and plaques *Multiple, purple papules and plaques become confluent in the groin and anterior thigh forming large plaques; associated edema was also present on the lower leg, ankle, and foot.*

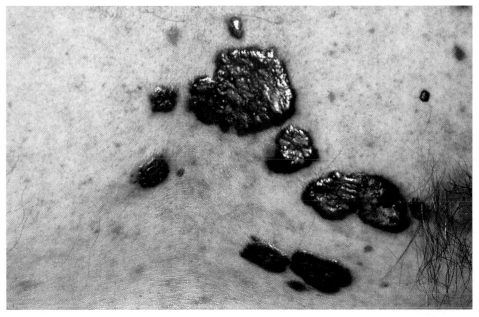

Figure 33-9 Kaposi's sarcoma, HIV-associated: plaques *Large, thick, deep purple plaques and nodules on the anterior chest.*

Dermatopathology   Discrete intradermal nodule with vascular channels lined by atypical endothelial cells among a network of reticulin fibers and extravasated erythrocytes with hemosiderin deposition. Three histologic stages are described:

> *Patch stage:* In the reticular dermis, proliferation of small, irregular, and jagged endothelial-lined spaces surrounding normal dermal vessels and adnexal structures; variable, inflammatory lymphocytic infiltrate (±plasma cells). Promontory sign: a normal vessel or adnexal structure protruding into an ectatic space.
>
> *Plaque stage:* Spindle cells expand throughout dermal collagen bundles forming irregular, cleftlike, angulated vascular channels that contain variable numbers of RBCs. Hemosiderin deposits; eosinophilic hyaline globules. Peripheral perivascular inflammatory infiltrate.
>
> *Nodular stage:* Spindle cells in sheets and fascicles with mild to moderate cytologic atypia, single cell necrosis, trapped RBCs within an extensive network of slitlike vascular spaces.

Culture   Rule out secondary infections

Chest X-Ray   Difficult to distinguish pulmonary KS from *Pneumocystis carinii* pneumonia. In KS, pulmonary nodules and pleural effusions more common.

Diagnosis

Confirmed on lesional skin biopsy

Pathophysiology

Likely that KS cells are derived from the endothelium of the blood/lymphatic microvasculature. Probably not a true malignancy but rather a widespread cellular proliferation in response to angiogenic substances. KS lesions produce factors that promote their own growth as well as the growth of other cells. A new member of the herpesvirus family, HHV8, has been implicated in the pathogenesis of KS.

Course and Prognosis

Classic KS   Average survival 10 to 15 years; usually die of unrelated causes. Secondary malignancies arise in >35 % of cases.

African-Endemic KS   Mean survival in young adults 5 to 8 years; young children, 2 to 3 years.

Immunosuppressive Drug–Associated KS Course may be chronic or rapidly progressive; KS usually resolves after immunosuppressive drugs are discontinued.

HIV-Associated KS   HIV-infected individuals with high CD4+ cell counts can have stable or slowly progressive disease for many years. Rapid progression of KS can occur after decline of CD4+ cell counts to low values, prolonged systemic corticosteroid therapy, or illness such as *P. carinii* pneumonia (PCP). KS of the bowel and/or lungs is the cause of death in 10 % to 20 % of patients.

Cutaneous KS lesions slowly increase in size, may become tuberous and confluent. Patients with only a few lesions, present for several months, without history of opportunistic infections, and CD4+ cell counts >200/μl tend to respond better to therapy and probably have a better overall prognosis. Immunosuppression caused by prednisone or methotrexate may precipitate appearance of KS, which may regress when these agents are withheld. At time of initial diagnosis, 40 % of KS cases have GI involvement; 80 % at autopsy. Reduced survival rate in patients with GI involvement. Pulmonary KS has high short-term mortality rate, i.e., median survival <6 months.

Management

The goal of therapy of KS is to control symptoms of the disease, not cure. A number of local and systemic therapeutic modalities are effective in controlling symptoms. Classic KS responds well to radiotherapy of involved sites. African-endemic KS, when symptomatic, responds best to systemic chemotherapy. Immunosuppressive drug–associated KS regresses or resolves when drug dosages are reduced or discontinued. HIV-associated KS usually responds to a variety of local therapies; for extensive mucocutaneous involvement or visceral involvement, chemotherapy is indicated.

Local therapy is usually directed at individual lesions that are cosmetically disturbing, bulky, bleeding, cause functional disturbance on the palms or soles, or cause lymphatic obstruction and lymphedema.

Limited Intervention

LOCAL THERAPY Effective for a variety of localized lesions; usually associated with mild to moderate discomfort for several days after therapy. The toxicity of systemic chemotherapy is avoided. Many patients with potentially cosmetically disfiguring facial lesions can be treated with a single or a combination of local therapies, minimizing the deformity of progressive KS. A significant percentage of locally treated lesions tend to gradually (months) recur.

Radiotherapy Indicated for tumorous lesions, confluent lesions with a large surface area, large lesions on distal extremity, large oropharyngeal lesions. Dosing: 8 Gy in a single fraction for small lesions, 800 to 3000 rads in single or divided dose.

Cryosurgery A cryospray device should be used. Indicated for deeply pigmented, protruding nodules. Best results with two freeze-thaw cycles. Pain is moderate during freeze cycle; little subsequent pain. Treated lesions heal with crust formation. Facial lesions heal most rapidly (1 to 2 weeks); trunkal and arm lesions in 2 to 4 weeks; lower extremity lesions in 3 to 6 weeks. KS often persists in deeper portions of lesion. Violaceous lesion is replaced with a white scar. Secondary infection is uncommon.

Laser Surgery Pulsed-dye laser effective for small superficial lesion, but expensive

Electrosurgery Effective for ulcerated, bleeding nodular lesion; must use a smoke evacuator in conjunction

Excisional Surgery Effective for selected small lesions. Not a realistic approach to the patient with many lesions.

INTRALESIONAL CYTOTOXIC CHEMOTHERAPY

Vinblastine 0.1 mg (0.5 ml of a 0.2 mg/ml solution) injected per square centimeter of lesion; for refractory lesions, incremental doses of up to 0.2 mg/cm^2 can be given. Most effective for small, early, papular lesions. Larger nodular lesions respond more slowly. For nodular oral lesions, which are usually highly vascular, the 0.2 mg/cm^2 solution is more effective. The maximal total vinblastine dose injected should not exceed 2 mg per clinic visit. The majority of individuals experience mild to moderate pain in the treated lesions lasting 2 to 7 days after injection. Some lesions heal with blister formation and crusting. Injection into hairy areas of the scalp, eyebrow, or beard results in transient alopecia. Inadvertent injection near a cutaneous sensory nerve can result in a neuritic pain that can last up to a month. For persistent lesion, injection can be repeated in 2 to 4 weeks. Secondary infection is uncommon.

Vincristine and Bleomycin Have also been used for intralesional therapy.

Aggressive Intervention

SINGLE-AGENT CHEMOTHERAPY

Adriamycin

Vinblastine IV bolus 0.1 mg/kg weekly

Lipid formulations of daunorubicin and doxirubicin (Daunosome and Doxol) are effective and less toxic than older formulation.

Etoposide (VP16) given orally

Paclitacel (Taxol) given intravenously every 3 weeks

COMBINATION CHEMOTHERAPY

Vincristine (2.0 mg) + bleomycin (15 units/m^2) + Adriamycin (20 mg/m^2) is given every other week in patients with relatively advanced KS.

Interferon-alpha (15 million units/day) + zidovudine (600 mg/day)

BACILLARY ANGIOMATOSIS

Bacillary angiomatosis (BA) is a systemic infection caused by *Bartonella* species, occurring nearly exclusively in HIV-infected individuals, characterized by cutaneous vascular tumors resembling Kaposi's sarcoma and symptomatic multisystemic infection, most commonly involving the liver (peliosis hepatis) and/or spleen (parenchymal bacillary peliosis).

Epidemiology and Etiology

Age Presumably an HIV-infected individual of any age

Etiology *B. henselae* and *B. quintana.* In immunocompetent individuals, *B. henselae* is also the agent of cat-scratch disease.

Reservoir *B. henselae* frequently causes asymptomatic bacteremia in kittens, which has been documented by isolation of the organism by blood cultures or anti-*B. henselae* antibodies. The reservoir for *B. quintana* is unknown.

Transmission Presumably enters percutaneously through minor breaks in the epidermis (scratches or bites). Latent human infection or person-to-person infection has not been documented. Fleas taken from infected cats have been shown by PCR to harbor *B. henselae* and may possibly transmit the organism from cat to human while biting.

Risk Factors BA occurs almost exclusively in HIV-infected individuals with advanced immunodeficiency. Uncommonly, in individuals who are immunocompetent, are immunocompromised for other reasons, and organ-transplant recipients.

Classification of Clinical Syndromes Associated with *Bartonella* Species Occurring in HIV Disease

Cutaneous BA
Peliosis hepatis (liver involvement)
Parenchymal bacillary peliosis (liver and spleen involvement)
Fever and bacteremia (*Bartonella* bacteremic syndrome)

History

Incubation Period Unknown, but probably days to weeks

History Of owning or having been scratched by a kitten. Patients with localized infection may be free of systemic symptoms. Those with more widespread disseminated infection have fever, malaise, weight loss.

CUTANEOUS BA Lesions may be painful, in contrast with Kaposi's sarcoma lesions, which are not painful.

PELIOSIS HEPATIS Presents with nausea, vomiting, diarrhea, fever, chills. Bony lesions may cause focal bone pain. The clinical picture can progress rapidly, in contrast with Kaposi's sarcoma, which usually progresses slowly.

BARTONELLA BACTEREMIC SYNDROME Symptoms develop insidiously (weeks to months): malaise, fatigue, anorexia, weight loss, recurring fevers of gradually higher elevations.

Physical Examination

Skin Lesions

TYPES Papules or nodules resembling angiomas (Figure 33-10A); up to 2 to 3 cm in diameter; usually situated in dermis with thinning or erosion of overlying epidermis surrounded by a collarette of scale. Pyogenic granuloma–like lesions (Figure 33-10B). Subcutaneous nodules, 1 to 2 cm in diameter, resembling cysts. Uncommonly, abscess formation.

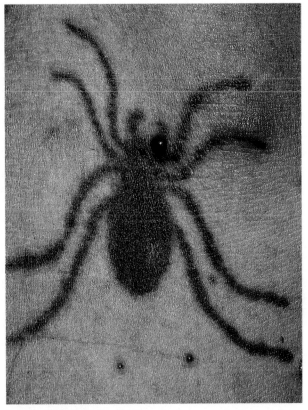

A

Figure 33-10 Bacillary angiomatosis   A. *Sharply demarcated cherry-red papules on the arm resembling cherry hemangioma, with similar lesions on the other arm, trunk, and thighs; the spider tattoo acquired a new red "eye."*

NUMBER Papules/nodules range from solitary lesions to >100 and, rarely, >1000.

COLOR Red, bright red, violaceous, or skin-colored

PALPATION Firm, nonblanching. Lesions may be nontender or painful, a finding not seen in nodular lesions of Kaposi's sarcoma.

DISTRIBUTION Any site, but palms and soles are usually spared. Occasionally, lesions occur at the site of a cat scratch. A solitary lesion presenting as a dactylitis.

Mucous Membranes Angioma-like lesions of lips and oral mucosa. Laryngeal involvement with obstruction.

Systemic Findings Infection may spread hematogenously or via lymphatics to become systemic, commonly involving the liver and spleen (hepatosplenomegaly, liver abscesses, necrotizing splenitis, hepatic/splenic necrotizing granulomata). Lesions also may occur in the heart (cardiac lesions, endocarditis), bone marrow, lymph nodes, muscles, and soft tissues, CNS (brain abscess, aseptic meningitis, encephalopathy).

Differential Diagnosis

Kaposi's sarcoma, pyogenic granuloma, epithelioid (histiocytoid) angioma, cherry angioma, sclerosing hemangioma, disseminated cryptococcosis

Laboratory and Special Examinations

Dermatopathology Lobular vascular proliferations composed of plump "epitheloid" cells. Neutrophils scattered throughout the lesion, especially around eosinophilic granular aggregates, which are masses of bacteria (visualized by Warthin-Starry staining or electron microscopy).

Liver Biopsy Associated with higher morbidity and mortality in that the lesions are vascular tumors. Dilated capillaries or multiple blood-filled cavernous spaces; myxoid stroma

containing an admixture of inflammatory cells and granular clumps *(Bartonella).*

Culture *Bartonella* can be isolated from lesional skin biopsy specimens, blood, or other infected tissues on endothelial-cell monolayer.

PCR Detects *Bartonella* DNA in tissue

Chemistry Bacillary peliosis hepatis associated with elevated gamma-glutamyltransferase, alkaline phosphatase

Serology Anti-*Bartonella* antibodies detected by indirect fluorescent-antibody testing (detected by the Centers for Disease Control and Prevention). Also, enzyme immunoassay for detection of IgG antibodies to *B. henselae* (Specialty Laboratories, Santa Monica, CA).

Imaging Lesions can be visualized by conventional radiographs and nuclear imaging. Lesions regress with appropriate therapy. CT scan shows hepatomegaly, ±splenomegaly.

Diagnosis

Clinical findings confirmed by demonstration of *Bartonella* bacilli on silver stain of lesional biopsy specimen or culture or antibody studies

Pathophysiology

Cutaneous lesions of BA resemble the bacterial infection verruga peruana, i.e., bartonellosis, the chronic cutaneous infection by *B. bacilliformis.* Vascular proliferation occurs in response to *Bartonella.*

Course and Prognosis

Course variable. In some individuals, lesions regress spontaneously. Untreated systemic infection causes significant morbidity and mortality. With effective antimicrobial therapy, lesions resolve within 1 to 2 weeks. As with other infections occurring in HIV disease, relapse may occur and require lifelong secondary prophylaxis.

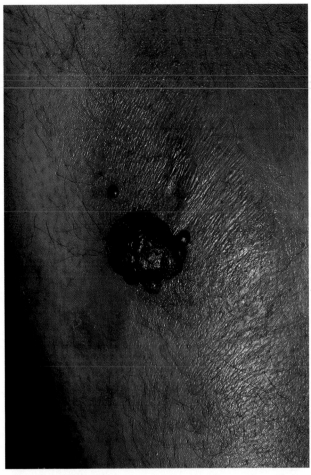

B

Figure 33-10 Bacillary angiomatosis B. *In the same patient, a large, ulcerated vascular tumor resembling a pyogenic granuloma on the right shin area.*

Management

Prevention HIV-infected individuals should avoid contact with cats, especially kittens, to minimize the risk for acquiring BA, as well as toxoplasmosis.

Antimicrobial Therapy Given for 8 to 12 weeks. A Jarisch-Herxheimer type reaction may occur shortly after beginning therapy.

ERYTHROMYCIN 500 mg PO q.i.d.

DOXYCYCLINE 100 mg PO b.i.d.

CIPROFLOXACIN 750 mg PO b.i.d.

AZITHROMYCIN 500 mg PO q.d.

Secondary Prophylaxis Lifelong maintenance if relapses occur

ORAL HAIRY LEUKOPLAKIA

Oral hairy leukoplakia (OHL) is a benign, virally induced hyperplasia of the oral mucosa, most commonly of the inferolateral surface of the tongue, characterized by white, corrugated, verrucous plaques, occurring in patients with progressive HIV-induced immunodeficiency.
Synonym: Oral viral leukoplakia.

Epidemiology and Etiology

Sex Males > females

Etiology Epstein-Barr virus (EBV)

History

Risk Groups Occurs almost exclusively in HIV-infected individuals. Rarely noted in immunosuppressed renal transplantation patients.

Incubation Period Usually >5 years after primary HIV infection

Symptoms Lesions are asymptomatic; uncommonly a cosmetic problem. Extent of lesions varies from day to day.

Physical Examination

Skin Findings

ORAL MUCOSA White or grayish white, well-demarcated verrucous plaque (Figure 33-11). Surface appears irregular, with corrugated or hairy texture. Often present bilaterally, but size of plaques usually not equal.

DISTRIBUTION OF LESIONS Most commonly on the lateral and inferior surface of the tongue. Less commonly seen on the buccal and soft palatal mucosa.

Differential Diagnosis

Hyperplastic oral candidiasis, condyloma acuminatum, geographic or migratory glossitis, lichen planus, tobacco-associated leukoplakia, mucous patch of secondary syphilis, squamous cell carcinoma either *in situ* or invasive, occlusal trauma

Laboratory and Special Examinations

Dermatopathology Acanthotic epithelium with hyperkeratosis, hairlike projections of keratin, areas of koilocytes (ballooned cells with clear cytoplasm)

Cultures Not helpful. *Candida albicans* is commonly isolated.

Electron Microscopy Herpes viral structures within epithelial cells; positive for Epstein-Barr virus markers; often also HPV viral particles.

Diagnosis

Clinical diagnosis. Does not rub off; does not clear with adequate anticandidal therapy.

Pathophysiology

Epstein-Barr viral infection of the oral mucosa appears to be responsible for the epidermal hyperplasia. In those patients who do not carry the diagnosis of AIDS at the time of detection of OHL, the probability of developing AIDS has been reported to be 48 % by 16 months after detection and 83 % by 31 months.

Course and Prognosis

The severity of OHL varies spontaneously from day to day. May clear completely during a course of treatment with zidovudine, acyclovir (oral or topical), IV ganciclovir, or foscarnet.

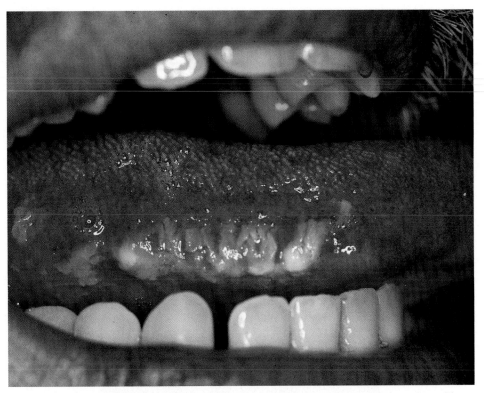

Figure 33-11 Oral hairy leukoplakia *White plaque on the lateral tongue with corduroy-like pattern.*

Management

OHL is asymptomatic, but its presence may cause anxiety in patients with the lesion. Reassurance that OHL is a benign viral infection is usually adequate to reduce patients' concerns.

Topical Therapy Podophyllin 25 % in tincture of benzoin applied to the lesion with a cotton-tipped applicator for 5 minutes is very ef-fective in most individuals. OHL usually recurs in weeks to months.

Systemic Antiviral Drugs Concomitant use of acyclovir, valacyclovir, famciclovir, ganciclovir, foscarnet for other indications often results in regression/clearing of OHL.

HERPES SIMPLEX VIRUS INFECTION

Herpes simplex virus infection (see also Herpes simplex virus: infections in the immunocompromised host, Section 29). Reactivated herpes simplex virus type 1 (HSV-1) or HSV-2 infection is one of the most common viral complications of HIV disease. In early HIV disease, HSV infection has a classic presentation, with grouped vesicles or erosions that heal in 1 to 2 weeks without treatment. With increasing immunodeficiency, early lesions present with erosions or ulcerations due to epidermal necrosis without vesicle formation. Untreated, these lesions may evolve to large, painful ulcers with raised margins. In contrast to healthy individuals, reactivated HSV in those with advanced HIV disease can cause large, chronic ulceration in the oropharynx, esophagus, and anogenitalia. HSV should be considered in the differential diagnosis of any ulcerative or crusted lesion occurring on the face or anogenitalia in an individual with advanced HIV disease. Ulcers persisting after adequate acyclovir therapy may be caused by acyclovir-resistant HSV strains.

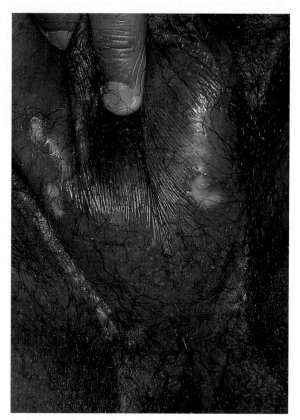

Figure 33-12 Chronic herpetic ulcers: inguinal fold, scrotum *Linear and oval ulcers of 6 week duration; this opportunistic infection was the presenting symptom of his HIV infection.*

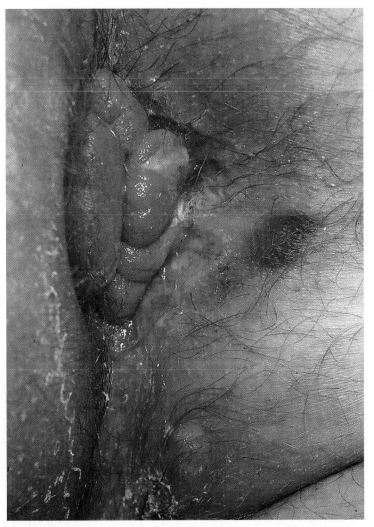

Figure 33-13 Chronic herpetic ulcers: perianal *Large, very painful ulcers with associated Kaposi's sarcoma.*

VARICELLA ZOSTER VIRUS INFECTION

Varicella-Zoster virus infection (see also VZV: Infections in the immunocompromised host, Section 29) Primary varicella-zoster virus (VZV) infection (chickenpox) in HIV-infected individuals can be severe, prolonged, and complicated by parenchymal infection, bacterial superinfection, and death. With increasing immunodeficiency, VZV infection can present clinically as chronic dermatomal verrucous lesions, one or more chronic painful ulcers or ecthymatous lesions within a dermatome, or disseminated infection presenting with vesicle(s)/bulla(e), ecthymatous lesion(s), ulcer(s), or nodule(s) resembling basal cell carcinoma or squamous cell carcinoma. Untreated these lesions persist for months or the lifetime of the patient. Herpes zoster can be recurrent within the same dermatome(s) or in other dermatomes. VZV can cause a rapidly progressive chorioretinitis with acute retinal necrosis, often bilaterally, in the absence of any cutaneus involvement and must be differentiated from cytomegalovirus (CMV) chorioretinitis.

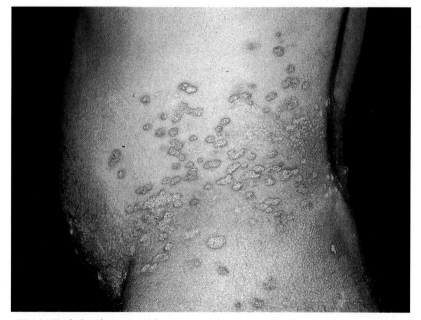

Figure 33-14 VZV infection: chronic verrucous zoster *Confluent warts, papules in several contiguous dermatomes, present for 2 years.*

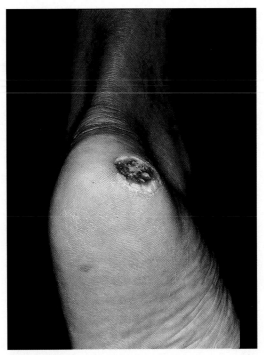

Figure 33-15 VZV infection: solitary ulcer on heel *The patient presented with a very painful bulla on the heel of 3 weeks duration. Debridement revealed a punched-out ulcer.*

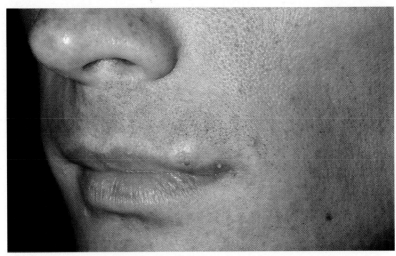

Figure 33-16 Molluscum contagiosum: giant *A large solitary skin-colored nodule with a central keratotic core or plug on the upper lip was the presenting symptom of this man's transfusion associated HIV infection.*

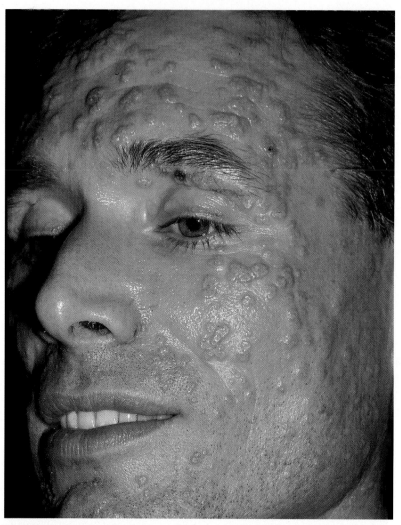

Figure 33-17 Molluscum contagiosum: multiple confluent   *Dozens of umbilicated skin-colored papules on the face of a male with advanced HIV disease. The lesions were successfully treated with aggressive electrodessication and curettage.*

CUTANEOUS SIGNS OF INJECTING DRUG USE

Injecting drug users usually attempt to inject drug into veins, which can result in "tracks" over accessible veins and scars at old injection sites. Injection of contaminated "drug" can produce sterile abscess formation or bacterial cellulitis.

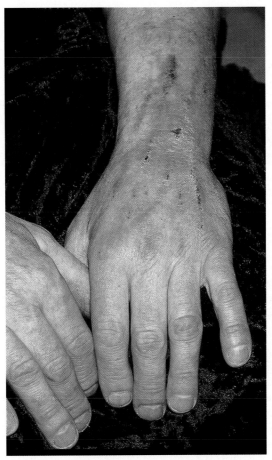

Figure 33-18 Injecting drug use: injection tracks over veins on the dorsum of the hand
Linear tracks with fibrosis and crusts were created by daily heroin injection into the superficial veins.

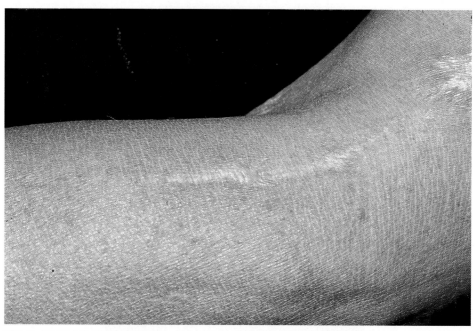

Figure 33-19 Injecting drug use: old injection sites in the anticubital fossa *Depressed white scars created ten years ago while injecting drugs intravenously in an HIV-infected individual.*

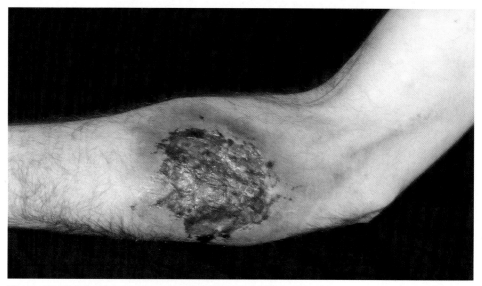

Figure 33-20 Injecting drug use: cellulitis at injection site *The patient injected illicit drug into the skin of the forearm causing an initial site of S. aureus cellulitis with associated bacteremia and infectious endocarditis and subsequent foreign body response at the site.*

VARIATIONS OF COMMON MUCOCUTANEOUS DISORDERS IN HIV DISEASE

Early in HIV disease when immune function is relatively intact, common dermatoses and infections present in typical ways, have the usual course, and respond to the treatments of choice. However, with progressive decline in immune function, each of these characteristics of a disease can be strikingly altered, such that the correct diagnosis is not considered nor correct treatment instituted.

Aphthous stomatitis (see also Aphthous ulcers, page 126) *Recurrent aphthous ulcerations occur more frequently and are larger (often >1 cm) in persons with advanced HIV disease. Ulcers may be quite extensive, commonly involving the tongue, gingiva, lips, and esophagus, at times causing severe odynophagia with rapid weight loss.*

Drug eruptions (see also Exanthematous drug eruption, page 576) *The incidence of cutaneous drug eruptions is greatly increased in HIV disease and may be correlated with the decline and dysregulation of immune function. Between 50 % and 60 % of patients with AIDS treated with trimethoprim-sulfamethoxazole develop a morbilliform eruption 1 to 2 weeks after starting therapy. Other drugs associated with an increased incidence of cutaneous reactions include sulfadiazine, trimethoprim-dapsone, and aminopenicillins. The incidence of toxic epidermal necrolysis caused by sulfonamides is also increased.*

Staphylococcus aureus Infection (see also Impetigo and ecthyma, page 604; Abscess, furuncle, and carbuncle, page 610; and Cellulitis, page 634) S. aureus *is the most common cutaneous bacterial pathogen in HIV disease. The nasal carriage rate of* S. aureus *is 50 %, twice that of HIV-seronegative control groups. In most instances,* S. aureus *infections are typical, presenting as primary infections (folliculitis, furuncles, carbuncles), secondarily impetiginized lesions (excoriations, eczema, scabies, herpetic ulcer, Kaposi's sarcoma), cellulitis, or venous access device infections, all of which can be complicated by bacteremia and disseminated infection.*

Dermatophytosis (see also Dermatophytoses, page 688) *Epidermal dermatophytosis in HIV-infected individuals can be extensive, recurrent, and difficult to eradicate. Tinea unguium is typically caused by* Trichophyton rubrum; *in HIV-infected patients, proximal white subungual onychomycosis, which is rare in non-HIV-infected individuals, is a common presentation of* T. rubrum *tinea unguium, appearing as a chalky-white proximal nail discoloration, and, when detected, is an indication for HIV serotesting.*

Human papilloma virus (HPV) infection (see also Human papilloma virus infections, page 766) *With advancing immunodeficiency, cutaneous and/or mucosal warts can become extensive and refractory to treatment. Of more concern, however, HPV-induced intraepithelial neoplasia, more recently termed* squamous intraepithelial lesion *(SIL), is a precursor to invasive squamous cell carcinoma (SCC), arising most often on the cervix, vulva, penis, perineum, and anus. In HIV-infected females, the incidence of cervical SIL is six to eight times that of controls. The current trend toward longer median survival of patients with advanced HIV disease may lead to an increased incidence of HPV-associated neoplasia and invasive SCC in the future. SIL on the external genitalia, perineum, or anus is best managed with local therapies such as 5-fluorouracil cream, cryosurgery, electrosurgery, or laser surgery rather than aggressive surgical excision.*

Molluscum contagiosum (see also Molluscum contagiosum, page 772)   *In HIV-infected individuals, molluscum contagiosum has up to an 18 % prevalence; the severity of the infection is a marker for advanced immunodeficiency. Patients may have multiple small papules or nodules or large tumors, >1 cm in diameter, most commonly arising on the face, especially the beard area, the neck, and intertriginous sites. Shaving is a major factor in the facial spread of mollusca and should be avoided if possible. Cystlike mollusca occur on the ears. Occasionally, mollusca can arise on the non-hair-bearing skin of the palms/soles. Multiple facial mollusca must be differentiated from the cutaneous lesions of disseminated fungal infection (cryptococcosis, histoplasmosis, coccidioidomycosis, and penicillinosis). Therapy is aimed at reducing the number of disfiguring lesions, rather than cure of the infection, and includes the use of cryosurgery, curettage, electrodesiccation, and laser ablation.*

Syphilis (see also Syphilis, page 877)   *The clinical course of syphilis in HIV-infected individuals is most often the same as in the normal host, with a painless chancre in primary syphilis or a macular or papular eruption is secondary syphilis. However, an accelerated course with the development of neurosyphilis or tertiary syphilis has been reported within months of initial syphilitic infection.*

Mucosal candidiasis (see also Mucosal candidiasis, page 724)   *Mucosal candidiasis affecting the upper aerodigestive tracts and vulvovagina is common in HIV disease. Oropharyngeal candidiasis, the most common presentation, is often the initial manifestation of HIV disease and a marker for disease progression. Four patterns are commonly seen: erythematous/atrophic, pseudomembranous/thrush, hyperplastic/Candida leukoplakia, and angular cheilitis. Esophageal and tracheobronchial candidiases occur in advance of HIV disease and are AIDS-defining conditions. The incidence of recurrent candidal vulvovaginitis appears to be increased in HIV-infected women compared with non-HIV-infected controls. The incidence of cutaneous candidiasis may be somewhat increased in HIV disease. In young children with HIV disease, chronic candidal paronychia and nail dystrophy are seen frequently.*

Invasive fungal infection with cutaneous dissemination (see also Disseminated cryptococcosis, page 744; Histoplasmosis, page 748; and Disseminated coccidioidomycosis, page 755)   *Latent pulmonary fungal infections with* Cryptococcus neoformans, Coccidioides immitis, Histoplasma capsulatum, *or* Penicillium marneffei *can reactivate in HIV-infected individuals and disseminate to the skin. The most common cutaneous presentation of disseminated infection is molluscum contagiosum–like lesions on the face; other lesions such as nodules, pustules, ulcers, abscesses, or a papulosquamous eruption resembling guttate psoriasis (seen with histoplasmosis) also occur.*

APPENDICES

APPENDIX A: TYPES OF SKIN LESIONS

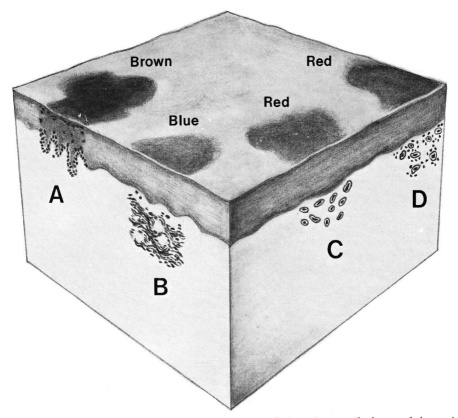

Figure A-1 Macule (*Latin:* macula, *"a spot"*) *A macule is a circumscribed area of change in normal skin color without elevation or depression. It is not palpable. Lesions may appear as macules but are shown to be elevated (i.e., papular) by oblique lighting. This may be important in pigmented lesions. Macules may be of any size and are the result of (1) hypopigmentation (e.g., vitiligo) or hyperpigmentation—melanin such as café-au-lait spots (A) and Mongolian spots (B) or hemosiderin D, (2) permanent vascular abnormalities of the skin, as in a capillary hemangioma, or (3) transient capillary dilatation (erythema) (C). Pressure of a glass slide (diascopy) on the border of a red lesion is a simple and reliable method for detecting the extravasation of red blood cells. If the redness remains under pressure from the slide, the lesion may be purpuric (D); if the redness disappears, the lesion is erythematous and is due to vascular dilatation (C).*

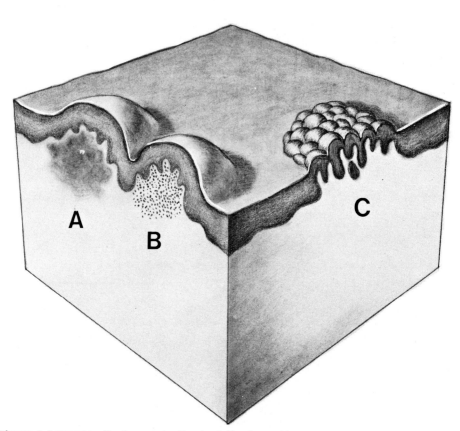

Figure A-2 Papule (*Latin:* papula, *"a pimple"*) *A papule is a superficial, solid lesion, generally considered less than 0.5 cm in diameter. Most of it is elevated above, rather than deep within, the plane of the surrounding skin. A papule is palpable. In papules the elevation is caused by metabolic, external or locally produced deposits (A) or by localized cellular infiltrates (B) or by hyperplasia of local cellular elements (C). Superficial papules are sharply defined. Deeper dermal papules resulting from cellular infiltrates have indistinct borders. Papules with distinct borders are seen when the lesion is the result of an increase in the number of epidermal cells (C) or melanocytes. The topography of a papule may consist of multiple, small, closely packed, projected elevations that are known as a* vegetation *(C). Confluence of papules leads to the development of larger, usually flat-topped, circumscribed, plateau-like elevations known as plaques (French;* plaque, *"plate"). See Figure A-3*

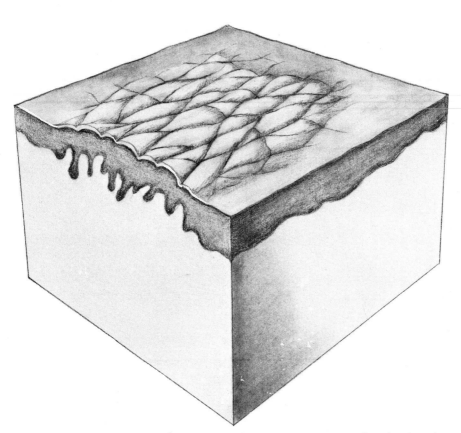

Figure A-3 Plaque *A plaque is a plateau-like elevation above the skin surface that occupies a relatively large surface area in comparison with its height above the skin. It is usually well-defined. Frequently it is formed by a confluence of papules as in psoriasis and mycosis fungoides. Lichenification is a less well-defined, large plaque where the skin appears thickened, and the skin markings are accentuated (as shown in this figure). The process results from repeated rubbing of the skin and most frequently develops in persons with atopy. Lichenification occurs also in eczematous dermatitis, psoriasis, and mycosis fungoides.*

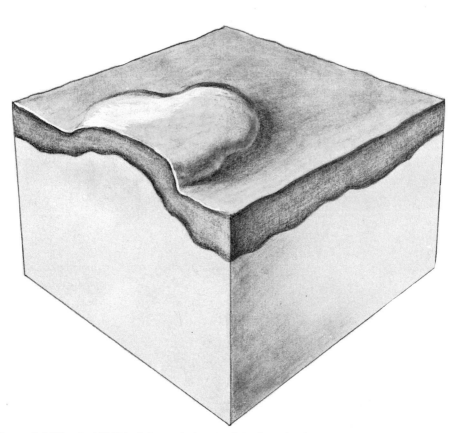

Figure A-4 Wheal (*Old English:* weal, *"a raised mark on the skin caused by the blow of a rod or lash"*) *A wheal is a rounded or flat-topped, pale-red papule or plaque that is characteristically evanescent, disappearing within hours. Wheals may be round, gyrate, or irregular with pseudopods—changing rapidly in size and shape due to shifting edema in the dermis.*

Wheals that do not disappear in 72 hours
are typical of *urticarial vasculitis*, and
a biopsy is indicated.

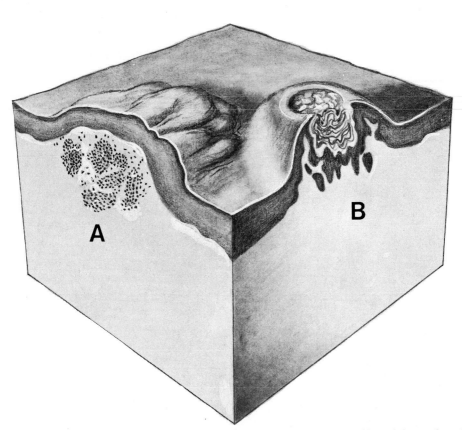

Figure A-5 Nodule *(Latin:* nodulus, *"small knot")* *A nodule is a palpable, solid, round or el-*
lipsoidal lesion and may involve the epidermis (B), dermis, or subcutaneous tissue (A). The depth
of involvement and the size differentiate a nodule from a papule. Nodules result from infiltrates
(A), neoplasms (B), or metabolic deposits in the dermis or subcutaneous tissue and often indicate
systemic disease. Tuberculosis, the deep mycoses, lymphoma, and metastatic neoplasms, for ex-
ample, can present as cutaneous nodules. Nodules can develop as a result of a benign or malig-
nant proliferation of keratinocytes, as in keratoacanthoma (B) and squamous cell and basal cell
carcinoma.

> Persistent nontender dermal nodules are
>   important signs of multisystem dis-
>   eases, and biopsy and cultures of
>   minced skin are necessary.

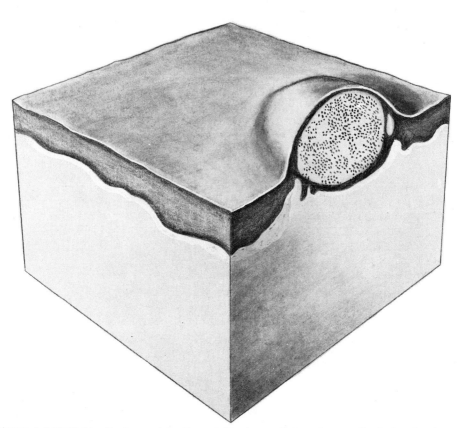

Figure A-6 Pustule (*Latin:* pustula, *"pustule"*) *A pustule is a circumscribed, superficial cavity of the skin that contains a purulent exudate that may be white, yellow, greenish yellow, or hemorrhagic. This process may arise in a hair follicle or independently. Pustules may vary in size and shape; follicular pustules, however, are always conical and usually contain a hair in the center. The vesicular lesions of herpes simplex and varicella zoster virus infections may become pustular.*

> A Gram's stain and culture should be done on all pustules for identification of bacteria and fungi.

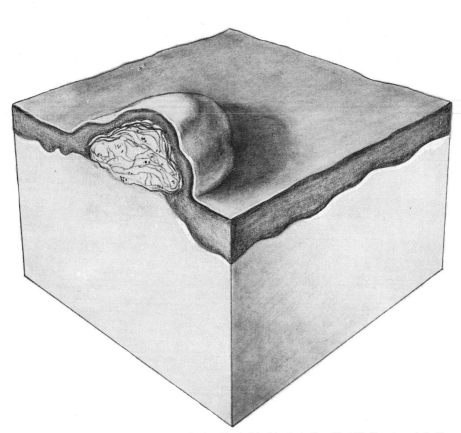

Figure A-7 Vesicle-Bulla (*Latin:* vesicula, *"little bladder"*; bulla, *"bubble"*) *A vesicle (less than 0.5 cm) or a bulla (more than 0.5 cm) is a circumscribed, elevated, superficial cavity containing fluid. Often the walls are so thin that they are translucent, and the serum, lymph fluid, blood, or extracellular fluid can be seen. Vesicles and bullae arise from a cleavage at various levels of the skin; the cleavage may be within the epidermis (i.e., intraepidermal vesication) or at the epidermal-dermal interface (i.e., subepidermal), as in this figure.*

> Grouped "herpetiform" vesicles are indications for the Tzanck test and/or viral cultures.

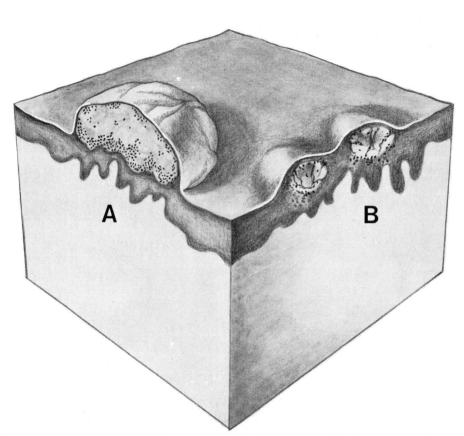

Figure A-8 Vesicle-Bulla [(A) Subcorneal, (B) Spongiotic] *When the cleavage is just beneath the stratum corneum, a subcorneal vesicle or bulla results (A), as in impetigo and subcorneal pustular dermatosis. Intraepidermal vesication may result from intercellular edema or spongiosis (B), as characteristically seen in delayed hypersensitivity reactions of the epidermis (e.g., in contact eczematous dermatitis) and in dyshidrotic eczema (B). Spongiotic vesicles may or may not be observed clinically as vesicles.*

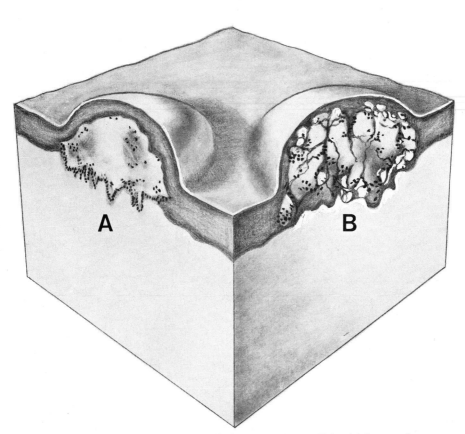

Figure A-9 Vesicle [(A) Acantholytic, (B) Viral] *Loss of intercellular bridges, or desmosomes, is known as* acantholysis *(A), and this type of intraepidermal vesication is seen in the vesicles or bullae of pemphigus. Viruses cause a curious "ballooning degneration" of epidermal cells (B) followed by acantholysis, as in herpes zoster, herpes simplex, and varicella.*

Viral bullae often have a depressed ("umbilicated") center. In older patients with multiple bullae, a biopsy and immunofluorescence are necessary for diagnosis of pemphigus or pemphigoid.

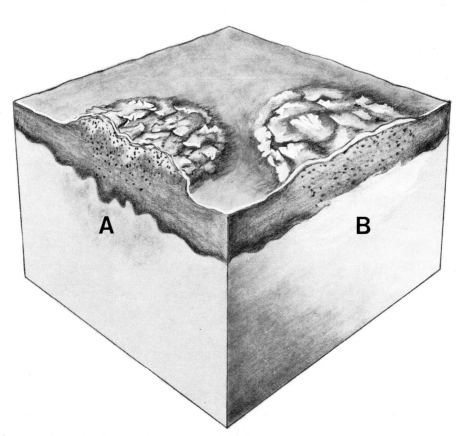

Figure A-10 Crusts [(A) Impetigo, (B) Ecthyma] (*Latin:* crusta, *"rind, bark, shell"*) *Crusts develop when serum, blood, or purulent exudate dries on the skin surface. Crusts may be thin, delicate, and friable (A) or thick and adherent (B). Crusts are yellow when formed from dried serum, green or yellow-green when formed from purulent exudate, or brown or dark red when formed from blood. Superficial crusts occur as honey-colored, delicate, glistening particulates on the surface (A) and are typically found in impetigo. When the exudate involves the entire epidermis, the crusts may be thick and adherent, and if it is accompanied by necrosis of the deeper tissues the condition is known as* ecthyma *(B).*

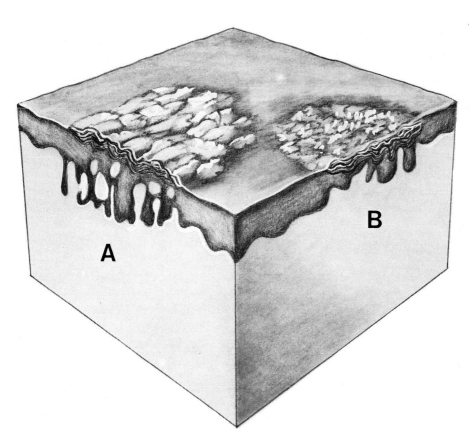

Figure A-11 Desquamation (scaling) [(A) Psoriasis, (B) Solar Keratosis] *Epidermal cells are replaced every 27 days. The end product of this holocrine process is the stratum corneum. This outermost layer of skin, the stratum corneum, normally does not contain nuclei and is imperceptibly lost. With an increased rate of proliferation of epidermal cells, as in psoriasis, the stratum corneum is not formed normally, and the outermost layers of the skin retain the nuclei (parakeratosis). These desquamating layers of skin are seen clinically as scales (A). Scales are thus flakes of stratum corneum. They may be large (like membranes) or tiny (like dust), adherent or loose. Densely adherent scales that have a gritty feel (like sandpaper) result from a localized increase in the stratum corneum and are a characteristic of solar keratosis (B).*

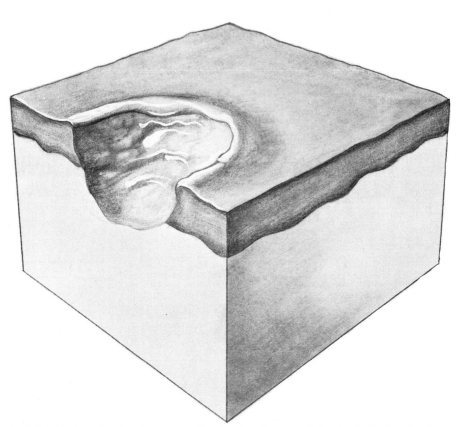

Figure A-12 Ulcer (*Latin:* ulcus, *"sore"*) *An ulcer is a skin defect in which there has been loss of epidermis and the upper papillary layer of the dermis. It may extend into the subcutis and always occurs within pathologically altered tissue. (This differentiates an ulcer from a wound which is a defect inflicted on normal tissue.) An erosion is a defect only of the epidermis, not involving the dermis; in contrast to an ulcer which always heals with scar formation, an erosion heals without a scar. Certain features that are helpful in determining the cause of ulcers include location, borders, base, discharge, and any associated topographic features, such as nodules, excoriations, varicosities, hair distribution, presence or absence of sweating, and pulses.*

In any ulcer not related to vascular disease, a wedge biopsy for histology and minced tissue for microbial culture is required.

APPENDIX B: SPECIAL CLINICAL AND LABORATORY AIDS TO DERMATOLOGIC DIAGNOSIS

Special Techniques Used in Clinical Examination

1. *Magnification with hand lens.* To examine lesions for fine morphologic detail, it is necessary to use a magnifying glass (hand lens) (7×) or a binocular microscope (5× to 40×). Magnification is especially helpful in the diagnosis of lupus erythematosus (follicular plugging), lichen planus (Wickham's striae), carcinomas (translucence and telangiectasia), and malignant melanoma (subtle changes in color, especially gray or blue; this is best visualized following application of a drop of mineral oil). Hand lenses with built-in lighting and a magnification of 10× to 30× (dermatoscope) are now available that permit observation of lesions covered with a drop of oil (oil-immersion effect) and thus allow inspection of deeper layers of the skin (dermal-epidermal junction.) This is called *epiluminescence microscopy* and allows the distinction of benign and malignant growth patterns, particularly in pigmented lesions.

2. *Oblique lighting* of the skin lesion, done in a darkened room, is often required to detect slight degrees of elevation or depression, and it is useful in the visualization of the surface configuration of lesions and in estimating the extent of the eruption.

3. *Subdued lighting* in the examining room enhances the contrast between circumscribed hypopigmented or hyperpigmented lesions and normal skin.

4. *Wood's lamp* (ultraviolet long-wave light, "black" light) is valuable in the diagnosis of certain skin and hair diseases and of porphyria. Long-wave ultraviolet radiation can be obtained by fitting a high-pressure mercury lamp with a specially compounded filter made of nickel oxide and silica (Wood's filter); this filter is very opaque to all light except for a band between 320 and 400 nm.

When the ultraviolet waves emitted by Wood's lamp (360 nm) impinge on the skin, fluorescent pigments and subtle color differences of melanin pigmentation can be visualized. Wood's lamp is particularly useful in the detection of the fluorescence of dermatophytosis in the hair shaft (green to yellow) and of erythrasma (coral red). A presumptive diagnosis of porphyria can be made if a pinkish red fluorescence is demonstrated in urine examined with the Wood's lamp; addition of dilute hydrochloric acid intensifies the fluorescence. Wood's lamp also helps to estimate variation in the lightness of lesions in relation to the normal skin color, in both dark-skinned and fair-skinned peoples; e.g., the lesions seen in tuberous sclerosis and tinea versicolor are hypomelanotic and are not as white as the lesions seen in vitiligo, which are amelanotic. Circumscribed hypermelanosis, such as a freckle and melasma, is much more evident (darker) under Wood's lamp. On the other hand, dermal melanin as in a Mongolian sacral spot does not become accentuated under Wood's lamp. Therefore, it is possible to localize the site of melanin by use of the Wood's lamp; this, however, is more difficult or not possible in patients with brown skin.

5. *Diascopy* consists of firmly pressing a microscopic slide over a skin lesion. The examiner will find this procedure of special value in determining whether the red color of a macule or papule is due to capillary dilatation (erythema) or to extravasation of blood (purpura) that does not blanch. Diascopy is also useful for the detection of the glassy yellow-brown appearance of papules in sarcoidosis, tuberculosis of the skin, lymphoma, and granuloma annulare.

6. *Acetowhitening* facilitates detection of subclinical penile warts. Male partners of HPV-infected females with genital warts may also be infected. Gauze saturated with

5 % acetic acid (white vinegar) is wrapped around the penis or placed between the labia. After 5 to 10 minutes the penis or vulva is inspected with a 10× hand lens. Warts appear as small white papules.

Clinical Tests

1. *Darier's sign* is "positive" when a brown macular or a slightly papular lesion of urticaria pigmentosa (mastocytosis) becomes a palpable wheal after being vigorously rubbed with the blunt end of an instrument such as a pen. The wheal may not appear for 5 to 10 minutes.
2. *Auspitz's sign* is "positive" when slight scratching or curetting of a scaly lesion reveals punctate bleeding points within the lesion. This suggests psoriasis, but it is not specific.
3. *Patch testing* is used to document and validate a diagnosis of allergic contact sensitization and identify the causative agent. It also may be of value as a screening procedure in some patients with chronic or bizarre eczematous eruptions (e.g., hand and foot dermatoses). Substances to be tested are applied to the skin in shallow cups (Finn chambers), affixed with a tape and left in place for 24 to 48 hours. Contact hypersensitivity will result in a papular-vesicular reaction that develops within 48 to 72 hours when the test is read. It is a unique means of in vivo reproduction of disease in diminutive proportions, for sensitization affects all the skin and may therefore be elicited at any cutaneous site. The patch test is easier and safer than a "use test" with a questionable allergen, for test items can be applied in low concentrations in small areas of skin for short periods of time. See textbooks on contact dermatitis for a list of antigens used in patch testing.
4. *Photopatch testing* is a combination of patch testing and UV irradiation of the test site and is used to document photoallergy.

Microscopic Examination of Scales, Crusts, Serum, and Hair

1. *Gram's stains* and *cultures of exudates and of tissue minces* should be made in lesions suspected of being bacterial or yeast *(Candida albicans)* infections. Ulcers and nodules require a scalpel biopsy in which a wedge of tissue consisting of all three layers of skin is obtained; the biopsy specimen is minced in a sterile mortar and is then cultured for bacteria (including typical and atypical mycobacteria) and fungi.
2. *Microscopic examination* for mycelia should be made of the roofs of vesicles or of the scales (the advancing borders are preferable) or of the hair. The tissue is cleared with 10 % to 30 % KOH and warmed gently (see Figure 25-2). Fungal cultures with Sabouraud's medium should be made.
3. *Microscopic examination of cells obtained from the base of vesicles* (Tzanck preparation) may reveal the presence of acantholytic cells in the acantholytic diseases (e.g., pemphigus or SSS syndrome) or of giant epithelial cells and multinucleated giant cells (containing 10 to 12 nuclei) in herpes simplex, herpes zoster, and varicella. Material from the base of a vesicle obtained by *gentle* curettage with a scalpel is smeared on a glass slide, stained with Giemsa's stain, Wright's stain, or methylene blue, and examined to determine whether there are acantholytic or giant epithelial cells, which are diagnostic. Culture of herpes simplex is now easily available.
4. *Laboratory diagnosis of scabies.* The diagnosis of scabies is usually considered immediately in a patient with intractable generalized pruritus and with papules and excoriations distributed in characteristic locations—on the flexor aspects of the wrists, in the finger webs, and on the buttocks and genitalia; the diagnosis is established by identification of the mite, or ova or feces, in skin scrapings removed from the papules or burrows (see Figure 30-8). The burrow,

a unique lesion, is a linear or serpiginous elevation of skin in the form of a ridge, 0.5 to 1.0 cm in length. These occur on the anterior surface of the wrists, in the webs of the fingers, or on the ulnar border of the hands. If burrows are not present, select a papule or the roof of a vesicle on the hand. The mineral oil technique is excellent for isolating the mite. Using a sterile scalpel blade on which a drop of sterile mineral oil has been placed, apply oil to the surface of the burrow or papule. Scrape the papule or burrow vigorously (about six times) in order to remove the entire top of the papule; tiny flecks of blood will appear in the oil. Transfer the oil to a microscopic slide and examine for mites, ova, and feces. The mites are 0.2 to 0.4 mm in size and have four pairs of legs (see Figure 30-8).

Biopsy of the Skin

Biopsy of the skin is one of the simplest, most rewarding diagnostic techniques in medical practice because of the easy accessibility of the skin and the variety of techniques for study of the excised specimen (e.g., histopathology, immunofluorescence, electron microscopy).

Selection of the site of the biopsy is based primarily on the stage of the eruption, and early lesions are usually more typical; this is especially important in vesiculobullous eruptions (e.g., pemphigus, herpes simplex), in which the lesion should be no more than 24 hours old. However, older lesions (2 to 6 weeks) are often more characteristic in discoid lupus erythematosus.

A common technique for diagnostic biopsy is the use of a 3.0- to 4.0-mm punch, a small tubular knife much like a corkscrew, which by rotating movements between the thumb and index finger cuts through the epidermis, dermis, and subcutaneous tissue; the base is cut off with scissors. If immunofluorescence is indicated (as, for example, in bullous diseases or lupus erythematosus), a special technique is necessary, and the laboratory should be consulted.

For nodules, however, a large wedge should be removed by excision including subcutaneous tissue. Furthermore, when indicated, lesions, regardless of size, should be bisected, one half for histology and the other half sent in a sterile container for bacterial and mycotic cultures or in special fixatives, cell culture media, or frozen for immunopathological examination.

Specimens for light microscopy should be fixed immediately in buffered neutral formalin. A brief but detailed summary of the clinical history and description of the lesions should accompany the specimen. Biopsy is indicated in *all* skin lesions that are suspected of being neoplasms, in all bullous disorders using immunofluoresence simultaneously, and in all dermatologic disorders in which a specific diagnosis is not possible by clinical examination alone.

APPENDIX C: GENERALIZED PRURITUS WITHOUT DIAGNOSTIC SKIN LESIONS

Persistent severe pruritus, like pain, is a dominating factor in existence; from day to day it takes over one's life. Intense pruritus may, in fact, be more maddening for the patient than pain because there is no effective medication to control the pruritus; pain usually can be controlled with analgesics. The physician, therefore, feels somewhat helpless in the management of these unfortunate patients. Pruritus leads to sleepless nights; a state of permanent fatigue ensues that precludes work and confounds family relationships. The approach to the patient with generalized pruritus without identifiable skin lesions is to consider this symptom in the same manner as a patient with factitious (i.e., not based on organic disease) dermatosis—*generalized pruritus and factitious dermatosis are both diagnoses of exclusion:* all organic causes must be excluded within reasonable limits.

The differential diagnosis of generalized pruritus is presented in Table C-1, the workup of these patients is presented in Table C-2, and pruritus ani is presented in Table C-3.

TABLE C-1   DIFFERENTIAL DIAGNOSIS OF PRURITUS

Metabolic and Endocrine Conditions	Malignant Neoplasms	Drug Ingestion	Infestations
Hyperthyroidism	Lymphoma and	Subclinical drug	Scabies[1]
Diabetes mellitus	leukemia	sensitivities:	Pediculosis corporis
Hypothyroidism	Other cancer (rare)	Aspirin, alcohol,	Hookworm
Chronic	Multiple myeloma	dextran, polymyxin	(ancylostomiasis)
renal failure		B, morphine, codeine,	Onchocerciasis
		scopolamine, D-	Ascariasis
		tubocurarine	

Hematologic Disease	Hepatic Disease	Psychogenic States	Miscellaneous Conditions
Polycythemia vera	Obstructive biliary	Transitory:	Dry skin (xerosis)
Paraproteinemia	disease	Periods of emotional	"Senile" pruritus[2]
Iron deficiency	Pregnancy (intrahepatic	stress	Pregnancy-related
	cholestasis)	Persistent:	disorders
		Delusions of parasitosis	Fiberglas exposure
		Psychogenic pruritus	Various primary skin
		Neurotic excoriations	diseases

[1]Diagnostic lesions may or may not present.
[2]Unexplained intense pruritus in patients over 70 years without obvious "dry skin" and with no apparent emotional stress.

TABLE C-2 APPROACH TO THE DIAGNOSIS OF GENERALIZED PRURITUS WITHOUT DIAGNOSTIC SKIN LESIONS

It is critical to recognize that nonspecific skin changes can be induced by rubbing and scratching. The false conclusion that a dermatologic cause for itching is necessarily present just because a rash can be seen is a trap that must be avoided.

The approach to the patient with persistent generalized pruritus begins with careful examination of the skin, followed by additional attention to the general history, review of systems, general physical examination, and investigations as outlined below.

Initial Visit

1. Detailed history of pruritus:
   - Are there any skin lesions that precede the itching?
   - Severity: Does the itching keep the patient awake?
2. History of constitutional symptoms, weight loss, fatigue, fever, malaise
3. Has there been a recent emotional stress situation?
4. History of oral or parenteral medication that can be a cause of generalized pruritus without a rash
5. Examine carefully for subtle primary skin disorders as a cause of the pruritus: xerosis or asteatosis, scabies, pediculosis (nits?)
6. General physical examination including *all* the lymph nodes; rectal examination and stool guaiac in adult patients (depending on the individual clinical situation, may be deferred to second or later visit)
7. If pruritus has been present for more than 2 weeks, obtain additional data (see nos. 1–4 below)
8. If dry skin or winter itch is a reasonable possible explanation, give the patient bath oil, followed by an emollient ointment. No soap; the bath is therapeutic, not for cleansing the skin; shower to clean.
9. Check for dermographism.
10. Follow-up appointment in 2 weeks

Subsequent Visit(s)

If no relief from symptomatic treatment given on the first visit, proceed as follows:
1. Refer patient to a dermatologist.
2. Obtain chest roentgenogram.
3. Detailed review of systems
4. Laboratory tests: complete blood tests including erythrocyte sedimentation rate, fasting blood sugar, renal function tests, liver function tests, hepatitis antigens, thyroid tests, stool for parasites
5. If the diagnosis has not been established at this point, the patient should be referred to an internist for complete workup including pelvic examination and Pap smear.

SOURCE: Bernhard JD, ed. *Itch Mechanisms and Management of Pruritis.* New York, McGraw-Hill, 1994, pp. 211–215.

TABLE C-3 PRURITUS ANI

Many patients, in desperation, become resigned to accepting pruritus ani as part of their lives and endure the embarrassment and the sleepless nights.

Pruritus ani is pruritus of the anal skin without evidence of a primary dermatologic disorder sometimes seen in this region, *viz.,* dermatophytosis, candidiasis, psoriasis, or seborrheic dermatitis. Pinworms are a rare cause and are seen usually only in children. The major factor in the pathogenesis of pruritus ani is irritation from the presence of fecal soiling on the anal skin; this is most often the result of incomplete cleansing of the area after defecation but also results in some persons from the weakness of the anal sphincter, which allows for fecal soiling when the rectum is distended by the arrival of feces or with flatus. The vicious cycle is irritation → itching → rubbing with the development of lichenification → more pruritus. When lichenification is present, control begins with a *very limited* course of potent topical corticosteroids to reduce lichenification. The main thrust of the management, however, must be directed at two provoking factors:

1. *Paroxysmal compulsive rubbing and scratching of the anal sphincter and skin around it.* Anxiety and stress appear to contribute to the itching. The "fits" of rubbing or scratching occur most often after defecation and at night, when the patient is often awakened by the itching. These bouts of pruritus can be somewhat relieved by menthol-camphor lotions.
2. *Poor anal hygiene.* Strict, "squeaky" clean anal cleansing with cotton pledgets soaked in witch hazel is ideal. Whenever possible, a shower or tub bath is the best method of cleansing; a more convenient method is with a bidet. After cleansing the area, liberal application of talcum powder helps absorb the fecal soiling that can occur during the day; ointments and oily lotions may actually aggravate the pruritus.

APPENDIX D: DIFFERENTIAL DIAGNOSIS OF RASHES IN THE ACUTELY ILL FEBRILE PATIENT

The sudden appearance of a rash and fever is frightening for the patient. Medical advice is sought immediately and often in the emergency units of hospitals; about 10% of all patients seeking emergency medical care have a dermatologic problem.

The diagnosis of an acute rash with a fever is a clinical challenge. Rarely do physicians have to "lean" on their eyes as much as when confronted by an acutely ill patient with fever and a skin eruption. If a diagnosis is not established promptly in certain patients (e.g., those having septicemia), lifesaving treatment may be delayed.

The cutaneous findings alone may be diagnostic before confirmatory laboratory data are available. As in problems of the acute abdomen, the results of some laboratory tests, such as microbiologic cultures, may not be available immediately. On the basis of a differential diagnosis, appropriate therapy—whether antibiotics or corticosteroids—may be started. Furthermore, prompt diagnosis and isolation of the patient with a contagious disease, which may have serious consequences, prevent spread to other persons. For example, varicella in adults rarely can be fatal. Contagious diseases presenting with rash and fever as the major findings include *viral infections* (rubella, enterovirus, and parvovirus infections) and *bacterial infections* (streptococcal, staphylococcal, meningococcal, typhoid, and syphilis).

The physical diagnosis of skin eruptions is a discipline mainly based on precise identification of the type of skin lesion. The physician must not only identify and classify the *type* of skin lesion but also look for additional morphologic clues such as the *configuration* (annular? iris?) of the individual lesion, the *arrangement* (zosteriform? linear?) of the lesions, the *distribution pattern* (exposed areas? centripetal or centrifugal? mucous membranes?). In the differential diagnosis of exanthems it is important to determine, by history, the *site of first appearance* (the rash of Rocky Mountain spotted fever characteristically appears first on the wrists and ankles), and very important is the *temporal evolution* of the rash (measles spreads from head to toes in a period of 3 days, while the rash of rubella spreads rapidly in 24 to 48 hours from head to toes and then sequentially clears—first face, then trunk, and then limbs).

Although there may be some overlap, the differential diagnostic possibilities may be grouped into four main categories according to the type of lesion (see Table D-1).

Laboratory Tests Available for Quick Diagnosis

The physician should make use of the following laboratory tests immediately or within 8 hours:

1. *Direct smear from the base of a vesicle.* This procedure, known as the *Tzanck test,* is performed by unroofing an intact vesicle, gently scraping the base with a curved scalpel blade, and smearing the contents on a slide. After air drying, the smear is stained with Wright's or Giemsa's stain and examined for acantholytic cells and multinucleated giant cells (see Appendix B).
2. *Viral culture,* especially for herpes simplex.
3. *Gram's stain of aspirates or scraping.* This is essential for proper diagnosis of pustules. Organisms can be seen in the lesions of acute meningococcemia, rarely in the skin lesions of gonococcemia and ecthyma gangrenosum.

4. *Touch preparation.* This is especially helpful in deep fungal infections and leishmaniasis. The dermal part of a skin biopsy specimen is touched repeatedly to a glass slice; the touch preparation is *immediately* fixed in 95% ethyl alcohol. Special stains are then performed and the slide examined for organisms in the cytology laboratory.
5. *Biopsy of the skin lesion.* All purpuric lesions should be biopsied. Inflammatory dermal nodules and most ulcers should be biopsied and a portion of tissue minced and cultured for bacteria and fungi. A 3.0- to 4.0-mm trephine and local anesthesia are used. In many laboratories the biopsy specimen can be processed within 8 hours if necessary.
6. *Blood and urine examinations.* Blood culture, rapid serologic tests for syphilis, and serology for lupus erythematosus require 24 hours. Examination of urine sediment may reveal red cell casts in allergic vasculitis.
7. *Dark-field examination.* In the skin lesions of secondary syphilis, repeated examination of papules may show *Treponema pallidum.* The dark-field examination is not reliable in the mouth because nonpathogenic organisms are almost impossible to differentiate from *T. pallidum.*

TABLE D-1 RASH AND FEVER IN THE ACUTELY ILL PATIENT: DIAGNOSIS ACCORDING TO TYPE OF LESION

Diseases Manifested by Macules, Papules, Nodules, or Plaques	Diseases Manifested by Vesicles, Bullae, or Pustules	Diseases Manifested by Purpuric Macules, Purpuric Papules, or Purpuric Vesicles	Diseases Manifested by Widespread Erythema ± Edema Followed by Desquamation
Drug hypersensitivities	Drug hypersensitivities	Drug hypersensitivities	Drug hypersensitivities
Sweet's syndrome	Allergic contact	Bacteremia[2]	Scarlet fever
Eosinophilia-myalgia syndrome	dermatitis from plants	Meningococcemia (acute or chronic)	Staphylococcal scalded-skin syndrome
Streptococcal cellulitis	Rickettsial pox	Gonococcemia[3]	Toxic shock syndrome
Erythema migrans of Lyme disease	Gonococcemia Varicella	Staphylococcemia *Pseudomonas*	Kawasaki's syndrome Toxic epidermal
Meningococcemia	(chickenpox)[1]	bacteremia	necrolysis
Human immunodeficiency virus, primary infection	Herpes zoster Herpes simplex[1] Eczema herpeticum[1]	Subacute bacterial endocarditis	Graft-versus-host reaction von Zumbusch
Erythema infectiosum (parvovirus B19)	Enterovirus infections (echovirus and coxsackie), including	Enterovirus infections (echovirus and coxsackie)	pustular psoriasis Erythroderma (exfoliative dermatitis)
Cytomegalovirus, primary infection	hand-foot-and-mouth disease	Rickettsial diseases: Rocky Mountain	
Epstein-Barr virus, primary infection	Toxic epidermal necrolysis	spotted fever Typhus, louse-	
Exanthem subitum (human herpesvirus type 6)	Staphylococcal scalded-skin syndrome Erythema multiforme	borne (epidemic) "Allergic" vasculitis[2] Disseminated	
Measles (rubeola)	bullosum	intravascular	
Measles (rubeola) atypical	Kawasaki's disease	coagulation (purpura fulminans[4])	

continued

TABLE D-1 RASH AND FEVER IN THE ACUTELY ILL PATIENT: DIAGNOSIS ACCORDING TO TYPE OF LESION (Continued)

Diseases Manifested by Macules, Papules, Nodules, or Plaques	Diseases Manifested by Vesicles, Bullae, or Pustules	Diseases Manifested by Purpuric Macules, Purpuric Papules, or Purpuric Vesicles	Diseases Manifested by Widespread Erythema ± Edema Followed by Desquamation
German measles (rubella)[3]			
Enterovirus infections (echo and Coxsackie)			
Adenovirus infections			
Typhoid fever			
Secondary syphilis			
Typhus, murine (endemic)			
Rocky Mountain spotted fever (early lesions)[3]			
Other spotted fevers			
Disseminated deep fungal infection in immunocompromised patients			
Pityriasis rosea (fever, rare)			
Erythema multiforme			
Erythema marginatum			
Systemic lupus erythematosus			
Dermatomyositis			
"Serum sickness" (manifested only as wheals and angioedema)			
Urticaria, acute (viral hepatitis)			
Gianotti-Crosti syndrome			

[1]One characteristic lesion of these exanthems is an umbilicated papule or vesicle.
[2]Often present as infarcts.
[3]May have arthralgia or musculoskeletal pain.
[4]Leading to large areas of black necrosis.

APPENDIX E: MALIGNANT MELANOMA

Screening Technique for Melanoma Risk in New Patients

1. *Ask about family history of melanoma or "atypical" nevi (irregular/prominent large moles).* Remember that the term *skin cancer* can be interpreted loosely to mean epithelial cancers rather than melanoma, and the history of melanoma therefore may be difficult or impossible to validate.
2. *Determine the skin phototype.* Ask only one question: "Do you tan easily?"

    *   If "Yes," the person is skin phototype III or IV
    *   If "No," the person is skin phototype I or II

    Skin phototypes I and II are considerably more at risk.

3. *Perform a full-body examination to determine the number of moles.* A count of more than 50 moles $\geq$ 2.0 mm in diameter indicates increased risk. (Note, however, that some people at risk may not have any moles, for example, persons with red hair or freckling.) Examine the fingers, toes, plantar and palmar surfaces, and mucocutaneous areas particularly in sub-Saharan Africans, African Americans, Asians, and Native Americans; and examine the scalp.
4. *Perform a full-body examination to determine types of moles.* The types of moles are:
    *   *Acquired common moles:* <5 mm in diameter and usually distinctly elevated.
    *   *Acquired "atypical" moles:* Often large (5.0 mm in diameter or larger), "flat" in appearance (but actually slightly elevated with side-lighting), and dark (often of variegated color patterns with irregular, indistinct, "fuzzy" borders or "fried egg" appearance).
    *   *Congenital melanocytic nevi:* Present in the first 2 weeks of life, verified by birth photograph or by direct or indirect report from patients. Elevated throughout the lesion and often with dark terminal hairs and a "pebbly" surface. Absolute size cannot be used to exclude a lesion as congenital

Recommendations for the Management of Pigmented Lesions to Facilitate Early Diagnosis of Malignant Melanoma

For the Examining Physician

1. Histologic diagnosis is necessary in all pigmented lesions with the following three physical characteristics—the hallmarks of atypicality in a pigmented lesion:
    a. Irregularity of the borders: with pseudopods, a notch, or even a "maple leaf" configuration (see Figures 9-8 and 9-9)
    b. An irregular array of colors: a gradation of red, gray, or blue, admixed with brown or black, displayed in a disorderly, haphazard pigment pattern. *Additional indications:* black nodules with uniform borders, irregularly pigmented lesions with uniform borders
    c. Increases in size
2. All congenital melanocytic nevi should be considered for excision, regardless of size. Lesions should be followed with photography until they can be excised some time before puberty. The timing of excision for small congenital lesions will depend on the clinical characteristics (light brown, uniform color is a sign of benignancy), or whether general anesthesia is needed, and on the disability that will result from surgery. All giant nevi should be removed if feasible.

3. Any pigmented lesion striking a physician's eye as "out of the ordinary" should be further evaluated (i.e., excision or referral for same).
4. All patients with a history of melanoma should be examined thoroughly for atypical melanocytic nevi (dysplastic nevi) and for the appearance of new primary melanomas. Patients with dysplastic nevi should be followed at 6-month intervals.
5. All blood relatives of patients with melanoma should be examined for dysplastic nevi and early primary melanoma. (The presence of a family history increases the risk 8- to 13-fold for an individual.)
6. All white patients presenting for any problem should be examined for the presence of large melanocytic nevi (greater than 1.0 cm), for dysplastic nevi, and for nevi on the scalp, mucous membrane, and anogenital area. All black persons should be examined for pigmented lesions of the soles, nail beds, and mucous membranes.

Advice to the Patient

The following advice should be made regarding pigmented lesions. Seek prompt examination for the following:

All persons with a family history of melanoma
All persons with skin phototype I or II, especially those with a history in youth of intense or prolonged sun exposure
Any pigmented mole that was present at birth
Any newly appearing mole after puberty
All persons with many (uncountable!) moles >2.0 mm in diameter and/or with any number of moles >5.0 mm in diameter
Any changing mole—in size, color, or border
Any mole that itches or is tender for more than 2 weeks
Any mole that is considered "ugly" because of its size, color, pattern, or borders

Persons with skin phototype I or II should *never* sunbathe. Persons with dysplastic nevi or a melanoma, regardless of skin phototype, should *never* sunbathe or do outdoor work without appropriate clothing. Sunscreens with a sun protection factor (SPF) of >30 should be used in all persons with dysplastic nevi or a previous history of melanoma and in persons with skin phototypes I and II. Avoid exposure to artificial forms of ultraviolet radiation (sunbeds and sunlamps).

TABLE E-1   AMERICAN JOINT COMMISSION ON CANCER (AJCC) STAGING SYSTEM (1992)

TNM STAGING OF MELANOMA

Primary tumor (pT)

pTX   Primary tumor cannot be assessed.

pTO   No evidence of primary tumor.

pTis   Melanoma *in situ* (atypical melanocytic hyperplasia, severe melanocytic dysplasia), not an invasive lesion (Clark Level I).

pT1   Tumor 0.75 mm or less in thickness and invading the papillary dermis (Clark Level II).

pT2   Tumor more than 0.75 mm but not more than 1.5 mm in thickness and/or invades the papillary-reticular dermal interface (Clark Level III).

pT3   Tumor more than 1.5 mm but not more than 4 mm in thickness and/or invades the reticular dermis (Clark Level IV).

pT3a   Tumor more than 1.5 mm but not more than 3 mm in thickness.

pT3b   Tumor more than 3 mm but not more than 4 mm in thickness.

pT4   Tumor more than 4 mm in thickness and/or invades the subcutaneous tissue (Clark Level V) and/or satellite(s) within 2 cm of the primary tumor.

pT4a   Tumor more than 4 mm in thickness and/or invades the subcutaneous tissue.

pT4b   Satellite(s) within 2 cm of the primary tumor.

Regional lymph nodes (N)

NX   Regional lymph nodes cannot be assessed.

N0   No regional lymph node metastasis.

N1   Metastasis 3 cm or less in greatest dimension in any regional lymph node(s).

N2   Metastasis more than 3 cm in greatest dimension in any regional lymph node(s) and/or in-transit metastasis.[1]

N2a   Metastasis more than 3 cm in greatest dimension in any regional lymph node(s).

N2b   In-transit metastasis.

N2c   Both (N2a and N2b).

Distant Metastasis

MX   Presence of distant metastasis cannot be assessed.

M0   No distant metastasis.

M1   Distant metastasis.

M1a   Metastasis in skin or subcutaneous tissue or lymph node(s) beyond the regional lymph nodes.

M1b   Visceral metastasis.

STAGE GROUPING

Stage I	pT1	N0	M0
	pT2	N0	M0
Stage II	pT3	N0	M0
	pT4	N0	M0
Stage III	Any pT	N1	M0
	Any pT	N2	M0
Stage IV	Any pT	Any N	M1

[1]In-transit metastasis involves skin or subcutaneous tissue more than 2 cm from the primary tumor not beyond the regional lymph nodes.

Primary Melanoma of the Skin: Three Major Types

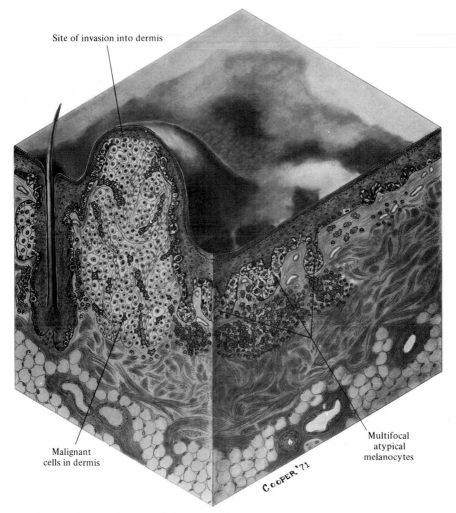

Site of invasion into dermis

Malignant
cells in dermis

Multifocal
atypical
melanocytes

COOPER '71

Figure E-1 Lentigo maligna melanoma *Illustrated is a large, flat, variegated, freckle-like macule (not elevated above the plane of the skin) with irregular borders. These areas show increased numbers of melanocytes, usually atypical and bizarre and distributed in a single layer along the basal layer; at certain places in the dermis, malignant malanocytes have invaded and formed huge nests. At the left is a large nodule that is composed of large epithelioid cells in this illustration; the nodules of all three types of melanoma are indistinguishable from each other.*

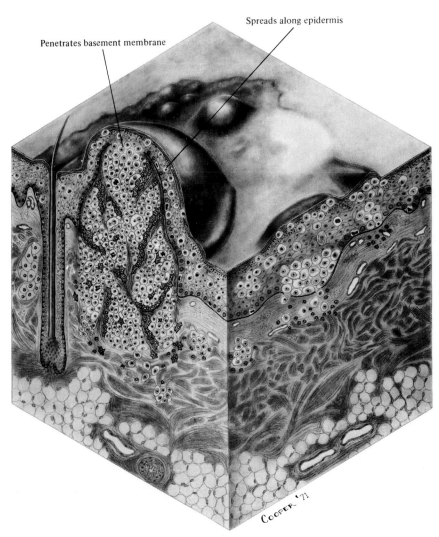

Penetrates basement membrane

Spreads along epidermis

COOPER '71

Figure E-2 Superficial spreading melanoma *The border is irregular and elevated through-out its entirety; biopsy of the area surrounding the large nodule shows a pagetoid distribution of large melanocytes throughout the epidermis in multiple layers, occurring singly or in nests, and uniformly atypical. On the left is a large nodule, and scattered throughout the surrounding por-tion of the nodule are smaller papular and nodular areas. The nodule on the left shows malig-nant melanocytes that are very large and have an abundance of cytoplasm. The melanocytes often have regularly dispersed fine particles of melanin. The nodules also may show spindle cells or small malignant melanocytes as in lentigo maligna melanoma and nodular melanoma.*

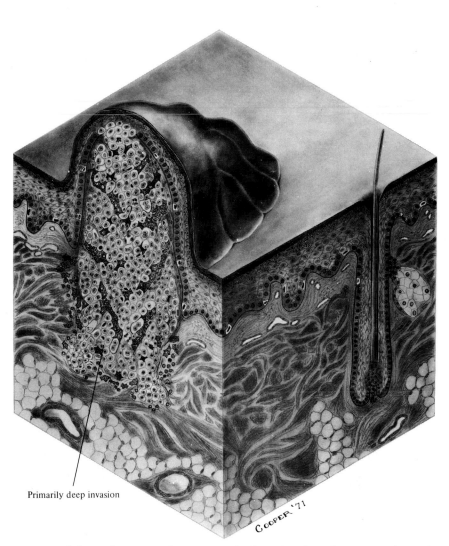

Primarily deep invasion

Figure E-3 Nodular melanoma *This arises at the dermal-epidermal junction and extends vertically in the dermis; intraepidermal growth is present only in a small group of tumor cells that conjointly are also invading the underlying dermis. The epidermis lateral to the areas of this invasion does not demonstrate atypical melanocytes. As in lentigo maligna melanoma and superficial spreading melanoma, the tumor may show large epithelioid cells, spindle cells, small malignant melanocytes, or mixtures of all three.*

Summary Data on Malignant Melanoma of Skin

I. **Incidence** (United States, 38,300* new cases in 1996)   Three percent of all cancers (excluding nonmelanoma skin cancer).

   A. Overall annual crude incidence rates (United States)

      Caucasians   10.4 per 100,000 population per year (1988)

   B. Increasing with time (U.S. whites) (SEER incidence rates, age-adjusted for U.S. whites), 1970–1992.

      1. 1970   4.5 per 100,000 population per year
      2. 1975   7.3 per 100,000 population per year
      3. 1980   10.0 per 100,000 population per year
      4. 1985   11.8 per 100,000 population per year
      5. 1990   12.9 per 100,000 population per year
      6. 1992   13.6 per 100,000 population per year

II. **Frequency for Type of Melanoma**

   A. Superficial spreading   70 %
   B. Nodular   16 %
   C. Lentigo maligna melanoma   5 %
   D. Unclassified (includes acral lentiginous type)   9 %

III. **Mortality** Overall deaths in 1995 (United States, 7300); melanoma represents 1 % to 2 % of all cancer deaths. In the period 1973 to 1992, there was a 34 % increase in the rate of deaths from melanoma; this was the third highest of all cancers. Over this period the percentage change in mortality rates for males exceeded that for females at 47.9 % and 16.9 %, respectively. In 1992, the death rate from melanoma was 5.9 times higher for whites than for blacks combined (2.5 and 0.4 per 100,000 population, respectively).

*Estimated [*CA Cancer J Clin* 46(1); Jan/Feb. 1996].

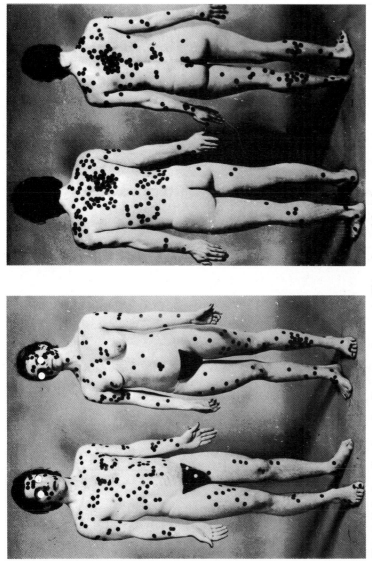

Figure E-4 *Localization of malignant melanoma in 731 males and females.*

Guidelines for Biopsy, Surgical Treatment, and Follow-Up of Patients with Melanoma

I. Biopsy

- Total excisional biopsy with narrow margins—optimal biopsy procedure, where possible
- Incisional or punch biopsy acceptable when total excisional biopsy cannot be performed or when lesion is large, requiring extensive surgery to remove the entire lesion
- When sampling the lesion: If raised, remove the most raised area; if flat, remove the darkest area.

II. Lentigo Maligna Melanoma

- Excise with a 1.0-cm margin beyond the clinically visible lesion or biopsy scar—unless the flat component involves a major organ (e.g., the eye), in which case lesser margins are acceptable. For lentigo maligna melanoma on areas other than the head and neck, the excision margins are the same as for superficial spreading melanoma, nodular melanoma, and acral melanoma.
- Excise down to the fascia or to the underlying muscle where fascia is absent. Skin flaps or skin grafts may be used for closure.
- No node dissection is recommended unless nodes are clinically palpable and suspicious for tumor.
- See recommendation for sentinel node studies for thickness >1.0 mm.

III. Superficial Spreading Melanoma, Nodular Melanoma, and Acral Melanoma

- Melanoma *in situ:* excise with a >0.5 cm margin from the lesion edge.

THICKNESS <1.0 MM

- Excise with a 1.0-cm margin from the lesion edge.
- Excise down to the fascia or to the underlying muscle where fascia is absent. Direct closure without graft is often possible.
- Node dissection is not recommended unless nodes are clinically palpable and suspicious for tumor.

THICKNESS 1.0 TO 4.0 MM

- Excise 2.0 cm from the edge of the lesion, except on the face, where narrower margins may be necessary.
- Excise down to the fascia or to the underlying muscle where fascia is absent. Graft may be required.
- The efficacy of elective lymph node dissection (ELND) remains controversial, with results from two prospective, randomized trials pending.
- The sentinel node procedure with injections of blue dye or, if available, technetium-99m with gamma-probe localization permits a minimally invasive technique for detecting melanoma metastasis in regional nodes.
- If the sentinel node (lymph node closest to the site of the primary melanoma) is positive, the regional lymphadenectomy is performed. If the sentinel node is negative, then the patient is spared an ELND.
- If regional node positive and completely resected with no evidence of distant disease, then adjuvant therapy with interferon-alfa-2b is discussed. In this setting, results of recent ECOG-Est 1689 trials have demonstrated improvement in median relapse-free survival and 5-year relapse-free survival of node-positive, resected patients compared with controls; also,

results of the Australian Cooperative Melanoma Group show significantly increased relapse-free 5-year survival rates in node-negative, no ELND treated >1.5 mm primary melanoma patients.

- Therapeutic nodal dissection is recommended if nodes are clinically palpable and suspicious for tumor and no evidence of distant disease is present.

THICKNESS >**4.0**

- Excise 3.0 cm from the edge of the lesion, except on the face, where narrower margins may be necessary.
- Excise down to the fascia or to the underlying muscle where fascia is absent. Graft may be required.
- Elective nodal dissection is not recommended.
- Therapeutic nodal dissection is recommended if nodes are clinically suspicious for tumor and no evidence of distant disease is present.

TABLE E-2 **EIGHT-YEAR SURVIVAL FOR PATIENTS WITH CLINICAL STAGE I MELANOMA IN THE VERTICAL GROWTH PHASE BASED ON SINGLE FACTOR ANALYSIS OF PROGNOSTIC VARIABLES**

Variable	Categories	% 8-Year Survival
Mitotic rate/mm^2	0.0	95.1
	0.1–6.0	79.4
	>6.0	38.2
TILs[1]	Brisk	88.5
	Nonbrisk	75.0
	Absent	59.3
Thickness	<0.76 mm	93.2
	0.76–1.69	85.6
	1.70–3.60	59.8
	>3.60	33.3
Anatomic site	Extremities	87.3
	Head, neck, and trunk	62.4
	Volar or subungual	46.2
Sex	Female	83.8
	Male	56.6
Regression	Absent	77.0
	Present	60.0

[1]Tumor-infiltrating lymphocytes.

SOURCE: Modified from Clark WH Jr, et al. Model predicting survival in stage I melanoma based on tumor progression. *J Natl Cancer Inst* 81:1893, 1989.

Differential Diagnosis of Melanoma: Masqueraders*

Melanocytic neoplasms

Melanoma *in situ*
Solar lentigo
Lentigo maligna
Dysplastic melanocytic nevus with marked atypia
Epithelioid and spindle cell nevus of Spitz
Pigmented spindle cell tumor of Reed
Recurring melanocytic nevus
Blue nevus, especially cellular type
Congenital nevomelanocytic nevus that is changing

Nonmelanocytic neoplasms

Pigmented actinic keratosis
Pigmented nodular basal cell carcinoma
Pyogenic granuloma
Atypical fibroxanthoma
Appendageal tumors (eccrine poroma?)
Seborrheic keratosis
Hemangioma pseudomelanoticum
Dermatofibroma
Large cell acanthoma

*Webster's: "a disguise or false outward show; have or put on a deceptive appearance."

APPENDIX F: SIX SIGNS OF MALIGNANT MELANOMA

ASYMMETRY in shape—one-half unlike the other half
BORDER is irregular—edges irregularly scalloped
COLOR is mottled—haphazard display of colors; shades of brown, black, gray, red, and white
DIAMETER is usually large—greater than the tip of a pencil eraser (6.0 mm)
ELEVATION is almost always present—surface distortion is assessed by side-lighting. Melanoma
   in situ and acral lentiginous lesions may be flat
ENLARGEMENT—a history of an increase in the size of lesion is perhaps one of the most im-
   portant signs of malignant melanoma

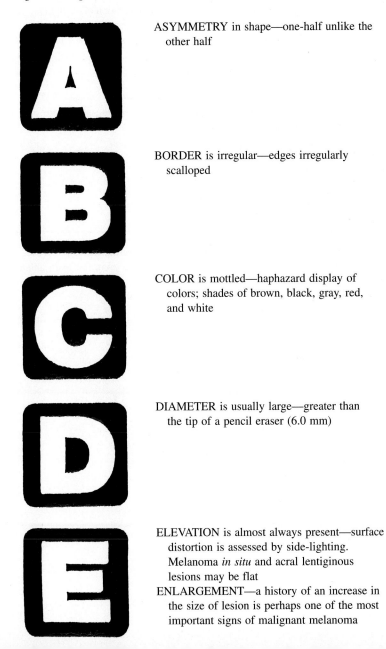

ASYMMETRY in shape—one-half unlike the
   other half

BORDER is irregular—edges irregularly
   scalloped

COLOR is mottled—haphazard display of
   colors; shades of brown, black, gray, red,
   and white

DIAMETER is usually large—greater than
   the tip of a pencil eraser (6.0 mm)

ELEVATION is almost always present—surface
   distortion is assessed by side-lighting.
   Melanoma *in situ* and acral lentiginous
   lesions may be flat
ENLARGEMENT—a history of an increase in
   the size of lesion is perhaps one of the most
   important signs of malignant melanoma

APPENDIX G: RISK FACTORS OF WHITE ADULTS FOR CUTANEOUS MELANOMA

Recent statistics show that melanoma incidence and mortality have continued to increase at an alarming rate—in some countries, as high as 4% a year—over the last decade.

At the same time, because melanoma can be cured when detected early enough, education has emerged as one of the weapons of choice in fighting the disease: education of consumers about the dangers of sun exposure and the importance of regular checkups, and education of physicians and healthcare professionals about how to recognize melanoma in its earliest, most treatable phases.

We believe it is time to add another weapon to the melanoma education arsenal: clear, simple, easily remembered definition of melanoma risk factors. Reliable epidemiologic studies have now identified six different risk factors associated with melanoma. These can be summarized with the mnemonic device **MMRISK,** as follows:

MMRISK*

A mnemonic device for promoting melanoma risk awareness among physicians and patients. Each letter represents one of the major risk factors for melanoma of the skin.

M Moles: atypical moles (more than 10)
M Moles: common moles (numerous)
R Red hair and freckling
I Inability to tan: skin phototypes I and II
S Sunburn: severe sunburn before age 14
K Kindred: family history of melanoma

A successful campaign to promote awareness of melanoma risk factors would greatly raise the emotional stake of the whole melanoma education process. "It is one thing if I learn about the vague threat of a 'melanoma epidemic'; it is quite another thing if I learn that, because I possess certain risk factors, I myself may be at increased risk of acquiring the disease."

Greater awareness of melanoma risk factors would inject a needed sense of urgency in the very population that needs it most.

*Mnemonic first presented on the internet: www.skindex.com on November 1, 1997

APPENDIX H: PHOTOSENSITIVITY

Diagnosis of Photosensitivity Syndromes (Table H-1)

History

The patient's history is often essential in making a diagnosis, especially because the eruption may have cleared by the time the patient is seen in consultation. The persons most easily recognized as photosensitive are those whose intermittent skin eruptions have an obvious temporal relationship to sun exposure. Others, who complain of an apparent allergic reaction to sunscreens, may instead be suffering from photosensitivity for which their sunscreens are not providing adequate protection— for example, a reaction to UVA exposure, against which most current sunscreens are not fully effective. A patient taking a thiazide diuretic might present with a chronic persistent rash on exposed sites, not recognizing it as light-induced. Much less commonly, generalized erythroderma might indicate UV exposure in the context of light-sensitive psoriasis or chronic actinic dermatitis.

The age of onset of the eruption is important because certain types of photosensitivity—for example, actinic prurigo—typically begin in childhood, whereas others, such as polymorphic light eruption, can occur at any age. It is also essential to ascertain the time course of the eruption, since reactions may occur minutes (e.g., solar urticaria) or days (e.g., polymorphic light eruption) after exposure; they may last only a few hours (e.g., solar urticaria) or several weeks (e.g., polymorphic light eruption). Symptoms such as itching (as in polymorphic light eruption, actinic prurigo, solar urticaria, eczema) or pain/burning (as in erythropoietic protoporphyria) should be noted. A rash that also occurs near an oven or open fire suggests that heat rather than UV radiation may be the exacerbating agent. A history of an eruption confined to the sunshine months is helpful when present, but some photodermatoses may occur at other times of the year. An eruption confined to the summer months suggests that UVB (290 to 320 nm) has a role; a perennial eruption suggests that UVA (320 to 400 nm) and/or visible radiation (400 to 800 nm) may be important. Another clue is to ask if the eruption can be induced by sunlight transmitted through window glass; if so, this suggests a UVA component; if not, UVB. [See Table H-1, from Fitzpatrick's J Clin Dermatol 1996; 3 (No. 3): 14.]

Other factors of importance in the history are exposure to chemicals and drugs (Table H-2)— systemic, such as certain antipsychotic medications or antibiotics, or topical, such as sunscreens or cosmetics. A careful drug history should include both current medications and drugs to which the patient was exposed at the time the photosensitivity started, since some degree of photosensitivity occasionally can persist for months after discontinuation of an offending agent. Also important is whether occupational or recreational exposure to UV radiation or plants has occurred. For example, a patient with lupus erythematosus who works as a welder or who sits in an office under fluorescent lighting may be chronically exposed to UV radiation if protection is not used. Questions should be asked about avocations such as gardening. Finally, a review of systems should include consideration of connective tissue disease symptoms and the neurologic signs occasionally associated with some of the porphyrias.

Physical Examination

DISTRIBUTION PATTERN   The most important clinical feature common to all the photosensitivity disorders is the distribution of skin lesions (Figure H-1). The eruption predominantly affects sun-exposed skin, generally sparing shaded sites. Classic photodermatoses involve the forehead, malar

TABLE H-1 CLINICAL EVALUATION FOR PHOTOSENSITIVITY SYNDROMES

	Actinic prurigo	Chronic actinic dermatitis	Hydroa vacciniforme	Polymorphic light eruption	Solar urticaria	Hereditary coproporphyria	Porphyria cutanea tarda	Variegate porphyria	Congenital porphyria	Erythropoietic protoporphyria	Bloom's syndrome	Cockayne's syndrome	Rothmund-Thompson syndrome	Xeroderma pigmentosum	Chemical/drug-induced
			Idiopathic						Metabolic						
SIGNS AND SYMPTOMS															
Pain alone					R					◆					O
Erythema				O	M					◆	◆	◆	◆	A	O
Swelling					S					◆				A	O
Papules	◆		E	◆											O
Wheals					◆										O
Petechiae									O						O
Vesicles			◆	O		◆	◆	◆	◆	S				A	O
Scarring	◆		◆			◆	◆	◆	◆	◆				◆	O
Scaly patches	◆	◆													O
Erythroderma		◆													O
Hyperpigmentation		◆				◆	◆	◆	◆					◆	O
Other morphology		◆								◆	◆	◆	◆	◆	
TIMING															
EXPOSURE INTERVAL															
Minutes				R	◆				A	◆					O
Hours				◆							◆	◆	◆	A	◆
Uncertain	◆	◆	◆	O		◆	◆	◆	◆		◆	◆	◆	◆	O
PERSISTENCE															
1 to 2 hours					◆										
Hours to days			◆	◆					A	◆					◆
Indefinite	◆	◆				◆	◆	◆	◆		◆	◆	◆	◆	
SEASON															
Spring/summer			◆	◆	O	◆	◆	◆	A	◆					
Year-round	◆	◆			O				◆	O					
HISTORY															
AGE OF ONSET															
Child	◆		◆						◆	◆	◆	◆	◆	◆	
Young adult				◆		◆		◆							
Older adult		◆					◆								
SEX															
Male		◆													
Female	◆			◆											
FAMILY HISTORY															
Usual						◆		◆	◆				O		
Sometimes				◆				◆		O					
CHEMICAL/DRUG EXPOSURE		O				◆	◆	◆							◆

◆ = many cases   A = acute cases   M = mild cases   S = severe cases

O = occasional cases   E = early cases   R = rare cases

CHART INFORMATION COMPILED BY JOHN L. M. HAWK, MD

TABLE H-2 DRUGS THAT CAUSE PHOTOSENSITIVITY

Antibiotics
Amoxicillin
Ciprofloxacin
Clofazimine
Dapsone
Demeclocycline
Doxycycline
Enoxacin
Flucytosine
Griseofulvin
Lomefloxacin
Minocycline
Nalidixic acid
Norfloxacin
Ofloxacin
Oxyfloxacin
Oxytetracycline
Pyrazinamide
Sulfonamide
Tetracycline
Trimethoprim

Anticancer drugs
Dacarbazine (DTIC)
Fluorouracil
Flutamide
Methotrexate
Vinblastine

Antidepressants
Amitriptyline
Amoxapine
Clomipramine
Desipramine
Doxepin
Fluoxetine
Imipramine
Maprotiline
Nortriptyline
Phenelzine
Protriptyline
Trazodone
Trimipramine

Antihistamines
Astemizole
Cimetidine
Cyproheptadine
Diphenhydramine
Ranitidine
Terfenadine

Antihypertensives
Beta-blockers
Captopril
Diltiazem
Methyldopa
Minoxidil
Nifedipine

Antiparasitics
Chloroquine
Quinine
Thiabendazole

Antipsychotic drugs
Chlorpromazine
Fluphenazine
Haloperidol
Perphenazine
Prochlorperazine
Thioridazine
Thiothixene
Trifluoperazine
Triflupromazine

Diuretics
Acetazolamide
Amiloride
Bendroflumethiazide
Benzthiazide
Chlorthiazide
Furosemide
Hydrochlorothiazide
Hydroflumethiazide
Methyclothiazide
Metolazone
Polythiazide
Triamterene
Trichlormethiazide

Hypoglycemics
Acetohexamide
Chlorpropamide
Glipizide
Glyburide
Tolazamide
Tolbutamide

Nonsteroidal anti-inflammatory drugs
Benoxaprofen
Diclofenac

Diflunisal
Fenbufen
Ibuprofen
Indomethacin
Ketoprofen
Nabumetone
Naproxen
Phenylbutazone
Piroxicam
Sulindac

Sunscreens
Aminobenzoic acid
Avobenzone
Benzophenones
Cinnamates
Homosalate
Menthyl anthranilate
PABA

Miscellaneous photosensitizing agents
Alprazolam
Amantadine
Amiodarone
Benzocaine
Benzoyl peroxide
Bergamot oil, oils of citron, lavender, lime, sandalwood, cedar
Carbamazepine
Chlordiazepoxide
Clofibrate
Contraceptives, oral
Desoximetasone
Disopyramide
Etretinate
Fluorescein
Gold salts
Griseofulvin
Hexachlorophene
Isotretinoin
6-methylcoumarin
Musk ambrette
Promethazine
Quinine sulfate and gluconate
Tretinoin
Trimeprazine

Adapted from: Drugs that cause photo-sensitivity. Med Lett Drugs Ther 1995; 37:35–36.

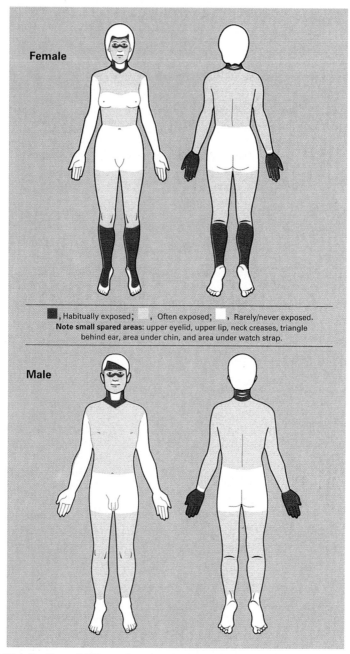

Figure H-1 Distribution of Skin Lesions in Photosensitivity Syndromes

region, nose, rim of the ears, sides and back of the neck, the V area of the chest, and the extensor surfaces of the extremities. Areas of sparing are also very important diagnostically. These usually include the recessed areas of the eyelids, the nasolabial lines, the web spaces of the fingers, and the areas behind the ears, under the nose, and under the chin. There may be a sharp cutoff at clothing margins or at sites of jewelry. However, although the distribution is often limited to sun-exposed areas, it may not involve all exposed areas, because of protection induced by chronic UV exposure and perhaps by consequent tanning or local immunologic tolerance. On the other hand, nonexposed areas sometimes may be affected, because clothing is not always completely protective or because the photosensitivity may be so severe that the disease extends beyond the exposed skin, in very rare cases to erythroderma. Usually patients with such extensive disease initially develop their eruption only on exposed areas.

TYPES OF LESIONS   The morphologic changes encountered with photosensitivity include combinations of erythema, papules, plaques, vesicles, urticaria, bullae, eczema, and altered pigmentation. Infrequently, petechiae, purpura, erythroderma, and scarring may be seen. Confluent erythema is typical of sunburn and occasionally may be the only sign of drug phototoxicity. Erythema and edema, especially if patchy on exposed sites, may suggest polymorphic light eruption—or, if they are confluent, solar urticaria or erythropoietic protoporphyria. Pruritic papules and less often plaques in a sun-exposed distribution, but often with sparing of some sun-exposed sites, are typical of polymorphic light eruption. Eczematous dermatitis may be seen in chronic actinic dermatitis, light-aggravated atopic or seborrheic dermatitis, photocontact dermatitis, or occasionally, photosensitivity induced by drugs (e.g., thiazides). Blistering may be seen with porphyria cutanea tarda, polymorphic light eruption, photocontact dermatitis, solar urticaria, and drug phototoxicity.

LABORATORY STUDIES (Table H-3)   First-line laboratory investigations for all photosensitive patients generally should include a routine assessment of complete blood count with platelets, liver function tests, renal function, and particularly serum ANA/Ro/La and possibly histology. Skin biopsy is adjunctive and often nondiagnostic, used mainly to confirm a suspected diagnosis or to classify a clinically atypical eruption. Usually these biopsies are from lesional skin, whether sun-exposed or not. If systemic lupus erythematosus is suspected, lesional biopsies from both sun-exposed and sun-protected skin may be needed, along with a nonlesional biopsy from a sun-protected area for histology and direct immunofluorescence.

Second-line investigations may be available only in specialized centers. In patients with a suggestive history or with signs of a porphyria—or in doubtful cases—screening of blood, urine, and stool porphyrins, or preferably of the plasma by spectrofluorometry, is necessary. If an abnormality is found, the porphyrin should then be quantified. Cutaneous phototesting is very important if photosensitivity is suspected but the diagnosis is not yet clear; monochromatic or broad-spectrum testing may be used—the former to define an abnormal action spectrum, most reliably in solar urticaria and chronic actinic dermatitis, and the latter to attempt to reproduce the eruption for diagnosis on clinical and histologic grounds, which is sometimes difficult. Patch and photopatch testing are indicated in an eczematous photosensitivity, particularly in chronic actinic dermatitis, where contact factors are often suspected of promoting the eruption.

Management

General treatment principles for all photosensitive patients require removal of any offending agent(s) such as the causative drug or allergen and instruction concerning restriction of sun exposure between the hours of 11 A.M. and 3 P.M., high sun protection factor sunscreens, and appropriate protective clothing, including a hat. Patients with UVA sensitivity need to be aware that many sunblocks have until recently provided only minimal protection in the UVA range and that there is thus

TABLE H-3 LABORATORY TESTS FOR PHOTOSENSITIVITY

The diagnosis of a photosensitivity syndrome is frequently made on the basis of a careful history and physical examination. Laboratory investigations serve to support the clinical suspicion. Generally, serology (ANA, Ro, La) is indicated for all patients with photosensitivity. Because of the possibility of overlapping syndromes (for example, solar urticaria and erythropoietic protoporphyria), many specialized centers will obtain the remaining laboratory studies and utilize the panel of positive and negative results to define the photosensitivity.

Blood, Urine, and Stool Porphyrin Testing

Useful in suspected light sensitivity.

Blood cell and plasma

- Congenital porphyria (raised uroporphyrin and coproporphyrin)
- Erythropoietic protoporphyria (raised protoporphyrin)

Urine

- Congenital porphyria (raised uroporphyrin and coproporphyrin)
- Hereditary coproporphyria (raised coproporphyrin; raised aminolevulinic acid and porphobilinogen during attacks only)
- Porphyria cutanea tarda (raised uroporphyrin)
- Variegate porphyria (raised aminolevulinic acid and porphobilinogen during attacks only)

Stool

- Congenital porphyria (raised uroporphyrin and coproporphyrin)
- Erythropoietic protoporphyria (raised protoporphyrin)
- Hereditary coproporphyria (raised coproporphyrin)

- Porphyria cutanea tarda (occasionally positive with coproporphyrin)
- Variegate porphyria (raised protoporphyrin and coproporphyrin)

Antinuclear Factor, Anti-SSA, and Anti-SSB Titer Estimations

Essential in inflammatory suspected light sensitivity.

Phototesting

Essential in suspected light sensitivity, especially eczematous variety.

Used to make diagnosis of chronic actinic dermatitis or eczematous chemical/drug-induced photosensitivity.

Determines action spectrum; broadbased testing may establish reduced minimal erythema dose photosensitivities; repeated photoprovocation testing may induce actual eruption, especially in polymorphic light eruption.

Helpful in suspected:

- Solar urticaria—to induce wheals and to determine action spectrum (preferably monochromatic testing); wheals induced by UVB, UVA, visible light, or combination

- Xeroderma pigmentosum, Cockayne's syndrome—to make diagnosis (delayed and persistent appearance of minimal erythema dose photosensitivity for 48 to 72 hours)

Often helpful in suspected:

- Actinic prurigo
- Hydroa vacciniforme
- Light-exacerbated dermatoses (preferably using a solar simulator)
- Polymorphic light eruption

Occasionally helpful in suspected:

- Cutaneous porphyrias, for which monochromator may induce erythema and, less often, wheal, pigmentation, or petechiae at 400 to 500 nm

Direct Immunofluorescence

May provide strong or supporting evidence for:

- Lupus erythematosus

Patch and Photopatch Testing

Essential in eczematous suspected light sensitivity.

Undertaken on clear skin of back to standard patch and photopatch test series; sometimes shows precipitating or exacerbating allergen or photoallergen.

- Chemical/drug-induced photosensitivity
- Chronic actinic dermatitis

Skin Biopsy

May provide supporting evidence for photosensitivity diagnosis.

- Cutaneous porphyrias
- Hydroa vacciniforme
- Lupus erythematosus
- Polymorphic light eruption

- Porphyria cutanea tarda
- Severe chronic actinic dermatitis

Assessment of DNA Repair

Useful for early diagnosis of xeroderma pigmentosum.

Other Highly Specialized Investigations

Spontaneous sister chromatid exchange levels

- Bloom's syndrome
- Cockayne's syndrome (possible)

Tissue enzyme measurements

- Porphyrias

In vitro assessment of cellular sensitivity to ultraviolet radiation

- Bloom's syndrome
- Cockayne's syndrome

Assessments of DNA and RNA synthesis

- Cockayne's syndrome (sometimes helpful)

a greater need to restrict sun exposure and use protective clothing. Therapy for the eruptions themselves is generally similar to that for other inflammatory dermatoses and involves topical steroids in mild cases and prophylactic courses of low-dose phototherapy, whether UVB or PUVA, systemic steroids, or immunosuppressive therapy, in more severe cases. The majority of patients can be helped significantly.

Summary

Recognition of photosensitivity requires an awareness of the problem by the clinician and a thorough history and physical examination along with the appropriate laboratory investigations, particularly assessment of serum ANA/Ro/La and, where necessary, histology, immunofluorescence, phototests, and patch and photopatch tests. A diagnosis can be achieved in the majority of patients; most young adults with a recurrent itchy photodermatosis have polymorphic light eruption, most elderly men with eczema have chronic actinic dermatitis, and most children have a DNA repair-defective disorder, erythropoietic protoporphyria, or actinic prurigo. As a better understanding of the mechanisms behind photosensitivity develops, it seems certain that more effective preventive and therapeutic approaches will evolve, whether as improved tolerance-inducing low-dose UV radiation therapy regimens, novel drugs, or better sunscreens.

APPENDIX I: ICHTHYOSIFORM DERMATOSES—
X-Linked Ichthyosis (XLI), Lamellar Ichthyosis (LI), and Epidermolytic Hyperkeratosis (EH)

X-LINKED ICHTHYOSIS

X-linked ichthyosis (XLI) occurs only in males and is characterized by prominent dirty brown scales occurring on the neck, extremities, trunk, and buttocks, with onset soon after birth.

Epidemiology

Age of Onset   Birth or infancy

Sex   Males

Mode of Inheritance   X-linked recessive; gene locus Xp22.32

Genetic Defect   Steroid sulfatase deficiency

Incidence   1:2000 to 1:6000

History

Age at Presentation   2 to 6 weeks of age. Corneal opacities develop during second to third week; also may be present in female carriers of XLI.

Symptoms   Discomfort due to xerosis. Cosmetic disfigurement of the dirty brown scales on the neck, ears, scalp, and arms; individuals appear to be dirty. Corneal opacities usually asymptomatic. Hypogonadism.

Physical Examination

Skin Lesions

TYPE   Large adherent scales (Figures I-1 and I-2) (not powdery as in ichthyosis vulgaris)

COLOR   Scales appear brown or dirty

DISTRIBUTION   Posterior neck, extensor arms, antecubital and popliteal fossae, trunk with relative sparing of flexural areas. Note absence of palm/sole and face involvement; follicular keratoses.

Eye Lesions   Comma-shaped stromal corneal opacities in 50 % of adult males. Present in some female carriers.

Genitourinary Abnormality   Cryptorchidism in 20 % of individuals

Differential Diagnosis

Lamellar ichthyosis, ichthyosis vulgaris, epidermolytic hyperkeratosis, contiguous gene syndromes

Laboratory and Special Examinations

Chemistry   Determine cholesterol sulfate level. Available via Cedric H. L. Shackleton, Ph.D., D.Sc., Children's Hospital Oakland, Research Institute, 747 52nd Street, Oakland, CA 94609; Tel: 510-428-3604; Fax: 510-428-3608.

Dermatopathology   Hyperkeratosis; granular layer present

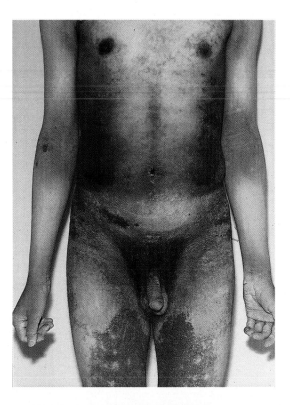

Figure I-1 X-linked ichthyosis *The scales are large and dark and most evident on the flexural areas.*

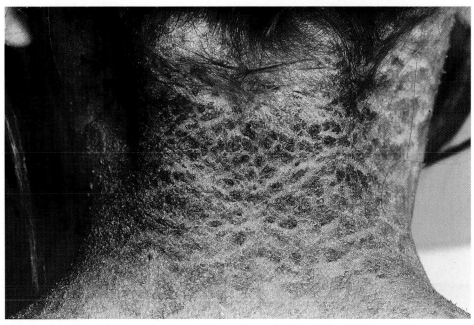

Figure I-2 X-linked ichthyosis *The scales are large, dark, and dirty ("dirty neck").*

Diagnosis

By family history and clinical findings

Prenatal Diagnosis Via amniocentesis and chorionic villus sampling; steroid sulfatase assay detects enzyme deficiency.

Pathogenesis

Steroid sulfatase deficiency is associated with failure to shed senescent keratinocytes normally, resulting clinically in retention hyperkeratosis associated with normal epidermal proliferation.

Course and Prognosis

No improvement with age. Usually worse in temperate climates and in winter season. With placental sulfatase deficiency, failure of labor to begin or progress may occur in mother carrying affected fetus.

Management

Support Group Foundation for Ichthyosis and Related Skin Types (FIRST), P. O. Box 20921, Raleigh, NC 27619; Tel: 800-545-3286; Fax: 919-781-0679.

Topical Therapy

EMOLLIENTS Hydrated petrolatum

KERATOLYTICS *Propylene Glycol* 44% to 60% in water applied h.s. after bath and occluded with a plastic suit worn as pajamas. When excess scaling has been removed, repeat once weekly as necessary.
  Others Salicylic acid, urea, and alphahydroxy acids (glycolic acid, lactic acid) in various vehicles

Systemic Treatment Etretinate or acitretin, 0.5 to 1.0 mg/kg orally until marked improvement, then taper dose to maintenance level. Continuous laboratory monitoring and, in long-term regimens, x-ray for calcifications and DISH syndrome are mandatory.

LAMELLAR ICHTHYOSIS

Lamellar ichthyosis often presents at birth with the infant encased in a collodion-like membrane (collodion baby) that is soon shed with subsequent formation of large, coarse scales involving all flexural areas as well as the palms and soles. During childhood and adulthood, the skin is encased in this platelike scale, which causes significant cosmetic disfigurement.

Epidemiology

Sex Equal

Mode of Inheritance Autosomal recessive; gene locus is 14q11 in some families.

Incidence <1:300,000

History

Age at Presentation Birth

Symptoms Hyperpyrexia: during exercise and hot weather because of inability to sweat. Water loss (excess)/dehydration: due to fissuring of stratum corneum. Increased nutritional requirements: for young children due to rapid growth and shedding of stratum corneum. Painful palmar/plantar fissures.

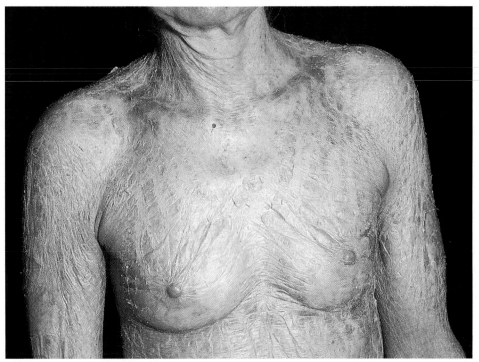

Figure I-3 Lamellar ichthyosis *Large, parchment-like scales over the entire body. Mild ectropion was also present in this patient.*

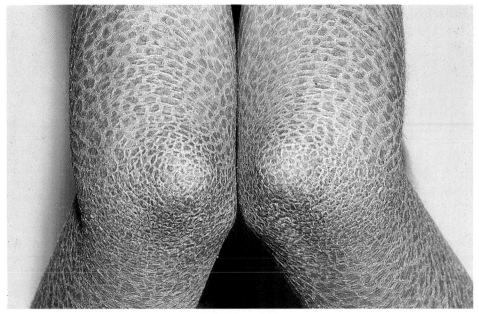

Figure I-4 Lamellar ichthyosis *Tessellated (tilelike) scales.*

Physical Examination

Skin Lesions

TYPE *Newborn* Collodion baby, encased in a translucent collodion-like membrane; shed in few weeks. Ectropion; eclabion. Generalized erythroderma.

Child/Adult Large parchment-like scales develop over the entire body (Figure I-3), and often fracturing of the hyperkeratin plate results in a tessellated (tile-like) pattern (Figure I-4). Scales are large and very thick. Hands/feet: keratoderma; fissures. At times, erythroderma. Secondary bacterial infections.

DISTRIBUTION Generalized. Hyperkeratosis around joints may be verrucous.

HAIR Bound down by scales; frequent infections result in scarring alopecia.

NAILS Dystrophy secondary to nail fold inflammation

MUCOUS MEMBRANES Usually spared. Ectropion may result in secondary infection.

Eye Lesions Ectropion

Differential Diagnosis

X-linked ichthyosis, epidermolytic hyperkeratosis, congenital ichthyosiform erythroderma, Netherton's syndrome, trichothiodystrophy

Laboratory and Special Examinations

Culture Rule out secondary infection and sepsis, especially in newborns.

Dermatopathology Hyperkeratosis; granular layer present; acanthosis variable

Course and Prognosis

Collodion membrane present at birth is shed within first few days to weeks. Newborns are at risk for hypernatremic dehydration, secondary infection, and sepsis. Disorder persists throughout life. No improvement with age. Hyperkeratosis results in obstruction of eccrine sweat glands with resultant impairment of sweating.

Management

Support Group Foundation for Ichthyosis and Related Skin Types (FIRST), P. O. Box 20921, Raleigh, NC 27619; Tel: 800-545-3286; Fax: 919-781-0679.

Newborn Care for in neonatal intensive care unit. High-humidity chamber. Emolliation. Monitor electrolytes, fluids. Follow for signs of local or systemic infection.

Child/Adult

EMOLLIENTS Hydrated petrolatum

KERATOLYTICS *Propylene Glycol* 44 % to 60 % in water applied h.s. after bath and occluded with a plastic suit worn as pajamas. When excess scaling has been removed, repeat once weekly as necessary
Other Salicylic acid, urea, and alpha-hydroxy acids (glycolic acid, lactic acid) in various vehicles

OVERHEATING Parents and affected individuals should be instructed about overheating and heat prostration that can follow exercise, high environmental temperatures, and fever. Repeated application of water to skin can replace function of sweating, cooling the body.

Retinoids Tretinoin, acitretin, and, to a lesser degree, isotretinoin (0.5 to 1.0 mg/kg) are effective as in XLI. High incidence of associated bony toxicities if given over prolonged period of time. Teratogenicity requires effective contraception.

EPIDERMOLYTIC HYPERKERATOSIS

Epidermolytic hyperkeratosis presents at or shortly after birth with blistering. With time, the skin becomes keratotic and even verrucous, particularly in the flexural areas, knees, and elbows.

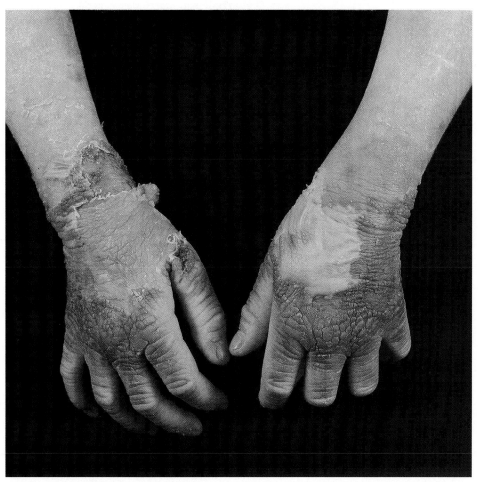

Figure I-5 Epidermolytic hyperkeratosis *Note massive hyperkeratosis and blisters within the hyperkeratotic areas.*

Epidemiology

Age of Onset Birth or shortly thereafter

Sex Equal incidence in males and in females

Mode of Inheritance Autosomal dominant

Incidence Rare

History

Blistering may recur periodically, leading to denuded areas, secondary infection, and sepsis. Hyperkeratotic lesions become verrucous, particularly in the flexural areas, and are associated with an unpleasant odor.

Physical Examination

Skin Lesions

TYPE Blistering at birth or shortly thereafter. Generalized or localized. Denuded areas develop that heal with normal-appearing skin. With time, the skin becomes keratotic and verrucous (Figures I-5 and I-6), particularly in the flexural areas, knees, and elbows. Hyperkeratotic scales adhere to underlying skin, often in a mountain range–like appearance; they are quite dark in color and are associated with an unpleasant odor. Recurrent blisters within hyperkeratotic areas and also shedding of hyperkeratotic masses result in circumscribed areas of skin that are relatively normal in appearance. This normal-appearing skin in hyperkeratotic areas is a valuable diagnostic sign. Secondary pyogenic infections.

DISTRIBUTION Generalized with prominent involvement of flexural areas. Palmar and plantar involvement. (*Note:* there is a variant of epidermolytic hyperkeratosis localized to palms and soles and genetically distinct from the generalized form.)

Hair and nails Hair is normal, but involvement of the nails may produce abnormal nail plates.

Mucous membranes Spared

Laboratory and Special Examinations

Dermatopathology Giant, coarse keratohyalin granules and vacuolization of the granular layer, resulting in cell lysis and subcorneal multiloculated blisters. Papillomatosis, acanthosis, and hyperkeratosis.

Course and Prognosis

Blister formation and massive hyperkeratosis are prone to bacterial superinfection, which is probably also responsible for the unpleasant odor. Palmar involvement can adversely affect manual dexterity.

Management

Topical application of alpha-hydroxy acids. Antimicrobial therapy. Systemic retinoids (etretinate, acitretin) may transiently lead to a worsening of the condition because of increased blister formation but later on improve the skin dramatically owing to a relative normalization of epidermal differentiation.

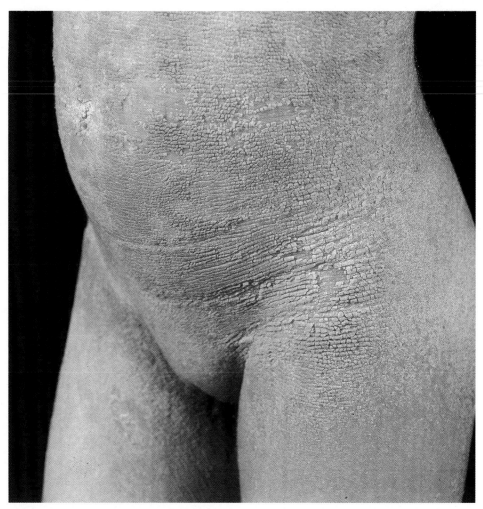

Figure I-6 Epidermolytic hyperkeratosis *The mountain-range like hyperkeratoses are characteristic as are the islands of almost normal skin where the horny materials have been shed.*

INDEXES

INDEX OF INFECTIOUS DISEASES WITH DERMATOLOGIC MANIFESTATIONS, LISTED BY GEOGRAPHIC AREA

With the marked increase in international travel in the past decade among all walks of life and all ages, it is necessary to ask a patient with skin lesions where he or she has lived and traveled. The following indexes of diseases with skin lesions are presented by areas of acquisition in order to facilitate diagnosis and thus appropriate treatment.

While there are many other infections associated with skin lesions that are found in the geographic areas listed here, the selected infections are rare or sporadic or are not uniformly distributed. The tables show sites of acquisition, not just where the diseases are diagnosed. The tables exclude diseases that have a worldwide distribution, those without skin manifestations, as well as sexually transmitted diseases that can be acquired in any geographic location. A more detailed description of geographic distribution of these and other infections can be found in M.E. Wilson, *A World Guide to Infections: Diseases, Distribution, Diagnosis* (New York, Oxford University Press, 1991).

It is important to keep in mind that a patient with an infection acquired in one geographic location may undergo medical evaluation in another location where the infection is not endemic. Also, many infections may be rare or sporadically acquired in regions outside of endemic areas. An example is anthrax. Sporadic infection may be acquired in any geographic location by way of contact with imported contaminated animal products.

Equally important to note is that infections that require a specific arthropod vector for transmission will have a distribution limited by the vector distribution. Presence of the vector is not sufficient for disease to occur. For example, a mosquito competent to transmit dengue is found in many states in the southern United States. In recent years, transmission of dengue has been documented only rarely within the United States (Texas).

These tables were compiled by Leslie C. Lucchina, M.D., and Mary E. Wilson, M.D.

INFECTIOUS DISEASES WITH DERMATOLOGIC MANIFESTATIONS IN THE UNITED STATES

	Northeast	South	Midwest	West
Anthrax	*	X	*	X
Blastomycosis	X	X	X	
Cercarial dermatitis	X	X	X	X
(*Note: Found in freshwater lakes and saltwater coast lines*)				
Coccidioidomycosis		X		X
Colorado tick fever			*	X
Cutaneous larva migrans	*	X	*	*
Dengue fever		*		
Dirofilariasis	*	*	*	*
(*Note: More cases reported from coastal areas*)				
Ehrlichiosis	X	X	X	X
Histoplasmosis	X	X	X	*
Hookworm		X	*	
Leishmaniasis (cutaneous)		*(Texas)		
Leprosy	*	*	*	*
(*Note: Most cases are imported*)				
Leptospirosis	X	X	X	X
(*Note: Especially Hawaii and warmer regions*)				
Lyme disease	X	X	X	X
Myiasis	*	*	*	*
Orf			X	X
Plague				X
Relapsing fever				X
Rhinoscleroma		*(Texas)		
Rickettsial infections:				
Rickettsialpox due to *Rickettsia akari*	*	*	*	*
Spotted fever due to *R. rickettsii* (Rocky Mountain spotted fever)	X	X	X	X
Typhus fever due to *R. prowazekii* (epidemic typhus)		X	*	*
Typhus fever due to *R. typhi* (murine or endemic typhus)	*	X	*	*
Seabather's eruption	X	X		
(*Note: Especially along Atlantic coast, though may be more widespread*)				
Sparganosis		X		
Strongyloidiasis	*	X	*	*
(*Note: Most cases are imported*)				
Trypanosomiasis (American)		*		*
Tularemia	*	X	X	*
Vibrio species infections of skin	X	X	X	X
(*Note: Especially associated with saltwater coast lines*)				

KEY: X = Infection may be acquired in this geographic location.

    * = Infection is rare and sporadic in this geographic location.

INFECTIOUS DISEASES WITH DERMATOLOGIC MANIFESTATIONS BY AREA OF ACQUISITION

	Africa	North America (except Mexico)	Mexico Central America
Anthrax	X	X	X
Bartonellosis due to *Bartonella bacilliformis*			*
Blastomycosis	*	X	*
Buruli ulcer due to *Mycobacterium ulcerans*	X		X
Cercarial dermatitis	X	X	X
Chancroid	X	X	X
Coccidioidomycosis		X	X
Colorado tick fever		X	
Cutaneous larva migrans	X	X	X
Dengue fever	X	*	X
Dirofilariasis	X	X	X
Ehrlichiosis	X	X	
Histoplasmosis	X	X	X
Hookworm	X	X	X
Leishmaniasis (cutaneous)	X	*	X
Leprosy	X	X	X
Leptospirosis	X	X	X
Loiasis	X		
Lyme disease	X	X	X
Myiasis	X	X	X
Onchocerciasis	X		X
Orf	X	X	X
Paracoccidioidomycosis	*		X
Penicilliosis marneffei			
Plague	X	X	*
Relapsing fever	X	X	X
Rhinoscleroma	X	X	X
Rickettsial infections			
Boutonneuse fever due to *Rickettsia conorii*	X		
Rickettsialpox due to *R. akari*	X	X	
Scrub typhus due to *R. tsutsugamushi*			
Spotted fever due to *R. rickettsii* (Rocky Mountain spotted fever)		X	X
Spotted fevers due to *R. australis, R. japonicum, R. sibirica*			
Typhus fever due to *R. prowazekii* (epidemic typhus)	X	X	X
Typhus fever due to *R. typhi* (murine or endemic typhus)	X	X	X
Schistosomiasis	X		
Seabather's eruption		X	X
Sparganosis	X	X	X
Strongyloidiasis	X	X	X
Trypanosomiasis (African)	X		
Trypanosomiasis (American)		*	X
Tularemia	X	X	X
Tungiasis	X		X
Vibrio species infections of skin	X	X	X

KEY: x = Infection may be acquired in this geographic location.   * = Infection is rare and sporadic in this geographic location.

Caribbean	South America	Asia	Europe	Australia New Zealand Oceania	Comment
X	X	X	X	X	
	X				See note below
		*	*	*	
	*	X		X	
X	X	X	X	X	Associated with fresh and salt water
X	X	X	X	X	More common in tropics
	X				
X	X	X	X	X	Especially tropics and subtropics
X	X	X		X	Especially tropics and subtropics
X	X	X	X	X	
		X	X		Probably more widespread than indicated
X	X	X	X	X	
X	X	X	X	X	Especially rural areas and tropics
X	X	X	X		
X	X	X	X	X	
X	X	X	X	X	Especially in tropics
		X	X	X	
X	X	X	X	X	Especially in tropics
	X	*			
X	X	X	X	X	Sheep and goat raising countries
	X				
		X			
	X	X	X		
	X	X	X		
	X	X	X	X	
		X	X		
		X	X		
		X		X	
	X				
		X	X	X	
	X	X	X	*	
X	X	X	X	X	
X	X	X	*		
X	X	X			May be more widespread than indicated
X	X	X	X	X	
X	X	X	X	X	Especially tropics and subtropics
*	X				
X		X	X		
X	X	X			
X	X	X	X	X	

Many of the infections listed may be acquired only in focal regions within the area indicated.

Note: *Bartonella henselae* and *B. quintana* have been associated with infection in the United States and in other geographic areas.

TABLE A CHRONIC LEG ULCERS: ETIOLOGY AND WORKUP*

Etiology	Workup
VASCULAR DISEASE	
Arteriosclerosis	Peripheral pulses, intermittent claudication, arterial vascular studies, pallor, cyanosis
Vasculitis Small or large vessel	History, biopsy
Hypertension	Ulcer location: lateral and medial ankle and shin; history of hypertension
Connective tissue disease SLE, RA, scleroderma, Behçet's	Biopsy, other systemic/cutaneous symptoms, livedo pattern, history, ANA, ESR
Venous stasis	Ulcer location: medial, lower third of shin; leg edema, stasis dermatitis
Lipodermatosclerosis	Induration, hyperpigmentation, "champagne bottle" legs
Cholesterol emboli	History of intravascular manipulation
Other insufficiency states: atrophie blanche, livedo reticularis, Raynaud's disease, thromboangiitis obliterans	History, smoker, biopsy
METABOLIC DISEASE	
Diabetes mellitus	
Small vessel disease	History, skin biopsy
Ulcers secondary to neuropathy	History
NEOPLASM	
Squamous cell carcinoma	Biopsy
Basal cell carcinoma	Biopsy
Melanoma	Biopsy
Metastatic disease	Biopsy
Leukemia/lymphoma	Biopsy
Kaposi's sarcoma	Biopsy
Mycosis fungoides	Biopsy
PHYSICAL TRAUMA	
Injury, pressure, neuropathies	History
Factitial	History
Radiation	History
Burn (heat, chemical)	History
Insect or animal bites	History
OTHER	
Drugs	History, biopsy
Panniculitis	History, biopsy
Pyoderma gangrenosum	History, associated underlying disease, biopsy
Nodular vasculitits (Erythema induratum)	History, biopsy

*This table was prepared by Daniella Duke, M.D.

Etiology	Workup

PAINFUL ULCERS

Etiology	Workup
Necrobiosis lipoidica	Skin biopsy
Gout	Serum uric acid, skin biopsy
Calcinosis cutis or calciphylaxis	Serum calcium, phosphate product, skin biopsy
Prolidase deficiency	Hypertelorism, saddle nose, respiratory infections corneal opacities, imidodipeptiduria
Arteriosclerosis	
Thromboangiitis obliterans	
Atrophie blanche	
Hypertension	
Pyoderma gangrenosum	
Raynaud's phenomenon/disease	
Vasculitis	

HEMATOLOGIC DISEASE

Etiology	Workup
Sickle cell anemia	Blood smear
Polycythemia vera	Red cell count
Leukemia	Blood smear, bone marrow, skin biopsy
Cryoglobulinemia	Serum cryoglobulin levels
Cryofibrinogenemia	Serum cryofibrinogen levels
Hypercoagulable states	Serum protein C, protein S, phospholipid antibodies, PT, PTT

INFECTION

Etiology	Workup
Bacterial	Biopsy, specimen culture of lesion and of minced biopsy
Ecthyma, *Pasteurella, Pseudomonas,* actinomycosis, anthrax, leprosy	
Acid-fast bacteria	Biopsy, specimen culture of lesion and of minced biopsy
Tuberculosis, atypical mycobacterial (*M. ulcerans*)	
Fungal	Biopsy, specimen culture of lesion and of minced biopsy
Blastomycosis, cryptococcis, histoplasmosis, sporotrichosis, coccidioidomycosis,	
Spirochetal Syphilis (gumma)	History, biopsy, special stains
Leishmaniasis	History, biopsy, special stains

INDEX OF DISORDERS IN WHICH THE DISTRIBUTION PATTERN OF THE LESIONS IS HELPFUL IN THE DIAGNOSIS

Common
  Atopic eczematous dermatitis
  Candidiasis
  Contact dermatitis
  Herpes zoster
  Pityriasis rosea
  Psoriasis
  Scabies
  Vitiligo

Less Common
  Acanthosis nigricans
  Dermatitis herpetiformis
  Erythema multiforme
  Eosinophilic folliculitis
  Gonococcemia (female)
  Ichthyosis, X-linked
  Lichen planus
  Lupus erythematosus, systemic
  Peutz-Jeghers syndrome
  Photosensitivity disorders
  Porphyria cutanea tarda
  Rocky Mountain spotted fever
  Syphilis, secondary
  Xanthoma, certain ones

INDEX OF GENERALIZED DISTRIBUTION INCLUDING CHARACTERISTIC PATTERNS

See also Distribution page xxv.

Macules

Drug eruption
Lupus erythematosus
Pityriasis rosea
Seborrheic dermatitis
Syphilis (secondary)
Vitiligo

Vesicles and Bullae

Bullous pemphigoid
Dermatitis herpetiformis
Drug eruption
Eczematous dermatitis, atopic
Eczematous dermatitis, contact
Erythema multiforme
Herpes simplex
Herpes zoster
Pemphigus vulgaris
Scabies

Pustules

Drug eruption
Generalized pustular psoriasis
  syndrome (von Zumbusch)

Papules

Atopic dermatitis
Drug eruption
Erythema multiforme
Lichen planus
Lupus erythematosus
Mycosis fungoides
Psoriasis
Secondary syphilis

Scales

Drug eruption
Ichthyosis vulgaris
Mycosis fungoides (Sézary's syndrome)

Wheals

Insect bites
Urticaria

Nodules

Mycosis fungoides
Neurofibromatosis

Lichenification

Atopic dermatitis

Recognize these skin alterations during the routine physical examination

(Numbers in parentheses refer to pages where disorder is discussed.)

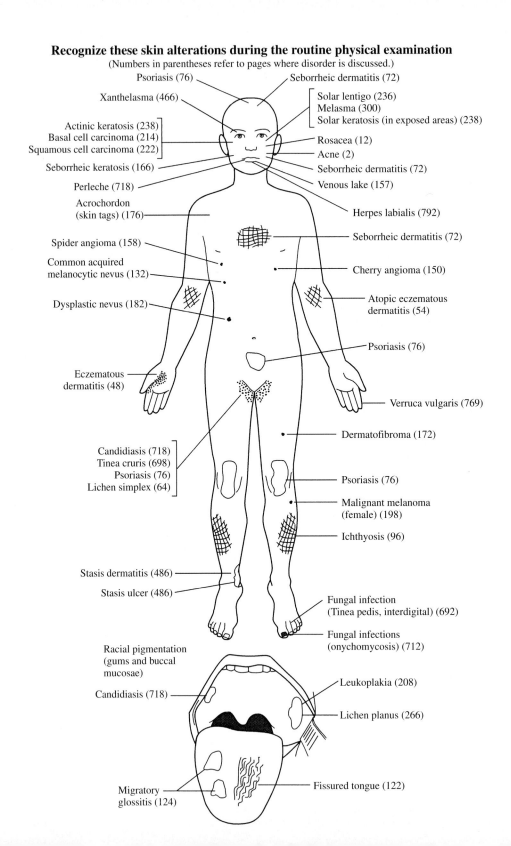

Psoriasis (76)

Seborrheic dermatitis (72)

Xanthelasma (466)

Solar lentigo (236)
Melasma (300)
Solar keratosis (in exposed areas) (238)

Actinic keratosis (238)
Basal cell carcinoma (214)
Squamous cell carcinoma (222)

Rosacea (12)
Acne (2)

Seborrheic keratosis (166)

Seborrheic dermatitis (72)

Perleche (718)

Venous lake (157)

Acrochordon
(skin tags) (176)

Herpes labialis (792)

Spider angioma (158)

Seborrheic dermatitis (72)

Common acquired
melanocytic nevus (132)

Cherry angioma (150)

Dysplastic nevus (182)

Atopic eczematous
dermatitis (54)

Psoriasis (76)

Eczematous
dermatitis (48)

Verruca vulgaris (769)

Dermatofibroma (172)

Candidiasis (718)
Tinea cruris (698)
Psoriasis (76)
Lichen simplex (64)

Psoriasis (76)

Malignant melanoma
(female) (198)

Ichthyosis (96)

Stasis dermatitis (486)

Stasis ulcer (486)

Fungal infection
(Tinea pedis, interdigital) (692)

Fungal infections
(onychomycosis) (712)

Racial pigmentation
(gums and buccal
mucosae)

Leukoplakia (208)

Candidiasis (718)

Lichen planus (266)

Migratory
glossitis (124)

Fissured tongue (122)

Recognize these skin alterations during the routine physical examination

(Numbers in parentheses refer to pages where disorder is discussed.)

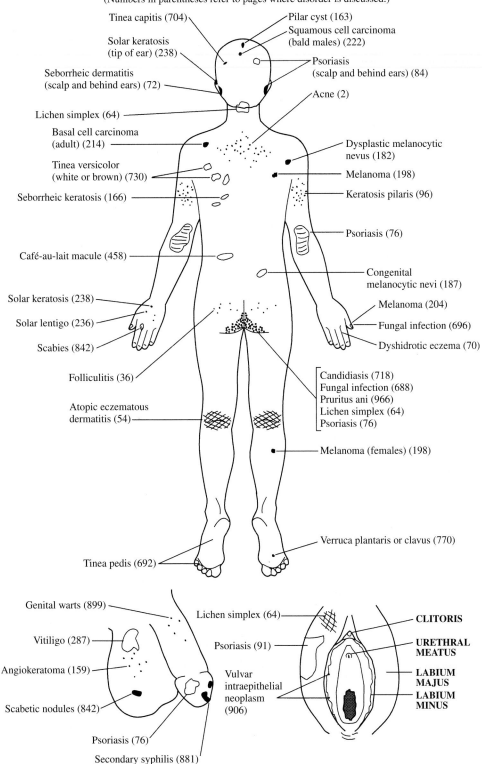

Tinea capitis (704)

Solar keratosis (tip of ear) (238)

Seborrheic dermatitis (scalp and behind ears) (72)

Lichen simplex (64)

Basal cell carcinoma (adult) (214)

Tinea versicolor (white or brown) (730)

Seborrheic keratosis (166)

Café-au-lait macule (458)

Solar keratosis (238)

Solar lentigo (236)

Scabies (842)

Folliculitis (36)

Atopic eczematous dermatitis (54)

Tinea pedis (692)

Pilar cyst (163)

Squamous cell carcinoma (bald males) (222)

Psoriasis (scalp and behind ears) (84)

Acne (2)

Dysplastic melanocytic nevus (182)

Melanoma (198)

Keratosis pilaris (96)

Psoriasis (76)

Congenital melanocytic nevi (187)

Melanoma (204)

Fungal infection (696)

Dyshidrotic eczema (70)

Candidiasis (718)
Fungal infection (688)
Pruritus ani (966)
Lichen simplex (64)
Psoriasis (76)

Melanoma (females) (198)

Verruca plantaris or clavus (770)

Genital warts (899)

Vitiligo (287)

Angiokeratoma (159)

Scabetic nodules (842)

Psoriasis (76)

Secondary syphilis (881)

Lichen simplex (64)

Psoriasis (91)

Vulvar intraepithelial neoplasm (906)

CLITORIS

URETHRAL MEATUS

LABIUM MAJUS

LABIUM MINUS

SUBJECT INDEX

Note: Page numbers followed by f indicate figures; page numbers followed by t indicate tables.

Cradle cap, 72
Cranial arteritis, 380–382, 381f, 383f
Creeping eruption, 853–854, 854f, 855f
CREST syndrome, 358, 363f
Cretinism, 437, 438
Crust, 958, 958f
Cryoglobulinemia, 388–390, 389f, 391f
  mixed (type II), 388, 390, 391f
  monoclonal (type I), 388, 389f, 390
  polyclonal (type III), 388, 390
Cryptococcosis
  cellulitis, 638
    treatment, 643t
  disseminated, 744–746, 745f, 747f
  and HIV infection, 948
Cushing's syndrome, 432–433, 433f
Cutaneous B-cell lymphoma, 552, 553f
Cutaneous larva migrans, 853–854, 854f, 855f
Cutaneous T-cell lymphoma, 544–548, 545f, 547f, 549f
  leonine facies, 549f
  patch phase, 545f
  plaque phase, 547f
  Sézary syndrome, 544, 550–551, 551f
  staging, 548t
  TNM classification, 548t
  tumor stage, 549f
Cutis rhomboidalis, 234
Cyclophosphamide, pigmentation effects of, 598
Cystic acne, 2, 5f
Cysts, 162–165
  digital myxoid (mucous; synovial), 164, 165f
  epidermal inclusion (traumatic epidermoid), 164, 164f
  epidermoid (sebaceous; infundibular; epidermal), 162f, 163
  milium, 165, 165f
  trichilemmal (pilar; isthmus catagen), 163, 163f

Darier's sign, 562, 563f, 962
Darling's disease, 748–751, 749f
Decubitus ulcers, 492–495, 493f, 495f
Defibrination syndrome, 536–538
Defluvium, 18
  telogen, 28–29, 29f
    drugs inducing, 30t–31t
Demodicidosis, 40, 42
Dercum's disease, 178
Dermal melanocytoma, 140, 141f
Dermatitis
  asteatotic, 75, 75f
  atopic, 54–63
    adult-type, 61–62, 62f, 63f

childhood-type, 57, 60f, 61f
  differential diagnosis, 55
  infantile, 57, 58f, 59f
  lichenification in, 64
  management, 56
berloque, 240
cercarial, 859, 859f
contact, 48–53, 49f
  allergic, 48, 50, 51t, 52t
  of the hands, 51f, 53
  nonallergic, 48, 50, 51t, 52t
crab, 618–619, 619f
eczematous, 48–75, 480, 482, 483f, 486, 490
  asteatotic dermatitis, 75
  atopic, 54–63
  contact, 48–53, 49f
  dyshidrotic eczematous dermatitis, 70–71
  leg, 480, 482, 483f, 486
  lichen simplex chronicus, 64–66
  of nipple, 526
  nummular eczema, 68–69
  from scabies, 842, 844, 846, 848
  seborrheic dermatitis, 72–74
herpetiformis, 325–326, 327f
  distribution, 327f
IgE, 54–63
lime, 240
phytophoto, 240, 241f
pigmented purpuric lichenoid, 306
radiation, 210–212, 211f, 213f
rosacea-like, 16–17, 17f
seborrheic, 72–74, 73f, 74f
Dermatofibroma, 172, 173f
  dimple sign, 172, 173f
Dermatoheliosis (photoaging), 228, 232–235, 233f, 235f
  advanced, 233f
  moderate, 235f
  prevention, 235
  solar keratosis, 232, 233f, 238, 239f
  solar lentigo, 232, 235f, 236, 237f
Dermatomes, 820, 820f–821f
Dermatomyositis, 328–330, 329f, 331f
Dermatophytic granuloma, 38
Dermatophytic onychomycoses, 712, 714
Dermatophytoses, 688–711
  epidermal, 691f, 692–703
  of hair, 704–711
  and HIV infection, 947
  laboratory diagnosis, 689
  management, 690, 691t
  pathogenesis, 689–690
  tinea barbae, 710, 711f
  tinea capitis, 704–708, 705f, 707f, 709f
  tinea corporis, 700, 701f

tinea cruris, 698–699, 699f
tinea facialis, 702, 703f
tinea manuum, 696–697, 697f
tinea pedis, 692–695, 693f, 695f
Dermatosis
acute febrile neutrophilic, 398–400, 399f, 400f
artefacta, 118, 119f
pigmented purpuric, 306–308, 307f, 309f
  differential diagnosis, 308
progressive pigmented purpuric, 306, 309f
transient acantholytic, 108–109, 109f
Desert fever, 755–756, 757f
Desmoplastic melanoma, 196–197, 197f
Desquamation, 959, 959f
Diabetes mellitus, 420–421, 455f
lower leg ischemia, 474
Diabetic bullae, 420, 421f
Diabetic ulcers, 488, 490
Diaper dermatitis, candidal, 718, 720, 722f, 723
Diascopy, 961
Digital myxoid cyst, 164, 165f
Discoid eczema, 68–69, 69f
Discoid lupus erythematosus
differential diagnosis, 238
and squamous cell carcinoma, 222
Disseminated intravascular coagulation,
  536–538, 537f, 539f
Donovanosis, 894–895, 895f
ulcerovegetative, 894, 895f
Drug-induced disorders
acanthosis nigricans, 505
adverse cutaneous reactions, 574–603
  classification, 574–575
  life threatening, 575
alopecia, 30t–31t
anaphylaxis, 580–583
angioedema, 580–583
in diabetes mellitus, 421
erythroderma, 285f
exanthemous eruptions, 576–579, 577f
fixed drug eruptions, 586–588, 587f, 589f
heparin necrosis, 600, 603f
and HIV infection, 947
hypersensitivity syndromes, 584–585, 585f
hypertrichosis, 46–47
lichen planus-like eruptions, 268t
pemphigus, 402
photosensitivity, 985t
  photoallergic, 246–248, 247f, 249f
  phototoxic, 242–244, 243f, 245f
pigmentation changes, 596–598, 597f, 599f
Stevens-Johnson syndrome, 590–594, 591f,
  593f
toxic epidermal necrolysis, 590–594, 591f,
  593f, 595f

urticaria, 580–583
warfarin necrosis, 600–602, 601f, 603f
Dyshidrotic eczematous dermatitis, 70–71, 71f
Dysmorphic syndrome, 119
Dysplastic (Clark) melanocytic nevus,
  182–186, 183f, 185f, 186t, 202
clinical features, 186t
melanoma evolving from, 185f, 201f

Ecthyma, 604–608, 609f
crust, 958, 958f
gangrenosum, 636, 655–657, 656f
and HIV infection, 947
Eczema
atopic, 54–63
craquelatum, 75, 75f
differential diagnosis, 531f
discoid, 68–69, 69f
herpeticum, 806–808, 807f, 809f
nummular, 68–69, 69f
pediculosis capitis, 836
vesicular palmar, 70–71, 71f
Eczematoid seborrhea, 72–74, 73f, 74f
Eczematous dermatitis, 48–75
asteatotic dermatitis, 75
atopic, 54–63
contact, 48–53, 49f
dyshidrotic eczematous dermatitis, 70–71
of leg, 480, 482, 483f, 486
lichen simplex chronicus, 64–66
of nipple, 526
nummular eczema, 68–69
from scabies, 842, 844, 846, 848
seborrheic dermatitis, 72–74
Effluvium, 18
anagen, 30, 31f
  drugs inducing, 30t–31t
telogen, 28–29, 29f
  drugs inducing, 30t–31t
Elephantiasis nostras verrucosa, 486
En cuirasse metastatic carcinoma, 520, 522
Endocarditis, infective, 622–625, 623f, 625f
acute, 622, 624
Janeway lesions, 623, 623f, 625t
Osler's nodes, 623, 625f, 625t
petechial lesions, 623, 625f, 625t
subacute, 622, 624
Eosinophilic folliculitis, in HIV infection,
  923–924, 925f
Eosinophilic granuloma, 556–560, 557f, 559f,
  561f
Epidermal cyst, 162f, 163
Epidermal inclusion cyst, 164, 164f
Epidermodysplasia verruciformis, 768
Epidermoid cyst, 162f, 163

traumatic, 164, 164f
Epidermophyton, 688, 698, 700
Epithelioid cell–spindle cell nevomelanocytic nevus, 142
Eruptive xanthomas, 463, 465t, 470, 471f
 in diabetes mellitus, 420
Erysipelas, 634–643, 635f, 637f
Erysipeloid, 618–619, 619f, 636
Erythema, migratory necrolytic, 512, 513f, 515f
Erythema induratum, 386
Erythema infectiosum, 828–830, 829f, 831f
 slapped cheeks, 828, 829f
Erythema migrans, 678, 679f, 680, 681f
Erythema multiforme syndrome, 332–334, 333f, 334f, 335f
 distribution, 334f
Erythema nodosum
 leprosum, 659
 syndrome, 336–337, 337f
Erythematous candidiasis, 724, 726
Erythrasma, 616, 617f
Erythroderma, 282–285
 differential diagnosis, 550
 drug-induced, 285f
 exfoliative, 282–284, 283f, 285f
Erythrohepatic protoporphyria, 254t, 263–264, 265f
Erythroplasia of Queyrat, 224f
Erythropoietic porphyria, congenital, 254t
Erythropoietic protoporphyria, 254t, 263–264, 265f
 erythema, 230
Escherichia coli cellulitis, 634, 637f
Espundia, 862, 864, 866, 869f
Esthiomene, 897
Estrogens, pigmentation effects of, 598
European blastomycosis, 744–746, 745f, 747f
Exanthem
 infectious, 776–778, 777f–779f
 subitum, 826–827, 827f
Exanthemous drug eruptions, 576–579, 577f
Excoriations, neurotic, 112–114, 113f, 115f
Extramammary Paget's disease, 528–530, 529f, 531f
 differential diagnosis, 528, 529f, 531f
Eyelid xanthoma, 463, 465t, 466, 467f

Fabry's disease, 159
Factitious syndromes, 118, 119f
Familial lipoma syndrome, 178
Fasciitis, necrotizing, 638, 641f
Favus, 38
Fever blister, 792–796, 793f, 795f
Fibroma
 oral (irritation; traumatic), 130, 131f

periungual, 499, 499f
 soft, 176, 176f
Fibrous nodule, 130, 131f
Fifth disease, 828–830, 829f, 831f
Fingers, clubbed, 501, 501f
Fish tank granuloma, 671–672, 673f
Fissured (scrotal) tongue, 122, 123f
Fixed drug eruptions, 586–588, 587f, 589f
 and HIV infection, 947
Flat warts, 766, 767–768, 771f
Flea bites, 850–852, 851f
Focal fibrous hyperplasia, 130, 131f
Fogo selvagem, 402
Follicular occlusion syndrome, 8
Folliculitis
 bacterial, 36, 37f
 of the beard, 710, 711f
 candidal, 36, 40, 718, 720
 decalvans, 32, 34f
 demodicidosis, 40, 42
 dermatophytic, 38
 eosinophilic, in HIV infection, 923–924, 925f
 fungal, 36, 40, 42
 gram-negative, 36, 38, 42
 herpetic, 36, 40, 43f
 "hot tub," 36, 38, 41f
 infectious, 36–42, 37f, 39f, 41f, 43f
  differential diagnosis, 40
  distribution, 38
  epidemiology and etiology, 36
  management, 42
  variants, 38, 40
 keloidal, 35f, 38
 Pityrosporum, 38, 39f
 Pseudomonas, 36, 38, 41f, 42
 staphylococcal, 36, 37f, 38, 39f, 42
 syphilitic, 36, 40
Fungal infections, 688–757. *See also specific infections*
 cutaneous, 688–733
  candidiasis, 718–729
  dermatophytoses, 688–711
  folliculitis, 36, 40, 42
  onychomycosis, 712–717
  pityriasis versicolor, 730–732
  tinea unguium, 712–717
 systemic, 734–757
  chromoblastomycosis, 738–739
  coccidioidomycosis, 755–756
  cryptococcosis, 744–746
  histoplasmosis, 748–751
  mycetoma, 734–736
  North American blastomycosis, 752–754
  sporotrichosis, 740–743

---

angioid streaks, 448, 451f
Psoriasiform lesions, migratory glossitis, 124, 125f
Psoriasis, 76–95
  arthritis and, 77
  classification, 76t
  desquamation, 959, 959f
  differential diagnosis, 77, 531f
  distribution, 78f
  epidemiology, 76–77
  generalized acute pustular (von Zumbusch), 93–95, 95f
  nonpustular, 76t
  palmoplantar pustulosis, 92, 93f
  pathophysiology, 78–79
  plaque, differential diagnosis, 352
  pustular, 76t
  trigger factors, 76–77
  vulgaris
    of elbows, knees, and isolated plaques, 80, 81f
    guttate type, 82, 83f
    inguinal, 91, 91f
    of nails, 89, 89f
    of palms and soles, 90, 90f
    of scalp, 84, 85f
    of trunk, 86–88, 87f
Psychiatric etiology, cutaneous disorders with, 112–119
  factitious syndromes, 118, 119f
  neurotic excoriations, 112–114, 113f, 115f
  parasitosis, delusions of, 116, 117f
Pubic lice, 839–840, 840f, 841f
Puerperal sepsis, 636
Purpura
  annularis telangiectodes, 306, 307f
  fulminans, 536–538, 537f, 539f, 648, 651f
  nonpalpable, differential diagnosis, 308
  palpable, differential diagnosis, 308
  pigmentosa chronica, 306
  progressive pigmentary, 306, 309f
  thrombocytopenic, in HIV infection, 533f
Purpuric dermatoses, pigmented, 306–308, 307f, 309f
  differential diagnosis, 308
Pustular psoriasis, generalized acute (von Zumbusch), 93–95, 95f
Pustule, 954, 954f
Pustulosis, palmoplantar, 92, 93f
PUVA photochemotherapy, and squamous cell carcinoma, 222
Pyoderma gangrenosum, 396, 397f
Pyogenic granuloma, 160f, 160–161

Radiation dermatitis, 210–212, 211f, 213f

acute, 210, 211f
chronic, 212, 213f
Ranula, 128–129
Rashes, differential diagnosis in acutely ill febrile patient, 967–968, 968t–969t
Raynaud's syndrome, 358, 359f, 364–366, 365f, 367f
  causes, 366t
Reiter's syndrome, 392–394, 393f, 395f
  circinate balanitis, 392, 395f
  keratoderma blennorrhagicum, 392, 393f
Reticuloendotheliosis, nonlipid, 556–560, 557f, 559f, 561f
Rheumatoid arthritis, and vasculitis, 368
Rhinophyma, 12, 14, 15f
Rickettsialpox, 758, 759t, 760, 761f
Rickettsial spotted fevers, 758–765
Ringworm, 700, 701f
  of the beard, 710, 711f
  of face, 702, 703f
Rocky Mountain spotted fever, 758, 759t, 762–765, 763f, 765f
  variants, 763
Rosacea, 12–14, 13f, 15f
  keratitis, 14
  stages, 14
Rosacea-like dermatitis, 16–17, 17f
Roseola infantum, 826–827, 827f
Rubella, 780–782, 781f, 783f
Rubeola, 784–786, 785f, 787f

Salmonella endocarditis, 622
San Joaquin Valley fever, 755–756, 757f
Sarcoidosis, 410–411, 411f–413f
  granulomatous dermatitis, 410, 411f
  scar, 410, 413f
Scabies, 842–848, 843f, 845f, 847f, 849f
  burrows, 844, 846, 847f
  differential diagnosis, 846
  distribution, 849f
  laboratory diagnosis, 962–963
  management, 846, 848
  nodules, 844, 845f, 846, 848
  Norwegian, 844, 846, 848
Scalp. See also under Hair
  giant cell arteritis, 380, 383f
  lichen planus, 267
  morphea, 274
  psoriasis vulgaris, 84, 85f
Scarlatiniform syndrome, 626
Scarlet fever, 644–646, 645f, 647f
  desquamation, 644, 647f
  enanthem, 644, 647f
  exanthem, 644
  Pastia's lines, 644, 645f

erysipelas, 634–643, 635f
impetigo, 604–608, 605f, 607f
scarlet fever, 644–646, 647f
toxic shock-like syndrome, 630
Sturge-Weber syndrome, port-wine stain in, 151
Subconjunctival hemorrhage, in endocarditis, 623, 625f
Sulfonamides, reactions to, 584–585, 585f, 586
Sunburn, 228, 229–231, 231f
confluent erythema, 230, 231f
differential diagnosis, 230
Sutton's disease, 126–128
Sutton's leukoderma acquisitum centrifugum, 138–139, 139f
Sweet's syndrome, 398–400, 399f, 400f
Swimmer's itch, 859, 859f
Swimming pool granuloma, 671–672, 673f
Synovial cyst, 164, 165f
Syphilides, noduloulcerative, 885, 886f
Syphilis, 877–889
course and prognosis, 888–889
folliculitis, 36, 40
and HIV infection, 887, 889, 948
laboratory examination, 887–889
latent, 885, 889
management, 889
primary, 877–878, 878f–880f, 887–888, 889
secondary, 881–883, 882f, 884f, 888, 889
condylomata lata, 881, 884f
papulosquamous lesions, 881, 882f, 883f
tertiary, 885, 886f, 888, 889
Syringoma, 177, 177f
Systemic lupus erythematosus (SLE), 346–348, 347f, 349f
alopecia, 32, 33f
sunburn-type erythema, 230
and vasculitis, 368
vitiligo vs., 288
Systemic sclerosis, progressive, 358–362

Tache bleue, 839
Tache noire, 758, 759f
T-cell leukemia/lymphoma, adult, 540–542, 541f, 543f
T-cell lymphoma
cutaneous, 544–548, 545f, 547f, 549f
erythroderma, 282, 283f
leonine facies, 549f
patch phase, 545f
plaque phase, 547f
Sézary syndrome, 544, 550–551, 551f
staging, 548t
TNM classification, 548t
tumor stage, 549f
large-cell anaplastic, 570

Telangiectasia, 500, 500f
hereditary hemorrhagic, 430–431, 431f
macularis eruptiva perstans, 562, 565f
spider, 158, 158f
Telangiectatic metastatic carcinoma, 522
Telogen effluvium, 28–29, 29f
drugs inducing, 30t–31t
Temporal arteritis, 380–382, 381f, 383f
Tendinous xanthoma, 463, 465t, 468, 469f
Tenosynovitis, gonococcal, 874
Terry's nails, 497, 497f
Thrombocytopenic purpura, in HIV infection, 533f
Thrush, 724, 725f
Tick-borne meningopolyneuritis of Garin-Bujadoux-Bannwarth, 682
Tick typhus, 758, 759t, 760
Tinea barbae, 710, 711f
Tinea capitis, 38, 704–708, 705f, 707f, 709f
black dot, 704, 705f, 706
ectothrix, 704, 705f, 706
entothrix, 704
favus, 704, 706, 707f
gray patch, 705f, 706
kerion, 704, 706, 707f
management, 708
Tinea corporis, 700, 701f
Tinea cruris, 698–699, 699f
Tinea facialis, 702, 703f, 711f
differential diagnosis, 352
Tinea manuum, 696–697, 697f
Tinea pedis, 692–695, 693f, 695f
dermatophytid, 692
inflammatory (bullous), 692, 694, 695, 695f
interdigital, 692, 693f, 694
moccasin type, 692, 693f, 694
ulcerative, 692, 694
Tinea unguium, 712–717, 715f
Tinea versicolor, 42f, 730–732, 733f
Tongue
fissured (scrotal), 122, 123f
hairy, 120, 121f
migratory glossitis (geographic tongue), 124, 125f
red strawberry, 644, 647f
Torulosis, 744–746, 745f, 747f
Toxemic rash of pregnancy, 414–416, 415f, 417f
Toxic epidermal necrolysis, 590–594, 591f, 593f, 595f
Toxic irritant contact dermatitis, 48, 50
vs. allergic, 51t
Toxic shock syndrome, 630–633, 631f, 632t
Transient acantholytic dermatosis, 108–109, 109f
Treponema pallidum, 877–889. *See also* Syphilis

Trichilemmal cyst, 163, 163f
Trichoepithelioma, 176, 177f
Tricholemmomas, 508, 509f, 510
Trichophyton, 688, 696, 698, 700, 702, 704, 712
Tuberculosis
  cutaneous, 664–668, 665f, 667f, 669f
    classification, 664
  metastatic abscess, 666, 668
  miliary, 666–667
  orificial, 667, 668, 669f
  primary inoculation, 664, 665f, 666, 667
  verrucosa cutis, 664, 665f, 666, 668
Tuberculous gumma, 666
Tuberous sclerosis, 452–454, 453f, 455f–457f
  angiofibromata, 452, 453f, 454
  ash-leaf macules, 452, 454, 455f
  confetti macules, 454, 457f
  hypopigmented macules, 452, 454, 455f, 456f
  vitiligo vs., 290
Tuberous xanthoma, 463, 465t, 468, 469f
Tungiasis, 856–857, 857f

Ulcers, 960, 960f
  aphthous, 126–128, 127f
  Buruli (Bairnsdale), 674–675, 675f
  chiclero, 862, 864, 869f
  decubitus, 492–495, 493f, 495f
  diabetic, 488, 490
  leg, 480, 486–491. *See also* Leg ulcers
  Martorell's, 488
  neuropathic, 488, 490, 491
  pressure, 492–495, 493f, 495f
  soft (chancroid), 890–892
Ulcus molle, 890–892
Ultraviolet radiation, 229, 286
  minimum erythema dose (MED), 229
  UVA and UVB, 229
Urticaria, 314–318
  acute, 315
  cholinergic, 314, 317, 317f, 320t
  chronic, 316, 318
    features, 320t
  cold, 314, 317, 320t
  complement-mediated, 314, 318
  dermographism, 314, 315f, 320t
  drug-induced, 580–583
  IgE-mediated, 314
  mast cell-releasing agents and, 314
  papular
    flea bites, 850, 851f
    pubic lice, 839, 841f
  perstans, 384–385, 385f
  pigmentosa, 562, 563f
  pressure, 320t
  solar, 314, 317, 320t

vascular/connective tissue autoimmune disease and, 314
vasculitis, 384–385, 385f
wheals, 317, 318, 321f

Vaginal candidiasis, 724, 726
Valley fever, 755–756, 757f
Varicella zoster virus, 810–825
  herpes zoster, 814–818, 817f, 819f
    in the immunocompromised, 822, 823f, 825f
    necrotizing ophthalmic, 815, 819f
  and HIV infection, 942, 942f, 943f
  in the immunocompromised, 822–825, 823f, 825f
  varicella, 810–813, 811f
Varicose veins, 480, 481f, 482, 484
Variegate porphyria, 254t, 259t, 260–262, 261f
  hazardous drugs, 262t
  laboratory differential diagnosis, 259t
Vascular "birthmarks," 148
Vascular hamartomas, 154
Vascular insufficiency, cutaneous manifestations of, 474–495
  atherosclerosis, 474–479
  leg ulcers, 486–491
  pressure ulcers, 492–495
  venous insufficiency, chronic, 480–484
Vascular malformations (nevus flammeus), 148, 151–152, 152f, 153f
Vascular spider, 158, 158f
Vasculitis, 368–387
  giant cell arteritis, 380–382, 381f, 383f
  hypersensitivity, 368–371, 369f, 371f
  nodular, 386–387, 387f
  polyarteritis nodosa, 372–376, 373f, 375f
  urticarial, 384–385, 385f
Vasculopathy, in diabetes mellitus, 420
Venereal warts, 766, 899–900, 901f, 902, 903f–905f
Venous insufficiency, 480–484, 481f, 482f, 484f, 485f
  differential diagnosis, 482
  and leg ulcers, 486–487, 487f, 490
  management, 490–491
Venous lake, 157, 157f
Venous malformations (cavernous hemangiomas), 148, 154–155, 155f
Venous ulcers, leg, 486
Verruca
  acuminata, 766, 899–900, 901f, 903f–905f
  plana, 766, 767–768, 771f
  plantaris, 766, 767, 769f, 770f
  vulgaris, 766, 767, 769f
Vesicle, 957, 957f
Vesicle-bulla, 955, 955f

ISBN 0-07-021388-7

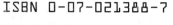